Nutrition and Metabolism

The Nutrition Society Textbook Series

Introduction to Human Nutrition

Introduction to Human Nutrition: a global
    perspective on food and nutrition
Body composition
Energy metabolism
Nutrition and metabolism of proteins and amino acids
Digestion and metabolism of carbohydrates
Nutrition and metabolism of lipids
Dietary reference standards
The vitamins
Minerals and trace elements
Measuring food intake
Food composition
Food and nutrition: policy and regulatory issues
Nutrition research methodology
Food safety: a public health issue of growing importance
Food and nutrition-related diseases: the global challenge

Nutrition and Metabolism

Core Concepts of Nutrition
Molecular Aspects of Nutrition
Integration of Metabolism 1: Energy
Integration of Metabolism 2: Macronutrients
Integration of Metabolism 3: Protein and Amino Acids
Pregnancy and Lactation
Growth and Aging
Nutrition and the Brain
The Sensory Systems and Food Palatability
The Gastrointestinal Tract
The Cardiovascular System
The Skeletal System
The Immune and Inflammatory Systems
Phytochemicals
The Control of Food Intake
Overnutrition
Undernutrition
Exercise Performance

Public Health Nutrition

An overview of public health nutrition
Nutrition epidemiology
Food choice
Assessment of nutritional status at individual and
    population level
Assessment of physical activity
Overnutrition
Undernutrition
Eating disorders, dieting and food fads
PHN strategies for nutrition: intervention at the level of
    individuals
PHN strategies for nutrition: intervention at the
    ecological level
Food and nutrition guidelines
Fetal programming
Cardiovascular disease
Cancer
Osteoporosis
Diabetes
Vitamin A deficiency
Iodine deficiency
Iron deficiency
Maternal and child health
Breast feeding
Adverse outcomes in pregnancy

Clinical Nutrition

General principles of clinical nutrition
Metabolic and nutritional assessment
Overnutrition
Undernutrition
Metabolic disorders
Eating disorders
Adverse reactions to foods
Nutritional support
Ethical and legal issues
Gastrointestinal tract
The liver
The pancreas
The kidney
Blood and bone marrow
The lung
Immune and inflammatory systems
Heart and blood vessels
The skeleton
Traumatic diseases
Infectious diseases
Malignant diseases
Pediatric nutrition
Cystic fibrosis
Clinical cases
Water and electrolytes

Nutrition and Metabolism

Second Edition

Edited on behalf of The Nutrition Society by

Susan A Lanham-New
Ian A Macdonald
Helen M Roche

A John Wiley & Sons, Ltd., Publication

This edition first published 2011
First edition published 2003
© 2011, 2003 by The Nutrition Society

Blackwell Publishing was acquired by John Wiley & Sons in February 2007. Blackwell's publishing program has been merged with Wiley's global Scientific, Technical and Medical business to form Wiley-Blackwell.

Registered Office
John Wiley & Sons Ltd, The Atrium, Southern Gate, Chichester, West Sussex, PO19 8SQ, UK

Editorial Offices
9600 Garsington Road, Oxford, OX4 2DQ, UK
The Atrium, Southern Gate, Chichester, West Sussex, PO19 8SQ, UK
2121 State Avenue, Ames, Iowa 50014-8300, USA

For details of our global editorial offices, for customer services and for information about how to apply for permission to reuse the copyright material in this book please see our website at www.wiley.com/wiley-blackwell.

Library of Congress Cataloging-in-Publication Data

Nutrition and metabolism / edited on behalf of the Nutrition Society by Susan A Lanham-New, Ian Macdonald, Helen Roche. – 2nd ed.
    p.   ;   cm. – (Nutrition Society textbook series)
  Includes bibliographical references and index.
  ISBN 978-1-4051-6808-3 (pbk. : alk. paper)   1. Nutrition.   2. Metabolism.   I. Lanham-New, S. (Susan)   II. Roche, Helen M.   III. Macdonald, Ian, 1921–   IV. Nutrition Society (Great Britain)   V. Series: Human nutrition textbook series.
  [DNLM: 1. Nutritional Physiological Phenomena.   2. Metabolism.   QU 145 N97546 2011]
  QP141.N7768 2011
  612.3–dc22

                              2010011217

A catalogue record for this book is available from the British Library.

This book is published in the following electronic formats: ePDF 9781444327786; Wiley Online Library 9781444327779

Set in 10/12pt Minion by SPi Publisher Services, Pondicherry, India

Printed and bound in Singapore by C.O.S. Printers Pte Ltd

5   2015

Contents

Additional resources are published on the book's website: www.wiley.com/go/nutmet

Contributors

Professor Abayomi O Akanji
Kuwait University
Kuwait

Associate Professor Linda Bandini
University of Massachusetts
USA

Dr France Bellisle
Institut National de la Recherche
    Agronomique
France

Professor John T Brosnan
University of Newfoundland
Canada

Dr Margaret E Brosnan
Memorial Hospital of Newfoundland
Canada

Dr Louise M Burke
Australian Institute of Sport
Australia

Professor Philip C Calder
University of Southampton
UK

Professor Aedín Cassidy
University of East Anglia
UK

Professor Peter Cleaton-Jones
University of Witwatersrand
South Africa

Dr Conor M Delahunty
CSIRO Food Science Australia
Australia

Dr Adam Drewnowski
University of Washington
USA

Professor John D Fernstrom
University of Pittsburgh
USA

Dr Madelyn H Fernstrom
University of Pittsburgh
USA

Professor Albert Flynn
University College Cork
Ireland

Professor Keith N Frayn
Oxford University
UK

Professor Michael J Gibney
University College Dublin
Ireland

Professor Angel Gil
Universidad de Granada
Spain

Dr Lisette CPGM de Groot
Wageningen Agricultural University
The Netherlands

Professor Asker E Jeukendrup
University of Birmingham
UK

Dr Colin D Kay
University of East Anglia
UK

Dr Paul Kelly
Barts and The London School of Medicine
    and Dentistry
UK

Dr Susan A Lanham-New
University of Surrey
UK

Dr Xavier M Leverve
Boenergetique Fonamentale et Appliquee
France

Professor Ian A Macdonald
University of Nottingham
UK

Professor Mariano Mañas
Universidad de Granada
Spain

Professor John C Mathers
University of Newcastle
UK

Professor Ronald P Mensink
Maastricht University
The Netherlands

Professor John M Pettifor
University of Witwatersrand
South Africa

Assistant Professor Herman E Popeijus
Maastricht University
The Netherlands

Dr Ann Prentice
Medical Research Council-Human Nutrition
   Research (MRC-HNR)
Cambridge

Dr Joop MA van Raaij
Wageningen Agricultural University
The Netherlands

Professor Gabriele Riccardi
University of Naples Federico II
Italy

Associate Professor Angela A Rivellese
University of Naples Federico II
Italy

Associate Professor Helen M Roche
University College Dublin
Ireland

Renee Scampini
UMASS Medical School
USA

Dr Prasong Tienboon
Chiang Mai University
Thailand

Professor Emilio Martínez de Victoria
Universidad de Granada
Spain

Professor Mark L Wahlqvist
National Health Research Institute
Taiwan

Dr Kate Ward
Medical Research Council-Human Nutrition
   Research (MRC-HNR)
Cambridge

Professor Christine M Williams
University of Reading
UK

Dr María D Yago
Universidad de Granada
Spain

Dr Parveen Yaqoob
University of Reading
UK

Dr Vernon R Young (deceased)
Formally of MIT
USA

Series Foreword

The early decades of the twentieth century were a period of intense research on constituents of food essential for normal growth and development, and saw the discovery of most of the vitamins, minerals, amino acids and essential fatty acids. In 1941, a group of leading physiologists, biochemists and medical scientists recognised that the emerging discipline of nutrition needed its own learned society and the Nutrition Society was established. Our mission was, and remains, 'to advance the scientific study of nutrition and its application to the maintenance of human and animal health'. The Nutrition Society is the largest learned society for nutrition in Europe and we have over 2000 members worldwide. You can find out more about the Society and how to become a member by visiting our website at www.nutsoc.org.uk.

The revolution in biology initiated by large-scale genome mapping and facilitated by the development of reliable, simple-to-use molecular biological tools makes this a very exciting time to be working in nutrition. We now have the opportunity to get a much better understanding of how specific genes interact with nutrient intake and other lifestyle factors to influence gene expression in individual cells and tissues and, ultimately, affect health. Knowledge of the polymorphisms in key genes carried by an individual will allow the prescription of more effective, and safe, dietary treatments. At the population level, molecular epidemiology is opening up much more incisive approaches to understanding the role of particular dietary patterns in disease causation. This excitement is reflected in the several scientific meetings which the Nutrition Society, often in collaboration with sister learned societies in Europe, Africa, Asia and the USA, organise each year. We provide travel grants and other assistance to encourage students and young researchers to attend and to participate in these meetings.

Throughout its history a primary objective of the Society has been to encourage nutrition research and to disseminate the results of such research. Our first journal, *The Proceedings of the Nutrition Society*, recorded, as it still does, the scientific presentations made to the Society. Shortly afterwards, *The British Journal of Nutrition* was established to provide a medium for the publication of primary research on all aspects of human and animal nutrition by scientists from around the world. Recognising the needs of students and their teachers for authoritative reviews on topical issues in nutrition, the Society began publishing *Nutrition Research Reviews* in 1988. We subsequently launched *Public Health Nutrition*, the first international journal dedicated to this important and growing area. These journals are available in electronic and conventional paper form, and we are exploring new opportunities to exploit the web to make the outcomes of nutritional research more quickly and readily accessible.

Just as in research, having the best possible tools is an enormous advantage in teaching and learning. This is the reasoning behind the initiative to launch this series of human nutrition textbooks designed for use worldwide. The Society is deeply indebted to the founding Editor-in-Chief, Professor Michael J Gibney (University College Dublin), for his foresight and hard work in bringing the first editions of this major publishing exercise to successful fruition and for overseeing the production of the second edition of the *Introduction to Nutrition* textbook. We are particularly grateful to Dr Susan A Lanham-New (University of Surrey) for agreeing to take on the challenge of being Editor-in-Chief for the second editions of the other three textbooks (*Nutrition and Metabolism*, *Public Health Nutrition* and *Clinical Nutrition*) and for also having the vision to add a fourth textbook, *Sports and Exercise Nutrition*. Read, learn and enjoy.

Ian A Macdonald
President of the Nutrition Society

Preface

More than a decade has passed since the idea of a Nutrition Society Textbook Series was first raised and it has proved to be an enormously successful venture. It is a great honour for me to be the new editor-in-chief of the series and credit should go to the first ever Editor-in-Chief, Professor Michael J Gibney (University College Dublin) for his tremendous vision and hard work in the early days of the Series' development.

Nutrition and Metabolism 2e is the second of this series of four textbooks: *Introduction to Human Nutrition 2e* was published last year and launched at the 2009 Nutrition Society Conference, held at the University of Surrey, Guildford. It was seen very much as an 'introductory' textbook and, as such, was designed not only for students of nutritional sciences but also for the many undergraduate and postgraduate students who have aspects of nutrition in their courses (e.g. medicine, pharmacy, nursing and food science). *Nutrition and Metabolism 2e* is aimed at the student (undergraduate and postgraduate) opting to pursue nutrition as a main academic subject. This textbook, as the title implies, has as its focus the physiological and biochemical basis for the role of nutrients in metabolism. The first seven chapters cover some core areas, some traditional areas, such as the integration of metabolic nutrition or areas related to stages of growth, and also focuses on molecular nutrition. This is an area of considerable growth and development. Following on from this, the chapters are organised in a slightly different manner, taking the view that the role of individual nutrients should be integrated into chapters on a 'systems' level rather than a specific nutrient one.

Plans are well underway for the second edition of *Public Health Nutrition*, and hence this topic is avoided in *Nutrition and Metabolism 2e*. The second edition of *Clinical Nutrition Textbook* will address the diet–disease links on a system-by-system basis.

The first edition of *Nutrition and Metabolism* was published in 2003 with Professor Ian A Macdonald (University of Nottingham) and Professor Helen M Roche (University College Dublin) as the specific N&M Textbook Editors, doing a splendid job. It has been a great pleasure to have had the opportunity to work with them again on the production of this new edition, and I thank them sincerely for all their hard work.

We have tried to minimise within-textbook overlap and have cross-referenced chapters where possible. However, some level of overlap across texts will undoubtedly occur, but from different perspectives. For example, *Nutrition and Metabolism 2e* introduces an analysis of how nutrients influence risk factors for coronary heart disease with a perspective on the metabolic dimension. Much of this will again arise in both *Public Health Nutrition 2e* and *Clinical Nutrition 2e*, from a population and preventive approach and from a patient and therapeutic approach, respectively.

Nutrition and Metabolism 2e is dedicated to Professor Vernon Young, who contributed greatly to the first edition and who sadly died in 2004. We acknowledge the tremendous contribution that he has made to our field of Nutritional Sciences.

There are plans for further titles in the Nutrition Society Textbook Series, which is certainly a fast-moving product, and it is a pleasure for me, as the new Editor-in-Chief, to be driving them.

The Nutrition Society Textbook Series is hugely indebted to Wiley-Blackwell, who have proved to be extremely supportive publishers. Special mention should go to Nigel Balmforth and Laura Price for their commitment to this Series. The Society is also indebted to Jennifer Norton, who is the new assistant editor of the textbooks. Her hard work, focus and organisation are first rate and we would certainly not be pressing ahead with such pace and efficiency without her input.

I hope that you will find the book of great use. Please enjoy!

Dr Susan A Lanham-New
University of Surrey and Editor-in-Chief,
Nutrition Society Textbook Series

First Edition Acknowledgements

The Nutrition Society would like to express its appreciation and thanks to all our Authors and Editors of the first edition of Nutrition and Metabolism

First Edition

Editor-in-Chief
Professor Michael J Gibney,
Trinity College Dublin, Ireland

Editors
Professor Ian A Macdonald
University of Nottingham, UK

Dr Helen M Roche
Trinity College Dublin, Ireland

Assistant Editor
Julie Dowsett
Trinity College Dublin, Ireland

Authors

Chapter one: Core Concepts of Nutrition
Professor Ian A Macdonald
University of Nottingham, UK

Professor Michael J Gibney
Trinity College Medical School, Ireland

Chapter two: Molecular Aspects of Nutrition
Professor Helen M Roche
Trinity College Medical School, Ireland

Professor Ronald P Mensink
Maastricht University, The Netherlands

Chapter three: Integration of Metabolism 1: Energy
Dr Xavier M Leverve
Bioenergetique Fonamentale et Appliquee, France

Chapter four: Integration of Metabolism 2: Protein and Amino Acids
Professor John T Brosnan
Memorial University of Newfoundland, Canada

Dr Vernon R Young
Massachusetts Institute of Technology, USA

Chapter five: Integration of Metabolism 3: Macronutrients
Professor Keith N Frayn
Oxford University, UK

Professor Abayomi O Akanji
Kuwait University, Kuwait

Chapter six: Pregnancy and Lactation
Dr Joop MA van Raaij
Wageningen Agricultural University, The Netherlands

Dr Lisette CPGM de Groot
Wageningen Agricultural University, The Netherlands

Chapter seven: Growth and Aging
Professor Mark L Wahlqvist
Monash University, Australia

Dr Prasong Tienboon
Chiang Mai University, Thailand

Dr Antigone Kouris-Blaszos
Monash University, Australia

Ms Katherine A Ross
Monash University, Australia

Ms Tracey L Setter
Monash University, Australia

Chapter eight: Nutrition and the Brain
Professor John D Fernstrom
University of Pittsburgh, USA

Dr Madelyn H Fernstrom
University of Pittsburgh, USA

**Chapter nine: The Sensory System:
Taste, Smell, Chemesthesis and Vision**
Dr Conor M Delahunty
University College Cork, Ireland

Professor Tom AB Sanders
King's College London, UK

Chapter ten: The Gastrointestinal Tract
Professor Mariano Mañas Almendros
Universidad de Granada, Spain

Professor Emilio Martínez-Victoria Munoz
Universidad de Granada, Spain

Professor Angel Gil
Universidad de Granada, Spain

Dr María D Yago
Universidad de Granada, Spain

Professor John C Mathers
University of Newcastle, UK

Chapter eleven: The Cardiovascular System
Professor Gabriele Riccardi
University of Naples Federico II, Italy

Dr Angela A Rivellese
University of Naples Federico II, Italy

Professor Christine M Williams
University of Reading, UK

Chapter twelve: The Skeletal System
Professor John M Pettifor
University of Witwatersrand, South Africa

Dr Ann Prentice
Elsie Widdowson Laboratory, UK

Professor Peter Cleaton-Jones
MRC/Wits Dental Research Institute, South Africa

**Chapter thirteen: The Immune
and Inflammatory Systems**
Dr Parveen Yaqoob
University of Reading, UK

Professor Philip C Calder
University of Southampton, UK

Chapter fourteen: Phytochemicals
Dr Aedín Cassidy
Unilever Research, UK

Dr Fabien S Dalais
Monash University, Australia

Chapter fifteen: The Control of Food Intake
Dr Adam Drewnowski
University of Washington, USA

Dr France Bellisle
*Institut National de la Recherche Agronomique,
France*

Chapter sixteen: Overnutrition
Professor Albert Flynn
University College Cork, Ireland

Associate Professor Linda Bandini
Boston University, USA

Chapter seventeen: Undernutrition
Dr Mario Vaz
St. John's Medical College, Bangalore, India

Chapter eighteen: Exercise Performance
Professor Asker E Jeukendrup
University of Birmingham, UK

Dr Louise M Burke
Australian Institute of Sport, Australia

To Vernon Young

1
Core Concepts of Nutrition

Ian A Macdonald and Michael J Gibney

Key messages

- The change in body reserves or stores of a nutrient is the difference between the intake of that nutrient and the body's utilisation of that nutrient. The time-frame necessary to assess the body's balance of a particular nutrient varies from one nutrient to another.
- The concept of turnover can be applied at various levels within the body (molecular, cellular, tissue/organs, whole body).
- The flux of a nutrient through a metabolic pathway is a measure of the rate of activity of the pathway. Flux is not necessarily related to the size of the pool or pathway through which the nutrient or metabolite flows.

- Nutrients and metabolites are present in several pools in the body. The size of these metabolic pools varies substantially for different nutrients/metabolites, and a knowledge of how these pools are interconnected greatly helps us to understand nutrition and metabolism.
- Darwinian theory of evolution implies a capacity to adapt to adverse conditions, including adverse dietary conditions. Many such examples can be cited. Some allow for long-term adaptation and others buy time until better conditions arrive.

1.1 Introduction

This textbook on nutrition and metabolism covers macronutrient aspects of nutrition in an integrated fashion. Thus, rather than considering the macronutrients separately, this book brings together information on macronutrients and energy in relation to specific states or topics (e.g. undernutrition, overnutrition, cardiovascular disease). Before considering these topics in detail it is necessary to outline the core concepts that underlie nutritional metabolism. The core concepts to be covered in this chapter are nutrient balance, turnover and flux, metabolic pools, and adaptation to altered nutrient supply.

1.2 Balance

As discussed in Chapter 3, nutrient balance must be considered separately from the concepts of metabolic equilibrium or steady state. In this chapter, the concept of balance is considered in the context of the classical meaning of that term, the long-term sum of all the forces of metabolic equilibrium for a given nutrient.

The concept of nutrient balance essentially restates the law of conservation of mass in terms of nutrient exchange in the body. It has become common practice to refer to the content of the nutrient within the body as a 'store' but in many cases this is not appropriate and the term 'reserve' is better. Thus, the idea of nutrient balance is summarised by the equation:

$$\begin{bmatrix} \text{nutrient} \\ \text{intake} \end{bmatrix} - \begin{bmatrix} \text{nutrient} \\ \text{utilisation} \end{bmatrix} = \begin{bmatrix} \text{change in body} \\ \text{nutrient reserves} \end{bmatrix}$$

The above equation can have three outcomes:

- zero balance (or nutrient balance): intake matches utilisation and reserves remain constant
- positive balance (or positive imbalance): intake exceeds utilisation and reserves expand
- negative balance (or negative imbalance): utilisation exceeds intake and reserves become depleted.

In relation to macronutrient metabolism, the concept of balance is most often applied to protein (nitrogen) and to energy. However, many research

---

Nutrition and Metabolism, Second Edition, edited by S. A. Lanham-New, I. A. Macdonald and H. M. Roche. © 2011 The Nutrition Society.

studies now subdivide energy into the three macronutrients and consider fat, carbohydrate and protein balance separately. This separation of the macronutrients is valuable in conditions of altered dietary composition (e.g. low-carbohydrate diets) where a state of energy balance might exist over a few days but be the result of negative carbohydrate balance (using the body's glycogen reserves to satisfy the brain's requirement for glucose) matched in energy terms by positive fat balance.

Balance is a function not only of nutrient intake but also of metabolically induced losses. Fat balance is generally driven by periods where energy intake exceeds energy expenditure (positive energy balance) and by periods when intakes are deliberately maintained below energy expenditure, such as in dieting (negative energy balance). However, nutrient balance can also be driven by metabolic regulators through hormones or cytokines. For example, the dominance of growth hormone during childhood ensures positive energy and nutrient balance. In pregnancy, a wide range of hormones lead to a positive balance of all nutrients in the overall placental, foetal and maternal tissues, although this may be associated with a redistribution of some nutrient reserves from the mother to the foetus (Chapter 6). By contrast, severe trauma or illness will dramatically increase energy and protein losses, an event unrelated to eating patterns.

Balance is not something to be thought of in the short term. Following each meal, there is either storage of absorbed nutrients [triacylglycerol (TAG) in adipose tissue or glucose in glycogen] or a cessation of nutrient losses (breakdown of stored TAG to non-esterified fatty acids or amino acid conversion to glucose via gluconeogenesis). As the period of post-prandial metabolism is extended, the recently stored nutrients are drawn upon and the catabolic state commences again. This is best reflected in the high glucagon to insulin ratio in the fasted state before the meal and the opposite high insulin to glucagon ratio during the meal and immediate post-prandial period. However, when balance is measured over a sufficient period, which varies from nutrient to nutrient, a stable pattern can be seen: zero, positive or negative (Figure 1.1). It is critically important with respect to obesity that

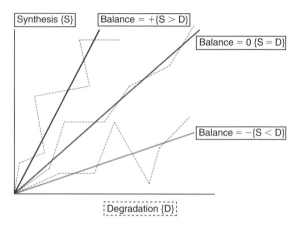

Figure 1.1 Positive, zero and negative nutrient balance over time with fluctuations upwards and downwards within that time.

the concept of balance is correctly considered. While at some stage energy balance must have been positive to reach an overweight or obese stage, once attained most people sustain a stable weight over quite long periods.

In the context of the present chapter, it is worth reflecting on the reasons why the period to assess energy balance correctly varies for different nutrients.

Fat and adipose tissue (Chapter 5)

- There is a very large capacity to vary the body's pool of adipose tissue. One can double or halve the level of the fat reserves in the body.
- The capacity to vary the level of TAG in blood en route to and from adipose tissue can vary considerably.
- Almost all of the TAG reserves in adipose tissue are exchangeable.

Calcium and bone (Chapter 12)

- The human being must maintain a large skeleton as the scaffold on which the musculature and organs are held.
- There is a very strict limit to the level of calcium that can be transported in blood. Excess or insufficient plasma calcium levels influence neural function and muscle function, since calcium is also centrally associated with both.

- Only a small fraction (the miscible pool) of bone is available for movement into plasma.

Because of these differences, calcium balance will require months of equilibrium while fat balance could be equilibrated in days or at most a few weeks.

1.3 Turnover

Although the composition of the body and of the constituents of the blood may appear constant, this does not mean that the component parts are static. In fact, most metabolic substrates are continually being utilised and replaced (i.e. they turn over). This process of turnover is well illustrated by considering protein metabolism in the body. Daily adult dietary protein intakes are in the region of 50–100 g, and the rates of urinary excretion of nitrogen match the protein intake. However, isotopically derived rates of protein degradation indicate that approximately 350 g is broken down per day. This is matched by an equivalent amount of protein synthesis per day, with most of this synthesis representing turnover of material (i.e. degradation and resynthesis) rather than being derived *de novo* from dietary protein (Chapter 4).

Similar metabolic turnover occurs with other nutrients; glucose is a good example, with a relatively constant blood glucose concentration arising from a matching between production by the liver and utilisation by the tissues (Chapter 3).

The concept of turnover can be applied at various levels within the body (molecular, cellular, tissue/organs, whole body). Thus, within a cell the concentration of adenosine triphosphate (ATP) remains relatively constant, with utilisation being matched by synthesis. Within most tissues and organs there is a continuous turnover of cells, with death and degradation of some cells matched by the production of new ones. Some cells, such as red blood cells, have a long lifespan (c. 120 days), while others, such as platelets, turn over in a matter of 1–2 days. In the case of proteins, those with very short half-lives have amino acid sequences that favour rapid proteolysis by the range of enzymes designed to hydrolyse proteins. Equally, those with longer half-lives have a more proteolytic-resistant structure.

A major advantage of this process of turnover is that the body is able to respond rapidly to a change in metabolic state by altering both synthesis and degradation to achieve the necessary response. One consequence of this turnover is the high energy cost of continuing synthesis. There is also the potential for dysfunction if the rates of synthesis and degradation do not match.

The consequences of a reduction in substrate synthesis will vary between the nutrients, depending on the half-life of the nutrient. The half-life is the time taken for half of the material to be used up, and is dependent on the rate of utilisation of the nutrient. Thus, if synthesis of a nutrient with a short half-life is stopped, the level of that nutrient will fall quickly. By contrast, a nutrient with a long half-life will disappear more slowly. Since proteins have the most complex of structures undergoing very significant turnover, it is worth dwelling on the mechanism of this turnover. Synthesis is fairly straightforward. Each protein has its own gene and the extent to which that gene is expressed will vary according to metabolic needs. In contrast to synthesis, a reasonably small array of lysosomal enzymes is responsible for protein degradation.

1.4 Flux

The flux of a nutrient through a metabolic pathway is a measure of the role of activity of the pathway. If one considers the flux of glucose from the blood to the tissues, the rate of utilisation is approximately 2 mg/kg body weight per minute at rest. However, this does not normally lead to a fall in blood glucose because it is balanced by an equivalent rate of glucose production by the liver, so the net flux is zero. This concept of flux can be applied at the cellular, tissue/organ or whole body level, and can also relate to the conversion of one substrate/nutrient to another (i.e. the movement between metabolic pathways). Flux is not necessarily related to the size of the pool or pathway through which the nutrient or metabolite flows. For example, the membrane of a cell will have several phospholipids present and each will have some level of arachidonic acid. The rate at which arachidonic acid enters one of the phospholipid pools and exits from that phospholipid pool is often higher in the smaller pools.

1.5 Metabolic pools

An important aspect of metabolism is that the nutrients and metabolites are present in several pools in the body (Figure 1.2). At the simplest level, for a given metabolite there are three pools, which will be illustrated using the role of dietary essential fatty acids in eicosanoid synthesis.

In the *functional pool*, the nutrient/metabolite has a direct involvement in one or more bodily functions. In the chosen example, intracellular free arachidonic acid, released from membrane-bound stores on stimulation with some extracellular signal, is the functional pool. It will be acted on by the key enzyme in eicosanoid synthesis, cyclo-oxygenase.

The *storage pool* provides a buffer of material that can be made available for the functional pool when required. Membrane phospholipids store arachidonic acid in the sn-2 position at quite high concentrations, simply to release this fatty acid when prostaglandin synthesis is needed. In the case of platelets, the eicosanoid thromboxane A_2 is synthesised from arachidonic acid released into the cytoplasm by stimuli such as collagen.

The *precursor pool* provides the substrate from which the nutrient/metabolite can be synthesised. Linoleic acid represents a good example of a precursor pool. It is elongated and desaturated in the liver to yield arachidonic acid. Thus, the hepatic pool of linoleic acid is the precursor pool in this regard. Not all nutrient pools should be thought of in the concept of the precursor, storage and functional pool model outlined above. The essential nutrients and the minerals and trace elements do not have a precursor pool. Nevertheless, no nutrient exists in a single homogeneous pool and an awareness of the existence of metabolic pools is essential to an understanding of human metabolism. For example, one might expect that a fasted individual would show a fall in all essential nutrient levels in the plasma pool. In many instances this is not the case initially because of the existence of storage pools, such as liver stores of iron or vitamin A. In the case of folic acid, fasting causes a rise in blood folic acid levels and this is explained by the concept of metabolic pools. A considerable amount of folic acid enters the gut via the bile duct and is reabsorbed further down the digestive tract. Thus there is an equilibrium between the blood folate pool and the gut folate pool. Fasting stops gallbladder contraction and thus the flow of folate to the gut, and hence folate is redistributed from one pool to another.

Another example of how an awareness of metabolic pools helps us to understand nutrition and metabolism is the intracellular free amino acid pool. This is the functional pool from which protein is synthesised. As this pool is depleted in the process of protein synthesis, it must be repleted, otherwise protein synthesis stops. Moreover, it is not just the intracellular pool of amino acids that matters but the intracellular pool of essential amino acids or, more precisely, the intracellular pool of the most limiting essential amino acid. Calculations show that if the pool of the most limiting amino acid in mammalian cells was not replenished, protein synthesis would cease in under 1 h. This highlights the need to transfer the limiting amino acid across the cell membrane, which raises the question of how that pool is repleted. Effectively, it can only be repleted if there is a comparable rate of protein degradation to provide the key amino acid, assuming the balance is zero. Thus there are links between the protein pool of amino acids and the extra- and intracellular pools of amino acids.

The size of these various pools varies substantially for different nutrients and metabolites. When studying the activities of metabolic processes within the body, it is often necessary to measure or estimate the size of the various pools in order to derive quantitative information about the overall rates of the processes. In addition, the actual situation may be more complex than the simple three-pool model described

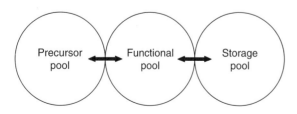

Figure 1.2 The pools in the body in which nutrients and metabolites may exist.

above. Nutritional assessment often involves some biochemical assessment of nutritional status. Blood is frequently the pool that is sampled and even there, blood can be separated into:

- erythrocytes, which have a long lifespan and are frequently used to assess folic acid status
- cells of the immune system, which can be used to measure zinc or ascorbic acid status
- plasma, which is used to ascertain the levels of many biomarkers
- fractions of plasma, such as cholesteryl esters used to ascertain long-term intake of polyunsaturated fatty acids.

In addition to sampling blood, nutritionists may take muscle or adipose tissue biopsies, or samples of saliva, buccal cells, hair and even toenails. A knowledge of how a nutrient behaves in different metabolic pools is critically important in assessing nutritional status. For example, the level of folic acid in plasma is determined by the most recent intake pattern and thus is subject to considerable fluctuation. However, since erythrocytes remain in the circulation for about 120 days, a sample of erythrocytes will represent very recently synthesised cells right through to erythrocytes ready for recycling through the turnover mechanism previously described. As erythrocytes do not have a nucleus, they cannot switch on genes that might influence folate levels, and so the cell retains the level of folate that prevailed at the time of synthesis. Thus, erythrocyte folate is a good marker of long-term intake. The free form of many minerals and trace elements is potentially toxic, and for this reason their level in the plasma is strictly regulated. Hence, blood levels are not used to assess long-term intake of selenium, but toenail clippings can be used.

1.6 Adaptation to altered nutrient supply

In many circumstances, the body is able to respond to altered metabolic and nutritional states in order to minimise the consequences of such alterations. For example, the brain has an obligatory requirement for glucose as a substrate for energy and it accounts for a significant part of resting energy expenditure. During undernutrition, where glu-

cose input does not match glucose needs, the first adaptation to the altered metabolic environment is to increase the process of gluconeogenesis, which involves the diversion of amino acids into glucose synthesis. That means less amino acid entering the protein synthesis cycle of protein turnover. Inevitably, protein reserves begin to fall. Thus, two further adaptations are made. The first is that the brain begins to use less glucose for energy (replacing it by ketones as an alternative metabolic fuel). The second is that overall, resting energy expenditure falls to help sustain a new balance if possible (Chapter 8). Stunting in infants and children, reflected in a low height for age, can be regarded as an example of successful adaptation to chronic low energy intake. If the period of energy deprivation is not too long, the child will subsequently exhibit a period of accelerated or catch-up growth (Chapter 7). If it is protracted, the stunting will lead to a permanent reprogramming of genetic balance. In many instances, the rate of absorption of nutrients may be enhanced as an adaptive mechanism to low intakes. Some adaptations appear to be unsuccessful but work for a period, effectively buying time in the hope that normal intakes will be resumed. In essential fatty acid deficiency the normal processes of elongation and desaturation of fatty acids take place but the emphasis is on the wrong fatty acid, that is, the non-essential 18-carbon monounsaturated fatty acid (oleic acid, C18:1 n-9) rather than the deficient dietary essential 18-carbon polyunsaturated fatty acid (linoleic acid, C18:2 n-6). The resultant 20-carbon fatty acid does not produce a functional eicosanoid. However, the body has significant reserves of linoleic acid which are also used for eicosanoid synthesis and so the machinery of this synthesis operates at a lower efficiency than normal. Eventually, if the dietary deficiency continues then pathological consequences ensue. In effect, adaptation to adverse metabolic and nutritional circumstances is a feature of survival until the crisis abates. The greater the capacity to mount adaptations to adverse nutritional circumstances the greater the capacity to survive.

1.7 Perspectives on the future

These basic concepts of nutrition will remain forever but they will be refined in detail by the emerging subject of nutrigenomics (Chapter 2). We will develop a greater understanding of how changes in the nutrient content of one pool will alter gene expression to influence events in another pool and how this influences the flux of nutrients between pools. We will better understand how common single nucleotide polymorphisms will determine the level of nutrient intake to achieve nutrient balance in different individuals.

Further reading

Frayn KN. Metabolic Regulation: a Human Perspective, 2nd edn. Oxford: Blackwell Publishing, 2003.

Websites

health.nih.gov/search.asp?category_id=29
http://themedicalbiochemistrypage.org/
www.nlm.nih.gov/medlineplus/foodnutritionandmetabolism.
  html

2
Molecular Aspects of Nutrition

Helen M Roche, Herman E Popeijus and Ronald P Mensink

Key messages

- The genome forms the information or blueprint to build up an organism and contains the full complement of genes (genotype) that when expressed determines the phenotype. The genome determines nutritional requirements and metabolic responses. Nutrients can modulate gene expression. These interactions between nutrition and the genome are referred to as *molecular nutrition* or *nutrigenomics*.
- The specific order of nucleotides within DNA forms the basis of genetic information. It is organised into chromosomes and every cell contains the full complement of chromosomes.
- Genetic variation can be the result of DNA alterations or damage that lead to genetic mutations. Genetic polymorphisms are common forms of genetic heterogeneity whereby there are several different forms of the sample allele in a population.

- Gene expression refers to the process whereby information encoded in the genes is converted into an observable phenotype.
- There are several tools to investigate molecular aspects of nutrition: animal models, cell/tissue-culture models, molecular cloning, gene expression analysis [polymerase chain reaction (PCR) and DNA microarrays], protein analysis, stable isotopes and metabolomics.
- Genetic background or common polymorphisms can determine nutrient requirements, the metabolic response to nutrients and/or susceptibility to diet-related diseases.
- Nutrients can interact with the genome and modulate gene expression. Hence, it is possible that nutrients could be used to manipulate an individual's metabolic response or to reduce their predisposition to diet-related diseases.

2.1 Introduction

Our genes determine every characteristic of life: gender, physical characteristics, metabolic functions, life stage and responses to external or environmental factors, which include nutrition. Nutrients have the ability to interact with the human genome to alter gene, protein and metabolite expression, which in turn can affect normal growth, health and disease. The human genome project has provided an enormous amount of genetic information and thus a greater understanding of our genetic background. It is true that we are only beginning to understand how nutrients interact with the genome. This aspect of nutritional science is known as *molecular nutrition or nutrigenomics*.

Molecular nutrition looks at the relationship between the human genome and nutrition from two perspectives. First, the genome determines every individual's genotype (or genetic background), which in turn can determine their nutrient state, metabolic response and/or genetic predisposition to diet-related disease. Secondly, nutrients have the ability to interact with the genome and alter gene, protein or metabolite expression. Gene expression is only the first stage of the whole-body or metabolic response to a nutrient and a number of post-translational events (e.g. enzyme activity, protein half-life, co-activators, co-repressors), but metabolomic events can also modify the ability of nutrients to alter an individual's phenotype. This chapter will review the core concepts in molecular biology, introduce the genome and discuss how we can characterise the effect of nutrition on gene, protein and metabolite expression using state-of-the-art transcriptomic, proteomic and metabolomic technologies, identifying some important research tools used to investigate these molecular aspects of nutrition, such as characterising how genetic background can determine nutrition and health. Some examples of how nutrients regulate gene, protein and metabolite expression will also be explored.

Nutrition and Metabolism, Second Edition, edited by S. A. Lanham-New, I. A. Macdonald and H. M. Roche.   © 2011 The Nutrition Society.

Overall the principal aim of nutrigenomics/molecular nutrition is to understand how the genome interacts with food, nutrients and non-nutrient food components, within the context of nutrition-related diseases. It attempts to determine nutrients that enhance the expression of gene, protein and metabolic pathways/networks that are associated with health and suppress those that predispose to disease. While it is unrealistic to assume that food intake and good nutrition can overcome our genetic fate, good nutrition can improve health and quality of life. Therefore, it is essential that we extend our understanding of the molecular interplay between the genome, food and nutrients; and therefore have a greater understanding of the molecular relationship between diet, health and disease.

2.2 Core concepts in molecular biology

The genome, DNA and the genetic code

The *genome* refers to the total genetic information carried by a cell or an organism. In very simple terms the genome (or DNA sequence) is the full complement of genes. The expression of each gene leads to the formation of a protein, which, together with many other proteins that are coded by other genes form tissues, organs and systems, constitute the whole organism. In complex multicellular organisms the information carried within the genome gives rise to multiple tissues (muscle, bone, adipose tissue, etc.). The characteristics of each cell type and tissue are dependent on differential gene expression by the genome, whereby only those genes are expressed that code for specific proteins to confer the individual characteristics of the cells that constitute each organ. For example, gene expression in muscle cells may result in the formation of muscle-specific proteins that are critical for the differentiation, development and maintenance of muscle tissue, and these genes are completely different from those expressed in osteoblasts, osteoclasts and osteocytes, which form bone. These differentially expressed proteins can have a wide variety of functions: as structural components of the cell or as regulatory proteins, including enzymes, hormones, receptors and intracellular signalling proteins that confer tissue specificity.

It is very important to understand the molecular basis of cellular metabolism because incorrect expression of genes at the cellular level can disrupt whole-body metabolism and lead to disease. Aberrant gene expression can lead to cellular disease when proteins are produced in the wrong place, at the wrong time, at abnormal levels or as a malfunctioning isoform that can compromise whole-body health. Furthermore, different nutritional states and intervention therapies can modulate the expression of cellular genes and thereby the formation of proteins. Therefore, the ultimate goal of molecular nutrition is to understand how nutrients interact with the genome and alter the expression of genes, and the formation and function of proteins that play a role in health and disease.

Deoxyribonucleic acid (DNA) is the most basic unit of genetic information, as the DNA sequence codes for the amino acids that form cellular proteins. Two individual DNA molecules are packaged as the chromosomes within the nucleus of animal and plant cells. The basic structure and composition of DNA are illustrated in Figure 2.1. DNA is composed of large polymers, with a linear backbone composed of residues of the five-carbon sugar residue deoxyribose, which are successively linked by covalent phosphodiester bonds. A nitrogenous base, either a *purine* [adenine (A) or *guanine* (G)] or a *pyrimidine* [cytosine (C) or *thymine* (T)], is attached to each deoxyribose. DNA forms *a double-stranded helical structure*, in which the two separate DNA polymers wind around each other. The two strands of DNA run *antiparallel*, such that the deoxyribose linkages of one strand runs in the 5′–3′ direction and the other strand in the opposite 3′–5′ direction. The double helix is mainly maintained by hydrogen bonds between nucleotide pairs. According to the *base-pair rules*, adenine always binds to thymine via two hydrogen bonds and guanine binds to cytosine via three hydrogen bonds. This complementary base-pair rule ensures that the sequence of one DNA strand specifies the sequence of the other.

The *nucleotide* is the basic repeat unit of the DNA strand and is composed of deoxyribose, a phosphate group and a base. The 5′–3′ sequential arrangement of the nucleotides in the polymeric chain of DNA contains the *genetic code* for the arrangement of amino acids in proteins. The genetic code is the universal language that translates the information stored within the DNA of genes into proteins. It is universal between species. The genetic code is read in groups of three nucleotides. These three nucleotides, called a

(a)

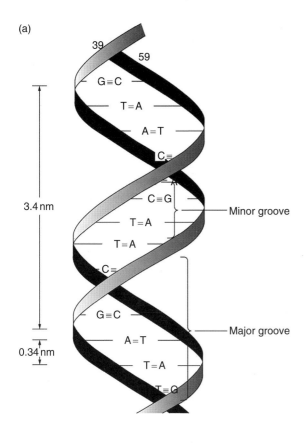

Minor groove

Major groove

(b)

Figure 2.1 Structure and composition of DNA. DNA contains deoxynucleotides consisting of a specific heterocyclic nitrogenous base (adenine, guanine, cytosine or thymine) joined to a deoxyribose phosphate moiety. Adjacent deoxynucleotides are linked through their phosphate groups to form long polynucleotide chains. (a) The DNA double helix; (b) a nucleotide; (c) the purine and pyrimidine bases. (Cox TM and Sinclair J, Molecular Biology in Medicine, 1997. Copyright © Wiley-Blackwell.)

Table 2.1 The genetic code

First base	Second base				Third base
	T	C	A	G	
T	TTT (Phe)	TCT (Ser)	TAT (Tyr)	TGT (Cys)	T
	TTC (Phe)	TCC (Ser)	TAC (Tyr)	TGC (Cys)	C
	TTA (Leu)	TCA (Ser)	TAA (Stop)	TGA (Stop)	A
	TTG (Leu)	TCG (Ser)	TAG (Stop)	TGG (Trp)	G
C	CTT (Leu)	CCT (Pro)	CAT (His)	CGT (Arg)	T

Ala, alanine; Arg, arginine; Asn, asparagine; Asp, aspartic acid; Cys, cysteine; Gln, glutamine; Glu, glutamic acid; Gly, glycine; His, histidine; Ile, isoleucine; Leu, leucine; Lys, lysine; Met, methionine; Phe, phenylalanine; Pro, proline; Ser, serine; Thr, threonine; Trp, tryptophan; Tyr, tyrosine; Val, valine.

codon, are specific for one particular amino acid. Table 2.1 shows the 64 possible codons, of which 61 specify for 22 different amino acids, while three sequences (TAA, TAG, TGA) are stop codons (i.e. do not code for an amino acid). Some amino acids are coded for by more than one codon; this is referred to as *redundancy*. For example, the amino acid isoleucine may be coded by the DNA sequence ATT, ATC or ATA. Each amino acid sequence of a protein always begins with a methionine residue because the start codon (ATG) codes for methionine. The three stop codons signal the end of the coding region of a gene and the resultant polypeptide sequence.

Chromosome (karyotype)

In eukaryotic cells, DNA is packaged as *chromosomes* and every cell contains a set of chromosomes (Figure 2.2). Each chromosome has a narrow waist known as the centromere, which divides each chromosome into a short and a long arm, labelled p and q, respectively. The tip of each chromosomal arm is known as the telomere. DNA is packaged in a very compact structure within the nucleus. Condensing of DNA is essential because the human cell contains approximately 4×10^9 nucleotide pairs, termed *base pairs (bp)* of DNA, whose extended length would approach more than 1 m. The most basic unit of the chromosome is the *nucleosome*, which is composed of a 145 bp linear strand of double-stranded DNA wound around a complex of *histone proteins* (H2a, H2b, H3 and H4). Nucleosomes are linked together by the histone protein H1 to form *chromatin*. During

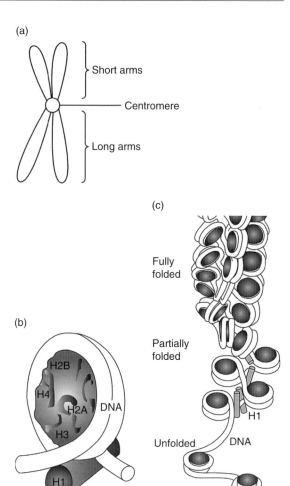

Figure 2.2 Structure of (a) a chromosome, (b) the nucleosome and (c) chromatin. (Cox TM and Sinclair J, Molecular Biology in Medicine, 1997. Copyright © Wiley–Blackwell.)

cell division this is then further compacted with the aid of non-histone chromosomal proteins to generate a chromosome. The structure of DNA in chromatin is important because it has profound effects on the ability of DNA to be transcribed.

The chromosomal complement or karyotype refers to the number, size and shape of the chromosomes. The human karyotype is composed of 22 pairs of autosomes and a pair of sex chromosomes: XX in the female and XY in the male. Most human cells contain 46 chromosomes, the *diploid* number. Chromosomal disorders are characterised by abnormalities of chromosomal number or structure. They may involve the autosomes or the sex chromosomes and may be the result of a *germ-cell mutation* in the parent (or a more distant ancestor) or a *somatic mutation* in which only a proportion of cells will be affected (mosaicism). The normal chromosome number is an exact multiple of the *haploid* number (23) and is referred to as the diploid number. A chromosomal number that exceeds the diploid number (46) is called *polyploidy*, and one that is not an exact multiple number is *aneuploidy*. Aneuploidy usually occurs when the pair of chromosomes fails to segregate (non-disjunction) during meiosis, which results in an extra copy of a chromosome (*trisomy*) or a missing copy of a chromosome (*monosomy*). Down's syndrome is a common example of trisomy, and is due to the presence of three copies of chromosome 21 (trisomy 21).

Structural abnormalities of chromosomes also occur. A *translocation* is the transfer of chromosomal material between chromosomes. Chronic myeloid leukaemia results from the translocation of genetic material between chromosome 8 and chromosome 22. This results in an abnormal chromosome, known as the Philadelphia chromosome, the expression of which results in leukaemia. *Chromosomal deletions* arise from the loss of a portion of the chromosome between two break points. *Inversions* arise from two chromosomal breaks with inversion through 180° of the chromosomal segment between the breaks.

Genotype, phenotype and allelic expression

The *genotype* of an organism is the total number of genes that make up a cell or organism. The term, however, is also used to refer to alleles present at one locus. Each diploid cell contains two copies of each gene; the individual copies of the gene are called *alleles*. The definition of an allele is one of two (or more) alternative forms of a gene located at the corresponding site (*locus*) on homologous chromosomes. One allele is inherited from the maternal gamete and the other from the paternal gamete, therefore the cell can contain the same or different alleles of every gene. *Homozygous* individuals carry two identical alleles of a particular gene. *Heterozygotes* have two different alleles of a particular gene. The term *haplotype* describes a cluster of alleles that occur together on a DNA segment and/or are inherited together. *Genetic linkage* is the tendency for alleles close together to be transmitted together through meiosis and hence be inherited together.

Genetic polymorphisms are different forms of the same allele in the population. The 'normal' allele is known as the *wild-type allele*, whereas the variant is known as the polymorphic or mutant allele. A polymorphism differs from a mutation because it occurs in a population at a frequency greater than a recurrent mutation. By convention, a polymorphic locus is one at which there are at least two alleles, each of which occurs with frequencies greater than 1%. Alleles with frequencies less than 1% are considered as a recurrent mutation. The alleles of the ABO blood group system are examples of genetic polymorphisms. The acronym *single nucleotide polymorphism* (*SNP*) is a common pattern of inherited genetic variation (or common mutation) that involves a single base change in the DNA. More recently *copy number variation* (*CNV*) has been identified as another common form of genetic variation, it is estimated that about 0.4% of the human genome differ with respect to CVN. As yet CNV has not been associated with susceptibility or resistance diet-related diseases but it is possible that this type of genetic variation may also be linked to nutrition and health. The traditional way of identifying genetic variants was as *restriction fragment length polymorphism* (*RFLP*). RFLPs result in different lengths of DNA fragments when restriction enzymes cleave – or do not cleave – DNA at specific target sites because of nucleotide changes in the DNA sequence at the site where the restriction enzyme would usually cleave DNA.

Epigenetics is a relatively new field of research which refers to changes in gene expression due to mechanisms other than changes in the underlying DNA sequence. The molecular basis of epigenetics is complex; put simply it refers to altered DNA structure. It involves modifications of the activation of certain genes, but not the basic DNA sequence. For example, DNA methylation refers to the addition of methyl groups to the DNA, which in turn affects transcriptional activity. Folate status can affect DNA methylation, which in turn can affect gene expression through mechanisms that are being actively researched.

There is a considerable amount of research investigating the relationships between common genetic polymorphisms and epigenetics with disease because certain genetic variations may predispose an individual to a greater risk of developing a disease. The effect of genetic variation in response to dietary change is also of great interest because some polymorphisms/epigenetic states may determine an individual's response to dietary change. Hence, genetic variation can determine the therapeutic efficacy of nutritional therapy, which may in turn determine the outcome of certain disease states. The interrelationship between diet, disease and genetic variation will be discussed in more detail in Section 2.5.

The *phenotype* is the observable biochemical, physiological or morphological characteristics of a cell or individual resulting from the expression of the cell's genotype, within the environment in which it is expressed. Allelic variation and expression can affect the phenotype of an organism. A *dominant allele* is the allele of a gene that contributes to the phenotype of a heterozygote. The non-expressing allele that makes no contribution to the phenotype is known as the *recessive allele*. The phenotype of the recessive allele is only demonstrated in homozygotes who carry both recessive alleles. *Codominant alleles* contribute equally to the phenotype. The ABO blood groups are an example of codominant alleles, where both alleles are expressed in an individual. In the case of *partial dominance* a combination of alleles is expressed simultaneously and the phenotype of the heterozygote is intermediate between that of the two homozygotes. For example, in the case of the snapdragon, a cross between red and white alleles will generate heterozygotes with pink flowers. *Genetic heterogeneity* refers to the phenomenon whereby a single phenotype can be caused by different allelic variants.

DNA damage, genetic mutations and heritability (monogenic and polygenic disorders)

Many agents can cause DNA damage, including ionising radiation, ultraviolet light, chemical mutagens and viruses. DNA can also change spontaneously under normal physiological conditions. For example, adenine and cytosine can spontaneously undergo deamination to produce hypoxanthine and uracil residues. A change in the nucleotide sequence is known as a *mutation*. A mutation may be defined as a permanent transmissible change in the nucleotide sequence of a chromosome, usually in a single gene, which may lead to loss or change of the normal function of the gene. A mutation can have a significant effect on protein production or function because it can alter the amino acid sequence of the protein that is coded by the DNA sequence in a gene. *Point mutations* include *insertions*, *deletions*, *transitions* and *transversions*. Two types of events can cause a point mutation: chemical modification of DNA, which directly changes one base into another, or a mistake during DNA replication that causes, for instance, the insertion of the wrong base into the polynucleotide during DNA synthesis. Transitions are the most common type of point mutations and result in the substitution of one pyrimidine (C–G) or one purine (A–T) by the other. Transversions are less common, where a purine is replaced by a pyrimidine or vice versa.

The functional outcome of mutations can vary very significantly. For example, a single-point mutation can change the third nucleotide in a codon and not change the amino acid that is translated, or it may cause the incorporation of another amino acid into the protein – this is known as a *missense mutation*. The functional effect of a missense mutation varies greatly depending on the site of the mutation and the importance of the protein in relation to health. A missense mutation can have no apparent effect on health or it can result in a serious medical condition. For example, sickle cell anaemia is due to a missense mutation of the β-globin gene: a glutamine is changed to valine in the amino acid sequence of the protein. This has drastic effects on the structure and function of the β-globin protein, which causes aggregation of deoxygenated haemoglobin and deformation of the red blood cell. A nucleotide change can also result in the generation of a stop codon (*nonsense mutation*) and no functional protein will be produced. *Frameshift mutations* refer to small deletions or insertions of bases that alter the reading frame of the nucleotide sequence; hence, the different codon sequence will affect the expression of amino acids in the peptide sequence.

Heritability refers to how much a disease can be ascribed to genetic rather than environmental factors. It is expressed as a percentage, a high value indicating that the genetic component is important in the aetiology of the disease. Genetic disorders can simply be classified as *monogenic* (or single-gene disorders) or *polygenic diseases* (multifactorial diseases). In general, we have a far greater understanding of the *single-gene disorders* because they are due to one or more mutant alleles at a single locus and most follow simple *Mendelian inheritance*. Examples of such disorders are:

- autosomal dominant: familial hypercholestrolaemia, von Willebrand's disease, achondroplasia
- autosomal recessive: cystic fibrosis, phenylketonuria, haemochromatosis, α-thalassaemia, β-thalassaemia
- X-linked dominant: vitamin D-resistant rickets
- X-linked recessive: Duchenne muscular dystrophy, haemophilia A, haemophilia B, glucose-6-phosphate dehydrogenase deficiency.

Some single-gene disorders show non-Mendelian patterns of inheritance, which are explained by different degrees of penetrance and variable gene expression. *Penetrance* means that a genetic lesion is expressed in some individuals but not in others. For example, people carrying a gene with high penetrance have a high probability of developing any associated disease. A low-penetrance gene will result in only a slight increase in disease risk. *Variable expression* occurs when a genetic mutation produces a range of phenotypes. *Anticipation* refers to the situation when a Mendelian trait manifests as a phenotype with decreasing age of onset and often with greater severity as it is inherited through subsequent generations (e.g. Huntington's chorea, myotonic dystrophy). *Imprinting* refers to the differential expression of a chromosome or allele depending on whether the allele has been inherited from the male or female gamete. This is due to selective inactivation of genes according to the paternal or maternal origin of the chromosomes. Although there are only a few examples of diseases that arise as a result of imprinting (e.g. Prader–Willi and Angelman's syndromes), it is thought that this form of gene inactivation may be more important than previously realised.

Polygenic (or multifactorial) diseases are those due to a number of genes (e.g. cancer, coronary heart disease, diabetes and obesity). Even though polygenic disorders are more common than monogenic disorders, we still do not understand the full genetic basis of any of these conditions. This reflects the fact that there is interaction between many candidate genes, that is, those genes that are thought to play an aetiological role in multifactorial conditions.

Furthermore, in polygenic inheritance, a trait is in general determined by a combination of both the gene and the environment.

The Human Genome Project

The Human Genome Project (HGP) is an important source of genetic information that will be a resource to molecular nutrition, especially in terms of understanding the interaction between nutrition and the human genome. The working draft sequence of the human genome was published in February 2001. The project showed that the size of the human genome is 30 times greater than that of the fruit fly and 250 times larger than yeast. Only 3% of the DNA in the human genome constitutes coding regions. Compared with the fruit fly, the human genome has much more non-coding or intronic regions. Although these intronic regions do not code for genes they may have a functional role, and these functional effects could, for example, include important promoter and/or repressor regions. The number of genes coded by the human genome was much less than expected. The human genome codes for approximately 25 000 genes. Indeed, a human has only two to three times as many genes as a fruit fly. The two- to three-fold difference between humans and fruit flies may largely be accounted for by the greater number of control genes (e.g. transcription factors) in the human genome.

In the future, we will have a greater understanding of the human genome and how it interacts with the environment. The HGP showed that humans are very alike: it estimated that humans are 99.8% genetically similar. Nevertheless, the implications of the HGP in relation to molecular nutrition are immense. The challenge is to identify the proportion of that genetic variation that is relevant to nutrition. The term 'gene mining' refers to the process that will identify the new genes involved in nutrition, health and disease. At the most basic level we already know that the human genome determines nutrient requirements, for example gender determines iron requirements – the iron requirement of menstruating women is greater than that of men of the same age. In the case of folate, research would suggest that the methylenetetrahydrofolate reductase (MTHFR) polymorphism could determine an individual's folate requirements. Since there are fewer genes than anticipated, it has been proposed that different isoforms of the same gene with different functionality are important. Already there are examples of this (e.g. the three isoforms of the apolipoprotein E (Apo E) gene determine the magnitude of postprandial triacylglycerol metabolism). Furthermore, it has been proposed that the interaction between the human genome and the environment is an important determinant of within- and between-individual variation. Within the context of molecular nutrition we will have to determine how nutrients alter gene expression and determine the functional consequences of genetic polymorphisms. With the information generated from the HGP we will have a more complete understanding and information in relation to the relevance of genetic variation, and how alterations in nutrient intake or nutritional status affect gene expression in a way that is relevant to human health and disease processes. In essence, the challenge is to bridge the gap between the genome sequence and whole-organism biology, nutritional status and intervention.

2.3 Gene expression: transcription and translation

Gene expression

Gene expression refers to the process whereby the information encoded in the DNA of a gene is converted into a protein, which confers the observable phenotype upon the cell. A *gene* may be defined as the nucleic acid sequence that is necessary for the synthesis of a functional peptide or protein in a temporal and tissue-specific manner. However, a gene is not directly translated into a protein; it is expressed via a nucleic acid intermediary called *messenger RNA (mRNA)*. The transcriptional unit of every gene is the sequence of DNA transcribed into a single mRNA molecule, starting at the promoter and ending at the terminator regions. The essential features of a gene and mRNA are presented in Figure 2.3. The DNA sequence of a gene comprises two non-coding (or untranslated) regions at the beginning and end of the gene coding region. The non-coding promoter and terminator regions of the DNA are partially transcribed, but not translated and therefore form the 5′ and 3′ *untranslated regions (UTR)* of mRNA. Although the non-coding regions of a gene and mRNA are not translated into the protein product of the gene, they contain critical parts of the genetic information involved in regulation of gene expression and the characteristics of the protein pro-

duction. The *promoter region* is located immediately upstream of the gene coding region; it contains DNA sequences, known as the TATA and CAAT boxes, which define the DNA binding sites at which transcription starts and regulate the rate of gene expression. The *TATA box* is an AT-rich sequence that occurs about 30 bp (−30 bp) upstream from the transcriptional start site. The *CAAT box* contains this short DNA sequence about 80 bp upstream (−80 bp) of the start site. These sequences, together with binding sites for other *transcription factors*, regulate the rate of tissue-specific gene expression. Transcription starts at the *CAP site*, so-called because following transcription the 5′ end of the mRNA molecule is capped at this site by the attachment of a specialised nucleotide (7-methyl guanosine). The CAP site is followed by the *initiation*, or *start codon* (ATG), which specifies the start of translation; hence, according to the genetic code every polypeptide begins with methionine. The DNA coding sequence for a gene in eukaryotes is not contiguous or uninterrupted. Each gene contains DNA sequences that code for the amino acid sequence of the protein, which are called *exons*. These exons are interrupted by non-coding DNA sequences, which are called *introns*. The last exon ends with a *stop codon* (TAA, TAG or TGA), which represents the end of the gene-coding region and it is followed by the terminator sequence in the DNA sequence that defines the end of the gene-coding region. The *3 UTR* of the mRNA molecule includes a *poly(A) signal (AATAAA)* that is added to the mRNA molecule following transcription.

Ribonucleic acid

RNA, like DNA, carries genetic information. The composition of RNA is very similar to DNA, and it plays a key role in all stages of gene expression. RNA is also a linear polynucleotide, but it differs from DNA in that it is single stranded and composed of polymers of ribose rather than deoxyribose, the pyrimidine base *uracil (U)* replaces thymine (T), and it is relatively unstable when compared to DNA. There are at least five different types of RNA in eukaryotic cells and all are involved in gene expression:

- Messenger RNA (mRNA) molecules are long, linear, single-stranded polynucleotides that are direct copies of DNA. mRNA is formed by transcription of DNA.
- Small nuclear RNA (snRNA) is a short, ±150 nucleotide (nt) RNA molecule that forms, together with

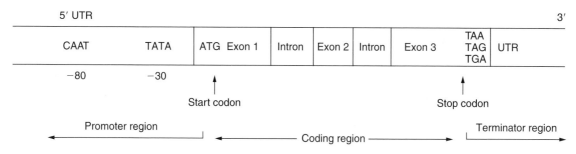

Figure 2.3 Essential features of the gene.

a protein, the small nuclear ribonucleoprotein (snRNP). Several of these snRNPs form with other proteins the splisosoom that facilitates the removal of introns from the precursor mRNA.

- Ribosomal RNA (rRNA) is a structural and functional component of ribosomes. Ribosomes, the cytoplasmic machines that synthesise mRNA into amino acid polypeptides, are present in the cytoplasm of the cell and are composed of rRNA and ribosomal proteins.
- Transfer RNA (tRNA) is a small RNA molecule that donates amino acids during translation or protein synthesis.
- A group of small RNAs such as microRNAs (miRNA), small interfering RNAs (siRNAs), Piwi-interacting RNAs (piRNAs) and repeat-associated siRNAs (rasiRNAs). These small RNA molecules have various functions at the transcriptional and/or post-transcriptional level, including the breakdown of mRNA, repression of transcription and chromatin remodelling.

RNA is about 10 times more abundant than DNA in eukaryotic cells; 80% is rRNA, 15% is tRNA and 5% is mRNA. In the cell mRNA is normally found associated with protein complexes called *messenger ribonucleoprotein* (*mRNP*), which package mRNA and aid its transport into the cytoplasm, where it is decoded into a protein.

Transcription

RNA transcription, which is the process whereby the genetic information encoded in DNA is transferred into mRNA, is the first step in the process of gene expression and occurs in the nucleus of the cell. It can be divided into four stages: template recognition, initiation, elongation and termination.

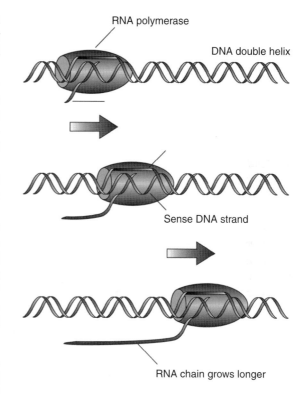

Figure 2.4 RNA polymerase II transcribes the information in DNA into RNA.

Transcription is catalysed by DNA-dependent *RNA polymerase* enzymes (Figure 2.4). In eukaryotic cells RNA polymerase II synthesises mRNA, while RNA polymerase I and RNA polymerase III synthesise tRNA and rRNA. RNA polymerase II is a complex 12-subunit enzyme and is associated with several transcription factors (TFs), including TFIIA, TFIIB, TFIIC, TFIID, TFIIE, TFIIF, TFIIH and TFIIJ. The strand of DNA that directs synthesis of mRNA via complementary base pairing is called the template

Figure 2.5 Transcription and processing of mRNA.

or *antisense strand*. The other DNA strand that bears the same nucleotide sequence is called the coding or *sense strand*. Therefore, RNA represents a copy of DNA. Transcription is a multistep process, initiated by the assembly of an initiation complex (TFIID, TFIIA, TFIIB, TFIIF, TFIIE, TFIIH) at the promoter, to which RNA polymerase II binds. TFIID recognises the promoter and binds to the TATA box at the start of the gene. TFIIH unwinds double-stranded DNA to expose the unpaired DNA nucleotide and the DNA sequence is used as a template from which RNA is synthesised. TFIIE and TFIIH are required for promoter clearance, allowing RNA polymerase II to commence movement away from the promoter. Initiation describes the synthesis of the first nine nucleotides of the RNA transcript. Elongation describes the phase during which RNA polymerase moves along the DNA and extends the growing RNA molecule. The RNA molecule is synthesised by adding nucleotides to the free 3′-OH end of the growing RNA chain. As only at this free 3′-OH end new nucleotides can be attached, RNA synthesis takes always place in the 5′-3′ direction. Growing of the RNA chain is ended by a process called *termination*, which involves recognition of the *terminator sequence* that signals the dissociation of the polymerase complex.

Post-transcriptional processing of RNA

After transcription of DNA into RNA, the newly synthesised RNA is modified. This process is called post-transcriptional processing of RNA (Figure 2.5). The *primary RNA transcript* synthesised by RNA polymerase II from genomic DNA is often called *heterogeneous nuclear RNA* (*hnRNA*) because of its considerable variation in size. Instead of hnRNA often the term *precursor mRNA* (*pre-mRNA*) is used to designate that it refers to unprocessed RNA. The primary transcript is an RNA molecule that represents a full copy of the gene extending from the promoter to the terminator region of the gene, and includes introns and exons. While still in the nucleus, the newly synthesised RNA is capped, polyadenylated and spliced. *Capping* refers to the addition of a modified guanine (G) nucleotide (7-methylguanosine) at the 5′ end of the mRNA. This 7-methylguanosine cap has three functions: it protects the synthesised RNA from enzymic attack, it aids pre-mRNA splicing and it enhances translation of the mRNA. *Polyadenylation* involves the addition of a string of adenosine (A) residues (a *poly-A tail*) to the 3′ end of the pre-mRNA. Then the pre-mRNA is spliced, which is performed by the spliceosome. This RNA–protein complex recognises the consensus sequences at each end of the intron (5′-GU and AG-3′) and

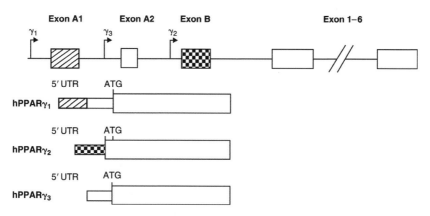

Figure 2.6 Alternative RNA splice variants of the peroxisome proliferator activator receptor-gamma (PPARγ) gene.

excises the introns so that the remaining exons are spliced together to form the mature mRNA molecule. After capping, polyadenylation and splicing, the mRNA is transported from the nucleus to the cytoplasm for translation.

Alternative splicing describes the process whereby other, alternative, splice recognition sites leads to the removal of certain exons, thereby generating different mature mRNA molecules and ultimately different proteins. As illustrated in Figure 2.6, one primary RNA transcript can be spliced in three different ways, leading to three mRNA isoforms, one with five exons or two with four exons. Upon translation the different mRNA isoforms will give rise to different isoforms of the protein product of the gene. This is a relatively common phenomenon and although the physiological or metabolic relevance of the different isoforms of many proteins is not fully understood it may be relevant to molecular nutrition. For example, the peroxisome proliferator activator receptor-gamma (PPARγ) gene can produce three different isoforms of mRNA (PPARγ$_1$, PPARγ$_2$, PPARγ$_3$) as a result of different promoters and alternative splicing. It would seem that the PPARγ$_2$ mRNA isoform is responsive to nutritional states. PPARγ$_2$ mRNA expression is increased in the fed state; its expression is positively related to adiposity and is reduced on weight loss. Therefore, PPARγ$_2$ mRNA may be the isoform that mediates nutrient regulation of gene expression. Besides alternative splicing, a peculiar way of splicing exists that occurs with introns that form a ribozyme. These special introns are RNA molecules that function as enzymes and catalyse their own excision, which is referred to as *self-splicing*.

RNA editing is another way in which the primary RNA transcript can be modified. Editing involves the binding of proteins or short RNA templates to specific regions of the primary transcript and subsequent alteration or editing of the RNA sequence, either by insertion of one or more different nucleotides or by base changes. This mechanism allows the production of different proteins from a single gene under different physiological conditions. The two isoforms of apo B are examples of RNA editing. In this case, RNA editing allows for tissue-specific expression of the apo B gene, such that the full protein apo B100 is produced in the liver and secreted on VLDL. By contrast, in the intestine the apo B48 isoform is produced because a premature stop codon is inserted so that transcription of the protein is halted and the resultant apoprotein is only 48% of that of the full-length apo B100 protein.

Control of gene expression and transcription

All individual cells of an organism contain the complete genetic blueprint of the organism. Therefore, it is of critical importance that the right genes are expressed in the correct tissue, at the proper level and at the correct time. Temporal and tissue-specific gene expression in eukaryotic cells is mostly controlled at the level of transcription initiation. Two types of factors regulate gene expression: *cis-acting control elements* and *trans-acting factors. Cis*-acting elements do not encode proteins; they influence gene transcription by acting as binding sites for proteins that regulate transcription. These DNA sequences are usually organised in clusters, located in the promoter region of the gene, that influence the transcription of genes. The TATA and CAAT boxes are examples of *cis*-acting elements.

The *trans*-acting factors are known as *transcription factors* or DNA binding proteins. Transcription factors are proteins that are encoded for by other genes, and include steroid hormone receptor complexes, vitamin-receptor proteins and mineral–protein complexes. These transcription factors bind to specific DNA sequences in the promoter region of the target gene and promote gene transcription. The precise mechanism(s) of how transcription factors influence gene transcription is not fully understood. However, transcription factors in general share some properties. They often have amino acid domains that contain one or more zinc ions, so-called zinc fingers that enable binding to DNA in a sequence-specific manner. Another type of domain contains predominantly the amino acid leucine, the leucine zipper, and has a function in binding ('zipping') to similar domains in other proteins based on the charge of the individual amino acids. Beside these domains, transcription factors often contain a nuclear localisation signal to direct the protein from the cytoplasm to the nucleus and specific amino acids that can be modified by, for instance, phosphorylation, ubiquitinylation or acetylation and thereby get activated or inactivated. These modifications enable fine-tuning of the action of transcription factors.

As mentioned, transcription factors play a key role in temporal and tissue-specific gene expression. On binding they are able to influence the transcription of usually more than one gene. There is ample evidence that transcription factors can remodel the chromatin structure in such a way that certain parts of the genome become available for transcription, while other parts of the chromosomes become tightly packed and inaccessible for transcription. For example, the genes for the enzymes of gluconeogenesis can be turned on in the hepatocyte, but not in the adipocyte. This is because the hepatocyte expresses the transcription factors that are required to initiate the expression of the gluconeogenic enzymes.

Master regulatory proteins regulate the expression of many genes of a single metabolic pathway. For example, in the lipogenic pathway the fatty acid synthase complex codes for seven distinct genes that have to be coordinately expressed to form the enzymes required for fatty acid synthesis. This ensures that

Figure 2.7 Three phases of translation. (a) Initiation: first codon methionine; (b) elongation: translation continues elongating the nascent peptide; (c) termination: translation ends on recognition of the stop codon.

sufficient levels of all of the enzymes of this metabolic pathway are available simultaneously.

RNA translation: protein synthesis

Translation is the process by which the genetic information coded in mRNA is converted into an amino acid sequence (polypeptide) through reading the mRNA coding sequence as a continuous, non-overlapping, tri-letter code (Figure 2.7). This three letter- or trinucleotide code (triplets or codons) can thus be read in three possible *reading frames* within a single-strand mRNA molecule. The five forms of RNA play an inherent role in this translation process. Small RNAs modulate the various processes, small nuclear RNAs help to remove the introns, mRNA represents the template from which the protein is synthesised, rRNA is the cytoplasmic machine that synthesises the protein product of the gene and tRNA donates the amino acids that are incorporated into the polypeptide during protein synthesis. The tRNA molecule has a very distinct structure that is used to deliver the amino acids of the nascent polypeptide. Protein synthesis occurs on the *ribosome* in the cytoplasm or on ribosomes attached to cytoplasmatic side of the rough endoplasmatic reticulum membrane. Ribosomes consist of two subunits, a 40S (small) and 60S (large), which combine to form the 80S particle. Protein synthesis begins by the formation of a complex involving a 40S ribosomal subunit carrying a methionine tRNA, which base pairs with the initiation codon AUG on the mRNA molecule. Translation is largely regulated by controlling the formation of the initiation complex, which is the 40S ribosomal subunit, the mRNA and specific regulatory proteins. The structure of the 5′ UTR is critical for determining whether mRNA is translated or sequestered in the untranslated ribonucleoprotein complex. Initiation of translation is also dependent on the presence of the 5′ cap structure and secondary structure of the mRNA next to the initiation codon. Secondary structures such as stem loops in the 5′ end of the mRNA inhibit the initiation of translation. Some of the translation regulatory proteins are cell specific and mRNA specific, allowing precise post-transcriptional control over the synthesis of specific proteins. The poly(A) tail also modulates translation. Although it is not essential for translation to occur, mRNA lacking the poly(A) tail is less efficiently translated.

Once the initiation complex has formed, synthesis of the polypeptide chain is driven by the interaction between *elongation factors* (elFs), the ribosome and tRNA along the length of the mRNA molecule. At each codon the ribosome and elFs promote the interaction between mRNA and tRNA. tRNA donates an amino acid, which is added to the newly synthesised polypeptide that corresponds to the codon in the mRNA. The tRNA achieves this because it bears a triplet of bases (*anti-codon*) that are complementary to the mRNA codon, and there is an amino acid attached to the acceptor arm of the tRNA that corresponds to the codon in the mRNA. When the anticodon of the tRNA matches the codon or trinucleotide sequence in the mRNA, the tRNA donates the amino acid to the newly synthesised polypeptide. For example, the first tRNA that carries methionine has the anticodon UAC; it recognises the methionine codon AUG on mRNA. Similarly, the anticodon AAC recognises the

leucine codon TTG on the mRNA. This process continues until the ribosome reaches a termination codon (UAA, UAG, UGA) and then the completed polypeptide is released from the ribosomal units.

Post-translational modification

Post-translational modification refers to the process that converts the pre-mature polypeptide into the mature protein product of the gene. The nascent polypeptide may start to form the complex structure of the protein as it is being synthesised directly in the cytoplasm or at the membrane of the rough endoplasmic reticulum. When formed at the ribosomes attached to the rough endosplasmatic membrane, the pre-mature polypeptide chain is likely to be transported to the Golgi body for further processing. The polypeptide may be modified further by hydroxylation, phosphorylation, glycosylation, or by proteolytic activities, which will confer functional characteristics to the protein. For example, the phosphorylation status of a protein can determine whether it is active or inactive.

2.4 Research tools to investigate molecular aspects of nutrition

For many reasons, it is not always possible to examine the molecular aspects of nutrition in humans. Such studies may be too expensive, while in many cases it is simply not possible to obtain the tissues or cells of interest. Another pragmatic problem is that responses to dietary interventions may vary widely between individuals owing to differences in genetic background and exposures to environmental factors. To overcome these problems, various approaches, such as animal and cell studies, are used to gain a better understanding of the effects of diet or specific dietary constituents at the cellular and molecular level. Although such approaches are valuable, it should always be kept in mind that each one has its strengths and limitations. Extrapolation to the human situation will always be a problem and questions that can be tackled in humans should therefore be addressed in humans.

Animal models

Dietary studies with animals have been carried out for many decades. One advantage of such studies is that they can be done in a highly controlled way. Food intake can easily be monitored and manipulated, while factors such as temperature, humidity and the stage of the disease can be controlled for. In addition, tissues and cells can be obtained that cannot be readily sampled in humans. It should be appreciated that each animal model has specific advantages and disadvantages, therefore many factors need to be considered before a model is chosen, including animal size, the time needed for breeding, litter size, costs of animal housing and the feasibility of performing blood sampling and vivisection. Then, as with human studies, it is possible to use techniques from the fields of genetics and molecular biology.

An important advantage of animal studies is that the effect of a nutrient can be investigated in animals with a similar genetic background. In this way, variation in responses between animals due to genetic heterogeneity is excluded. Genetic homogeneity can be obtained by inbreeding. For this, genetically related animals, such as brothers and sisters, are mated for many generations. The overall result will be that heterozygosity between animals will reduce and that in the end an inbred strain is obtained with a similar genetic, homozygous background. Genetic homogeneity, however, is not always an advantage. If, for example, the mode of action of a food component is not known or if the main purpose is to test the safety of nutrients or drugs, genetic heterogeneity may be preferable because it increases the extrapolation of results. In addition, differences in responses between various strains can be helpful for elucidating the responses at the molecular level. Thus, it is evident that a clear research question is needed before the choice of animal model can be made.

Using molecular tools applied to the germ cells of animals, it is possible to insert an isolated (foreign) gene sequence into an animal's genomic material. The resultant animals that carry such a foreign gene are called transgenic animals and have traits coded by these genes. Another approach is to knock out a certain endogenous gene. With this technique, a specific gene is modified, which results in a loss of function of that specific gene. With these approaches it is possible to test candidate genes for their effects on the parameters of interest. Transgenic and knockout animals are valuable models for nutrition research. For example, mice have been generated that express human Apo AI. In this way, it was possible to examine in

detail the role of this apolipoprotein in atherogenesis. By inserting or knocking out genes, the importance of specific genes on the genesis of disease and on complex biological pathways in various tissues can be addressed. Finally, by interbreeding mouse strains with different genetic backgrounds, the interaction between genes and the relative contribution of genes and diet on phenotype can be unravelled.

Another tool involves the generation of transgenic mice with tissue-specific expression of a particular gene. This can be accomplished in several ways. It is, for example, possible to insert a tissue-specific promoter before the foreign gene of interest. This DNA construct can then be used to create a transgenic animal. It is possible to make genes whose expression is dependent on the presence or absence of dietary components, such as tetracycline. In this way, it is even possible to switch on the expression of a gene in a specific tissue at any stage of the disease just by taking away tetracycline from (or adding it to) the diet. Alternatively, the so-called Cre–Lox recombination system is widely used to control tissue-specific expression of knockout of genes. In this system, the enzyme Cre-recombinase is used to recognise specific DNA sequences, the so-called LoxP sites. When two LoxP sites flank a certain DNA code, this DNA code is removed by the Cre-recombinase. Using this system, tissue-specific expression, knockout or even replacement of the gene of interest can be achieved by crossing animals that contain a LoxP cassette with animals that express Cre-recombinase in a tissue-specific manner. Alternatively, the Cre-recombinase mRNA can be delivered by injection or using viruses to the animal. Other ways to manipulate gene expression in the intact animal can also be manipulated by DNA electroporation or with adenovirus-mediated gene delivery. With these methods, DNA can also be inserted into a specific tissue. This results in increased levels of mRNA expression and subsequent protein synthesis from the gene of interest. Another way to study the function of specific genes is through the use of tissue or cell transplantation. For example, apoE gene expression in macrophages, which are made by bone marrow, can be studied *in vivo* by bone-marrow transplantation. For these experiments two strains of inbred mice with similar genetic background are used: one strain has no functional apoE gene locus (apoE knockout mice) but the other strain has. After lethal irradiation of the bone marrow of the apoE knockout mice, a bone-marrow cell suspension from the wild-type animal is injected. Within about 4 weeks, the knockout animals are completely reconstituted with the bone marrow from the wild-type animals. As a consequence, their macrophages do not contain apoE and the specific effects of macrophage apoE production can be studied.

Tissue cultures

In vitro studies with intact tissues or isolated cells are an alternative to *in vivo* human and animal studies. If conditions are optimal, cells survive, multiply and may even differentiate after isolation. Tissue cultures can be divided into two categories: organ cultures and cell cultures. An organ culture is composed of a complete or a small part of an intact organ or tissue that is brought into the culture medium. The advantage is that, at least to some extent, the normal biochemical and morphological differentiation and communication routes between the various cell types of a tissue are maintained. Furthermore, it is possible to mimic closely the physiological environment. The survival time of organ cultures, however, is limited and generally not more than 24 h. In addition, it is not possible to culture the cells further and fresh material is needed for each set of experiments.

Cell suspensions are different to tissue cultures in that the extracellular matrix and intercellular junctions between cells are disrupted. For this, tissues are first treated with proteolytic enzymes and with components that bind calcium. The proteolytic enzymes cut the proteins that hold together the tissue in which the cells are embedded whereas chelating agents, like EDTA, capture di- and tri-cationic metal ions like calcium to prevent cadherin binding between cells. The tissue is then mechanically dispersed into single cells. By doing this, a suspension is obtained that is composed of various cell types. If necessary, it is possible to isolate further one specific cell type that can be used for experiments or serve as starting material for a cell culture.

Cell cultures prepared directly from the organs or tissues of an organism are referred to as primary cultures. These cells may still have the potential to divide and in this way secondary and tertiary cell cultures are obtained. Depending on the type of cell and technique used, these cells can be cultured in a suspension or as a monolayer. As for tissue cultures, survival time is limited. However, cell lines can be

Table 2.2 Common tissue-culture models

Cell line	Organism	Tissue	Morphology
HUVEC	Human	Umbilical vein, vascular endothelium	Epithelial
HepG2	Human	Liver, hepatocellular carcinoma	Epithelial
Caco-2	Human	Colon, colorectal adenocarcinoma	Epithelial
CV-1	African green monkey	Kidney	Fibroblast
293	Human	Kidney	Epithelial
HeLa	Human	Cervical adenocarcinoma	Epithelial
THP-1	Human	Monocyte, acute monocytic leukaemia	Suspension culture

used that have obtained the ability to replicate indefinitely. Such cells are frequently derived from cancerous tissue and are all derived from the same stem cell, therefore they have a similar genetic make-up. It should be emphasised, however, that after each cell passage these cells lose some of their biochemical and morphological characteristics: the older they are, the more differences can exist from the original stem cell. However, it is feasible to freeze cells after each passage. After thawing properly, these cells can be cultured further from the point where they were frozen, which makes it possible to go back to a previous passage.

Studies with isolated tissue or cell models are very useful for mechanistical studies. Table 2.2 details common tissue-culture models. The effects of adding nutrients or combinations of nutrients can be studied in detail. The responses of cells to these stimuli can be examined under the microscope or biochemically. It is also possible to examine the effects on mRNA or protein expression, and interactions between two or more different cell types. Finally, it is possible to insert isolated (foreign) gene sequences into the cells or to down-regulate gene expression of specific genes using RNA interference. However, extrapolation of the results to the intact animal or to the human situation is always a problem.

Molecular cloning

Molecular cloning refers to the process of making copies of a DNA segment, which is not necessarily the entire gene. This segment can be a piece of genomic DNA, but also complementary DNA (cDNA) derived from mRNA. After isolating the

DNA fragment, it is inserted into a plasmid that serves as a vector. A plasmid is a circular double-stranded, relatively small (1–1000 kb) DNA molecule that can replicate independently of the bacterial chromosome. The vector with its piece of foreign DNA is subsequently inserted into bacterial cells. As a vector has the capability to replicate autonomously in its host and the host itself can also be grown indefinitely in the laboratory, huge amounts of the plasmids containing the DNA segment of interest can be obtained. Many vectors are available and the selection of the vector depends, among other things, on the size of the DNA fragment, whether it is genomic DNA or cDNA, and on the host to be used. The purpose of cloning is to generate sufficient amounts of a particular DNA sequence for further study.

Molecular cloning has important applications in a number of areas of molecular nutrition. For example, this method could be used to test the functionality of an SNP and determine whether or not the SNP is differentially affected by a nutrient. In this case, two DNA constructs could be made, one with and the other without the SNP. Each construct can be inserted into a vector that can be used to transfect a cell line of interest. After exposure of these cells to different nutritional interventions, it is, for instance, possible to determine whether dietary effects on mRNA or protein expression are affected by this particular SNP.

DNA libraries have been generated to facilitate faster gene research. These libraries, which are widely available nowadays, are collections of bacterial or fungal clones in which each individual clone contains a vector with a piece of foreign DNA inserted. To construct a genomic library, the genomic DNA is first partially digested with restriction enzymes, as the genomic DNA as a whole is too large to be inserted into a vector. These so-formed DNA fragments are then inserted into the proper vector and cloned by a suitable host (e.g. *Escherichia coli*). An efficient way to limit the total number of clones is first to isolate the chromosomes and then to construct a library for that particular chromosome. Similarly, cDNA libraries have been constructed. Such libraries are constructed from the mRNA population present within a particular cell at the exact moment of mRNA isolation. A potential advantage of a cDNA library over a genomic library is that the cloned material does not contain the non-coding regions and the introns as present in the genomic DNA. Furthermore, it is possible to make cDNA libraries from specific tissues or cells. In this way, cDNA libraries can be constructed that are enriched with clones for genes that are expressed preferentially in a certain tissue, or during a specific disease or state of development.

Quantification of gene expression: single-gene mRNA expression

Single-gene expression is measured by quantification of the mRNA transcripts of a specific gene. It mainly gives information on the effects of, for example, nutrients at the transcriptional level. mRNA quantification can also provide a good estimate of the level of protein present in a sample, at least when production of the protein is transcriptionally regulated. Since only very small amounts of mRNA are present and mRNA is relatively unstable, mRNA samples are first translated into cDNA with the reverse transcriptase (RT) enzyme. To make detection possible, cDNA molecules corresponding to the transcribed gene of interest need to be amplified by the polymerase chain reaction (PCR). To control for experimental variation in the RT and the PCR step, an internal control RNA can be used in the entire RT-PCR or a DNA competitor in the PCR only. The total procedure is then called competitive RT-PCR or, when a DNA competitor is used, RT-competitive-PCR. For mRNA analyses, several procedures are available to extract RNA from lysed cells. With most methods, total RNA is isolated that consists of rRNA, mRNA and tRNA. Only approximately 5% of total RNA is mRNA. As eukaryotic cells contain natural RNAses, which are liberated during cell lysis, it is important to ensure that activity of these RNAses is minimised in order to avoid digestion of the isolated RNA. Therefore, it is essential to use RNAse inhibitors during RNA extraction and the following analytical steps. Glassware and plasticware should be RNAse free or be treated with RNAse inhibitors. After isolation, concentrations of RNA can be determined by measuring the optical density at 260 nm.

After RNA isolation, cDNA is synthesised from mRNA with the RT step. As described previously, cDNA differs from genomic DNA in that it only contains the exons from DNA. RT or first strand synthesis can be done by several protocols. One possibility is to use random hexamers. These hexamers bind at many places to the RNA, while the gaps in between are filled with nucleotides by the enzyme reverse transcriptase. It is also possible to make use of the poly(A) tail, which is present on the 3′ UTR of nearly all mRNA molecules. With both procedures, all mRNA present in the sample is copied into cDNA. It is also possible to make only cDNA for one gene in particular during the RT reaction. In this case, the first strand synthesis can be performed by the use of a primer that is specific for this particular gene.

The RT step has variable reproducibility and quality control for this step is crucial. Each difference in RT efficiency is augmented in the following exponential PCR. To overcome these problems, a known amount of a competitive RNA template can be added to the RNA sample as an internal control. The size of the internal standard is in general 20–30 bp longer or shorter than the gene of interest. This RNA standard is also copied into cDNA during the RT step with the same efficiency as the normal RNA transcripts present in the RNA sample. Both the standard derived cDNA and the mRNA derived cDNA are amplified in the following PCR. Separation, however, is always possible, as the two RT-PCR products differ in size.

After the RT step, specific cDNA molecules are amplified by Taq DNA polymerase. For this reaction two primers are used, which are complementary to both ends of the targeted product. The primers are the starting points for the Taq DNA polymerase enzyme. The Taq polymerase reads the cDNA strand from the 3′ side to 5′, thus forming a complementary strand from 5′ to 3′ by incorporating the four available nucleotides A, T, G and C. This process of amplification requires a specific-temperature programme, which is referred to as a PCR cycle. First, the double-stranded cDNA is denatured at 95°C. The temperature is then decreased to the annealing temperature, which is the temperature at which the primers bind to the individual strands, normally at about 60°C. Next, the temperature is increased to 72°C, the optimum temperature for Taq polymerase to incorporate nucleotides at the 3′-OH end of the growing DNA sequence using the complementary strand as template. This is called extension. Thus, during one PCR cycle the number of the targeted product is doubled. This means that after n cycles the number of copies of only one cDNA molecule is 2^n. After 25 cycles 2^{25} (33×10^6) copies are formed from each cDNA molecule. Such a quantity can be visualised using a detection system.

If an internal control is used during the RT-PCR, the original number of mRNA molecules can be calculated by comparing the intensity of the PCR product of the mRNA of interest with the intensity of the PCR product from the internal control. Since the initial amount of the internal standard is known, the unknown amount of mRNA can be calculated.

If no internal control is used, expression of a gene is related to the expression of a constitutive gene such as β-actin or GAPDH. These housekeeping genes are always expressed to the same extent and can therefore be used as a measure for the amount of RNA used in the reaction as well as for cDNA synthesis. The PCR for the housekeeping genes needs to be performed from the same cDNA as that for the gene of interest.

Detection of the PCR products formed is carried out by different methods. A frequently used method in the past was separation of the multiplied DNA fragments by gel electrophoresis followed by visualising the fragments with ethidium bromide staining using ultraviolet (UV) light. Several other stains can be used, such as cybr green or gelstar. The intensities of the bands on the gels are analysed by densitometry, which is proportional to the concentration. Alternatively, it is also possible to use a labelled (radioactive, biotin or digoxigenin) probe, which is complementary to the amplified gene of interest. After gel electrophoresis, blotting and denaturation these probes hybridise with the PCR product, which can be visualised and quantified.

Currently, most methods make use of intercalating agents (like cyber green) of fluorescent-labelled primers during the PCR in conjunction with PCR equipment with an optical detection system. When the fluorochromes in the labelled primers are excited using light with the proper wavelength, they emit light that can be quantified using a light-sensitive sensor. The amount of fluorescent signal emitted correlates linearly with the amount of product formed in the RT-PCR reaction. Therefore this method is also referred to as quantitative PCR (Q-PCR) or real-time PCR (RT-PCR). Here Q-PCR is preferred as RT-PCR might introduce some confusion with reverse transcriptase PCR. Q-PCR enables continued measurement of the newly formed PCR product in each cycle. The advantage of this way of quantifying the amount of PCR product is that it is more reliable and much more sensitive than PCR endpoint measurements using densiometry.

(Q-)PCR techniques are particularly useful for the quantification of mRNAs that are present at low concentrations. At higher concentrations, mRNA can also be identified by a technique called Northern blotting. For this, RNA or purified mRNA is first separated according to size by electrophoresis, transferred to a filter and denaturated. This filter is then incubated with a labelled probe, which specifically binds to the mRNAs of interest. After washing to remove the non-hybridised probe, the specific RNA transcript can be detected. When the probe hybridises with more than one transcript (e.g. splice variants), more bands will appear on the filter. Today, Northern blotting is still used to determine the existence of various mRNA splice-variants, but for standard quantifications Q-PCR has become the standard method.

Quantification of gene expression: multiple-gene mRNA expression

In general, the expression of large numbers of genes (i.e. an expression profile) changes when environmental conditions, such as nutrient exposure or nutritional status, are altered. For example, dietary interventions known to up-regulate the expression of the low-density lipoprotein (LDL) receptor may also change the expression of genes coding for cholesterol-synthesising enzymes. Furthermore, expression profiles may vary between tissues, and also it is known that not all individuals respond in a similar way to changing conditions. This may be due to differences in genetic background and variables such gender, age, amount of physical activity or state of the disease. DNA microarrays are useful to understand better the interactions between a large number of genes and to examine events at a transcriptional level.

DNA microarrays or chips are used as a tool to detect differences in the expression level of a large number of genes between two or more samples in a single assay. The concept behind this technique is comparable to that underlying Northern blotting. First, gene-specific oligonucleotides are individually spotted or printed on a flat solid support at designated places. These polynucleotides, which may be from known and unknown genes, are then probed with cDNA from both the test and reference material. These two sources of cDNA, which each has its own specific label, compete for binding on the array. The intensity of the signal from the label can now be measured and gives a global indication of the amount of cDNA present in the test sample relative to that in the reference sample. For example, the test material can be fluorescence labelled with a red tag and the control material with a green tag. If expression of a certain gene is similar in the test and reference samples, a yellow signal will appear. The final step is to interpret the expression profiles for which computer software is available. Likewise, arrays exist that measure gene expression levels of one sample at a time.

In principle, it is possible to obtain with DNA microarrays information on the expression profiles of numerous known and unknown genes at the same time in different tissues at various stages of a disease. Such studies will give an enormous amount of data, which need to be analysed in a meaningful way. For this, use is made of bioinformatics tools, such as clustering analysis and principal component analysis, which integrate multiple gene expression profiles. Bioinformatic approaches that look at the effect of nutrients on metabolic/biochemical pathways and networks are also of use, as they allow the integration of genes that are functionally related to each other. These approaches facilitate characterisation of a 'transcriptomic signature' that describes the effect of a nutrient or metabolic state of a cell/tissue.

Quantification of protein synthesis

Proteins fulfil a very diverse role, which varies from being structural and contractile components to being essential regulatory elements in many cellular processes in the form of enzymes or hormones. Although mRNA serves as a template for protein, it is important to realise that the amount of mRNA is not necessarily correlated with the amount of protein. For example, mRNA can be degraded without being translated. In addition, proteins can be modified after translation in such a way that their half-life, functions or activities are altered. Finally, genetic variation may also result in different molecular forms of the protein. It is therefore important to obtain information not only on gene expression, but also on protein synthesis, modification and activity.

Various techniques are used for protein analysis. The most sensitive techniques are a combination of one or two methods that make use of differences in molecular weight, electric charge, size, shape or interactions with specific antibodies. A frequently used technique is Western blotting in combination with specific protein detection using antibodies. Proteins are first isolated from a tissue or cell extract and then separated according to size by electrophoresis. Proteins are transferred and permanently bound to a filter, which is subsequently incubated with one or two antibodies. At least one antibody is raised against this protein. This first or second antibody that recognises the first antibody is tagged with a detectable component, which makes it possible to quantify the amount of protein present in the sample. It is also possible to detect and quantify amounts of protein using enzyme-linked immunosorbent assays (ELISAs) or radioimmunoassays (RIAs). These techniques are mainly based on immunoreactivity and can detect many proteins at physiological concentrations. However, they do not make use of differences in molecular weight, as with Western blotting, and may therefore be less specific for determining post-translational modification of proteins. Furthermore, unknown proteins may also be present on a Western blot that shows changes in expression profile using general protein staining [e.g. silver or Coomassie Brilliant Blue (CBB) staining). The most direct approach to identify these unknown proteins is to determine the amino acid sequence. Typically, a purified protein is first cleaved into a number of large peptide fragments, which are isolated. The next step is to determine the amino acid sequence of each fragment. If a part of or the total amino sequence is known, this amino acid sequence is compared to a library of known protein stretches to identify the protein. Alternatively, the amino acid sequence can be reverse translated to the mRNA and the exon sequence of the corresponding gene can be generated as information on the amino acid sequence provides information on the nucleotide sequence. This can then be used to synthesise probes to build libraries or to synthesise these proteins on a large scale for further studies or for the production of drugs such as insulin.

Cleavage of the protein into fragments and then into amino acids is also helpful to determine those parts of the protein that are transformed after translation. In this way, for example, it is possible to identify sides and the degree of phosphorylation or glycosylation. Comparable to DNA microarrays, arrays have also been developed for protein profiling. Instead of gene-specific polynucleotides, antibodies raised against proteins are spotted on a flat solid support.

Stable isotopes: a tool to integrate cellular metabolism and whole-body physiology

With DNA arrays and protein arrays it is possible to obtain information on the expression and formation of many genes and proteins, respectively. This provides valuable information for delineating how patterns are influenced by internal and external stimuli. It does not, however, provide information on enzyme activity or quantify metabolic events *in vivo*. For example, an increase in the synthesis of a certain protein for gluconeogenesis does not necessarily mean that glucose production is also increases. Glucose production is very complex and controlled at many levels. To address such issues, stable isotope technology is helpful, with which quantitative information can be obtained in humans on *in vivo* rates of synthesis, degradation, turnover, fluxes between cells and tissues, and so on.

Stable isotopes are molecules that differ slightly in weight owing to differences in the number of neutrons of one or more atoms. For example, ^{12}C and ^{13}C refer to carbon atoms with atomic masses of 12 and 13, respectively, which behave similarly metabolically. In nature, about 99% of carbon atoms are ^{12}C and only 1% ^{13}C. As ^{13}C atoms are non-radioactive, they can be used safely in human experiments. In contrast, radioactive isotopes are frequently used in animal or cell studies.

These characteristics make stable isotopes useful tools to integrate cellular metabolism and whole-body physiology. With the appropriate analytical techniques, it is possible to separate atoms and molecules based on differences in mass. Experiments are based on the low natural abundance of one of the isotopes. To use a very simplistic example, if one is interested in the rate of appearance in breath of $^{13}CO_2$ from the oxidation of an oral dose of glucose, ^{13}C-labelled glucose (which is prepared on a commercial scale) can be given. The expired air will become enriched with $^{13}CO_2$, which can be measured. One now has the certainty that this $^{13}CO_2$ is derived from ^{13}C-labelled glucose. Ultimately, this gives information on the rate, proportion and amount of glucose oxidised. Such an approach is instrumental in increasing our understanding of the metabolic consequences of the effects found at the cellular and molecular level.

Metabolomics: the most recent tool for nutrigenomics

Metabolomics represents the newest 'omics' technology being applied within molecular nutrition and nutrigenomics. It utilises analytical chemistry technologies such as nuclear magnetic resonance (NMR) spectroscopy and mass spectrometry (MS) to capture complete data on the low molecular weight metabolites, nutrients and other compounds in various human biofluids, cells and tissues. This chemical fingerprint/small molecule metabolite profile that reflects cellular processes is referred to as the metabolome. The metabolome is viewed as the functional outcome of all metabolites that are the end product of gene and protein expression. The opportunities and challenges associated with the application of metabolomics in nutrition research is the subject of a recent review (Gibney *et al.*, 2005). The main opportunity is that metabolomics may provide the comprehensive biomarker of multiple metabolites to assess nutrient status, metabolic responses, disease predisposition, etc. Although the metabolome can be readily defined, it is not possible to analyse the entire range of metabolites by a single analytical method. In addressing this limitation the Human Metabolome Database has been established wherein more than 2500 metabolites, 1200 drugs and 3500 food components that can found in the human body are documented. The biological interpretation of metabolomic data is also a great challenge within the context of human nutrition. It can be difficult to directly relate metabolites to specific biomarkers of nutritional status.

2.5 Genetic variability: determinants of health and response to nutrients

Nutrigenetics is a common term which describes how genetic variation determines an individual's risk of a diet-related disease, their nutrient requirement and metabolic response, as well as responsiveness to a bioactive dietary component or nutritional intervention. Genetic polymorphisms may affect metabolic responses to diet by influencing the production, composition and/or activity of proteins. A considerable amount of research has therefore been conducted on the effects of common genetic polymorphisms on the response to nutrients. This is of great interest

for at least two reasons. First, such studies provide information on specific molecular process underlying dietary responsiveness. Secondly, if a common genetic polymorphism determines the dietary response, then people can be identified who will, or will not, benefit from specific dietary recommendations. This *personalised nutrition* approach allows targeted dietary treatment for specific metabolic aberrations and ultimately the outcome of certain disease states.

Several general criteria can be formulated to assess the impact of the results of *genetic association* studies which attempt to link genetic variation and dietary responses. First of all, the polymorphism should affect the metabolic response by influencing the production, composition and/or activity of the protein. Mutations/polymorphisms in the promoter region will not necessarily affect the composition of the protein, but may affect its production. In contrast, mutations in an exon may not affect the production, but can change the composition and consequently the structure or activity of a protein. However, it is also possible that mutations in introns are associated with dietary responses. In such cases, it is very likely that this mutation is in *linkage disequilibrium* or associated with another functional genetic variation that is directly responsible for the effect observed. Essentially there should be pronounced, biologically relevant, effects of the polymorphism on dietary responses. In terms of the practical applicability of a gene-nutrient interaction, it is important that sufficient subjects in the population carry the variant, for example >10%. Finally, there should be a plausible biological mechanism or, ideally, well-characterised functional studies to explain the association and demonstrate the gene–nutrient interaction.

To date most studies have focused on single genetic variants (SNPs) in individual genes, examples of which are described below. The challenge will be to identify the other candidate genes involved in each diet-related disease (obesity, the metabolic syndrome, T2DM, CVD, cancers, etc.). This is not easy given the complex polygenetic nature of these disorders, which involve perturbations in multiple metabolic pathways. Also, within any pathway there might be several genes involved, for example there are more than 50 involved in lipid metabolism. *Genome wide association studies* (*GWAS*) is a new approach that attempts to screen the whole genome to identify new genetic variants associated with disease. This approach identified a new candidate gene, TCF7L2, associated with greater risk of type 2 diabetes. There is no doubt that this approach will identify new candidates for diet-related diseases in the future.

Common polymorphisms and disease: the cholesteryl ester transfer protein Taq IB polymorphism

Cholesteryl ester transfer protein (CETP) is an important protein that regulates cholesterol metabolism, therefore genetic and nutritional factors that affect this protein are important with respect to coronary heart disease. In human plasma CETP facilitates the transfer of cholesteryl ester from high-density lipoprotein (HDL) to apo B-containing lipoproteins such as LDL and very low-density lipoproteins (VLDL). As high LDL and VLDL cholesterol concentration and low HDL cholesterol concentrations are related to increased cardiovascular risk, CETP could be regarded as a potentially atherogenic factor. Worldwide, a few people have been identified with no CETP activity. From *in vitro* studies it appeared that these subjects have a defect in the transfer of cholesteryl ester from HDL to LDL or VLDL. These patients also have increased HDL cholesterol and lowered HDL triacylglycerol levels. Animals with no plasma CETP activity are relatively resistant to atherosclerosis, while CETP transgenic mice have decreased HDL cholesterol levels. Specific CETP inhibitors increase HDL cholesterol and slow down the progression of atherosclerosis in rabbits. All of these findings are in agreement with the predicted metabolic and functional effects of CETP *in vivo*.

The primary structure of human plasma CETP is known. The initial studies used a human liver library, in which CETP cDNA was identified, isolated and cloned using a partial amino acid sequence from purified CETP. Further studies demonstrated that the gene is located on chromosome 16. Several DNA polymorphisms for the CETP gene have been described. One of these polymorphisms, the *Taq* IB, has been identified in intron 1 by the restriction enzyme *Taq* I. The presence of this DNA variation is frequently referred to as B1 and its absence as B2. The B1 allele frequency varies between populations, but is in general somewhere between 0.4 and 0.6. This means that 16–36% of the population has the CETP *Taq* IB-1/1 genotype. Cross-sectional epidemiological

studies in various population groups have shown that the presence of the B2 allele is associated with decreased CETP activity and increased HDL cholesterol levels. Furthermore, it has been reported that subjects with the B2 allele have a lower cardiovascular risk.

Although this CETP polymorphism determines HDL cholesterol levels, effects on dietary responses are less evident. Several studies did not see any effect at all, but other studies have suggested that this polymorphism modulates the HDL or LDL cholesterol response to alcohol and fat intake. Effects, however, are small and not found in all studies. Furthermore, it should be realised that the CETP *Taq* IB mutation is situated in intron 1 and it is not very likely that this mutation is functional. This suggests that this mutation in the CETP gene is a marker for a mutation in another part of the same gene or in another gene involved in lipid metabolism. Indeed, it has been found that the *Taq* IB mutation is in linkage disequilibrium with a functional mutation in the CETP promoter region.

Gly972Arg polymorphism in insulin receptor substrate-1

Insulin is well known for its role in glucose and lipid metabolism. After binding of insulin to the insulin receptor, insulin receptor substrate-1 (IRS-1) is activated by phosphorylation. In this way, the signal from plasma insulin is mediated in a variety of insulin-responsive cells and tissues, through the insulin receptor at the cell surface, towards intracellular enzymes. Because of this central role in the signal transduction pathway, IRS-1 may be involved in the decreased insulin sensitivity observed in patients with non-insulin-dependent diabetes mellitus.

The IRS-1 gene was cloned from a human male placenta library and found to be located on chromosome 2. Mice with no functional IRS-1 gene have been bred. These animals have a clustering of metabolic abnormalities characteristic for diabetic subjects. The sensitivity of IRS-1-deficient cells for insulin could be partially restored by transfecting these cells with IRS-1. Such studies clearly demonstrate the importance of IRS-1 in the insulin signalling cascade and insulin secretion pathways. However, disruption of the IRS-1 gene is not lethal in mice, which suggests that other pathways exist that can pass the signal of plasma insulin.

There are several amino acid polymorphisms in IRS-1, one of which, a glycine to arginine substitution at amino acid 972 (Gly972Arg mutation), is quite common. In the heterozygous form, the codon-972 variant of IRS-1 is present in about 10% of the population, but may be more prevalent in subjects with non-insulin-dependent diabetes mellitus or dyslipi-demia. Carriers of the Gly972Arg allele have lower fasting insulin concentrations and a less favourable plasma lipoprotein profile than non-carriers. Furthermore, cultured cells transfected with either wild-type human IRS-1 or the Gly972Arg variant showed that this mutation impaired insulin-stimulated signalling. From these studies, it appears that this polymorphism may contribute to insulin resistance.

More interestingly from a nutritional point of view, an interaction between this Gly972Arg mutation of IRS-1 and body mass has been suggested. The already increased frequency of the Gly972Arg mutation in patients with coronary heart disease was even further increased in obese subjects. The results of the intravenous glucose tolerance test were less favourable in moderately overweight heterozygous carriers of this polymorphism than in wild-type subjects. These findings suggest that only overweight subjects with this Gly972Arg variant would benefit from weight loss with respect to improved insulin sensitivity. It should be noted that this interaction with obesity has not been observed in all studies.

677C–T polymorphism of methylene-tetrahydrofolate reductase

Increased levels of plasma homocysteine, a sulphur-containing amino acid, are associated with an increased risk of various disorders such as neural tube defects, thrombotic disease and vascular disease. These associations do not prove a causal role for homocysteine in these diseases, but they do indicate that homocysteine plays an important role in many physiological processes. In homocysteine metabolism, a crucial role is fulfiled by the enzyme methylene-tetrahydrofolate reductase (MTHFR). The MTHFR gene is located on chromosome 1. Some subjects with MTHFR deficiency have been identified and they all have increased homocysteine levels. To study the *in vivo* pathogenetic and metabolic consequences of MTHFR deficiency, an MTHFR knockout mouse

model has been generated. Homocysteine levels are slightly elevated in heterozygous animals and are increased 10-fold in homozygous knockout mice. The homozygous animals show similar diseases to human MTHFR patients, supporting a causal role of hyper-homocystinaemia in these diseases. Nevertheless, extrapolation from animal studies to the human situation remains a problem.

A common DNA polymorphism in the MTHFR gene is a C-to-T substitution at nucleotide 677, which results in the replacement of alanine for valine. The allelic frequency of the 677C–T genotype, which can be identified with the restriction enzyme *Hinf*I, is as high as 35% in some populations, but the allelic frequency of the 677C–T polymorphism varies widely between populations. Substitution of the alanine for valine results in a reduced enzyme activity and individuals homozygous for this polymorphism have significantly increased plasma homocysteine concentrations. Thus, the 677C–T mutation may have functional consequences. An increased frequency of the 677T allele in patients with pre-eclampsia, neural tube defects and cardiovascular disease has been claimed by some studies, but refuted by others.

It has been hypothesised that the lack of association between MTHFR polymorphisms and disease in certain populations may be due to differences in dietary status. Homocysteine metabolism requires the participation of folate and vitamin B_{12}. In the plasma, a negative relationship exists between homocysteine levels and those of folate and vitamin B_{12}. Moreover, supplementation with folate in particular, but also with vitamin B_{12}, reduced fasting homocysteine levels. In this respect, subjects carrying the 677C–T mutation were more responsive. Thus, a daily low-dose supplement of folic acid will reduce, and in many cases normalise, slightly increased homocysteine levels, which is explained by a possible effect on the stability of folate on MTHFR. Whether this will result in a reduced disease risk or whether certain population groups are more responsive to folate intervention needs to be established.

Methyl-malonic aciduria cblB type: result from GWAS

In genome-wide association studies (GWAS), large numbers of genetic markers such as SNPs are screened that cover (a large part of) the total genome ('genome wide') of a species. The aim of this approach is to discover a group of genetic markers that are associated with a certain trait, for example the risk of developing type 2 diabetes, blood pressure, weight gain, or abnormalities in serum lipid and lipoprotein concentrations. Groups of markers that associate with the trait can then be investigated further. Ultimately, results should be used to predict long-term outcomes early in life and to enable personal (nutritional) advice to prevent possible adverse effects.

Using GWAS it has been found that SNPs within the gene methyl-malonic aciduria cbIB type (MMAB) are associated with serum lipid and lipoprotein concentrations. This gene encodes a protein that catalyses the final step in the conversion of vitamin B12 into adenosylcobalamin. Adenosylcobalamin is an active form of vitamin B12 and is a cofactor for the enzyme methylmalonyl-CoA mutase. Mutations in the MMAB gene could result in diminished adenosylcobalamin levels and causes accumulation of methyl-malonic acid. Consequently, patients with a defect in the gene MMAB are prone to life-threatening acidosis. MMAB defects are treated by vitamin B12 supplementation, although this is successful in only one-third of MMAB patients.

Why SNPs within the MMAB gene were related to abnormalities in serum lipid and lipoprotein concentrations is currently unknown. What is known is that these SNPs together with several other SNPs are associated with higher LDL cholesterol and lower HDL cholesterol concentrations on a carbohydrate-rich diet even when corrected for differences in fat and protein intake. However, to determine whether these relationships are truly causal requires further study. For instance, in a GWAS using a Japanese genetic SNP database no associations were found between MMAB with serum lipoprotein concentrations. This may suggests that ethnic background may modulate the outcome of such studies. Another explanation is of course that – as GWAS only reveal associations – the observed relationships were due to chance. Thus, it is evident that associations found using GWAS always need to be verified using other approaches.

Conclusions

Results of studies on the effects of genetic polymorphisms on the response to dietary interventions are often inconsistent. Several explanations can be offered for this. First of all, many of the earlier, pioneering studies were carried out in retrospect. This means that genotyping was performed after the study had ended and that groups were not well balanced. For example, if a study is carried out with 150 subjects and the allele frequency of a certain mutation is 10%, then the expected number of subjects homozygous or even heterozygous for that mutation will be too low. As a consequence, groups will be small and it will be difficult to find any differences between the groups with respect to differences in responses to the diets, simply because of a lack of statistical power. Another explanation is that the effects of the polymorphism of interest depend on the make-up of other genes (gene–gene interaction). Human studies on gene–gene interaction are even more difficult to design. Suppose that the frequency of a certain polymorphism is 10% and that of another is 20%. Such values are not uncommon, but it means that only 2% of the subjects may have the combination of the two mutations of interest. Thus, one needs to screen many subjects to find appropriate numbers. Similarly, effects may depend on gender, age or other factors, such as body mass index, smoking or state of the disease. Without doubt, studies on gene–gene or environment–gene interaction will expand our knowledge of the effects of the genetic code on the response to nutrients. Finally, it is possible that in a certain population the polymorphism is a marker for another, unknown, genetic defect. Ideally, results should therefore always be confirmed in different, independent populations with different genetic backgrounds.

As already mentioned, one of the rationales for studies on genetic polymorphisms in relation to dietary responses is that people can be identified who will, or will not, benefit from specific dietary recommendations – often referred to as *personalised nutrition*. However it has become clear that dietary responses are a complex combination of genetic and environmental factors. In general, the known relationships between responses to diet with genetic polymorphisms are not very strong and different combinations of genetic and environmental factors may ultimately lead to a similar response. To address such issues, cell and animal studies are also relevant. Another approach is to make a complete inventory of differences in gene expression or protein synthesis in a particular organ or cell type after changing dietary intake. For this, microarray analyses can be useful. It is clear that there is still a long way to go, but studies on specific molecular processes underlying dietary responsiveness remain a major challenge.

2.6 Nutrient regulation of gene expression

While nutritional recommendations strive to promote good health through good nutrition, it is clear that such population-based strategies do not account for variations in an individual's nutritional requirements. These variations are due to our genetic background and environmental factors, including nutrition. The previous section showed how different genetic variations or polymorphisms can alter an individual's nutritional responses to diet. This section will examine how nutrients affect gene, protein and metabolite expression. The expression of a gene that results in an active protein can be regulated at any number of points between transcription and the synthesis of the final protein product. While the process of gene expression is well understood, as detailed in Section 2.3, relatively little is known about how nutrients affect gene expression at the level of mRNA, protein and/or metabolite. Nevertheless, there are a few examples of nutrients that affect gene expression to alter mRNA and/or active protein levels by interacting with transcriptional, post-transcriptional and post-translational events. The effect of nutrients on gene expression is a very intensive area of research. In light of the technological advances in molecular biology, as detailed in Section 2.4, the number of examples of nutrient regulation of gene expression will expand rapidly over the next few years. Ultimately, it is important not only to understand the concept of nutrient regulation of gene expression (at the mRNA, protein and metabolite level), but also to know how changes at the level of the gene relate to whole-body metabolism and health.

Nutrient regulation of gene transcription

Theoretically, gene expression can be regulated at many points between the conversion of a gene sequence into mRNA and into protein. For most genes, the control of transcription is stronger than that of translation. As reviewed in Section 2.3, this is

Table 2.3 Effect of nutrients on gene transcription

Nutrient	Gene	Transcriptional effect
Glucose	Glucokinase	Increase
Retinoic acid	Retinoic acid receptor	Increase
Vitamin B$_6$	Steroid hormone receptor	Decrease
Zinc	Zinc-dependent enzymes	Increase
Vitamin C	Procollagen	Increase
Cholesterol	HMG CoA reductase	Decrease
Fatty acids	SREBP	Increase

HMG CoA, 3-hydroxy-3-methylglutaryl-coenzyme A; SREBP, sterol regulatory response element binding protein.

achieved by specific regulatory sequences, known as *cis*-acting control elements, in the promoter region of the gene, and *trans*-acting factors, known as transcription factors or DNA-binding proteins, that interact with the promoter region of genes and modulate gene expression. Nutrients can alter the transcription of target genes; some examples of this are detailed in Table 2.3.

Direct and indirect nutrient regulation of gene transcription

Certain dietary constituents can influence gene expression by direct interaction with regulatory elements in the genome, altering the transcription of a given gene. Examples include retinoic acid, vitamin D, fatty acids and zinc. However, nutrients can also have an indirect effect on gene transcription. It is often difficult to discern whether a gene–nutrient interaction is a direct effect of a particular nutrient, or an indirect effect of a metabolite or a secondary mediator such as a hormone, eicosanoid or a secondary cell message that alters transcription. For example, many genes involved in fat and carbohydrate metabolism have genes that have an insulin response element in their promoter region. Hence, a particular fatty acid or carbohydrate could mediate its effect via insulin. The indirect route may be particularly important for the more complex dietary components because they have a number of bioactive constituents. For example, part of dietary fibre is metabolised by the colonic flora to produce butyric acid. Butyric acid, in turn, may affect gene expression by selective effects on G-proteins (which are intracellular messengers) or by direct interactions with DNA regulatory sequences.

Nutrient regulation of transcription factors

Nutrients can also regulate transcription factor activity and thereby alter gene expression. The peroxisome proliferator activated receptors (PPARs) are a good example of *trans*-acting transcription factors that can be modulated by nutritional factors. PPARs are members of the nuclear hormone receptor superfamily and these regulate the expression of many genes involved in cellular differentiation, proliferation, apoptosis, fatty acid metabolism, lipoprotein metabolism and inflammation. PPARs are ligand-dependent transcription factors, which are activated by a number of compounds, including fatty acids. There are several members of the PPAR family, PPARα, PPARγ and PPARδ (β), each with multiple isoforms. PPARα is primarily expressed in the liver, PPARγ in adipose tissue and PPARδ (β) is ubiquitously expressed. When activated by fatty acids (or eicosanoids and pharmacological PPAR agonists) the PPARs dimerise with the retinoid X receptor (RXR). This PPAR–RXR heterodimer binds to a PPAR response element (PPRE) in the promoter region of the target gene and induces transcription of the target gene. Many genes involved in lipid and glucose metabolism have PPRE, some of which are listed in Table 2.4. Therefore, the PPARs represent an example of how nutrients can regulate gene expression through transcription factors. Sterol regulatory response element binding proteins (SREBPs) are another group of transcription factors that mediate the effects of dietary fatty acids on gene expression. There are two forms of SREBP: SREBP-1 regulates fatty acid and triacylglycerol synthesis, whereas SREBP-2 regulates the genes involved in cholesterol metabolism. Therefore, the SREBPs modulate the expression of the genes involved in cholesterol and fatty acid metabolism, in response to different fatty acid treatments.

Nutrients and post-transcriptional control of gene expression

It is generally accepted that the initiation of transcription is the primary mode of regulating gene expression, and there are good examples of different nutrients increasing and decreasing mRNA expression. However, there is increasing evidence that the response of gene expression to nutrients involves control of post-transcriptional events. Much of the evidence for post-transcriptional control comes from observed discrepancies between mRNA abundance and transcriptional rates (altered mRNA abundance associated with unchanged gene transcription implies altered mRNA stability). In addition, mRNA abundance is not necessarily correlated to protein concentration (altered protein concentration in the absence of any changes in mRNA abundance implies either altered translation of the mRNA or changes in the proteolytic breakdown of the protein). Since nutrients can regulate mRNA translation and stability, mRNA abundance may not reflect amounts of protein or rates of synthesis. Therefore, it is incorrect to assume that if a nutrient alters the level of mRNA then there is a concomitant change in protein levels. To assess with confidence the effect of a nutrient on gene expression, mRNA analysis should be accompanied by measurements of the protein product.

Some examples of post-transcriptional control of gene–nutrient interactions are presented in Table 2.5.

Table 2.4 PPAR-responsive genes and their metabolic effect

PPAR target genes	Target cell	Metabolic effect
aP2	Adipocyte	Adipogenesis
FABP, ACS	Adipocyte	Fatty acid synthesis
Apo CIII, LPL	Hepatocyte	VLDL metabolism
Apo AI, Apo AII	Hepatocyte	HDL metabolism

PPAR, peroxisome proliferator activator receptor; VLDL, very low-density lipoprotein; HDL, high-density lipoprotein; FABP, fatty acid binding protein; ACS, acyl-CoA synthetase; LPL, lipoprotein lipase.

Table 2.5 Nutrient regulation of gene expression: post-transcriptional control

Gene	Nutritional factor	Control point	Regulatory element
Ferritin	Iron	Translation	5′ UTR
Transferrin receptor	Iron	Stability	3′ UTR
Glutathione peroxidase	Selenium	Translation	3′ UTR
Glucose transporter-1	Fed/fasted state	Translation	5′ UTR
Lipoprotein lipase	Fatty acid supply	Translation	3′ UTR
Apolipoprotein CIII	Hyperlipidaemia	Unknown	3′ UTR

Figure 2.8 Iron regulates its own metabolism through post-transcriptional regulation of transferrin and ferritin.

It is important to note that often the non-coding region of the gene may play a key role in the regulation of gene expression whereby nutrients interact with regulatory elements located in the 5′ and the 3′ UTRs of a range of target genes, mediating the effect of nutrients on gene expression.

Iron is a classical example of how a nutrient regulates the expression of the genes involved in its metabolism (Figure 2.8). Transferrin and ferritin are key proteins involved in iron metabolism, and the expression of each is determined by the non-coding region of transferrin and ferritin mRNA. The transferrin receptor is required for the uptake of iron in cells. Transferrin receptor has five regulatory sequences, known as the iron response elements (IREs) in the 3′ UTR. In the absence of iron, *trans*-acting transcription repressor proteins, the iron regulatory proteins (IRPs), bind to the IRE and protect the mRNA from degradation. In the presence of iron, the IRPs are removed from the transferrin receptor mRNA, leading to mRNA destabilisation, decreased translation of mRNA and decreased transferrin receptor synthesis. This mechanism therefore prevents excessive amounts of iron being taken up by a cell.

Ferritin is required for the storage of iron. It sequesters cellular iron, which would otherwise be toxic. The expression of ferritin is also regulated post-transcriptionally. This controls the supply of free iron within the cell according to cellular iron levels. Ferritin has an IRE in the 5′ UTR that regulates transcription. When cellular iron levels are low the IRP binds the IRE and represses translation of ferritin, thus supplying free iron as required for cell metabolism. In the presence of iron the IRP does not bind the IRE and ferritin translation is increased to allow storage of iron. The presence of similar IREs in the transferrin receptor and ferritin mRNA is important because it allows coordinated regulation of the synthesis of the two proteins according to different cellular levels and requirements for protein.

Nutrient regulation of translation and post-translational protein modification

Hypothetically, a nutrient could regulate the translation of mRNA into protein. However, to date there are no examples of a direct effect of a nutrient on protein translation that is independent of alterations in mRNA. Similarly, there is little information on the effects of nutrients on post-translational protein modification. Vitamin K is one of the very few examples of nutrient regulation of post-translational protein modification, and it has this effect by regulating the activation of prothrombin. Prothrombin is an essential protein involved in the coagulation system. It is the proenzyme for thrombin, which is an inherent component of the clot. Prothrombin cannot function correctly unless its glutamic acid residues are carboxylated. Carboxylation of prothrombin allows it to bind to calcium, and prothrombin can only participate in the clotting process if it can bind to calcium. This post-translational modification means that the nascent prothrombin protein is dependent on the supply of vitamin K. Apart from the effect of overt vitamin K deficiency on coagulation, the extent to which an individual's vitamin K status affects clotting is unknown. Further research that specifically addresses whether and/or how nutrients modulate protein expression is required to gain a greater understanding of this aspect of molecular nutrition.

Metabolomic signatures of nutritional intervention

Nutritional metabolomics attempts to characterise the metabolome that reflects a certain nutritional status/sensitivity at the whole organism, tissue, cellular and biochemical process levels. It needs to be appreciated that an individual metabolomic profile represents highly complex regulation of many simultaneous biochemical pathways in different organs. As a consequence inter-individual metabolomic variation is very high, therefore nutritional metabolomics needs to account for the multifactorial nature of an individual's metabolomic phenotype. For example, the gut microflora can have a huge impact on individual metabolomic profiles. Consequently it is advised that within dietary intervention trials to characterise the nutritional metabolome the subjects should consume a defined diet with/without the nutritional intervention to exclude the effect of other non-diet-related complex interactions. To date there are very few studies that have employed metabolomics to characterise the human metabolic phenotype. However, there is no doubt that there will be a wealth of data generated in the near future characterising the nutritional metabolome.

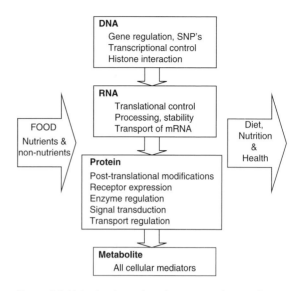

Figure 2.9 Molecular interactions between nutrients and nonnutrient food components with the genome, transcriptome, proteome and metabolome as predictors of nutrition and health. (Roche HM. Nutrigenomics – new approaches for human nutrition research, J Sci Food Agri 2006; 86: 1156–63. Copyright © Wiley–Blackwell.)

2.7 Perspectives on the future

Molecular nutrition and nutrigenomics represent a new phase of nutrition research that will provide a much greater understanding of the interactions between nutrients and the human genome. This chapter has explored the technological opportunities in molecular biology that can be applied to nutrition research. These rapidly advancing technologies present tremendous opportunities for improving our understanding of nutritional science. The Human Genome Project will undoubtedly improve our understanding of genetic background and diversity. From the perspective of nutrition, we should be able to develop a greater understanding of how nutrients interact with genetic destiny, alter disease processes and promote health. Within the context of human nutrition, probably the greatest challenge is to develop experimental models that mimic the *in vivo* response and whole-body metabolism. These models are needed in order to maximise the potential of the novel molecular technologies that then can investigate the molecular and cellular effects of nutrients wherein the results can be extrapolated and applied to human health. No doubt the next decade will be very exciting in terms of applying the novel molecular technologies in an intelligent and meaningful way to nutrition research. One of the greatest challenges for nutrigenomics will be to characterise the nutritional phenotype. This will require a systems biology and functional genomics approach to integrate genetic, transcriptomic, proteomic and metabolomic information to give a more complete picture of human nutrition and health (Figure 2.9). It is hoped that the next phase of molecular nutrition research will generate a more comprehensive understanding of the cellular and molecular effects of nutrients and improve our understanding of whether and how nutrients modulate disease processes. In the future this *personalised nutrition approach* might provide the ability to define scientifically sound, evidence-based and effective nutritional strategies to promote health.

Reference

Gibney MJ, Walsh M, Brennan L, Roche HM, German B, van Ommen B. Metabolomics in Human Nutrition: Opportunities and challenges. Am J Clin Nutr 2005; 82: 497–503.

Further reading

Anon. Nutrition in the post-genomic era. Proc Nutr Soc 2002; 61(4): 401–463.

Anon. Personalised Nutrition. Proc Nutr Soc 2008; 67(4): 390–408.

Berdanier CD, ed. Nutrient Regulation of Gene Expression: Clinical Aspects. Boca Raton: CRC Press, 1996.

Cox TM, Sinclair J. Molecular Biology in Medicine. Oxford: Blackwell, 1997.

Hanash SM. Operomics: molecular analysis of tissues from DNA to RNA to protein. Clin Chem Lab Med 2000; 38: 805–813.

Hirschi KD, Kreps JA, Hirschi KK. Molecular approaches to studying nutrient metabolism and function: an array of possibilities. J Nutr 2001; 131: 1605S–1609S.

Luscombe NM, Greenbaum D, Gerstein M. What is bioinformatics? A proposed definition and overview of the field. Meth Inf Med 2001; 40: 346–358.

3
Integration of Metabolism 1: Energy

Xavier M Leverve

Key messages

- Energy metabolism refers to the ways in which the body obtains and spends energy from food. In terms of energy transduction, part of nutrient energy is converted into chemical, mechanical, electrical or osmotic forms of energy.
- The steady state refers to when the production of final metabolites equals the consumption of the initial precursors: exactly the same amount of matter enters and leaves the system.
- The mitochondrion is the key cellular organelle involved in energy metabolism. The mitochondrion is also involved in other key cellular processes, including apoptosis, calcium signalling and reactive oxygen species production.
- The chemical energy in nutrients (redox energy) is converted into adenosine triphosphate (ATP). ATP is the universal currency of cellular energy metabolism; it is formed from adenosine diphosphate (ADP), essentially by oxidative phosphorylation.
- At a given cellular level, ATP can be synthesised aerobically or anaerobically, that is in the presence or absence of oxygen. When considering the whole organism, interorgan aerobic and anaerobic energy metabolism must be complementary and steady-state energy metabolism must be completely aerobic.
- Energy metabolism for the whole body is primarily due to resting energy expenditure. The thermic effects of food and physical activity are also important components of energy expenditure.

3.1 Introduction

From an energy point of view, life is a succession of transfers that obey the second law of thermodynamics, which states that the entropy of the universe is steadily increasing. But, when considering living organisms as isolated systems, they appear to be a kind of exception to this principle since. By definition, a biosynthetic pathway would decrease the entropy of the newly synthesised biomolecules, at the expense of the universe free energy, through catabolism of nutrients. Unlike plants, animals, including humans, are unable to use light directly as a source of energy. Hence, these living organisms must use another source of energy, provided from the catabolism of nutrients, the synthesis of which is directly or indirectly permitted via plant photosynthesis. Our life is therefore indirectly but totally dependent on sunlight, as the unique energy source for plants, and on the complex, but highly regulated, pathways that link nutrient degradation to adenosine triphosphate (ATP) synthesis.

All kinds of biochemical reactions are linked to energy transfer, therefore each physiological function, as well as each pathological disorder or therapy, must have a consequence for biological energy. It is probable that further investigation of energy disorders in pathological states will lead to a better understanding of the underlying pathophysiological mechanisms and to new therapeutic tools. Living systems must be efficient in situations of both abundance and penury, therefore two distinct classes of diseases can be proposed. On the one hand are diseases of excess nutrients. For example, excess energy intake is associated with obesity, diabetes, hyperlipidaemia and atherosclerosis. On the other hand, diseases related to a deficit of nutrients can occur at the level of the whole body, individual organs or discrete

Nutrition and Metabolism, Second Edition, edited by S. A. Lanham-New, I. A. Macdonald and H. M. Roche. © 2011 The Nutrition Society.

cells. Diseases of scarcity include anorexia, cachexia, shock, hypoxia and ischaemia, which can lead to acute or chronic nutrient imbalance.

The last introductory remark concerning energy metabolism is related to the fact that there is a peril to life related to respiratory chain activity. Indeed, energy metabolism is mainly based on redox reactions involving molecular oxygen as the final electron acceptor, and reactive oxygen species (ROS) represent a major danger to many biomolecules and therefore to life. ROS are probably one of the major determinants of the process of ageing. In this view, understanding the mechanisms for sensing and transducing the surrounding oxygen concentrations, based on the flux of ROS production, represents a major field of research for possible applications oriented towards new therapies for several diseases such as anoxia, ischaemia, diabetes, atherosclerosis, cancer and degenerative pathologies.

3.2 Energy metabolism at the cellular level

Thermodynamics

Energy is a property of the matter permitting it to be transformed, either as the result of work or as achieving work. The common use of terms such as 'energy consumption' or 'energy production' is not proper. Indeed, in accordance with the first law of thermodynamics the amount of energy in the universe remains constant, so it is only possible to convert energy from one form to another, but not to produce or to consume it. This is known as energy transduction. Hence, humans transform nutrient-contained energy into chemical, mechanical, electrical or osmotic forms of energy. The second law of thermodynamic indicates that the transformation of energy is always in the direction of continuous increased universe entropy, which is the ultimate form of energy that cannot be used for any further work. In simple terms entropy can be viewed as the degree of disorder of matter; it is a kind of waste after a work achievement. Whatever biochemical reactions are, fast or not, probable or not, reversible or not, they must always follow energy transfers and the general direction of metabolism always obeys the laws of thermodynamics.

'Our world is the location of permanent energy exchanges between systems, which have different potentials. These energy exchanges are performed in strict accordance with two principles called thermodynamics laws.' This statement, proposed by the French scientist Carnot more than a century ago, was never really demonstrated but so far it has never failed! The first law states that the total energy of the universe is constant: '*Rien ne se perd, rien ne se crée, tout se transforme*', while the second gives the direction of the exchanges: universe entropy must always increase.

The consequences of the second law may be illustrated by a simple example. According to this second law, entropy can never decrease. However, when a litre of water freezes, the degree of organisation of its constitutive molecules increases and therefore entropy decreases. To achieve this result, the freezer produces heat in such a way that the overall result (water in and freezer out) is increased entropy according to the second law. Life can be compared to this: although it leads to the organisation of molecules, thus decreasing their own entropy, the degradation of nutrients initially produced from the energy of the light of the sun results in an increased entropy of the universe.

Equilibrium, steady state, metabolic control and metabolic regulation

One of the main features of any living system is represented by the achievement of real steady states. Metabolic reactions are completed close to or far from the equilibrium, leading to the definition of two different fields of thermodynamics: equilibrium thermodynamics and non-equilibrium thermodynamics. It is therefore important to realise that the actual meaning of equilibrium is often misused. Equilibrium means that both forward and reverse reactions are strictly equal in such a way that the net flux is equal to zero and reactant concentrations are constant. Such a state is incompatible with life and might be viewed as a definition of death: no change, no past, no future, but only an endless stable state. In the state of equilibrium, every event is completely reversible, leading to a total lack of evolution. In living organisms many of the biochemical reactions are not really at equilibrium but occur close to it. In terms of energy metabolism, this near state of equilibrium is often referred to as energy balance. However, it is important to realise that energy balance is not a state of equilibrium but is a steady state. Indeed, maintaining the energy content of the body depends on energy intake (in) and energy dissipation (out), so strictly speaking body composition (or its energy content) is maintained constant but at the expense of substrate supply and product removal, which is the definition of a steady state. In these near-equilibrium reactions both forward and reverse reactions are of large magnitude, but one of them is slightly greater than the other. This permits a real net flux to be achieved, while reactant concentrations are quickly equilibrated after any change in the concentration of the others. Thermodynamic strengths impose the direction of the reactions according to the second law of thermodynamics.

> • Equilibrium equals death: no net flux, no work and definitive immobility.
> • Steady state: constant renewal, characteristics of life, but exogenous systems are required for sustaining it with both input (nutrients and oxygen entering the system) and exit (wastage).

In any living system, the maintenance of a single metabolic parameter (blood glucose, cellular ATP, oxygen concentration, etc.) at a constant level can be referred to as substrate balance. It is important to appreciate that this is a limited part of a metabolic pathway, within the context of whole-body metabolism, which in turn has its metabolic steady state. The metabolic 'steady state' is also often referred to as 'metabolic balance'. For examples of this relating to fat and carbohydrate metabolism, refer to Chapter 5. Such a metabolic state can be defined as a peculiar condition where both net resulting flux and related intermediates are constant, meaning that production of final metabolite(s) equals consumption of initial precursor(s) (Figure 3.1). In this view, the '*milieu intérieur*', as denominated by Bernard more than a century ago, is the result of the metabolism of every cell from every organ in a whole organism. Its steady-state composition can be viewed as the best compromise between cell priorities and needs for cellular or interorgan cooperation. Hence, each cell can theoretically interfere with the metabolism of every cell. The transition between different steady states is initiated by changes in intermediates and/or fluxes (pre-steady states) allowing the new steady state to be reached, as a consequence of the new physiological (i.e. fed versus fasted, sleep, physical activity, pregnancy, growth, etc.) or pathological states. The meta-

bolic fluxes (e.g. ATP synthesis, oxygen consumption, gluconeogenesis, glycolysis, β-oxidation) are dependent on two different kinds of parameter:

• one pertaining to the thermodynamic strengths, which is the energetic result of reactant concentrations (i.e. substrates versus products) pushing the conversion of a precursor into a product.
• the second pertaining to kinetic constraints, which might be viewed as the ability of a metabolic machinery (e.g. enzyme, carrier) to achieve the conversion (transport) of a substrate into a product.

When a system is in a steady state, any change in a given kinetic parameter (e.g. increase in enzymic activity or supply of a nutrient) will affect the entire network, causing it to achieve a new steady state. The information as to the 'new' rules of the system resulting from the change in one parameter can be relayed in two separate, but not mutually exclusive, ways.

First, any change in one of the kinetic constraints of the system will in turn affect the different intermediates, upstream and/or downstream, of the modified step (Figure 3.2). The magnitude of the transmitted effect on the different intermediates depends on the characteristics of each step. This parameter is called elasticity. This form of information transmitted by the changes in intermediate concentrations is called *metabolic control*.

Secondly, a given change in one of the intermediates can trigger a signal (e.g. hormonal or cellular signalling), which in turn affects the kinetics of one or more step(s) of the pathway. Such a mechanism is referred to as *metabolic regulation*.

> • Metabolic control: a modification occurring on a step of a given pathway can be transmitted by adjacent modifications of all reactants involved in the pathway in order to affect the whole pathway.
> • Metabolic regulation: a modification occurring on a step of a pathway can be transmitted to an effector, external to the system (any kind of signalling), which in turn can affect one or more step(s) of the pathway or of other pathways.

Cellular and mitochondrial aerobic energy metabolism

The transformation of a part of the energy contained in nutrients into a form that can be used by the cells for different types of work can be divided into two

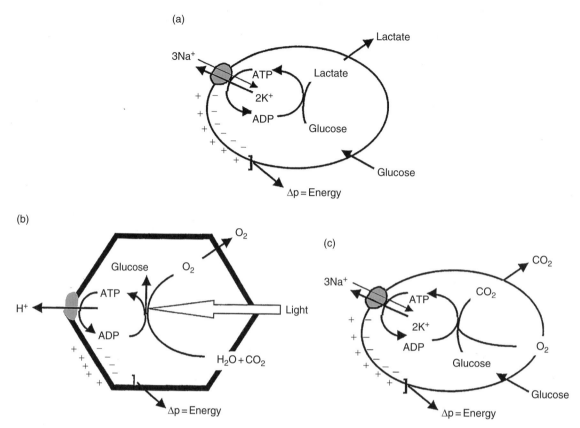

Figure 3.1 Examples of living energy transducing systems. (a) Anaerobic system: the energy source is provided by organic nutrients (i.e. made by a living system) converted through a pathway (fermentation), resulting in ATP generation (phosphate potential or ATP/ADP · Pi ratio). The plasma membrane ATPase (Na$^+$/K$^+$-ATPase) allows the conversion of this phosphate potential into a membrane potential (Δp) because of the electrogenic exchange of 3 Na$^+$ with 2 K$^+$ and permits the cell to generate some work. The erythrocyte represents a good example of a completely anaerobic cell, where the unique source of energy is glucose and the unique energy wastage is lactate, with a stoichiometry of 2 moles of ATP for 1 mole of glucose. (b) Phototrophic system: the energy source is light, which enables the extraction of hydrogen from water. The transduction of energy into ATP and then into membrane potential is similar to the anaerobic system except that Na$^+$/K$^+$-ATPase is replaced by a proton ATPase. (c) Aerobic system: the source of energy is the redox power contained in the nutrients (carbohydrates or lipids), electrons from hydrogen finally being transferred to oxygen, permitting the formation of water. The successive energy transduction processes are similar to those of the anaerobic system (a), but the production of ATP is much higher. The stoichiometry of ATP synthesis depends on the substrates used, and the waste products are water and carbon dioxide.

successive steps. First, the chemical energy contained in the nutrient must be converted into a redox form and then this redox potential must be transduced as a phosphate potential [ATP/(ADP · Pi, where ADP is adenosine diphosphate and Pi is inorganic phosphate)] by ATP synthesis.

From macronutrient to redox potential

The macronutrients, carbohydrates (glucose), amino acids and fatty acids are catabolised by different pathways, including glycolysis, β-oxidation and amino acid pathways. However, all of them converge towards a common intermediate: acetyl-coenzyme A (acetyl-CoA). Glycolysis is the only energy-yielding pathway capable of producing ATP independently of the mitochondrion and without oxygen. This process is referred to as anaerobic metabolism (see later section). In the mitochondrial matrix, the tricarboxylic acid cycle, also known as the Krebs cycle, leads to a complete oxidation of acetyl-CoA, resulting in the formation of reducing equivalents (three NADH, H$^+$ and one FADH$_2$) and carbon dioxide (CO_2). The

(a)

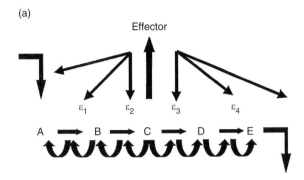

(b)
Steady state:

$$[A] = [B] = [C] = [D] = [E] = \text{constant}$$

(c)
$$J_{A \to E} = J\varepsilon_1 = J\varepsilon_2 = J\varepsilon_3 = J\varepsilon_4$$

Figure 3.2 Metabolic regulation, metabolic control and steady state: a schematic view. Capital letters (A, B, C, D, E) represent intermediates, ε_1, ε_2, ε_3, ε_4 are enzymes and J means flux. (a, b) Schematic representations of metabolic regulation and metabolic control, respectively; (c) metabolic characteristics of a steady state. In this view any metabolic intermediate (glucose, lactate, ATP, etc.) could be viewed as the intermediate B and ε_2 is a part of the downstream pathway (glycolysis, gluconeogenesis, ATPase, etc.).

A potential is the amount of a given form of energy that can be *potentially* used for work. On top of a mountain, a litre of water represents a given amount of energy. If this water falls from the top of the mountain through a waterfall, a part of this energy is progressively converted into kinetic potential during the fall. At the bottom of the waterfall, when the water crashes on a rock, the kinetic potential is then converted to heat, that is to entropy. In this case some of the initial potential is directly converted to heat. If the waterfall is equipped with a turbine, some of the kinetic energy can be converted to electrical energy: this is an example of coupling machinery. But when the electrical energy is converted to light, it will result in an increase in entropy. In this case the potential energy is also finally converted to heat, but on the way it also provides light.

- Redox potential [$(NADH \times H^+)/NAD^+$]: the amount of energy that can be released when one (or often two) electron(s) jump(s) from one compound (which will be oxidised) to another (which will be reduced).
- Phosphate potential [$ATP/(ADP \cdot Pi)$]: the amount of energy that can be released when ATP is converted to ADP and Pi.

main result of the Krebs cycle activity is to provide reducing power to the respiratory chain in the form of NADH/NAD$^+$ or FADH$_2$/FAD, rather than ATP formation. (NAD$^+$ is nicotinamide adenine dinucleotide, NADH its reduced form and NAD$^+$ its oxidised form; FAD is flavin adenine dinucleotide.) Only one ATP, or guanosine triphosphate (GTP), is formed per mole of oxidised acetyl-CoA, compared with 14 ATP molecules that can result from reducing equivalent reoxidation.[1] Oxygen is not directly involved in this part of the pathway. However, the dehydrogenases that oxidise acetyl-CoA work at near-equilibrium and the accumulation of NADH, due to lack of oxygen, inhibits the net flux of acetyl-CoA through the Krebs cycle. Hence, although not directly involved, oxygen plays a crucial role in the Krebs cycle activity by maintaining adequate reducing potential.

From redox potential to ATP synthesis

Mitochondrial energy is supplied by proton oxidation, oxygen being the final electron acceptor:

$$4H^+ + 4e^- + O_2 \to 2H_2O + \text{energy}$$

This reaction leads to a large release of energy, which is normally dissipated as heat, pressure or an increase in volume. The unique property of the mitochondrial respiratory chain is to convert, with high efficiency, energy towards ADP phosphorylation. As first proposed by Mitchell, and now generally accepted, energy release during oxidation in the respiratory chain results in active proton transport outside the mitochondrial matrix. Hence, owing to the sequence of the respiratory chain complexes, the redox energy is converted into another form of potential: the mitochondrial inner membrane potential or proton-motive force. The next step in the oxidative phosphorylation pathway is to use this proton-motive force for ATP synthesis. The enzymic complex of mitochondrial ATP synthase (Figure 3.3) achieves this. It is important to note that oxidation (also known as respiration) and phosphorylation (or ATP synthesis) are connected through a common intermediate, the proton-motive force.

This proton-motive force depends on:

- the activity of the respiratory chain by pumping protons out of the matrix
- the ATPase by transferring protons back in the matrix when ATP is synthesised
- the properties of the inner membrane, creating a barrier that is impermeable to protons.

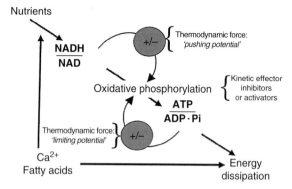

Figure 3.3 Regulation of oxidative phosphorylation flux. The control of oxidative phosphorylation is exerted by two different factors: kinetic parameters (i.e. kinetic properties of the different enzymes) and thermodynamic factors (i.e. forces exerted on the system). A dramatic change in the flux without a large change in either redox potential or phosphate potential implies subtle co-ordinated mechanisms, as is done, for instance, by calcium or fatty acids, which affect the oxidative phosphorylation pathway simultaneously upstream and downstream.

Practical assessment of oxidative phosphorylation

Although it is relatively simple to investigate the oxidative phosphorylation pathway in isolated mitochondria, this is much more difficult in an intact system or *in vivo*. The whole pathway of oxidative phosphorylation can be divided schematically into several steps:

(1) Cytosolic pathways that result in cytosolic redox potential.
(2) Mitochondrial oxidation of acetyl-CoA (Krebs cycle), which results in mitochondrial redox potential.
(3) Respiratory chain activity and its resultant proton-motive force.
(4) ATP synthesis and resultant mitochondrial phosphate potential.
(5) Electrogenic ATP–ADP exchanges across the mitochondrial inner membrane (adenine nucleotide translocator) and resultant cytosolic phosphate potential.

The electrochemical potential across the inner mitochondrial membrane is of crucial importance for each of these steps. Therefore, any phenomenon that could affect it (e.g. proton leak, see below) would affect the complete pathway of ATP synthesis.

Cytosolic lactate dehydrogenase and mitochondrial 3-hydroxybutyrate dehydrogenase work at near-equilibrium state, therefore the cytosolic and mitochondrial redox state can be evaluated by measuring lactate-to-pyruvate and 3-hydroxybutyrate-to-acetoacetate ratios.[2] These measurements are useful tools that can be used to evaluate any defects in the oxidative pathway *in vivo*. The activity of the respiratory chain can be assessed by measuring the rate of oxygen consumption either at the level of the whole body or in an isolated organ, cell(s) or mitochondrion. The most difficult parameters of oxidative phosphorylation to assess are phosphate potential, ATP synthesis (or turnover rate) and the yield of ATP synthesis, that is of oxidative pathway. Indeed, if ATP concentration could be calculated *in vivo* by nuclear magnetic resonance (NMR), then phosphate potential could be determined if the concentration of ADP was known. However, ADP concentration cannot be obtained directly. Moreover, since adenine nucleotides are highly compartmentalised in the cell (see below), average values for intracellular or tissue ATP levels are of limited interest.

Regulation of the flux through oxidative phosphorylation

Although much is known concerning the regulation of the different enzymes of the oxidative phosphorylation pathway, the actual regulation of mitochondrial respiration and the rate of ATP synthesis are not fully understood. The sophisticated machinery of this pathway can be simplified as a single step catalysing the following reaction:

$$2NADH + 2H^+ + O_2 + 6ADP + 6Pi$$
$$\rightarrow 2NAD^+ + 2H_2O + 6ATP$$

As for any biochemical reaction, its rate is dependent on kinetic and thermodynamic parameters: the activity and affinity of enzymes and resulting thermodynamic strength applied to the system (i.e. the difference between upstream and downstream potentials). In the case of oxidative phosphorylation, redox potential (NADH/NAD) represents upstream potential and *pushes* the flux; while downstream, opposed to the redox potential and *limiting* the flux, is the phosphate potential (ATP/ADP · Pi) (Figure 3.3). Thus, an increased NADH/NAD ratio and/or a decreased ATP/ADP · Pi ratio will increase the flux.

Conversely, a decrease in NADH/NAD and/or an increased ATP/ADP · Pi ratio will reduce oxidative phosphorylation flux. The mitochondrial redox potential depends on several factors. These include Krebs cycle activity, leading to NADH production, and phosphate potential, which depends on ATP hydrolysis (i.e. the cellular work). From these considerations it appears that a large change in flux of ATP synthesis must be accompanied by a large change in the related forces, resulting in a paradox: a high flux of ATP synthesis can be achieved only if mitochondrial ATP concentration is very low. The regulation of oxidative phosphorylation is much subtler and achieves a very large change in ATP synthesis at nearly constant forces. As an example, during myofibrillar contraction increased calcium concentration promotes energy dissipation by simultaneously activating several dehydrogenases, particularly those involved in the Krebs cycle. Hence, the increase in calcium results in coordinated changes affecting energy metabolism via a simultaneous increase in both the NADH supply system (Krebs cycle) and the ATP consuming processes (muscle contraction). With this mechanism of a simultaneous push and pull, a large change in the oxygen consumption–ATP synthesis pathway is possible without a major change in the related forces: redox or phosphate potentials.

Yield of ATP synthesis (ATP/O ratio)

The yield of oxidative phosphorylation can be expressed as the ratio between ATP synthesis rate and the number of atoms of oxygen consumed (ATP/O). This ratio is of major importance to life and it can be modified by several parameters, therefore its regulation is finely tuned. Three main mechanisms modify the fluxes of oxidation and phosphorylation. Although both oxidation and phosphorylation are considered as one pathway, they can be independently and differentially regulated by:

- the number of coupling sites at the level of the respiratory chain
- the stoichiometry of the coupling process at the level of the proton pumps (slipping)
- the proton permeability across the mitochondrial inner membrane (proton leak).

The number of coupling sites located on the electron pathway towards molecular oxygen depends on the nature of the redox carrier (NADH or $FADH_2$). For NADH three coupling sites are successively involved (complexes 1, 3 and 4), while there are only two coupling sites for $FADH_2$ (complexes 3 and 4). Hence, the yield of ATP synthesis is roughly 30% lower when $FADH_2$ is oxidised, compared with NADH. The glycolytic pathway results in NADH formation, while the fatty acid β-oxidation results in equimolar formation of NADH and $FADH_2$. Hence, the stoichiometry of ATP synthesis to oxygen consumption is lower when lipids are oxidised, compared with carbohydrates.[3] Since the mitochondrial inner membrane is impermeable to NADH, cytoplasmic NADH donates reducing equivalents to the mitochondrial electron transport chain through two shuttle systems, the malate/aspartate shuttle and the glycerol-3-phosphate/dihydroxyacetone-phosphate shuttle. Although the first one gives electrons to complex I (i.e. as NADH), the second shuttle gives electrons directly to complex II. Subsequently, by tuning the respective proportion of flux through the two shuttles, the yield of oxidative phosphorylation can be regulated. This target is one of the major effects of thyroid hormones on mitochondrial energy metabolism. These hormones affect the transcription of mitochondrial glycerol-3-phosphate dehydrogenase, which regulates the flux through the glycerol-3-phosphate/dihydroxyacetone-phosphate shuttle.

The modulation of the coupling between proton transport (proton pump slipping) and redox reaction (respiratory chain) or ATP synthesis (ATP synthase) is another possibility to adjust the flux of oxidation and phosphorylation. The coupling between the two vectorial reactions (proton transport and oxidation or phosphorylation) is not fixed and several experiments have shown some variations in this coupling. For example, general anaesthetics or the lipid composition of the mitochondrial membrane can alter this.

The inner mitochondrial membrane is not completely impermeable to protons, and proton leak results in uncoupling between respiratory rate and phosphorylation. This energy is dissipated as heat. This phenomenon, first described in brown adipose tissue, is probably a general feature of all kinds of mitochondria. It results in slight disconnection between the rate of oxidation and phosphorylation, and therefore alters the yield of oxidative phosphorylation. This mechanism should not be viewed as a negative event leading to less efficient ATP synthesis. It allows independent adaptation of oxygen consumption/reoxidation of reducing equivalents and ATP synthesis. Indeed, the discovery of this function in brown adipose tissue in mammals, which is related to an uncoupling protein (UCP), has opened a new era in our understanding of the regulation of oxidative phosphorylation by describing a physiological role for energy wastage. Several other UCPs have been described recently, and UCP1 mediates this effect in brown adipose tissue. Homologues, including UCP2 and UCP3, are expressed in most tissues, including white adipose tissue, muscle, macrophages, spleen, thymus and Kupffer's cells. However, their role in energy metabolism is less defined than that for UCP1. The complementary DNA (cDNA) encoding brain mitochondrial carrier protein has also been cloned. This protein (BMCP1) is also homologous to the UCPs; when expressed in yeast it is a potent uncoupler, so it could be a new member of the UCP family. The physiological function of UCP1 in brown fat is well recognised as a heat-producing mechanism. The presence of homologous uncoupling proteins (UCP2 and UCP3) in white adipose tissue and skeletal muscle suggests that they may also influence whole-body energy metabolism and may play a role in the pathogenesis of obesity. However, not all studies support this hypothesis. For example, overexpression of UCP3 in skeletal muscle reduces white adipose tissue mass, but adipose tissue is not altered in UCP2 and UCP3 knockout mice. It has also been proposed that mitochondrial uncoupling regulates mitochondrial ROS production. Moreover, it is becoming clear that the mitochondrial membrane potential plays a role in the regulation of many important cellular functions, including calcium signalling, permeability of the transitional mitochondrial pore [permeability transition pore (PTP)], fatty acid oxidation and apoptosis. It is therefore likely that the role of mitochondrial uncoupling in cellular homeostasis is not limited to energy metabolism. It has recently been proposed that efficiency mitochondrial oxidative phosphorylation plays a key role in insulin secretion by pancreatic β-cell islets.

ATP distribution: cellular energy circuits

It is not yet known how ATP distribution among the different cellular sites of energy dissipation (e.g. biosynthetic pathways, muscle contraction, metabolite transport and membrane potential maintenance, gene transcription and translation, protein synthesis and degradation) is regulated. Indeed, all of these processes compete with each other, and a very precise regulation of energy distribution is mandatory. In many textbooks it is tacitly supposed that ATP and ADP simply diffuse in the cell, except for crossing intracellular membranes where specific carriers are involved. Such a simple view cannot hold when considering that a simple diffusion through the cytoplasm would not be compatible with a specific energy supply to a given step. Several experimental studies have addressed this problem and investigated the role of the phosphocreatine/creatine shuttle in the transfer of energy in muscle and cardiac cells. It was proposed that cytosolic and mitochondrial creatine kinases act as an energy shuttle (see Figure 3.4), permitting the channelling of energy from one cellular location (a part of the mitochondrion membrane) to a precise site of energy utilisation (myofibrillar ATPase, Na^+/K^+-ATPase, endoplasmic reticulum ATPase, biosynthetic pathway, etc.). In such a view the 'energy-rich bond' is transported rather than ATP or creatine phosphate molecules per se. Hence, by playing with the location of creatine kinase (e.g. by the transcription of different isoforms), the cell can build several tracks for energy channelling that can be used according to the cellular priorities for energy. This feature of cellular energy channelling and compartmentation has been recently conceptualised as IntraCellular Energy Units (ICEU).

Mitochondrial metabolism and cell signalling

Mitochondria have many specific functions related to some peculiar enzymic equipment. For instance, they play a major role in fatty acid β-oxidation, as well as in urea synthesis and gluconeogenesis. Recently, the role of mitochondria in cellular calcium homeostasis has been extended by the discovery of transitional permeability, mediated by the PTP, which mediates calcium uptake across the inner mitochondrial membrane. This phenomenon, which is blocked specifically by cyclosporin A, appears to be involved in the trigger of cellular death pathways, necrosis or

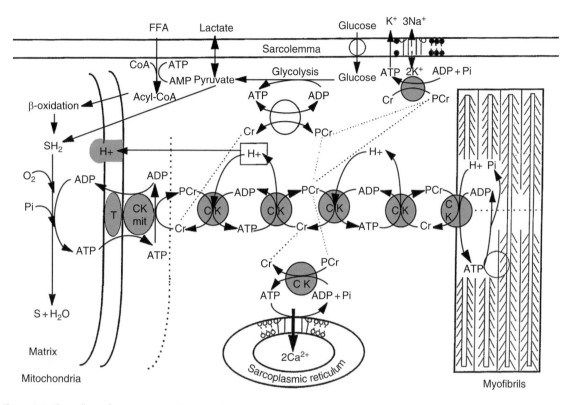

Figure 3.4 Channelling of energy in a cardiac cell. The pathway for intracellular energy transport and the corresponding feedback signal conduction in muscle, brain and many other types of cells (but excluding liver cells) is the phosphocreatine pathway (energy circuit or energy shuttle). This channelling enables a wave of energy to be transferred from a precise location in the mitochondrial membrane to a precise site of dissipation (myofibrils, Ca^{2+} ATPase in the sarcoplasmic reticulum, sodium ATPase, etc.). Conversely, the signal given by a rise in ADP, due to mechanical work for instance, is channelled to the mitochondrial matrix without effective transportation of the ADP molecule. From this picture it is clear that the meaning of an average cellular ATP or ADP concentration becomes limited. (With kind permission from Springer Science + Business Media: Molecular and cellular biochemistry, metabolic compartmentation and substrate channelling in muscle, Sak VA. 133 (1994) 155–192.)

apoptosis. Mitochondria regulate cell death, or apoptosis, by releasing cytochrome c into the cytosol when mitochondria swell after PTP opening. Mitochondria also play a major role in cellular calcium homeostasis, by a mechanism called calcium uptake–calcium release. Mitochondria achieve this because they are able to take up free calcium from the cytoplasm, owing to their specific channels and very high membrane potential, and to release it when the PTP opens.

The mitochondrion has other effects on cellular signalling. It is a major site for ROS formation. Indeed, two specific complexes of the respiratory chain are largely recognised as sites for ROS production: complex 1 or NADH reductase and complex 3 or bc_1-complex, with the latter being quantitatively the most important site. The production of mitochondrial ROS seems to represent not only a negative event leading to irreversible mitochondrial DNA damage and to ageing, but also a main signalling pathway both in physiology (oxygen and substrate sensing) and pathology. The subtle mechanism of cellular oxygen sensing (see below) is based on superoxide production by membrane-bound NADPH-oxidase and involves a cytoplasmic dimerisation of specific transcriptional factors ([Hypoxia Inducible Factor] HIF-1 α and β), which are subsequently translocated into the nucleus. The combination of superoxide and nitric oxide results in peroxinitrite formation, which represents another example of ROS-based signalling pathway.

Cellular anaerobic metabolism

In the absence of oxygen, there are in principle three possibilities for ATP synthesis:

- adenylate kinase
- creatine kinase
- lactate production from glucose.

Although the first two possibilities are qualitatively important as ATP synthetic pathways, their significance is quantitatively very limited and could only meet the energy needs for a few seconds or minutes. Conversely, glycolysis is a more powerful and sustained pathway for ATP synthesis in the absence of oxygen when substrate supply (glucose) and wastage disposal (reducing equivalent and proton) as lactate are sufficient. In this pathway, two ATPs are produced from one glucose molecule, whereas three ATPs are formed when glucose is provided from glycogen stores. The net result of glycolysis is the formation of pyruvate, ATP, NADH and H^+. The pool of NAD^+–NADH is very small, so the maintenance of a sustained glycolytic flux even in the presence of sufficient amounts of glucose is possible only when NAD^+ is regenerated from NADH reoxidation. Since in the absence of oxygen this cannot be achieved by mitochondrial metabolism, the unique way to remove the excess of reducing equivalents, in lactic organisms, is to convert pyruvate into lactate (yeast can produce ethanol or glycerol for the same purpose). Lactic acid production allows the release of reducing potential, together with protons and carbons. Hence, ATP production by anaerobic glycolysis is mainly controlled by:

- the phosphate potential [ATP/(ADP · Pi)]
- the pH
- the level of cytosolic redox state (NADH/NAD ratio).

Adaptation to energy deficit

The consequences of cellular energy deficit and the mechanisms underlying adaptation to this situation can be understood from the results of numerous studies, in both hypoxia and ischaemia. Such adaptation must rely on a permanent adjustment between energy demand and ATP synthesis. When oxygen and ATP are decreasing, energy-dissipating processes must also be reduced to the same extent and according to several priorities. Therefore, energy demand has to adapt to match oxygen supply and ATP production capacity. This needs a sensitive oxygen-sensing system, associated with the possibility of a cellular metabolic conformance to oxygen disposal. Oxygen conformance means that cells can anticipate any possible lack or excess of oxygen by sensing the oxygen tension in the surroundings. The pathway of cellular oxygen signalling is now understood, especially the role of ROS production on gene expression via HIF. The adaptive changes related to hypoxia or energy deficit have been divided into defence and rescue phases. The defence phase occurs immediately after a decline in oxygen and consists of channel arrest, decreased Na^+/K^+-ATPase activity, urea synthesis, gluconeogenesis, protein synthesis and proteolysis (a highly ATP-consuming process), in such a way that ATP demand equals ATP production. Then, the rescue phase involves transcriptional effects, particularly involving HIF, wherein HIF-mediated activation of genes is required for sustained survival at low ATP turnover (increased glycolytic enzymes, decreased enzymes involved in aerobic-linked metabolism) and, finally, production of tertiary cell signalling messengers (fos and jun).

3.3 Energy metabolism in the body as a whole

General considerations

Energy in the body is mainly utilised for active transport across cellular membranes, synthesis of new molecules and contraction of contractile fibres. Whole-body energy metabolism is expressed as resting energy expenditure (REE), which is much easier to determine than the classical basal energy expenditure (BEE). In healthy adults, it is estimated as 40 kcal h^{-1} m^{-2}, the body surface being determined as follows:

$$S\,(m^2) = 71.84 \times H^{0.725}(cm) \times W^{0.425}(kg)$$

As shown in Table 3.1, REE is predominantly related to the metabolism of four main organs: liver, brain, heart and kidneys. Although these organs represent only 5.5% of total body mass, they account for almost 60% of total body energy expenditure. REE is influenced by many factors, such as age (55 kcal h^{-1} m^{-2} for the newborn versus 35 kcal h^{-1} m^{-2} in the elderly),

Table 3.1 Respective contribution of the different organs to oxygen consumption and body mass

	Oxygen consumption (%)	Mass (%)
Liver	20	2.5
Brain	20	2.0
Heart	10	0.5
Kidneys	10	0.5
Muscles	20	40.0
Others	20	54.5

gender (10% higher in males as compared to females), food intake, pregnancy and several diseases.

Energy metabolism can be investigated by several means. The most common way to determine energy expenditure is based on measurements by indirect calorimetry that assess energy dissipation from oxygen consumption (Vo_2). Moreover, by determining the respiratory quotient ($RQ = Vco_2/Vo_2$, where Vco_2 is carbon dioxide production) and the excretion of urea, it is possible to determine the nature of the oxidised substrates (carbohydrates versus lipids).[4] As described above, energy metabolism (i.e. the transduction of energy contained in nutrients to ATP synthesis) involves many steps, and some of them can be investigated in clinical practice by measuring lactate/pyruvate or β-hydroxybutyrate/acetoacetate ratios and oxygen consumption. The other methods are limited to clinical research. Examples of these include intracellular ATP by NMR or by biopsy, infrared spectroscopy for *in situ* redox potential determination and doubly labelled water.

Interplay between aerobic and anaerobic energy metabolism

The amount of ATP produced from nutrients by mitochondrial oxidative phosphorylation is far higher than that occurring in anaerobic conditions. A healthy adult human produces, and therefore consumes, a mass of ATP approximately equivalent to his or her body mass every day. Total ATP body content is about 100–200 g. Assuming for simplification that ATP synthesis is achieved only from glucose metabolism, 650 g of glucose is required for the aerobic synthesis of 70 kg of ATP. In comparison, 13 kg of glucose would be necessary to produce the same quantity of ATP by the anaerobic pathway. But, besides the indisputable quantitative advantages of

aerobic metabolism, the anaerobic pathway is qualitatively of great importance.

Tissue anaerobic metabolism

In several tissues anaerobic energy metabolism is predominant even in the presence of sufficient oxygen concentration. This is the case in red blood cells, which completely lack mitochondria. It is interesting to consider that although these cells contain probably the highest amount of oxygen, their energy needs are completely met anaerobically. Erythrocyte anaerobic energy metabolism is not marginal, when considering that red blood cells represent a completely anaerobic organ of almost 2.5 kg (≈40 g of glucose-lactate/day, i.e. 20% of total glucose turnover). Epithelial cells of the cornea are also dependent on anaerobic glycolysis as their unique energy source. The kidney medulla is another example of a physiological advantage of anaerobic energy production despite the low rate of ATP synthesis. In this tissue a very high osmotic pressure is maintained in the extracellular fluid as the result of tubular cell activity of ion transport. A rich vascularisation would lead to a high energetic cost to maintain such a gradient because of efficient exchanges between cells and plasma. However, owing to the poor blood supply to these cells, their energy metabolism is achieved mainly via the anaerobic pathway occurring from the glucose present in the tubular ultrafiltrate.

Energy metabolism is compartmentalised in the cell. Glycolytic ATP resulting in lactate formation even in fully aerobic experimental conditions probably predominantly supports the plasma membrane-linked ATPase activities. Hence, in cardiac cells, which are fully aerobic in physiological conditions, lactate release is very low or absent, but a specific role of glycolytic ATP meets the energy requirements of plasma membrane active transport, while the energy required for contraction comes from mitochondrial oxidative phosphorylation. This example illustrates the complementary aspects of aerobic and anaerobic energy metabolism even in a well-oxygenated organ.

Energy metabolism in the brain: neurone astrocyte cooperation

The brain is very sensitive to hypoxia because of its high metabolic rate. A moderate degree of hypoxia results in brain lactate accumulation. Some recent experimental data lead to a very fascinating hypothesis, known as the activity-dependent astrocyte–neurone lactate shuttle. It is proposed that the main energy substrate for neurones is not glucose but lactate, provided by astrocyte anaerobic glycolysis. In astrocytes, ATP provided by glycolysis is functionally linked to the plasma membrane Na-ATPase. After glutamate activation, the reuptake of glutamate by astrocytes is associated with sodium, and the active pumping of sodium out of the cell is then linked to glycolysis activation. The lactate produced is used as the energy substrate for activated neurones. In this view there is a functional coupling between astrocyte and neurone energy metabolism. The upper part of glucose oxidation (i.e. from glucose to lactate) occurs in astrocytes, while the lower part (i.e. pyruvate oxidation) occurs in neurones, in such a way that brain metabolism as a whole is permitted by complete glucose oxidation into water and carbon dioxide. A similar feature of glucose-lactate cooperation in tissue energy metabolism has been also shown in other coordinated cell metabolism, such as Sertoli's cells and spermatozoa, Henle's and proximal tubular cells in the kidney and probably in many other situations.

Aerobic–anaerobic metabolism: perspectives in whole-body integrated metabolism

Except for the initial substrates (nutrients, oxygen) and the final waste products (water, carbon dioxide, urea, etc.), every metabolite is a substrate for some cells, while it is a product for others. Hence, although anaerobic ATP production is a reality at cellular level, this is not the case when the whole-body integrated metabolism is considered at steady state. In this latter case, energy metabolism is always purely aerobic. Indeed, anaerobic metabolism implies that the end-product of glycolysis must be excreted as lactate in human cells, or as ethanol or glycerol in yeast, for instance. This can be the case for isolated cells or organs, but since lactate excretion from the body is negligible, lactate is ultimately metabolised or oxidised. Therefore, when considering the body as a whole, energy metabolism is fully aerobic and lactate is not a waste end-product, but a metabolite that is an alternative substrate and product. When lactate accumulates in the body, such as during a short bout of high-intensity exercise, anaerobic metabolism contributes to net ATP synthesis. However, during the recovery process, lactate is metabolised and disappears from the body without significant net excre-

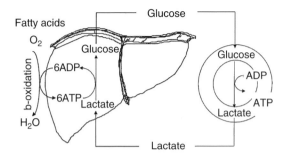

Figure 3.5 Combination of anaerobic and aerobic pathways results in a fully aerobic life. The glucose recycled via lactate creates a futile cycle between three- and six-carbon compounds. On the one hand this dissipates directly two-thirds of the energy as heat (since six ATP are needed to build one glucose from two lactate, whereas only two ATP are produced when splitting glucose into lactate), but on the other hand the source of energy in liver mainly comes from fatty acid oxidation. Hence, glucose recycling provides 'glycolytic ATP' to several peripheral cells (e.g. erythrocytes) while this ATP is formed from energy coming from lipid oxidation. In other words, one can say that 'the liver respires for anaerobic tissues like erythrocytes'.

tion. Accordingly, when considering both exercise and recovery periods, energy metabolism is completely aerobic. Similarly, in pathological diseases, if blood lactate concentration is stable, whatever its concentration, energy metabolism is fully aerobic.

> All metabolism is ultimately aerobic, and anaerobic metabolism exists in certain tissues and in certain metabolic states for defined and logical reasons.

The glucose–lactate cycle, initially described by Cori as substrate recycling between erythrocytes and the liver, can be extended to nearly all organs and cells. This recycling has important metabolic implications for both qualitative and quantitative aspects of whole-body energy homeostasis. On the one hand, only 2 moles of ATP result from the fermentation of 1 mole of glucose, whereas 6 moles of ATP are needed to give back 1 mole of glucose (Figure 3.5). Hence, when considering the *overall yield*[5] of glucose–lactate cycling, one-third of the ATP synthesised aerobically in the liver is used anaerobically in the erythrocytes. On the other hand, glycolysis provides glycolytic ATP to cells, whereas glucose is built with an energy source provided by fatty-acid aerobic oxidation, since this source is largely predominant, if not exclusive, in the liver.

Hence, the metabolic result of glucose–lactate recycling is the transfer of aerobically synthesised

ATP from lipid oxidation in the liver to anaerobic glycolytic ATP in peripheral cells. This is achieved by a decrease in *efficiency* (but see note 5), which is compensated for by qualitative metabolic advantages. The large mass of lipid stores compared with the limited amount of carbohydrates or the metabolic cost of the use of gluconeogenic amino acids provided from protein breakdown might represent one of these advantages. A second advantage is related to the possibility of sharing between organs or cells a part of the aerobic energy metabolism pathway. For example, erythrocyte energy metabolism is entirely anaerobic owing to the lack of mitochondria, but since lactate is further metabolised by the liver, the erythrocyte and liver work as a fully aerobic system. Hence, the liver respires for red blood cells and, except for the situation when lactate is accumulating or excreted, energy metabolism is entirely aerobic whatever the lactate concentration. Therefore, lactate plays a pivotal role not only in anaerobic metabolism but also in aerobic metabolism by providing reduced substrates from one cell to the respiratory chain of another. Lactate–pyruvate interconversion may also be viewed as a shuttle for transporting reducing equivalents from one organ to another or from one cell to another, as it has been described during prolonged submaximal exercise. Such redox shuttle is not limited to interorgan exchanges but also concerns intraorgan metabolism, that is, intercellular shuttle (Figure 3.6), and any reduced compound released by one cell and taken up by another can play the role of a redox shuttle. A large increase in the interconversion of lactate to pyruvate and pyruvate to lactate has been recently reported in type 2 diabetes. Such a phenomenon could explain a regional lactate production and utilisation in critically ill patients.

Role of lactate in ischaemia–reperfusion injury

The succession of aerobic–anaerobic phases that results in deleterious events is known as ischaemia–reperfusion injury. This occurs in various cell types, but some, including the brain, are especially sensitive to this kind of injury. In experimental conditions, as well as in clinical practice, an increased brain lactate is always interpreted as proof of brain hypoxia. It is believed that lactate is not only a marker of hypoxia but also a causal pejorative event. Lactic acid is interpreted as a toxic metabolite for neurons. This leads to

(a)

(b)

Figure 3.6 Role of lactate/pyruvate interconversion as a reducing equivalent shuttle. Lactate-to-pyruvate exchange and vice versa could be viewed as a reducing equivalent shuttle (a) from one organ to another or (b) from one cell to another, depending on the oxygen tension in the immediate cell vicinity. This mechanism enables the oxidative energy metabolism to be shared between cells, one cell being able to respire for another.

the acceptance that hyperglycaemia exacerbates the brain ischaemia–reperfusion injury. It was recently proposed that lactate is in fact an adequate substrate for aerobic energy production during the initial stage of recovery after transient ischaemia or hypoxia. Monocarboxylate anions (i.e. lactate or ketones) prevent cerebral dysfunction during hypoglycaemia and the protective effect of lactate is also present in patients with insulin-dependent diabetes.

3.4 Perspectives on the future

Several key questions regarding cellular energy metabolism are still poorly understood as yet and further investigations are mandatory for a better understanding of the pathogenesis of several diseases. So far, our view of the mechanisms and the consequences of the metabolic compartmentation is very limited. It is probable that this field of investigation will explode in the future. The relationship between cellular death and mitochondrial metabolism represents a new direction that might lead to significant therapeutic advances. Nevertheless, it is clear that the most difficult achievement is to obtain a real integrative view of the energy metabolism. How are the hierarchy and priorities of the different ATP-utilising pathways defined? Shall we be able to manipulate this hierarchy using new drugs in the future?

Notes

1 The complete oxidation of one acetyl-CoA in the Krebs cycle results in three NADH, H$^+$ and one FADH$_2$, leading to the formation of $(3 \times 3\ ATP) + 2\ ATP = 11\ ATP$; since pyruvate oxidation results in the formation of one NADH, H$^+$ ($= 3\ ATP$) the net result of pyruvate oxidation is 14 ATP, while glycolysis produces 4 NADH, H$^+$ ($= 12\ ATP$). Hence, the result of the complete oxidation of one glucose molecule is $(2 \times 14) + 12 + 2$ (produced at the levels of the Kreb's cycle). Hence, the ATP actually produced at the level of the Krebs cycle represents only 2/38, that is 5%, of total ATP. It must be realised that these calculations require a fixed stoichiometry of ATP synthesis from respiration, which is not completely true (see below).

2 Plasma lactate/pyruvate and 3-hydroxybutyrate/acetoacetate ratios reflect schematically cytoplasmic and mitochondrial redox states, respectively. They can be used to assess disorders in the redox pathway: lactate/pyruval increase may indicate a deficit in oxidation and 3-hydroxybutyrate/acetoacetate a deficit in liver mitochondrial function, since the liver plays a major role in ketone metabolism. However, it must be kept in mind that these parameters in the blood reflect an averaged value between several tissues, organs, cells and mitochondria (see *milieu intérieur*) and therefore one value may hide the opposite change in the various organs.

3 When a fatty acid is oxidised through mitochondrial β-oxidation (1 NADH, H$^+$ and 1 FADH$_2$ = 5 ATP) and acetyl-CoA in the Krebs cycle $(11 + 1\ ATP)$ it leads to the formation of 17 ATP per two-carbon fragment, but since fatty acids require an activation ($ATP \rightarrow AMP$) it represents a cost equivalent to 2 ATP per chain of fatty acid. This explains why the actual yield of ATP production is dependent on the length of the chain (see note 1).

4 The actual metabolic reflect of the respiratory quotient is limited by the fact that the kinetics of the changes are not of the same order of magnitude between oxygen and carbon dioxide. Indeed, oxygen storage is very limited in the body and any metabolic change at the level of cellular respiration is reflected by the body respiratory exchanges. By contrast, regarding carbon dioxide, owing to extremely broad storage, mainly as bicarbonate, there is latency between the changes occurring at the cellular level and the total body respiratory exchanges. Therefore, any statement concerning non-steady state conditions must be interpreted with extreme caution. This is the reason why some authors propose calling the parameter the respiratory exchange ratio (RER) rather than the respiratory quotient (RQ).

5 The notion of yield in this sense is not really proper. Indeed, *sensu stricto* yield means the proportion of energy converted from one form to another. For example, one can speak of the yield of mechanical work, which is the percentage of energy converted to work, the difference being heat loss in this example. Concerning the body as a whole in steady state, if no net mechanical or biological (pregnancy, lactation, growth, increase in body weight, etc.) work is achieved, the actual yield is always zero: the entirety of energy is dissipated as heat. In the case of glucose–lactate cycling, yield is taken as the sense of metabolic efficiency: only one-third of the energy derived from aerobic ATP synthesis is ultimately used in erythrocyte metabolism.

Further reading

Boss O, Muzzin P, Giacobino J-P. The uncoupling proteins, a review. Eur J Endocrinol 1998; 139: 1–9.

De Duwe CR. Vital Dust. Life as a Cosmic Imperative. Glasgow: Harper Collins, 1995.

Newsholme E, Leech A. Biochemistry for the Medical Sciences. Chichester: John Wiley, 1983.

Nicholls DG. Bioenergetics: an Introduction to the Chemiosmotic Theory. London: Academic Press, 1982.

Saks, VA *et al.* Metabolic compartmentation and substrate channelling. Mol Cell Biochem 1994; 133(134): 155–192.

Westerhoff HV, Groen AK, Wanders RJ. Modern theories of metabolic control and their applications (Review). Biosci Rep 1984; 4: 1–22.

4
Integration of Metabolism 2: Macronutrients

Keith N Frayn and Abayomi O Akanji

Key messages

- We take in carbohydrate, fat and protein; ultimately (if we are not growing) we oxidise them, liberating energy, but they may be directed to storage pools before this happens.
- The metabolism of each of these macronutrients is highly regulated, partly by direct metabolic interactions between them, but largely through the secretion of hormones.
- In particular, the metabolic fates of fat and carbohydrate are intimately related: when one is predominant, the other tends

to be minimised. This is achieved both by hormonal effects (e.g. insulin suppresses fat mobilisation) and by metabolic interaction (e.g. fatty acids tend to inhibit glucose oxidation in muscle).
- The interplay of these various regulatory systems in different tissues enables humans, as intact organisms, to adapt to a wide variety of metabolic demands: starvation, overfeeding or a sudden increase in energy expenditure during exercise.

4.1 Introduction: fuel intake and fuel utilisation

The human body as a machine

The human body is a type of machine. It takes in fuel (chemical energy in food) and converts this to useful forms of energy: heat, physical work and other forms of chemical energy, including biosynthesis and pumping of substances across membranes. The chemical energy is liberated from the fuels by oxidation.

The fuels that we take in are the macronutrients: carbohydrate, fat and protein. Each of these may be burned in a bomb calorimeter. The products are carbon dioxide, water and oxides of nitrogen from the nitrogen content of the protein. Their combustion also liberates heat. Similarly, after their oxidation in the body, waste products are excreted. These are essentially carbon dioxide, water and urea (which contain the nitrogen from the protein). Within the body these macronutrients may be partially oxidised (e.g. glucose to pyruvic acid) or converted to other substances, but essentially in the end they are either oxidised completely in the body or stored: humans do not excrete significant amounts

of lactate, ketone bodies, amino acids or other products of their metabolism. It is often useful to maintain this 'global' view of the body's metabolic activities (Figure 4.1).

The pattern of energy intake is sporadic: people usually take in regular, discrete meals, which are digested and absorbed into the circulation over discrete periods. Even though the pattern of food consumption in developed countries may be approaching one of continuous 'grazing', the pattern of energy intake is not geared in general to the pattern of energy expenditure. Therefore, the body must be able to take in fuels (macronutrients), store them as necessary and oxidise them when required. This clearly requires control mechanisms that are similar to the throttle that determines when gasoline (petrol) is used from the storage tank in a car. The situation is more complex than the flow of gasoline, however. In the car there is just one engine demanding fuel. In the human body there are multiple organs, each with its own requirements that vary with time on an individual basis. Furthermore, whereas we fill up our car tank with just one fuel, as humans we take in the three macronutrients. Each

Nutrition and Metabolism, Second Edition, edited by S. A. Lanham-New, I. A. Macdonald and H. M. Roche. © 2011 The Nutrition Society.

Fat 100 g/day
Carbohydrate 300 g/day
Protein 100 g/day
O_2 500 l/day

CO_2 450 l/day
Urea, NH_3: ~15 g N/day
H_2O 320 g/day

Figure 4.1 Global view of the body's macronutrient utilisation. Figures are approximate and refer to a 70 kg person. Note that, ultimately, combustion of the dietary macronutrients is complete except for the conversion of protein–nitrogen to urea and ammonia.

Table 4.1 The body's macronutrient stores in relation to daily intake

Macronutrient	Total amount in body (kg)	Energy equivalent (MJ)	Days' supply if the only energy source	Daily intake (g)	Daily intake as % of store
Carbohydrate	0.5	8.5	<1	300	60
Fat	12–18	550	56	100	0.7
Protein	12	200	(20)	100	0.8

These are very much typical, round figures. Days' supply is the length of time this store would last if it were the only fuel for oxidation at an energy expenditure of 10 MJ/day: the figure for protein is given in parentheses since protein does not fulfil the role of energy store in this way.

of the body's organs has its own particular requirements for these macronutrients, and so the flow of individual substrates into and out of storage pools must be regulated in a complex, highly coordinated way. This regulated flow of 'energy substrates', and the way in which it is achieved, is the theme of this chapter.

Macronutrient stores and the daily flow of fuel

The body's macronutrient stores are summarised in Table 4.1. Also summarised are the daily intakes (in very round figures) of the macronutrients, for comparison. It will immediately be obvious that the store of carbohydrate, glycogen, is very limited in relation to the daily turnover. In comparison, most people have vast stores of fat and protein.

The concept of energy balance was introduced in Chapters 1 and 3. Here, the concept of substrate balance is introduced (Figure 4.2). It is less clear-cut than that of energy balance because of potential interconversion of substrates. However, if someone is in a steady state of body weight, then the amount of each macronutrient completely disposed of each day must equal that ingested (on average: there will be fluctuations from day to day).

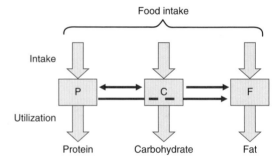

Figure 4.2 Concept of macronutrient balance. As with energy balance, what goes in must come out, with the exception of what is stored. In the case of macronutrients, however, some interconversions are possible. (Reprinted by permission from Macmillan Publishers Ltd: [Nature] Frayn KN. Physiological regulation of macronutrient balance. Int J Obes 1995; 19 (Suppl 5): S4–S10. Permission conveyed through the Copyright Clearance Center, Inc.)

It is useful here to think of the body's 'strategy' in using its fuel stores. The term 'strategy' has to be interpreted carefully. It does not imply that someone is directing substrate flows, rather that these are the patterns that have evolved because they have survival benefits. Some important organs can, under normal circumstances, only use carbohydrate as a fuel source. The brain is the best example. The adult brain requires

Table 4.2 Fat and carbohydrate as fuel stores

	Energy liberated on oxidation (kJ/g)	Water associated (g/g of fuel)	Energy stored (MJ)/kg carried
Carbohydrate	17	3	4.3
Fat	37	0.2	31

Carbohydrate (glycogen) is stored with about three times its own weight of water; fat with only a small amount of adipocyte cytoplasm.

about 100 g glucose per day, close to the amount of glycogen stored in the liver. (As we will see, glycogen stored in skeletal muscles has a local role as a fuel source for the muscles themselves.) Therefore, the glycogen store may be regarded more as a daily buffer than as a long-term fuel reserve. Although there appears to be plenty of protein, there is no specific storage form of protein. All proteins in the body have a defined role: structural, enzymic and so on. Therefore, to use protein as a fuel involves some loss of bodily function. Hence, it is not surprising that protein is relatively well protected and the body's protein is not, in general, used as a fuel for energy beyond an amount equivalent to the daily intake. In contrast, the body's fat stores are there primarily as a source of energy. There is a very clear reason why fat (triacylglycerol, TAG) is the major energy store in mammals. Because TAG molecules are hydrophobic, they coalesce into lipid droplets that are stored, in adipocytes, with only a small amount of cytoplasm. The efficiency of energy storage in terms of kilojoules stored per gram is around eight times that for carbohydrate (Table 4.2). Protein is similar to carbohydrate, although some proteins may be less heavily hydrated. During starvation, the body's strategy is to minimise the use of carbohydrate and protein, and to obtain as much energy as possible from fat stores.

4.2 Regulatory mechanisms

The body needs mechanisms for regulating the flow of individual macronutrients in and out of storage pools. There are various ways in which this regulation is achieved.

It is useful to think of short-term and longer-term mechanisms. Short-term means minutes or hours and covers what might happen in between meals or

during a bout of exercise. Longer term is taken to mean a period of several hours or days.

Short-term regulation of macronutrient flux

In the short term, some regulation is achieved simply by substrate availability affecting rates of reaction by 'mass action' effects. There is an old observation that if an unusual excess of protein is ingested, it will be oxidised over the next 24 h or so. Krebs investigated the means by which this is achieved and concluded that it reflects the kinetic properties of the initial enzymes of amino acid degradation, including the aminotransferases (transaminases), which have a high K_m (typically several mmol/l, but for alanine aminotransferase 34 mmol/l). A high K_m means that the higher the concentration of substrate, the faster will be the reaction. Similarly, the first steps in glucose uptake and metabolism in the liver, transport across the cell membrane by the facilitated transporter GLUT2 and phosphorylation by hexokinase IV (glucokinase), are both characterised by a high K_m and high capacity. Therefore, glucose will be taken up and enter metabolic pathways in the liver according to its extracellular concentration. As glucose is absorbed from the small intestine and reaches the liver via the hepatic portal vein, so it will be taken out of the bloodstream (thus helping to minimise fluctuations in blood glucose concentration). Another example is that of ethanol: the first enzyme in the metabolism of ethanol has a low K_m but high capacity, and ethanol will be oxidised at a constant rate when it is available from the diet.

Beyond that, many pathways are regulated by the effects of pathway products or intermediates on the enzymes of that pathway. Often this is achieved by binding of substrates to enzymes, causing allosteric effects that regulate enzyme activity. One example is that of phosphofructokinase in the pathway of glycolysis. The activity of this enzyme is regulated by a number of compounds related to the pathway, including activation by adenosine monophosphate (AMP) and inhibition by adenosine triphosphate (ATP) and citrate. It is also activated by the compound fructose-2,6-bisphosphate, a by-product of the pathway of glycolysis (note that fructose-1,6-bisphosphate is the product of phosphofructokinase), generated by a separate enzyme apparently purely for regulatory purposes.

Table 4.3 Some response elements in the promoter regions of genes regulating macronutrient metabolism that are affected by dietary macronutrients

Response element	Examples of genes with this element	Notes
Carbohydrate response element	Pyruvate kinase (glycolysis) Pyruvate dehydrogenase E1 subunit Fatty acid synthase	The transcription factor is ChREBP. It is activated by a product of glucose metabolism, possibly xylulose 5-phosphate (pentose phosphate pathway).
Insulin response element	Hexokinase II (+ve) Acetyl-CoA carboxylase (+ve) Glucose-6-phosphatase (−ve) Carnitine palmitoyltransferase (−ve)	May be positive (stimulates transcription) or negative (suppresses transcription)
PPAR-response element	α: Enzymes of peroxisomal fatty acid oxidation in liver β or δ: Enzymes for fatty acid oxidation in muscle γ: Factors leading to adipocyte proliferation	There are three major isoforms of the transcription factor PPAR: α, (β or δ) and γ. The ligand for PPAR is a fatty acid or a lipid derivative, perhaps an eicosanoid
Sterol regulatory element	LDL receptor HMG-CoA reductase (cholesterol synthesis)	The transcription factor is SREBP; it is activated by a low cellular cholesterol concentration

ChREBP, carbohydrate response element binding protein; PPAR, peroxisome proliferator-activated receptor; acetyl-CoA, acetyl-coenzyme A; LDL, low-density lipoprotein; HMG-CoA, 3-hydroxy-3-methylglutaryl-coenzyme A; SREBP, sterol regulatory element binding protein.

These examples help to explain the regulation of pathways within cells. When considering the regulation of macronutrient-derived substrates in the body, one often has to think of effects that involve more than one tissue. For instance, the use of fatty acids as a fuel by skeletal muscle during exercise requires that adipocytes increase the release of fatty acids as muscle uses them. Such inter-tissue coordination is brought about largely through the nervous and hormonal systems. Hormones are released from the endocrine glands in response to a signal, transmitted either through the blood (e.g. an increase in the blood glucose concentration stimulates insulin secretion from the pancreas) or through the nervous system [e.g. release of epinephrine (adrenaline) from the adrenal medulla is brought about by nerve stimulation]. The hormone travels through the circulation to transmit a signal to another tissue, by binding to a specific receptor (a protein), which may be on the cell surface (this is the case for epinephrine, and for peptide hormones such as insulin and glucagon) or within the cell (steroid hormones, thyroid hormones). Binding of hormone to receptor brings about changes in signal transduction pathways, often involving reversible phosphorylation of proteins (see Table 4.3), and ultimately changes in enzyme activity. Short-term changes in enzyme activity are themselves often the result of reversible phosphorylation or

dephosphorylation (e.g. epinephrine stimulates fatty acid release from adipocytes by phosphorylation of the enzyme hormone-sensitive lipase, causing its activity to increase many-fold).

Longer-term regulation of macronutrient flux

In the longer term, regulation is achieved in many cases by alteration of gene expression, usually increased or decreased transcription, but sometimes via alterations in the stability of messenger RNA (mRNA). This would be the case, for instance, if someone switches from a high-fat to a high-carbohydrate diet. Adaptation, through alterations of gene expression, will occur over a period of days. This form of regulation will also operate during a normal day – for instance, the expression of the lipoprotein lipase gene alters during the day in response to fasting overnight and feeding during the day – but usually the acute effects of hormones are more dominant over this period.

Alterations in gene expression can be brought about by both substrates and hormones. This is a field where knowledge has expanded rapidly in recent years. It is now recognised that the genes for many enzymes concerned with energy metabolism have specific promoter sequences that recognise the availability of carbohydrate, fatty acids and related hormones (e.g. insulin-response elements). Some of these response elements are listed in Table 4.3. See also Tables 2.3 to 2.5 in Chapter 2 for more information.

4.3 Hormones that regulate macronutrient metabolism

Pancreatic hormones

The pancreas is mainly an exocrine organ, producing digestive juices that are discharged into the small intestine. Only 1–2% of the volume of the pancreas is occupied by endocrine (hormone-producing) cells, arranged in groups (the islets of Langerhans) surrounded by exocrine tissue. Nevertheless, the products of these endocrine cells are of enormous importance for the regulation of macronutrient metabolism according to nutritional state. Each islet is supplied with blood through a small arterial vessel, and drained by veins that lead to the hepatic portal vein. The islet cells can therefore respond to changing concentrations of substrates in the blood (e.g. blood glucose) and the hormones they release act first on the liver. The liver extracts a large proportion (40–50%) of insulin and glucagon, so other tissues are exposed to lower concentrations.

Insulin

Insulin is produced by the β-cells of the pancreatic islets. The insulin molecule is synthesised as one polypeptide chain, but during processing in the β-cell it is cleaved to produce two peptide chains linked by disulphide bonds. Although the β-cell responds to concentrations of various macronutrients in the blood (Table 4.4), the major factor regulating insulin secretion under most circumstances is the blood glucose concentration. Thus, insulin responds to nutritional state: in the fed state, since most meals contain carbohydrate, insulin secretion is stimulated, and during fasting, when glucose concentrations fall, insulin secretion is low. It is now recognised that insulin secretion after a meal that contains carbohydrate is potentiated by hormones released from the gut called 'incretins'. They are described in more detail below.

Insulin exerts its effects on other tissues by binding to specific receptors in the plasma membrane. These receptors are composed of four protein subunits, two α- and two β-subunits. (The α- and β-subunits are

Table 4.4 Macronutrients in the circulation and their effects on insulin and glucagon secretion

	Insulin	Glucagon	Comments
Glucose	Stimulates	Inhibits	
Amino acids	Stimulates	Stimulates	Some amino acids are more potent than others
Non-esterified fatty acids	Short-term: potentiates glucose stimulation Long-term: inhibits glucose stimulation	No effect	

synthesised initially as one polypeptide chain.) When insulin binds to the cytoplasmic face of the insulin receptor, the intracellular domains become activated and initiate phosphorylation of tyrosine residues, both in themselves and in other proteins. Among these other proteins are a family known as insulin receptor substrate (IRS) proteins, particularly IRS-1 and IRS-2. This initiates a chain of events, which for metabolic signals includes activation of the enzyme phosphatidylinositide-3-kinase. The signal passes via other steps to the enzyme to be regulated. Enzymes are regulated in the short term by insulin, usually by dephosphorylation. Insulin also brings about longer term regulation by alteration of gene transcription. Some of the important effects of insulin on macronutrient metabolism are summarised in Table 4.5.

Overall, the metabolic effects of insulin may be summarised as anabolic. It brings about a net deposition of glycogen in liver and muscle, a net storage of fat in adipose tissue and a net synthesis of protein, especially in skeletal muscle. Note that these effects are brought about at least as much by inhibition of breakdown as by stimulation of synthesis: in the case of muscle protein, this is probably the major mechanism for the anabolic effect of insulin. Patients with untreated type I diabetes mellitus, who lack insulin, display marked wasting, which is reversed when insulin is given.

Glucagon

Glucagon is a single polypeptide chain of 29 amino acids, secreted from the α-cells of the islets. Its main metabolic effects are on the liver: in fact, it is debatable whether glucagon has metabolic effects outside

Table 4.5 Major metabolic effects of insulin

Tissue	Pathway/enzyme	Short or long term?	Key enzyme	Comments
Liver	Stimulation of glycogen synthesis/suppression of glycogen breakdown	Short	Glycogen synthase/glycogen phosphorylase	Regulates glucose storage in liver
	Stimulation of glycolysis/ suppression of gluconeogenesis	Short and long	Short term mainly via fructose 2,6-bisphosphate Long term via altered expression of a number of enzymes	Regulates hepatic glucose output
	Stimulation of *de novo* lipogenesis	Short and long	Acetyl-CoA carboxylase	*De novo* lipogenesis does not (under most circumstances tested) make a major contribution to triacylglycerol synthesis in liver, but this pathway is important for regulation of fatty acid oxidation
	Stimulation of triacylglycerol synthesis	Short and long	Phosphatidic acid phosphohydrolase, diacylglycerol acyltransferase (and others)	
	Stimulation of cholesterol synthesis	Short and long	3-Hydroxy-3-methyl- glutaryl-CoA reductase	
	Suppression of fatty acid oxidation/ketogenesis	Short	Carnitine palmitoyl transferase-1	Via malonyl-CoA (product of acetyl-CoA carboxylase)
Skeletal muscle	Stimulation of glucose uptake	Short	Glucose transporter GLUT4	Regulates glucose uptake by muscle (GLUT4 is translocated to the cell membrane upon stimulation by insulin)
	Stimulation of glycogen synthesis	Short	Glycogen synthase	
	Net protein anabolic effect	Short	Not clear	Insulin may suppress protein breakdown more than stimulation of protein synthesis
Adipose tissue	Stimulation of triacylglycerol removal from plasma	Short and medium	Lipoprotein lipase	'Medium term' is during periods between meals, by increased transcription plus altered intracellular processing
	Stimulation of triacylglycerol synthesis	Short and long	Phosphatidic acid phosphohydrolase, diacylglycerol acyltransferase (and others)	
	Suppression of fat mobilization	Short	Hormone-sensitive lipase	Suppresses release of non-esterified fatty acids

the liver. Its major role is to maintain glucose output during fasting, and its secretion is stimulated when the plasma glucose concentration falls. In many respects hepatic glucose output is regulated by the ratio of insulin to glucagon (insulin/glucagon high, glucose output suppressed; insulin/glucagon low, glucose output increased). Glucagon secretion is also stimulated by amino acids (Table 4.4). It has been suggested that this is important if a meal of pure protein is eaten (as might have been the case after a hunt, for our hunter–gatherer ancestors), as glucagon would then prevent hypoglycaemia caused by amino acids stimulating insulin secretion.

Incretins

Incretin is a term used to describe a peptide hormone released from the gut that potentiates the secretion of insulin after a meal containing carbohydrate. It has long been recognised that if glucose is given by mouth, the insulin response is considerably greater than if the same amount of glucose is given intravenously. That led to the discovery of the incretins. There are two major incretins in humans: glucagon-like peptide-1 (GLP-1) and gastric inhibitory polypeptide (GIP) (also known as glucose-dependent insulinotrophic polypeptide). GLP-1 is a fragment of a larger prohormone, actually proglucagon, the precursor of pancreatic glucagon (see above). Cleavage of proglucagon in the enteroendocrine cells of the intestine gives rise to two active products, known as GLP-1 and GLP-2. (They get their name because they are similar in sequence to glucagon.) The incretin system is of interest because it is the target of novel treatments for type 2 diabetes. GLP-1 itself will improve insulin secretion if given by injection, but its half-life in blood is very short because it is degraded by a specific peptidase. New treatments include analogues of GLP-1 that are resistant to degradation, which have to be injected, and small molecular-weight inhibitors of the peptidase, which prolong the action of the body's own GLP-1 and can be given by mouth.

Catecholamines

The catecholamines that are relevant to macronutrient metabolism are epinephrine (adrenaline) and norepinephrine (noradrenaline). Epinephrine is a hormone released from the central part (medulla) of the adrenal glands, which sit over the kidneys. Its release is initiated by nervous signals that come from the hypothalamus, the integrating centre of the brain. Stimuli for epinephrine release include stress and anxiety, exercise, a fall in the blood glucose concentration and a loss of blood. Epinephrine acts on tissues through adrenergic receptors (sometimes called adrenoceptors) in cell membranes. These receptors are again proteins. The family of adrenergic receptors is summarised in Table 4.6. They are linked with

Table 4.6 Adrenergic receptors

	Receptor subtype		
	β	α_1	α_2
Second messenger system	Adenylate cyclase/cAMP	Phospholipase C/ intracellular [Ca^{2+}]	Inhibition of adenylate cyclase
Metabolic effects	Glycogen breakdown Fat mobilisation	Glycogen breakdown	Inhibition of lipolysis

There are at least three subtypes of β-adrenergic receptor, not distinguished here.
Based on Frayn (2010).

metabolic processes through a signal chain. For certain types of adrenergic receptor, the first step is the interaction of the receptor with a trimeric protein that can bind guanosine triphosphate, called a G-protein. There are inhibitory and stimulatory G-proteins, named for their effects on the next step in the sequence, the enzyme adenylate cyclase. Adenylate cyclase produces cyclic 3′,5′-adenosine monophosphate (cAMP), which then acts on the cAMP-dependent protein kinase (protein kinase A) to bring about phosphorylation of key proteins, including glycogen phosphorylase and hormone-sensitive lipase. (In the case of glycogen phosphorylase, there is another step, protein kinase A phosphorylates phosphorylase kinase, which then acts on glycogen phosphorylase.) Therefore, epinephrine acting on β-receptors will cause mobilisation of stored fuels, glycogen and TAG, raising plasma concentrations of glucose and non-esterified fatty acids (NEFA). This was termed by the American physiologist Walter Cannon in 1915 the 'fight or flight' response, implying that epinephrine, released in response to stress or anxiety, produces fuels that may be used to run away or stand up to an aggressor.

The inhibitory effects of epinephrine, mediated by α_2-adrenergic receptors, may be seen as moderating the effects of overstimulation via β-receptors. For instance, adipocytes have both β- and α_2-adrenergic receptors, the latter presumably opposing excessive lipolysis that might be brought about by high concentrations of (nor)epinephrine.

Norepinephrine is not strictly a hormone, at least under normal circumstances. It is a neurotransmitter. It is released at the ends of sympathetic nerves (nerve terminals) in tissues. It acts on adrenergic receptors, which are identical to those acted on by epinephrine and listed in Table 4.6. The stimuli for norepinephrine release are similar to those for epinephrine, and in many cases it is not clear which exerts the more important effect. Most of the norepinephrine released from sympathetic nerve terminals is taken up again by the nerve ending for degradation or resecretion, but some always escapes or spills over, and may reach the plasma. Plasma concentrations of norepinephrine are usually higher than those of epinephrine, and when norepinephrine is present at elevated concentrations (e.g. during strenuous exercise) it is believed to act as a hormone as well.

Cortisol

Cortisol is a steroid hormone, released from the outer layer (cortex) of the adrenal glands. It responds to stress in a similar way to epinephrine. Its secretion is stimulated by another hormone, adrenocorticotrophic hormone (ACTH), which in turn is released from the pituitary gland at the base of the brain. About 95% of circulating cortisol is bound to plasma proteins, especially cortisol binding globulin (CBG or transcortin). Thus, only a relatively small fraction (~5%) circulates free; however, it is this free fraction that is the physiologically active form. As will be discussed in further detail later, in relation to thyroid hormones, the highly significant protein binding of cortisol has important implications.

Cortisol acts on receptors, but these are not in the cell membrane: they are within the cell, and once cortisol is bound, they migrate and bind to the chromosomes where they regulate gene transcription. Therefore, the metabolic effects of cortisol are all long term, mediated by increased gene expression. Its metabolic effects are generally catabolic, including increased fat mobilisation, stimulation of gluconeogenesis and increased breakdown of muscle protein.

Growth hormone and insulin-like growth factors

Growth hormone is a peptide hormone released from the pituitary gland, and has some direct metabolic effects on tissues. These include increased fat mobilisation and stimulation of hepatic glucose output. Its secretion is stimulated by stress, including a fall in the plasma glucose concentration. However, the main effect of growth hormone, as its name suggests, is an anabolic one, promoting growth, especially through increased cartilage synthesis, an important aspect of longitudinal growth (lengthening of bones). It was shown in the 1960s that this is not a direct effect; rather growth hormone acts on the liver to stimulate production of further peptide hormones, the insulin-like growth factors (IGF-1 and IGF-2) that directly mediate these effects. IGF-1 and -2 have structural similarities to insulin, as their name suggests, and they act via similar (but specific) receptors. However, it has been proposed that when insulin is present at abnormally high concentrations, it can bind to and activate IGF receptors, and vice versa.

Thyroid hormones

The thyroid hormones, thyroxine (also known as T_4 since it contains four atoms of iodine per molecule) and triiodothyronine (T_3), are produced by the thyroid gland in the neck, responding in turn to the peptide hormone thyroid-stimulating hormone (TSH) released from the pituitary. Most (about 80%) of the circulating T_3 concentration is derived from deiodination of T_4 in peripheral tissues, especially the liver and the kidney. T_3 is a significantly more potent thyroid hormone than T_4; many would indeed consider T_4 as only a prohormone for T_3. Deiodination may also produce another thyroid hormone, called reverse triiodothyronine (rT_3); this hormone is essentially metabolically inactive. Its levels increase particularly during stressful situations, for example major surgery, starvation and severe sepsis. Increased production of rT_3 in these situations may be considered part of the adaptive energy-conserving response to stress.

More than 99% of the circulating thyroid hormones, T_3 and T_4, is bound to plasma proteins, especially thyroxine binding globulin (TBG), thyroxine binding prealbumin (TBPA) and albumin. Only a tiny fraction (<1%) circulates free; however, it is this free fraction, designated as free T_4 or free T_3 that is the physiologically active form that promotes thyroid hormone activity at the peripheral tissues. The highly significant protein binding of the thyroid hormones (as with cortisol) has two important implications: (1) variations in plasma protein concentrations will affect the plasma levels of these hormones, for example the hypoproteinaemia of severe protein malnutrition is associated with low total thyroid hormone levels, but free hormones are retained at normal levels by the action of pituitary TSH, and (2) certain important drugs such as salicylates and phenytoin can displace thyroid hormones from binding sites on plasma proteins; this may also reduce the total but not free hormone levels.

The action of free thyroid hormones on other tissues is mediated via nuclear receptors, as described for cortisol, and therefore again thyroid hormones have long-term rather than short-term effects. Their effects are again mainly catabolic, and include net breakdown of muscle protein. However, their most important metabolic effect is stimulation of energy expenditure. People with elevated thyroid hormone concentrations have elevated metabolic rate and may become thin, whereas people deficient in thyroid hormone concentrations have a low metabolic rate and easily gain weight. It should be added here that alterations in thyroid function are not considered to be responsible for the vast majority of cases of human obesity, and treatment with thyroid hormones is not useful in weight reduction (unless there is a deficiency) as the system is highly regulated and administration of thyroid hormones simply leads the thyroid gland to produce less.

The metabolic explanation for the increased energy expenditure brought about by thyroid hormones is not entirely clear, but is usually considered to represent some effect on the efficiency of coupling respiration with ATP synthesis in mitochondria.

Leptin and other peptides secreted by adipose tissue

The peptide hormone leptin was only discovered at the end of 1994, although its existence had been postulated much earlier. It is produced almost exclusively by adipocytes in white adipose tissue. Traces are produced in other tissues, including placenta and stomach, but their function is not clear and they do not appear to contribute significantly to plasma concentrations. It is secreted in amounts that correspond to the degree of fat storage in the adipocyte: bigger fat cells secrete more leptin. It acts on receptors that are present in a number of tissues, although probably the most important are in the brain, particularly the hypothalamus. A short isoform of the leptin receptor is expressed in the choroid plexus, the region that governs the blood–brain barrier and is believed to transport leptin into the brain.

In the brain, leptin signals a decrease in appetite and, in small animals, an increase in energy expenditure. The latter does not seem to be true in humans. This constitutes an important system for regulation of energy stores. When fat stores are low, leptin levels are low and this alters signals in the hypothalamus with the net result of an increase in appetite. When fat stores are high, leptin levels are increased and the hypothalamic signals tend to lead to a net reduction in food intake. The system is summarised in Figure 4.3.

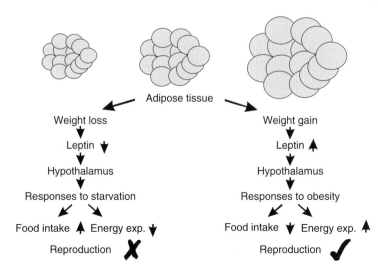

Figure 4.3 Leptin system and energy balance. Well-filled adipocytes secrete leptin, which signals to the hypothalamus to decrease food intake and increase energy expenditure (the latter only in rodents, not humans). They also signal to the reproductive system that energy reserves are sufficient. (Reprinted by permission from Macmillan Publishers Ltd: [Nature] Friedman JM. The alphabet of Weight Control, 1997; 385: 119–120.)

The power of this system is seen when it is disturbed. It was discovered through genetic work on the *ob/ob* mouse, a mutant mouse with spontaneous high food intake, low energy expenditure and massive obesity that leads to diabetes. This mouse is homozygous for a mutation in the *ob* gene, now known to code for the protein leptin. Treatment of *ob/ob* mice with synthetic leptin leads to a reduction in body weight through decreased food intake and increased energy expenditure. The *db/db* (diabetic) mouse is another mutant with identical phenotype: it has a mutation in the leptin receptor and cannot be treated with synthetic leptin. A small number of people have been found with mutations in either the leptin gene or the leptin receptor. They all display massive obesity, associated with an intense drive to eat. Some people with mutations in the leptin gene have now been treated with synthetic leptin and have shown reductions in weight for the first time in their lives. However, the vast majority of obese humans have a normal leptin gene and leptin secretion that appears to be operating normally, in that they have high levels of leptin in the blood. It has been postulated that these people suffer from 'leptin resistance', implying that there is some problem with access of leptin to the brain or with its function within the brain. In one sense this must be true, but a precise molecular explanation has not yet been found. It seems that in humans, low or absent leptin levels are a potent stimulus for appetite, whereas high levels have less effect: the system operates to protect against starvation rather than against over-consumption.

The leptin system also has an important role in reproduction. The *ob/ob* mouse is sterile, and people with mutations in leptin or its receptor have delayed sexual maturity. Leptin seems to be a signal from adipose tissue to the reproductive organs, relaying that there are sufficient energy reserves to begin the energy-demanding processes of reproduction and nurturing children (Figure 4.3). Leptin also affects the immune system. Leptin-deficient humans treated with leptin have shown improvements in reproductive and immune function.

It is now recognised that adipose tissue secretes a number of peptides other than leptin. These are known as 'adipokines'. Some are secreted by the adipocytes themselves, some by other cells in the tissue, for instance macrophages. Adiponectin is a protein secreted from adipocytes, which appears to confer protection against insulin resistance and cardiovascular disease. It is unusual in that, as adipocytes grow larger, they secrete less adiponectin. Therefore, in general, plasma adiponectin concentrations are higher in lean than in overweight people. Other adipokines have been suggested to be associated with, and perhaps causes of, insulin resistance and metabolic disturbances associated with adipose tissue accumulation. These include resistin, retinol binding protein 4 and some inflammation-related cytokines such as tumour necrosis factor-alpha (TNF-α) and interleukin-6.

4.4 Macronutrient metabolism in the major organs and tissues

As mentioned in the introduction, different tissues have their own characteristic requirements, or preferences, for metabolic fuels, and their demand for fuel may vary from time to time. Some of the major consumers of metabolic energy will be discussed in this section. Many of these tissues or organs also play roles in energy metabolism other than simply consuming fuel. Often they need energy derived from oxidative metabolism to support these activities.

Brain

The brain is a large organ (1.5 kg in an adult) and has a high requirement for oxidative metabolism to support its continuous electrical activity. This is usually met almost entirely by glucose. Fatty acids cannot cross the blood–brain barrier in significant amounts for use as an energy substrate, although the brain also has a large need for fatty acids for structural purposes, especially during development. Brain glucose consumption has been estimated by drawing blood from the carotid artery (supplying the brain) and the jugular vein (draining the brain). It is around 100–120 g/day. In the overnight fasted state the liver produces about 2 mg glucose/kg body weight per minute which, for a 70 kg person, is equivalent to about 200 g/24 h. Thus, the brain would consume about half of the liver's glucose output after an overnight fast.

The brain can use other water-soluble fuels, notably the ketone bodies, 3-hydroxybutyrate and acetoacetate. When their concentration rises during starvation, they displace glucose as a fuel and can sustain about two-thirds of the brain's oxidative fuel requirement during prolonged starvation.

Within the hypothalamus, the blood–brain barrier operates differently, and signals from blood may enter and play regulatory roles. For instance, although insulin does not regulate brain glucose utilisation to any significant extent, there are insulin receptors in the hypothalamus which regulate appetite and energy metabolism. There are also sites where fatty acids are oxidised, again leading to regulation of energy metabolism in the whole-body.

Liver

The adult human liver weighs about 1.5 kg and is a highly active organ in the regulation of carbohydrate, fat and amino acid metabolism. To support its metabolic activities, it has a large requirement for oxidative fuel metabolism (its oxygen consumption is about 20% of the whole body's at rest, the largest of any single organ or tissue, excluding skeletal muscle during exercise). The fuels used by the liver are amino acids, fatty acids and glucose, usually in that order of importance.

However, the liver's importance in energy metabolism is more as a regulatory organ, controlling the uptake and release of compounds to maintain homeostasis. The best example is that of blood glucose. When the glucose concentration in the blood is high, the liver takes up glucose and phosphorylates it to glucose-6-phosphate. The fate of that glucose-6-phosphate is determined by hormones, particularly the balance of insulin and glucagon, which stimulate glycogen synthesis and degradation, respectively. When the glucose concentration is low, the liver will release glucose, formed from glycogen breakdown and from gluconeogenesis. The liver is the major organ releasing glucose into the blood, although the kidney plays an increasing role during starvation. Thus, the liver plays a major role in keeping blood glucose concentrations relatively constant throughout the day. Major control points for glucose metabolism in the liver are illustrated in Figure 4.4.

The liver is a major site for fatty acid oxidation. It derives fatty acids from plasma NEFA (released from adipose tissue) and from the uptake of lipoprotein particles that carry TAG and cholesteryl esters. Fatty

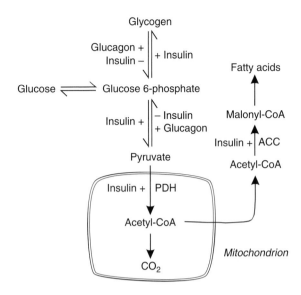

Figure 4.4 Regulation of glucose metabolism by the liver. When blood glucose concentrations are elevated, the liver extracts glucose from the circulation and phosphorylates it to glucose-6-phosphate. The metabolic fate of glucose-6-phosphate is determined by the balance of insulin and glucagon. Conversely, when blood glucose levels fall, the liver releases glucose from stored glycogen or from gluconeogenesis. PDH, pyruvate dehydrogenase; ACC, acetyl-coenzyme A carboxylase.

acid oxidation leads directly to production of acetyl-coenzyme A (acetyl-CoA), but in the liver this may be converted to ketone bodies, 3-hydroxybutyrate and acetoacetate. The liver is the only organ producing ketone bodies, which, as mentioned above, are an important fuel for the brain during starvation. The alternative fate for fatty acids in the liver is esterification, especially to form TAG. The balance between fatty acid oxidation and esterification is regulated by the mechanism shown in Figure 4.5. This mechanism, involving malonyl-CoA, is central to the integration of carbohydrate and fat metabolism in liver and skeletal muscle.

The liver is the only site of urea production. Amino acids derived from dietary protein, and from protein breakdown in peripheral tissues, are oxidised and their nitrogen is transferred to the urea cycle. As well as providing a route for disposal of excess amino acids and their nitrogen content, this provides the major source of oxidative fuel for the liver under most circumstances. The rate of amino acid oxidation is largely determined by amino acid availability, as mentioned earlier. See Chapter 5 for more information on amino acid metabolism in the liver.

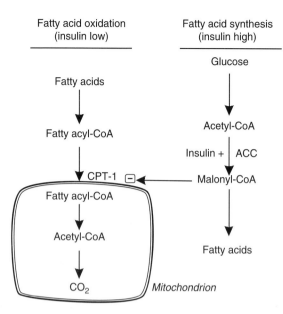

Figure 4.5 Regulation of fatty acid oxidation in liver and other tissues by malonyl-coenzyme A (CoA). Insulin stimulates synthesis of malonyl-CoA (see Figure 5.4) and this inhibits fatty acid entry into the mitochondrion for oxidation. In tissues other than liver (e.g. skeletal muscle) this system operates to regulate fatty acid oxidation, although the later part of the pathway of fatty acid synthesis (beyond malonyl-CoA) is absent. ACC, acetyl-CoA carboxylase; CPT-1, carnitine-palmitoyl transferase-1 (sometimes called carnitine-acyl transferase-1).

Kidneys

Each kidney, weighing about 150 g in an adult, is composed of many cell types. However, a broad distinction can be made between the outer layer, or cortex, and the inner part, or medulla. Most of the metabolic activity involved in pumping substances back from the tubules after filtration goes on in the cortex. The cortex, therefore, has a larger requirement for oxidative fuel, and appears able to oxidise most fuels (fatty acids, ketone bodies, glucose). It has a correspondingly high blood flow and oxygen consumption: the oxygen consumption of the two kidneys is about 10% of the whole body's at rest. The major role of the renal cortex in energy metabolism in the body is as a relatively large consumer. The medulla, in contrast, has a rather poor blood supply and an anaerobic pattern of metabolism.

The kidneys also play a specific role in amino acid metabolism. Glutamine is used by the kidney, especially during starvation, and ammonia is liberated during its metabolism and excreted into the renal tubules (see

Chapter 5, Figure 5.10). This can be an important means of reducing an acid load in the circulation which, as shown later, is a potential problem during starvation.

Adipose tissue

There are two types of adipose tissue, white and brown. The metabolic function of brown adipose tissue is to generate heat, largely by oxidation of fatty acids. It is important in small animals, especially the newborn, and in animals that hibernate. Until recently, brown adipose tissue was considered unimportant in adult humans. However, this view has recently been challenged. 'Hot spots' of metabolism in the neck region in some people, visualised using the technique of positron-emission tomography (PET), which detects regions with a high rate of glucose utilisation, have been shown to represent brown fat depots. They become activated especially when the person is exposed to cold. Their significance for energy balance is, however, not yet clear.

This section will concentrate on white adipose tissue, the major site for storage of excess dietary energy in the form of TAG. The amount of TAG stored within each adipocyte is large in comparison to daily turnover, so the half-life for turning over adipocyte TAG stores is around 1 year. This, coupled with the fact that the requirement of white adipose tissue for oxidative fuel consumption is very low, led to the view that white adipose tissue is rather inert metabolically. It has been recognised in recent years, however, that white adipose tissue has a highly active pattern of metabolism. Adipose tissue is the only site of release into the circulation of NEFA, a major metabolic fuel for many tissues, and it controls the flow of NEFA on a minute-by-minute basis. To match this, it is also responsible for a large proportion of the uptake of dietary fatty acids via the enzyme lipoprotein lipase (LPL), situated in adipose tissue capillaries, and the pathway of TAG synthesis within adipocytes. All this is achieved with a very small consumption of fuel, which in white adipose tissue appears to be mainly glucose. Regulation of the major pathways of fat mobilisation and storage is shown in Figure 4.6.

Skeletal muscle

Skeletal muscle constitutes typically 40% of body weight. Resting muscle has a rather low blood flow and metabolic activity, but because of its bulk it makes a significant contribution to whole-body

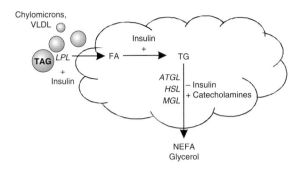

Figure 4.6 Regulation of the major pathways of fat mobilisation and storage in white adipose tissue. + denotes stimulation. Of the three enzymes that sequentially bring about complete hydrolysis of stored TAG, HSL is subject to short-term regulation as shown. The activity of ATGL is also regulated, although mechanisms are not yet clear. Insulin and catecholamines also affect the phosphorylation of proteins, including perilipin, that coat the lipid droplet in the cell, and this may regulate the access of the lipases. ATGL, adipose triglyceride lipase; FA, fatty acids; HSL, hormone-sensitive lipase; LPL, lipoprotein lipase; MGL, monoacylglycerol lipase; NEFA, non-esterified fatty acids; TAG, triacylglycerol; VLDL, very low-density lipoprotein particles.

Table 4.7 Metabolic characteristics of different muscle fibre types

	Type I Red	Type IIa White	Type IIb White
Other names	Slow-twitch oxidative (SO)	Fast-twitch oxidative/ glycolytic (FOG)	Fast-twitch glycolytic (FG)
Speed of contraction	Slow	Fast	Fast
Myoglobin content	High	Low	Low
Capillary density	High	Low	Low
Mitochondrial (oxidative) enzyme activity	High	Low	Low
Triacylglycerol content	High	Low	Low
Myofibrillar ATPase activity	Low	High	High
Glycogenolytic enzyme activity	Low	High	High

fluxes of the macronutrients. During exercise, however, the metabolic activity of skeletal muscle can increase 1000-fold, and it may dominate the body's metabolic activities.

Skeletal muscle is composed of fibres, or multinucleate cells. There are different types of fibre, adapted for either short-duration, rapid contractions, using fuels present within the fibre, or slower, rhythmic contractions that can be continued for long periods, largely using fuels and oxygen supplied from the blood. The differences between these fibre types are summarised in Table 4.7.

The oxidative fuels used by skeletal muscle are mainly fatty acids and glucose. Amino acid oxidation typically accounts for around 15% of muscle fuel oxidation, similar to the whole body, and this figure does not increase appreciably with exercise. Skeletal muscle plays important roles in whole-body macronutrient metabolism, both as a consumer (glucose, fatty acids, amino acids) and as a supplier (lactate, particular amino acids, especially glutamine and alanine).

The main factors regulating muscle fuel utilisation are nutritional state (feeding and fasting) and exercise. In the fed state, insulin stimulates glucose uptake and utilisation, by recruitment of the insulin-regulated glucose transporter GLUT4 to the cell membrane and by activation of glycolysis and glycogen synthesis.

When fatty acids are available at high concentrations (e.g. during fasting, when insulin concentrations will also be low), they will be used as the preferred fuel. The reciprocal utilisation of glucose and fatty acids by muscle is therefore determined partly by extracellular factors (substrate availability, insulin), but also by mechanisms within the cell. Oxidation of fatty acids, when available, will suppress glucose oxidation, but a high rate of glucose utilisation (and high insulin) will suppress fatty acid oxidation via the malonyl-CoA/ CPT-1 system, which operates in both muscle and liver (see the section on the liver, above).

The store of glycogen in muscle is large, typically 300–500 g in the whole body, compared with 100 g or so in the liver. However, because muscle lacks the enzyme glucose-6-phosphatase, this cannot be delivered as glucose into the blood. It cannot therefore be used as a fuel by the brain, except by conversion to lactate and export to the liver, where lactate can be converted to glucose. It seems to be present primarily as a fuel for local utilisation, especially in fast-twitch (type II) fibres.

There are different patterns of macronutrient utilisation in skeletal muscle during brief, intense exercise (anaerobic exercise, involving mainly type II fibres) and during sustained exercise (aerobic exercise, involving mainly type I fibres). In either case the primary requirement of metabolism is to generate ATP, which fuels the sliding of myosin along actin filaments, which underlies muscle contraction.

Aerobic metabolism (e.g. oxidation of glucose or fatty acids) is efficient: about 30 ATP molecules are produced per molecule of glucose completely oxidised. In contrast, anaerobic metabolism is inefficient (3 molecules of ATP per molecule of glucose from glycogen). One might imagine that skeletal muscle would only use the former, but aerobic metabolism requires the diffusion of substrates and oxygen from the blood into the muscle fibres, and the diffusion of carbon dioxide back to the blood. The rates of these diffusion processes are low in comparison with the need to generate ATP during intense exercise. Therefore, during brief, intense (anaerobic) exercise (e.g. weight-lifting, high-jumping, sprinting 100 m), ATP is generated by anaerobic metabolism of glucose-6-phosphate derived from intracellular glycogen. The stimulus for glycogen breakdown is not initially hormonal (that would also require time for movement through the blood), instead the processes of muscle contraction and glycogen breakdown are coordinated. The mechanism is release of Ca^{2+} from the sarcoplasmic reticulum, which initiates muscle contraction and also activates glycogen breakdown. At the same time, allosteric mechanisms activate glycolysis and the net flux through this pathway may increase 1000-fold within a few seconds.

Despite the rapid utilisation of ATP during intense exercise, the concentration of ATP in muscle only falls slightly. This is because of the existence of a reservoir of energy in the form of creatine phosphate (also called phosphocreatine). There is about four times as much creatine phosphate as ATP in skeletal muscle. As ATP is hydrolysed, so it is re-formed from creatine phosphate (with the formation of creatine). The activity of the enzyme concerned, creatine kinase, is high and it operates close to equilibrium. At rest, creatine phosphate is re-formed from creatine and ATP. Gradual non-enzymic breakdown of creatine forms creatinine, which is excreted in the urine at a remarkably constant rate, proportional to muscle mass.

During sustained exercise, blood-borne fuels and oxygen are used to regenerate ATP through aerobic metabolism. This requires coordinated adjustments in other tissues (e.g. adipose tissue must increase fatty acid release; the heart must deliver more blood) and this is brought about by the hormonal and nervous systems. Fatty acids predominate as the oxidative fuel in low- or moderate-intensity sustained exercise, but carbohydrate is the predominant fuel for high-inten-

sity exercise (e.g. elite long-distance running). Although most of the fuel is blood-borne, still the intramuscular glycogen store seems essential for maximal energy output, and when this is depleted the athlete feels a sensation of sudden intense fatigue or 'hitting the wall'. Dietary preparation to maximise muscle glycogen stores before an event is now common practice.

Gut

The primary role of the intestinal tract in macronutrient metabolism is to ensure the uptake of dietary nutrients into the body. However, the intestinal tract has its own requirements for energy. There is a high rate of cell turnover, especially in the small intestine, and this requires a supply of amino acids to act as substrates for protein synthesis and for purine and pyrimidine synthesis (to make DNA and RNA). In addition, there are active transport mechanisms (e.g. for glucose absorption) that require energy. A major metabolic fuel for the small intestine appears to be the amino acid glutamine. This can be partially oxidised to produce ATP, and at the same time acts as a precursor for purine and pyrimidine synthesis. In fact, glutamine appears to be a major fuel for most tissues that have the capacity for rapid rates of cell division (e.g. lymphocytes and other cells of the immune system).

In the colon the situation is somewhat different. Bacterial fermentation of non-starch polysaccharides and resistant starch in the colon produces the short-chain fatty acids, acetic, propionic and butyric acids. Acetic and propionic acids are absorbed and used by tissues in the body (propionic mainly in the liver), but a large proportion of the butyric acid is used as an oxidative fuel by the colonocytes. The supply of butyric acid to the colonocytes appears to protect them against neoplastic change.

4.5 Substrate fluxes in the overnight fasting state

The nutritional state of the human body typically cycles through feeding and fasting over each 24 h period. The macronutrients of the three or more meals eaten during the day enter the system over a period of several hours, and are either oxidised or sent into stores. By about 8 h after a meal (variable, depending on the size and the nature of the meal) the macronutrients have been fully absorbed from the

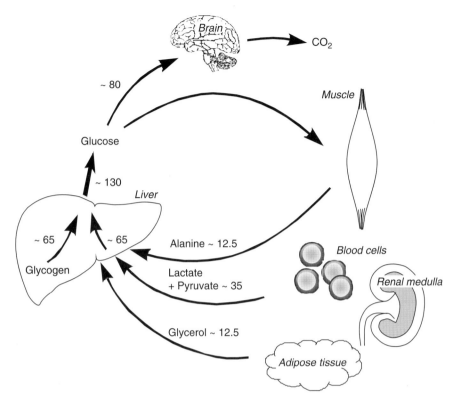

Figure 4.7 Glucose metabolism after an overnight fast. Numbers are approximate values in milligrams per minute for a typical person. From Frayn (2010).

gastrointestinal tract and the body enters the postabsorptive state. This lasts until a further meal is eaten or, if no further food is forthcoming, the body gradually enters a state of early starvation. Many studies of nutritional physiology are conducted after an overnight fast (typically around 10 h after last eating), when there is a relatively steady metabolic state.

The regulation of macronutrient flux through the circulation during these different periods of the 24-h cycle is brought about by a number of mechanisms, as outlined in Section 4.2. After an overnight fast, the concentration of insulin will be relatively low, and the glucagon/insulin ratio reaching the liver will be high.

Carbohydrate metabolism after an overnight fast

After an overnight fast, no new dietary glucose is entering the circulation, and yet the glucose in the blood is turning over at a rate of about 2 mg/min per kilogram of body weight (equivalent to around 200 g/24 h, see Section 4.4). The concentration will be

steady at about 5 mmol/l. New glucose is coming almost entirely from the liver, partly from glycogen breakdown (stimulated by the high glucagon/insulin ratio reaching the liver) and partly from gluconeogenesis. Substrates for the latter will include lactate and pyruvate coming from blood cells and from peripheral tissues (muscle, adipose tissue), the amino acid alanine released from muscle and adipose tissue, and glycerol, released from adipose tissue as a product of lipolysis. A major consumer of glucose at this time will be the brain, with skeletal muscle, renal medulla and blood cells also using significant amounts. (Skeletal muscle glucose utilisation after an overnight fast, at rest, is low per gram of muscle, but because of its large mass this becomes significant.) The pattern of glucose metabolism is illustrated in Figure 4.7.

Note that, of the tissues using glucose, only those carrying out complete oxidation lead to irreversible loss of glucose from the body. In other tissues a proportion (muscle, kidney) or all (red blood cells) of

Figure 4.8 Summary of regulation of pyruvate dehydrogenase (PDH). PDH is a multienzyme complex associated with the inner mitochondrial membrane. The dehydrogenase subunit is subject to both allosteric and covalent regulation in accordance with nutritional state. Covalent modification is brought about by reversible phosphorylation, catalysed by the enzyme PDH kinase. PDH is inactivated by phosphorylation by PDH kinase, which occurs when cellular energy status is high (e.g. during rapid oxidation of fatty acids). PDH is activated by dephosphorylation, brought about by a specific PDH phosphatase, stimulated by insulin.

the glucose is released again as three-carbon compounds (mainly lactate) and can be taken up by the liver for gluconeogenesis. This gives the enzyme pyruvate dehydrogenase (PDH) a key role in regulating loss of glucose from the body. Not surprisingly perhaps, PDH is controlled by many factors reflecting the nutritional state of the body, including insulin, which activates it (Figure 4.8).

There is a potential metabolic cycle between peripheral tissues and the liver: muscle, for instance, releases lactate, the liver converts it to glucose, muscle can take this up and produce lactate. This is known as the Cori cycle, after its discoverer. It will be discussed again and illustrated below.

Fat metabolism after an overnight fast

Fatty acids in the circulation are present in a number of forms: NEFA, TAG, phospholipids and cholesteryl esters. In all cases these molecules are hydrophobic or at most somewhat amphipathic (having both hydrophobic and hydrophilic qualities), therefore they cannot circulate in solution in the blood plasma.

NEFAs are carried bound to albumin. Each molecule of albumin has around three high-affinity binding sites for fatty acids. Albumin, in a partially delipidated state, arrives in the capillaries of adipose tissue, and picks up NEFA released from adipocytes. It arrives in

the capillaries of another tissue (e.g. skeletal muscle or liver) and, because of a concentration gradient between plasma and tissue, fatty acids tend to leave it and diffuse into the tissue. A typical plasma albumin concentration is 40 g/l; with a relative molecular mass of 66 kDa, that is about 0.6 mmol/l. There is therefore an upper limit under many physiological conditions of about 2 mmol/l for NEFA. After an overnight fast their concentration is typically 0.5–1.0 mmol/l. They enter the circulation only from adipose tissue, where fat mobilisation is stimulated after overnight fast mainly, it seems, by the fall in insulin concentration compared with the fed state. Catecholamines and other hormones, such as growth hormone and cortisol, may exert short- or longer term stimulatory effects.

NEFA are removed from the circulation by tissues that can use them as an energy source, such as liver and skeletal muscle. Fatty acid utilisation in these tissues is stimulated after an overnight fast (compared with the fed state) by the increased NEFA concentration in plasma. Within the tissues, fatty acid oxidation is stimulated by the low insulin concentration and low glucose utilisation, leading to a low intracellular malonyl-CoA concentration, so that fatty acids enter mitochondria for oxidation (see Figure 4.5).

The other forms of fatty acids in the circulation, TAG, phospholipids and cholesteryl esters, are transported in specialised macromolecular aggregates, known as 'lipoprotein particles'. Phospholipids are also carried as components of blood cell membranes. The lipoprotein particles are like droplets in an emulsion. They consist of a core of hydrophobic lipid (TAG and cholesteryl esters) stabilised by an outer shell, which is a monolayer of phospholipid molecules with their polar head groups facing outwards into the aqueous plasma and their tails pointing into the hydrophobic core. There are various classes of lipoprotein particle. A detailed description is outside the scope of this chapter but important characteristics are given in Table 4.8. Phospholipids and cholesteryl esters will not be discussed further because they are not directly relevant to macronutrient metabolism, although cholesteryl esters are highly relevant to cardiovascular disease.

In the overnight fasted state most TAG are carried in the very low-density lipoprotein (VLDL) particles secreted from the liver. A typical concentration would be 0.5–1.5 mmol/l in plasma, but this is very variable from person to person. Since each TAG molecule contains three fatty acids, this is potentially a much greater source

Table 4.8 Major lipoprotein fractions in plasma

	Density range (g/ml)	Major lipids	Function, comments
Chylomicrons	<0.950	Dietary TAG	Transport dietary TAG from small intestine to peripheral tissues
Very-low-density lipoproteins (VLDL)	0.950–1.006	Endogenous TAG	Transport hepatic TAG to peripheral tissues
Low-density lipoproteins (LDL)	1.019–1.063	Cholesterol/ cholesteryl esters	Remnants remaining after removal of TAG from VLDL: main carriers of cholesterol in the circulation; elevated levels are a risk factor for atherosclerosis
High-density lipoproteins (HDL)	1.063–1.210	Cholesteryl esters/ phospholipids	Transport of excess cholesterol from peripheral tissues back to liver for excretion (protective against atherosclerosis)

TAG, triacylglycerol.

of energy than the plasma NEFA pool (TAG-fatty acid concentration 1.5–4.5 mmol/l). However, the turnover is slower, and in practice plasma NEFA is the predominant substrate for fatty acid oxidation in tissues.

VLDL-TAG derives within the liver from a number of sources: plasma NEFA taken up by the hepatocytes, plasma cholesteryl esters and TAG taken up by the hepatocytes, and TAG stored within the cells. In the fasting state, plasma NEFA is the major source, although they are processed through a pool of TAG within the hepatocyte.

VLDL particles give up their TAG-fatty acids to tissues through the action of the enzyme LPL. LPL is expressed in many extrahepatic tissues, especially muscle, adipose tissue and mammary gland, where it is increased enormously during lactation. Within these tissues it is bound to the luminal aspect of the capillary endothelium. Here it can interact with the VLDL particles as they pass through the capillaries, hydrolyzing their TAG and releasing fatty acids that diffuse into the tissues down a concentration gradient. This concentration gradient is generated by the binding of fatty acids to intracellular fatty acid binding proteins, and then their subsequent metabolism. After hydrolysis of some of its core TAG, the VLDL particle may recirculate a number of times through capillary beds, losing TAG until it has a core composed almost entirely of cholesteryl esters. Then it is called a low-density lipoprotein (LDL) particle.

The distribution of TAG-fatty acids to tissues is regulated by the tissue-specific regulation of LPL expression in the capillaries. In turn, this is achieved through effects on gene transcription (mRNA abundance) and on intracellular, post-translational processing of the immature enzyme. In adipocytes in particular, a significant proportion of LPL molecules is degraded without reaching the capillary endothelium, and nutritional regulation of adipose tissue LPL expression largely involves switching between these pathways. A summary of tissue-specific regulation of LPL is given in Figure 4.9. It is relatively inactive in adipose tissue after an overnight fast, which makes good sense because in that state adipose tissue is a net exporter of NEFA and has no need to take up additional fatty acids.

Amino acid metabolism after an overnight fast

There is a complex pattern of flow of amino acids into and out of the circulation, covered in detail in Chapter 5. Some general points are relevant here. As shown in Figure 5.9, glutamine and alanine predominate amongst the amino acids released from skeletal muscle after an overnight fast, much more than would be predicted from their abundance in muscle protein. This shows that other amino acids 'donate' their amino groups to form glutamine and alanine, which are exported from the muscle. Similarly, the uptake of amino acids across the abdominal tissues (liver and gut) shows almost the exact counterpart: the greatest removal is of glutamine and alanine. Hence, muscles and probably other tissue, including adipose tissue, are using glutamine and alanine as 'export vehicles' for their amino acid nitrogen, sending it to the liver, where urea can be formed.

The pathway whereby alanine comes to play such a prominent role will be outlined here, since it is

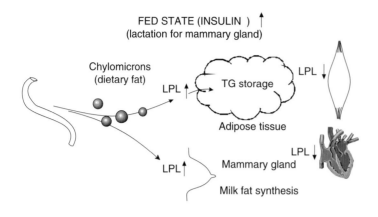

FED STATE (INSULIN) ↑
(lactation for mammary gland)

Chylomicrons
(dietary fat)

LPL ↑

TG storage

LPL ↓

Adipose tissue

LPL ↑

LPL ↓

Mammary gland

Milk fat synthesis

FASTED STATE (INSULIN) ↓
(also physical training for skeletal muscle)

Skeletal
muscle

LPL ↑

CO_2

Adipose tissue

LPL ↓

VLDL
(endogenous fat)

LPL ↑

Myocardium

CO_2

Figure 4.9 Tissue-specific regulation of lipoprotein lipase (LPL) according to the needs of the tissue for fatty acids. LPL, lipoprotein lipase; TAG, triacylglycerol; VLDL, very low-density lipoprotein. (Gurr MI *et al.* Lipid Biochemistry: An Introduction, 5th edn. Copyright © Wiley–Blackwell.)

Figure 4.10 Transamination (aminotransferase) reaction involving pyruvate/alanine and 2-oxoglutarate/glutamate. All amino acids can participate in transamination reactions, which are usually the first step in their degradation.

relatively well understood. Alanine is formed by transamination of pyruvate (Figure 4.10). Hence, other amino acids can donate their amino group to pyruvate, a substantial proportion of which is formed from the pathway of glycolysis. The remaining carbon skeleton can be oxidised in the muscle. The branched-chain amino acids (leucine, isoleucine, valine) play a

predominant role in skeletal muscle amino acid metabolism. Their corresponding carbon skeletons, the branched-chain 2-oxo acids, are oxidised by an enzyme, the branched-chain 2-oxo acid dehydrogenase, which is similar in many ways to PDH (which is also a 2-oxo acid dehydrogenase). Thus, they contribute to oxidative fuel metabolism in muscle.

The production of alanine by transamination of pyruvate gives rise to a metabolic cycle that has been termed the glucose–alanine cycle. It operates in parallel with the Cori cycle, as illustrated in Figure 4.11.

4.6 Postprandial substrate disposal

This section examines how the relatively steady metabolic state after an overnight fast is disturbed when macronutrients are ingested and enter the circulation. This will demonstrate clearly some of the ways in which the metabolism of the different macronutrients is coordinated. It is unusual to eat a meal that

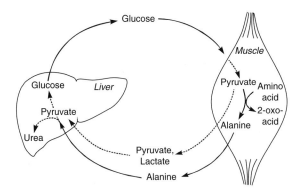

Figure 4.11 The glucose–alanine and Cori cycles operate in parallel. Note that peripheral tissues other than muscle may be involved (e.g. adipose tissue). [Reproduced from Frayn (2010).]

contains only fat, and since both glucose and amino acids will stimulate the secretion of insulin, this is an important signal of the transition from postabsorptive to fed, or postprandial, state.

Impact on endogenous metabolism

Among the most rapid changes detectable in macronutrient metabolism following ingestion of a meal is the suppression of mobilisation of endogenous fuels. The production of glucose by the liver is switched off, as is the release of NEFA from adipose tissue. Therefore, the body preserves its endogenous macronutrient stores, and switches to using incoming macronutrients and storing any excess.

Glucose

Glucose enters the circulation through the hepatic portal vein. Hence, it reaches the liver in high concentrations: concentrations of almost 10 mmol/l have been measured in the portal vein when the systemic concentration is still only 4–5 mmol/l. Glucose will enter hepatocytes and be phosphorylated, as described in Section 4.4. Nevertheless, despite a high capacity of the liver for soaking up glucose, much will still pass though into the systemic circulation, otherwise there would be no rise in glucose concentration and no stimulation of insulin secretion. Within the liver, the rise in insulin/glucagon ratio switches off gluconeogenesis and glycogenolysis, and stimulates glycogen synthesis. Until recently these were considered as 'on-off' switches: either gluconeogenesis or glycolysis operated; glycogen synthesis and glycogen breakdown

operated at different times. Now it is recognised that the system is more fluid; there appears always to be some glycogen synthesis and breakdown, so there is cycling between glycogen and glucose-6-phosphate. The nutritional state determines which pathway predominates. Similarly, it is now recognised that gluconeogenesis must continue in the postprandial period. Studies with isotopic tracers show that a significant proportion of liver glycogen laid down in the period following a meal is not synthesised directly from blood glucose. Instead, the glucose is first converted to three-carbon compounds (lactate, pyruvate, alanine) and then, via pyruvate, converted by the gluconeogenic pathway to glycogen. The latter is known as the indirect pathway for glycogen synthesis and, depending on the experimental design, accounts for around 25–40% of liver glycogen synthesis.

Skeletal muscle will also take up glucose, insulin activating the glucose transporter GLUT4 (recruiting it to the plasma membrane) and, within the cell, insulin stimulating both glycogen synthesis and glucose oxidation. This is aided by the fall in plasma NEFA concentration (see below), so removing competition for oxidative disposal. There is no indirect glycogen synthesis in muscle since the gluconeogenic pathway does not operate. Other insulin-responsive tissues such as adipose tissue also increase their glucose uptake: although this does not make a major contribution to glucose disposal from the plasma, it has important effects within the adipocytes (Section 4.3). The brain, and the red blood cells, continue to use glucose at the same rate as before, since their glucose uptake is not regulated by insulin.

Lipids

NEFA release from adipose tissue is suppressed very effectively by insulin. Thus, the body's fat stores are 'spared' at a time when there are plenty of dietary nutrients available. This suppression is brought about by the mechanisms shown in Figure 4.6. Because the flux of NEFA to muscle is reduced, competition for glucose uptake is removed. The reduced delivery of NEFA to the liver will tend to suppress the secretion of VLDL-TAG. In addition, insulin seems to suppress this directly. However, the short-term regulation of VLDL-TAG secretion is not clearly understood *in vivo*; it has been studied mainly in isolated hepatocytes.

Dietary TAG is absorbed into the enterocytes, and packaged into large, TAG-rich lipoprotein particles,

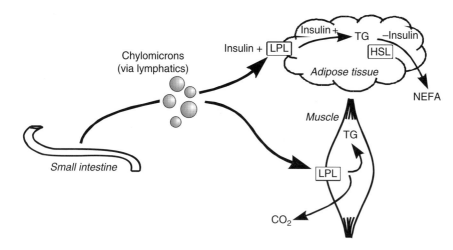

Figure 4.12 Most direct pathway for storage of dietary fat as adipose tissue triacylglycerol (TAG). Skeletal muscle is also shown as this will be the destination of some of the dietary fat. HSL, hormone-sensitive lipase; LPL, lipoprotein lipase; NEFA, non-esterified fatty acids.

the chylomicrons. These enter the circulation relatively slowly (peak concentrations after a meal are typically reached at 3–4 h) and give the plasma a turbid appearance (postprandial lipaemia). It seems beneficial for the body to be able to remove chylomicron-TAG from the circulation quickly; there is considerable evidence that delayed removal of chylomicrons is associated with an increased risk of developing coronary heart disease. Rapid removal is achieved by insulin activation of adipose tissue LPL. Chylomicrons and VLDL compete for clearance by LPL, but chylomicrons are the preferred substrate, perhaps because their larger size enables them to interact with a larger number of LPL molecules at once. Nevertheless, it would make good physiological sense if VLDL-TAG secretion were suppressed after a meal, as discussed above, to minimise competition and allow rapid clearance of chylomicron-TAG. Because of the tissue-specific activation of LPL by insulin (Figure 4.9), adipose tissue plays an important role in clearance of chylomicron-TAG, although muscle, because of its sheer mass, is also important; and in a physically trained person, muscle LPL will itself be up-regulated (compared with a sedentary person), so making a greater contribution to minimising postprandial lipaemia.

Within adipose tissue, the fatty acids released from chylomicron-TAG by LPL in the capillaries diffuse into the adipocytes: this is aided by the suppression of intracellular lipolysis, reducing intracellular NEFA concentrations. Insulin also acts to stimulate the pathway of TAG synthesis from fatty acids and glycerol phosphate. The precise steps at

which insulin acts are not entirely clear, but it may be that a number of enzymes of fatty acid esterification are activated. In addition, increased glucose uptake will produce more glycerol-3-phosphate (from dihydroxyacetone phosphate, an intermediate in glycolysis), and this itself will stimulate TAG synthesis. Thus, dietary fatty acids can be stored as adipose tissue TAG by a short and energy-efficient pathway (Figure 4.12).

Amino acids

Again, the pattern of amino acid metabolism is complex (with 20 different amino acids, each having its own pathways), but some generalisations can be drawn. Further detail is given in Chapter 5. The small intestine itself may remove some amino acids such as glutamine for use as a metabolic fuel. A further selection of amino acids is removed by the liver, and the mixture of amino acids entering the systemic circulation is depleted of glutamine and enriched in the branched-chain amino acids. These will be taken up largely by muscle, where they play a special role in oxidative metabolism. Amino acids are secretagogues for (i.e. they stimulate secretion of) both insulin and glucagon (Table 4.4).

The rate of protein synthesis in muscle, the largest single reservoir of protein in the body, is regulated by many factors, including anabolic hormones (androgens, growth hormone), physical activity of the muscle and catabolic hormones (e.g. thyroid hormones, cortisol). In the short term, insulin also has a net anabolic effect. Measurements made using isotopic tracers suggest that this reflects not so much a stimulation of muscle protein synthesis as an inhibition of muscle protein breakdown. Nevertheless, the net effect is an increased sequestration of amino acids in muscle in the fed state.

Cardiovascular changes

The regulation of the metabolic disposal of the macronutrients in the period following a meal was discussed above. It is important to realise that eating a meal leads to a series of coordinated changes. As well as the purely metabolic responses, there are changes in the cardiovascular system. Cardiac output will rise (slightly, this a relatively small effect compared with physical exercise) and the distribution of blood flow to different tissues will change. There is an increase in blood flow to the abdominal viscera to help in the process of absorption and transport of nutrients into the circulation. The blood flow through certain tissues also increases: skeletal muscle blood flow is stimulated by insulin (there is some debate about the physiological relevance of this, although it is certainly seen when insulin is infused at high concentrations) and adipose tissue blood flow rises after a meal. These changes may help to deliver substrates to the tissues where they will be used.

4.7 Short-term and longer-term starvation

Starvation: general aspects

Earlier, the postabsorptive state was defined as that in which the absorption of nutrients from the gastrointestinal tract is essentially complete and the body is in a relatively stable metabolic state (typically, after an overnight fast in humans). In addition, the events were described that occur when this state is interrupted, as it usually is, by ingestion of a meal. Another possible outcome is that no meal is forthcoming, perhaps because of food shortage or for therapeutic reasons (to achieve rapid weight loss or in preparation for surgery), or perhaps because the individual chooses not to eat, for instance for religious reasons. In that case the body gradually enters a state of early starvation, progressing eventually to a relatively steady metabolic state of complete starvation, which can last for a matter of several weeks. Some initially obese people, starved under close medical supervision and with supplementation with vitamins and minerals, have survived several months of starvation. The ability of the human body to cope with long periods of starvation illustrates perfectly the interaction and coordination of metabolism in different organs and tissues.

Starvation may be total or partial (when energy intake is not sufficient to maintain a steady body mass). Our understanding of complete starvation largely comes from detailed studies carried out in the 1960s on obese women fasting under medical supervision to lose weight. There is a worry that the responses observed may not be typical because the excess initial fat stores of the subjects may have produced a different set of responses from those of initially slimmer people. There are some observations of normal-weight people starved for various reasons: during periods of famine in Europe in World War II, during periods of famine elsewhere in the world today and people who have chosen to starve themselves, for instance for political reasons. Tragic though these cases are, the observations that have been made help us to understand the adaptations of the body to deprivation and may in the future help those whose access to food, or ability to consume it, is limited. Our understanding of partial starvation was increased enormously by studies carried out in Minnesota, USA, during World War II, by the celebrated nutritionist Ancel Keys (1904–2004). The volunteers were conscientious objectors. They were fed for a period of 24 weeks on about 40% of their estimated energy requirements and they were carefully monitored during this time. Noticeable features of starvation were lethargy and depression. These were rapidly reversed when full feeding was resumed. The data from these studies were published in full and papers are still being written on them today. The responses to partial starvation seem essentially to be similar to those to total starvation, albeit somewhat less marked.

If no carbohydrate is entering the body from the gut, then the body's limited carbohydrate reserves (Table 4.1) become very precious, and much of the metabolic pattern in starvation can be understood in terms of preservation of carbohydrate. Some tissues have a continual need for glucose. If the glucose is oxidised, specifically if its carbon atoms in the form of pyruvic acid go through the PDH reaction, then it is irreversibly lost to the body. Glucose can then be generated *de novo* only from non-carbohydrate precursors: glycerol from lipolysis and the carbon skeletons of some amino acids. While TAG stores may be used without detriment to the organism, all the body's protein, as discussed earlier, has some specific function other than as a fuel for oxidation. As discussed later, the pattern of metabolism adapts to starvation in such a way that protein oxidation is minimised, so far as possible, and as much energy as possible derived from fat.

Short-term starvation

A rapid response to starvation is loss of the liver glycogen store: this is virtually completely depleted within 24 h. At this stage there is still a need for generation of glucose at a high rate for oxidation in the brain. Net protein breakdown may be relatively rapid. This is sometimes called the gluconeogenic phase. Because of the lack of incoming glucose, plasma glucose concentrations will fall slightly, insulin concentrations will fall and glucagon secretion will increase. These changes reduce glucose utilisation by tissues such as skeletal muscle, which can use fatty acids instead, and in particular suppression of PDH activity in tissues that are responsive to insulin will reduce irreversible disposal of glucose. There will be stimulation of lipolysis in adipose tissue, and of hepatic glucose production through gluconeogenesis. At this stage gluconeogenesis is largely proceeding at the expense of muscle protein. This phase may last for 3–4 days.

Longer term starvation

At around 1 week, short-term starvation merges into a period when glucose and insulin concentrations fall further, lipolysis increases still further and a sparing of protein breakdown is observed. This sparing of protein oxidation is reflected in a gradual decrease in the excretion of nitrogen in the urine. It is understandable in terms of the body's need to protect its protein, but the mechanism is not fully clear. Some features of this phase are clear. Increased lipolysis leads to increased delivery of NEFA and glycerol from adipose tissue. Since glycerol is a gluconeogenic precursor, the need for amino acids is reduced. Furthermore, the oxidation of fatty acids within the liver is increased by the high glucagon/insulin ratio, and ketone bodies are produced in high concentrations in the circulation. Although the brain cannot use NEFA, it can use the water-soluble

ketone bodies that are derived from them. In the phase of adapted starvation, say from 2–3 weeks of starvation onwards, ketone bodies reach a relatively steady concentration around 7–9 mmol/l (compared with less than 0.2 mmol/l typically after an overnight fast) and largely replace glucose as the oxidative fuel for the brain: they have been shown to meet about two-thirds of brain oxidative fuel requirements. The need for protein breakdown to feed gluconeogenesis is therefore again reduced. Because of the inactivation of pyruvate dehydrogenase (by the low insulin concentration), much of the glucose that is used by tissues outside the brain is only partially broken down, to pyruvate and lactate, which can then be recycled in the liver through gluconeogenesis. Thus, red blood cells, for instance, which have an obligatory requirement for glucose, are not depleting the body of glucose.

Although this shows how the need for protein oxidation is reduced, the cellular mechanism by which this is achieved also needs to be understood. There are several suggestions. Energy expenditure (metabolic rate) falls during starvation, sparing the body's fuel stores for as long as possible. The main mechanism is a fall in concentration of the active thyroid hormone, T_3 (with increased production of the inactive form, rT_3; see Section 4.3). The reduction in protein breakdown has been suggested simply to reflect this overall slowing of metabolism. Since thyroid hormones have a catabolic effect on muscle protein, the fall in their concentration may in itself spare muscle protein. In addition, it has been suggested that the high concentrations of ketone bodies exert a protein-sparing effect, possibly through suppression of the activity of the branched-chain 2-oxo acid dehydrogenase in skeletal muscle that is responsible for irreversible breakdown of the branched-chain amino acids.

The high concentrations of NEFA and ketone bodies (note that both 3-hydroxybutyric acid and acetoacetic acid are acids) might cause a metabolic acidosis (low blood pH), but this is corrected in part by the mechanism described earlier, whereby glutamine is metabolised in the kidney, releasing ammonia that is excreted along with H^+ ions. Urinary nitrogen excretion is normally largely in the form of urea, but during starvation the relative amount of ammonia increases, as does the contribution of the kidney to gluconeogenesis (the carbon skeleton of glutamine will contribute to this).

Ultimately, the body's fat store limits the length of survival. It appears that once the fat store is essentially depleted, then there is a phase of rapid protein breakdown that leads quickly to death. Thus, fatness is a useful adaptation when food is plentiful, if there are likely to be long periods of famine. In present-day industrialised societies, the latter is not a feature of life, but it may explain why there is such a strong tendency for people to become obese.

4.8 Perspectives on the future

The Human Genome Project has now sequenced the entire human genome. It encodes about 25 000 genes, each of which may lead to several different protein products by differential splicing and post-translational modifications. The function of most of these proteins is unknown. A major challenge for the next few decades will be to bridge the gap between molecular biology and whole-body function. Many new techniques will be required. For instance, proteomics is the determination of the proteins expressed in any one cell or tissue: the proteome is the protein equivalent of the genome. No-one has yet deciphered the proteome of any human cell. Once this has been done, it will be an enormous task to determine how all these proteins interact within one cell to produce the mixture of metabolites that we now call the metabolome. Then we will still need to determine how cells interact within tissues and how tissues and organs interact in the whole body. The science of integrative physiology, well known in the early to middle part of the twentieth century, will have to be resurrected to make this possible.

Nutrition is a prime example of a science in which an integrated approach is necessary. We can study the nutritional needs of a single cell, but most cells require a constant supply of nutrients to keep them alive in cell-culture systems. They will die within a day or two if nutrients are not provided. A human being, in contrast, can survive for perhaps 2 months without food because of the coordination that occurs between different cells. This chapter has described metabolism at the level of the cell, the tissues and organs, and the whole body. It is hoped that this approach will help the reader to see the grander picture of life: there is more to it than molecules!

Further reading

Frayn KN. Physiological regulation of macronutrient balance. Int J Obes 1995; 19 (Suppl 5): S4–S10.

Frayn KN. Metabolic Regulation: A Human Perspective, 3rd edn. Oxford: Wiley–Blackwell, 2010.

Friedman JM. The alphabet of weight control. Nature 1997; 385: 119–120.

Friedman JM, Halaas JL. Leptin and the regulation of body weight in mammals. Nature 1998; 395: 763–770.

Gurr MI, Harwood JL, Frayn KN. Lipid Biochemistry: An Introduction, 5th edn. Oxford: Blackwell Science, 2002.

Murray RK, Granner DK, Rodwell VW. Harper's Illustrated Biochemistry, 27th edn. New York: Lange Medical Books/ McGraw-Hill, 2006.

Salway JG. Metabolism at a Glance, 3rd edn. Oxford: Blackwell Publishing, 2004.

5
Integration of Metabolism 3: Protein and Amino Acids

Margaret E Brosnan, John T Brosnan and Vernon R Young

Key messages

- Protein and amino acid metabolism are large-scale, dynamic and regulated processes that accomplish a variety of physiological functions. Their measurement, in living animals, requires the application of sophisticated methodology involving isotopic tracers. In a healthy adult human, some 300 g of protein are synthesised and degraded each day; some 100 g of amino acids are consumed, as dietary protein, on a typical Western diet.
- Protein synthesis and degradation (or turnover) play a critical role in determining the levels of the many proteins in organisms, for example enzymes, contractile proteins, membrane proteins, plasma proteins, peptide hormones and regulatory proteins. Protein synthesis and turnover are, therefore, of the most fundamental importance.
- The synthesis of different proteins may be regulated both by the expression of individual genes and also by a variety of other regulatory processes, especially at the initiation of messenger RNA translation.
- Protein breakdown is a stochastic process, such that newly synthesised proteins are as likely to be degraded as older proteins. Protein degradation has the additional function of promptly removing damaged or mutant proteins. The rate of protein turnover is heterogeneous, thus different proteins are degraded at varying rates, from a half-life in minutes for ornithine decarboxylase to a half-life of years for mature collagen.

- Muscle, the largest protein mass in the body, plays an important role as a source of amino acids in a number of situations, for example as a source of amino acids for gluconeogenesis during starvation and for the synthesis of defence proteins (acute phase proteins, immunoglobulins) during catabolic illness.
- Amino acids are the most versatile of nutrients. In addition to their primary role as precursors for protein synthesis, they play a variety of other roles such as serving as neurotransmitters (e.g. glutamate and glycine) and precursors for neurotransmitters (e.g. serotonin and dopamine), for signalling molecules (e.g. nitric oxide and epinephrine) and for the synthesis of a variety of small molecules (e.g. creatine and glutathione). Methionine plays a major role in the provision of methyl groups for methylation reactions. The metabolic disposal of dietary amino acids and, in particular, of the nutritionally indispensable (or essential) amino acids, is tightly regulated.
- There is a considerable flux of amino acids between tissues. This interorgan metabolism is facilitated by amino acid transporters and accomplishes a variety of physiological roles such as supplying amino acids to the liver for gluconeogenesis, to the kidney for acid–base balance, and the synthesis of dispensable amino acids. This interorgan amino acid metabolism can vary during development and between species and in different metabolic states.

5.1 Introduction

This chapter is concerned with the integration of amino acid and protein metabolism within the organism. Chapter 4 of the first volume of this series (*Introduction to Human Nutrition*) deals, in large part, with the dietary requirement for protein and amino acids, determination of their requirements, as well as the means of meeting them. The present chapter builds on these themes and examines the functions, mechanisms and regulation of protein and amino acid metabolism that underlie their nutritional requirements. It also attempts to integrate this metabolism so as to provide an understanding of the roles played by different tissues in different circumstances.

Proteins are major functional molecules of cells and it follows that normal body function depends, in

Nutrition and Metabolism, Second Edition, edited by S. A. Lanham-New, I. A. Macdonald and H. M. Roche.   © 2011 The Nutrition Society.

a profound way, on the expression of a myriad of specific proteins. Although current estimates of the human genome suggest a gene complement of about 26 000, it is estimated that we express as many as 100 000 different proteins because of such mechanisms as differentially spliced RNAs. The precise quantity of each protein in a cell depends on its rate of synthesis and degradation. Accordingly, the mechanisms and regulation of protein synthesis and turnover are major topics in this chapter. Furthermore, it is clear that although the outlines of these processes are common from tissue to tissue, their regulation occurs in a tissue-specific and protein-specific manner. Thus, during catabolic illnesses there is a net loss of muscle protein; at the same time, there is an increased hepatic synthesis of a set of defence molecules, known as positive acute-phase proteins. Decreased availability of a specific amino acid will result in a generalised decrease in protein synthesis, although the synthesis of the specific amino acid transporter that imports this amino acid into cells may be enhanced. Indeed, an appreciation of the differences between the metabolism of amino acids and proteins in different tissues is the key to an understanding of the integration of this process within the body. Amino acid metabolism provides one of the best examples of an interorgan process in which events in different tissues combine and collaborate to bring about overall physiological goals. Thus, the concentrations of amino acids circulating in the blood are normally maintained within certain limits, and this ensures a supply of these key substrates for protein synthesis to all tissues and organs. The synthesis of individual amino acids is the responsibility of specific tissues. During starvation, many amino acids released as a result of muscle proteolysis are converted to glucose in the liver and thus provide a key energy fuel to the brain. The earlier view of the role of the intestine in amino acid metabolism has been transformed from an organ that is involved only in digestion and absorption to one that obtains a substantial fraction of its metabolic energy from the catabolism of dietary amino acids and undertakes a significant metabolic processing of absorbed amino acids before their entry into the portal circulation. The liver is the major organ for the catabolism of amino acids and as such it plays a major role in determining dietary amino acid requirements. The fact that the rate of amino acid catabolism is never zero is

one of the principal reasons why adults require a continuous supply of dietary nitrogen and of indispensable (essential) amino acids.

This chapter provides the reader with an understanding of the nature and regulation of protein synthesis and turnover, and an appreciation of how these occur in a tissue-specific manner. It will also discuss the techniques that are available to determine the rates of protein synthesis, protein turnover and amino acid oxidation, both on a whole-body basis and in some individual organs, and give an appreciation of the magnitude of these fluxes. The regulation of amino acid metabolism will be discussed, in particular amino acid catabolism and the many metabolic roles played by amino acids. By the end of this chapter you should have an understanding of how these different processes occur in an organ-specific manner (including amino acid fluxes between organs) and appreciate the integration of amino acid and protein metabolism, both under physiological situations (e.g. fed versus fasted states) and during pathological challenges (e.g. catabolic illnesses and genetic diseases of amino acid transport).

5.2 Protein and amino acid turnover

The proteins of cells and organs and those in the circulation play various roles (Table 5.1); they are the 'workhorses' and serve in such roles as biological catalysts (enzymes), regulators of gene expression and components of molecular structures, such as the cell membrane, endoplasmic reticulum, the contractile apparatus of smooth, striated and cardiac muscle and the multifunctional proteolytic complex (proteasome) that is responsible for a major fraction of cellular protein breakdown. In most cells and tissues, proteins are being continually synthesised and degraded. The overall process of synthesis and degradation, or of anabolism and catabolism, is referred to as protein turnover. Each component of turnover consists of a complex organisation of proteins and other molecules that are subject to regulation. Hence, rates of synthesis and degradation of proteins may vary depending on the intracellular and extracellular environmental conditions. These include the availability and balance of nutrients to which cells are exposed, and the hormones and other peptide factors that bind to receptors on cell surfaces or within the

Table 5.1 Some functions of proteins

Function	Examples
Enzymic catalysis	Branched-chain ketoacid dehydrogenase
Plasma transport	Vitamin B_{12} binding proteins, ceruloplasmin, apolipoproteins, albumin
Membrane transport	Na^+/K^+-ATPase, glucose transporters
Messengers/signals	Insulin, growth hormone
Movement	Kinesin, actin
Structure	Collagens, elastin
Protein folding	Chaperonins
Storage/sequestration	Ferritin (for iron), metallothionein (for zinc)
Immunity	Antibodies, tumour necrosis factor, interleukins
Growth, differentiation, gene expression	Peptide growth factors, transcription factors

cell, causing changes in turnover. This continuous, variable-rate, cycle of protein synthesis and breakdown permits the organism to:

- adjust to changes in the internal environment
- remodel tissues during growth or repair
- remove mutant, damaged and misfolded proteins selectively.

About 30% or more of protein production is faulty and these defective products are removed by the mechanisms described below. Turnover serves a critical role in multiple cell functions, including cell cycle progression, oncogenesis, apoptosis (programmed cell death), regulation of gene expression, inflammation and immune surveillance, and the regulation of metabolic pathways. It is hardly surprising, therefore, that malfunctions in protein turnover are associated with human diseases, including neurodegenerative disorders and cancer. The magnitude of the apoptotic process may be readily appreciated by imagining the outcome if apoptosis were prevented owing to a defect in the turnover of one or more of the many enzyme proteins involved in this process, such as the caspases (a group of cysteine proteases that are one of the main effectors of apoptosis), but mitosis (cell division) proceeded at a normal rate. It has been estimated that an 80-year-old person would have 2 tonnes of bone marrow and lymph nodes and a gut that was about 16 km long!

The amino acids serve as the currency of protein metabolism. In addition to serving as the building blocks for proteins they meet many other functions,

some of which will be considered later in this chapter. However, at this stage it is important to appreciate that there is an intimate relationship between the rates of protein synthesis and breakdown and the status of cellular and organ amino acid metabolism, making it somewhat difficult to separate a discussion of each of these major components of the nitrogen economy of the organism. Nevertheless, the mechanisms of protein synthesis and degradation or breakdown will be considered first. An examination of how these processes are regulated will follow, before turning to the metabolism of amino acids. Subsequently, those factors of nutritional importance that influence the rates of protein synthesis and breakdown, the mechanisms involved, the organs affected and the impact of these factors on and interactions with amino acid metabolism will be considered.

5.3 Protein synthesis

In a healthy adult human, about 300 g of new protein is synthesised per day and, for a maintenance condition, an equivalent amount of protein is degraded to its amino acids. The synthesis of proteins consists of many different patterns and amounts depending on the type of cell and its condition at that time. The production of proteins follows the synthesis of messenger RNA (mRNA) via the process of *transcription* of a gene's nucleotide sequence, which involves several steps. The first are transcription initiation and elongation. These steps are followed by RNA-processing reactions such as capping, splicing and transcription termination. Transcription and its control are discussed in Chapter 2 of this volume.

With the appearance of the mRNA in the cytosol the *translational* phase of protein synthesis takes place, although it should be noted that about 23 proteins are made within the mitochondrion. All mammalian organisms initially construct proteins from a set of 20 amino acids (the only known variants being formyl-methionine in mitochondria and selenocysteine) via the translation of mRNA that codes for a predetermined sequence of amino acids in the polypeptide chain. The major stages of translation are:

(1) initiation
(2) elongation
(3) termination
(4) ribosome recycling.

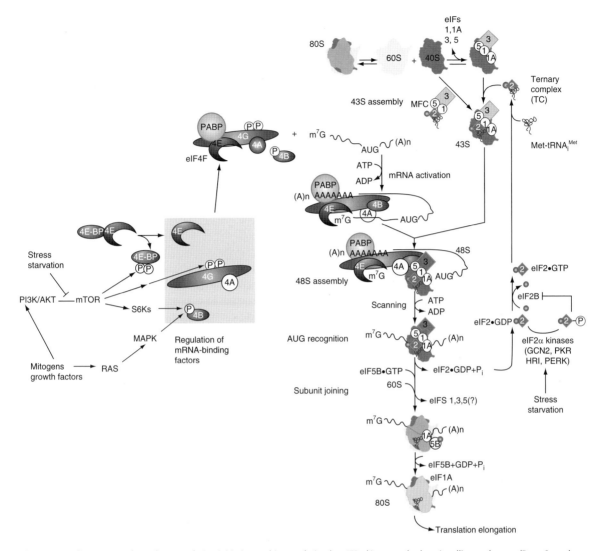

Figure 5.1 Eukaryotic cap-dependent translation initiation and its regulation by eIF2a kinase and other signalling pathways. (From Sonenberg and Hinnebusch, 2009, with permission.)

Initiation

The *initiation* of translation occurs via a complex process in which initiator methionyl transfer RNA (met-tRNAi), 40S and 60S ribosomal subunits are assembled, with the aid of eukaryotic initiation factors (eIFs), into an 80S ribosome at the initiation codon of the mRNA (Figure 5.1). There are several linked stages involved in this process:

(1) selection of met-tRNAi from the pool of tRNAs by eukaryotic initiation factor eIF2 and binding of an eIF2/GTP/Met-tRNAi ternary complex and other eIFs to the 40S ribosomal subunit, with the formation of a 43S preinitiation complex

(2) binding of the 43S complex to mRNA, which has been activated by binding of eIF4F to the m7G cap at the mRNA 5′-terminus and poly A binding protein (PABP) to the poly(A) tail of the mRNA

(3) ATP-dependent scanning of the mRNA-bound ribosomal complex along the 5′-non-translated region (5′NTR) from its initial binding site to the initiation codon (AUG), to form a 48S initiation

complex, where the initiation codon is base-paired to the anticodon of met-tRNAi,

(4) displacement of factors from the 48S complex and the joining of the 60S ribosomal subunit to form an 80S initiation complex, leaving met-tRNAi in the ribosomal P site. This process may be seen in Figure 5.1 and further information is available in Sonenberg and Hinnebusch (2009).

Elongation

The *elongation* phase proceeds following the formation of the initiation complex. It involves three distinct steps that are repeated many times during the formation of a polypeptide. These include:

(1) transfer of an appropriate aminoacyl-tRNA from cytoplasm to the A-site of the ribosome
(2) covalent linkage of a new amino acid to the growing polypeptide chain, or peptidyl transfer
(3) movement of tRNA from the A-site to P-site and with simultaneous translocation of mRNA by three nucleotides.

The formation of the aminoacyl-tRNA involves the hydrolysis of high-energy phosphate bonds and the cycle is repeated and proceeds at a rate of about 18–20 amino acids incorporated per second. The binding of the aminoacyl-tRNA to the ribosome and the translocation of the peptidyl-tRNA require energy that is obtained via the hydrolysis of two guanosine tri-sphosphates (GTPs) per cycle.

Termination

Two release factors, eRF1 and eRF3, and one GTP are required. When one of the stop codons (UAA, UAG or UGA) enters the A site of the ribosome, GTP is hydrolysed and eRF1.eRF3 catalyse peptidyl-tRNA cleavage.

Ribosome recycling

When translation stops, mRNA and deacylated tRNA are still associated with the ribosome. At least two factors, eIF3 and eIF1, are required to split off the 60S ribosomal subunit and to dissociate the deacylated tRNA and mRNA from the 40S subunit. This integrated process of initiation, elongation, termination and ribosome recycling is the *translational phase* of protein synthesis. More detailed reviews may be found in the reading list.

5.4 Regulation of the translation phase of protein synthesis

Our bodies are composed of more than 200 distinct types of differentiated cells and, with few exceptions, all cells contain identical genetic information. Thus, at the most basic level, the pattern and content of the different proteins in cells are determined by their patterns of gene expression, by regulation of transcription. However, an important site of regulation may occur at the level of mRNA translation in some tissues and/or for some proteins.

The rate-limiting step in translation is usually, but not always, located within the initiation phase, with the intrinsic activity or strength of most mRNAs determined by:

- the accessibility of the capped 5′-terminus and poly(A) tail to initiation factors
- the ability of the 40S ribosomal subunit to bind and scan the mRNA distally
- the frequency of recognition of the initiator codon and surrounding context.

A major mechanism of control of global protein synthesis is via phosphorylation/dephosphorylation of the translation components, primarily of initiation and elongation factors. Phosphorylation of the α-subunit of eIF2 may cause a repression of protein synthesis by decreasing formation of the ternary complex (Figure 5.1). Alternatively, phosphorylation of 4E-BP by mTOR in response to insulin or amino acids will increase binding of eIF-4F to the cap structure which recognises the mRNA 5′ cap, thus increasing the rate of translational initiation. The kinase, mTOR, is also involved in phosphorylation of other factors which increase translation, including eIF4G, S6 kinase and eEF-2 kinase. Thus, a complex set of interactions, some redundant or overlapping, serve to link the rate of translation to the overall metabolic needs and state of the cell. More detailed reviews of this topic may be found in Sonenberg and Hinnebusch (2009).

In addition to the more general regulation of translation, important regulators of specific mRNA translation are the large family of miRNAs, ~22 nt non-coding RNAs which bind to proteins (Apo, GW182) to form an miRNP (miRNA-induced silencing complex or miRISC) that binds to specific sites in the 3′ UTR of mRNAs. Such binding promotes repression of mRNA translation and, in some cases, also activates mRNA degradation. More detailed information may be found in Carthew and Sontheimer (2009).

5.5 Post-translational events

While the process of polypeptide synthesis, as outlined above, is limited essentially to the incorporation of the common 20 amino acids, chemical analysis of proteins for their constituent amino acids often reveals many more than just these 20 amino acids. Although it is impossible to propose a precise number of amino acids and their derivatives actually present in proteins in the biosphere, the number may be quite high. There are about 1000 amino acids or more in nature, although not all of these occur as protein-bound amino acids. Furthermore, the final polypeptide produced may differ from that specified by the gene through modifications of the number of peptide bonds. Shortening of the polypeptide chain by proteolytic cleavage or, in other cases, lengthening of the chain by addition of one or more amino acids to the carboxyl- (C-) or amino- (N-) terminal ends may occur. For example, the initiator methionyl residue is often removed from the amino terminal of newly synthesised proteins.

The secondary, or derived, amino acids found in proteins arise by chemical modification of the primary amino acid during, or after, its gene-specified insertion into the polypeptide. This process is termed the 'post-translational' phase and it has been estimated that 50–90% of proteins are modified in this way. Some of the more common enzyme-catalysed post-translational modifications are listed in Table 5.2. A few protein modifications can occur spontaneously, as in the addition of glucose residues to give glycosylated haemoglobin (HbA_{1C}); this is especially marked when blood glucose concentration is elevated in diabetes mellitus.

Post-translational modifications add versatility to the genome. Such changes may affect protein–protein interactions, protein–nucleic acid interactions, protein stability, subcellular location of some proteins, enzymatic activity of modified proteins and protein function. Post-translational events can often carry the same significance for production of functional proteins as do the transcriptional and

Table 5.2 Examples of common enzyme-catalysed post-translational modifications

Modification[a]	Residue modified	Example of modified protein
Glycosylation	Asparagine	Integrin
Hydroxylation	Proline, lysine	Collagen
Phosphorylation	Serine	eIF-2α
Methylation	Lysine	Histone H4
Acylation	N-terminal glycine	Glutamate cysteine ligase
Acetylation	Lysine	Histone H3
ADP ribosylation	Arginine	Tubulin
Ubiquitination[b]	Lysine	Histone H2

[a] These modifications are mediated by specific enzymes, which for the sake of clarity are omitted from this table.
[b] There are a number of proteins in the ubiquitin protein family (e.g., ubiquitin, Sumo, Nedd8).

translational phases that are responsible for the formation of proteins in the first instance.

5.6 Protein degradation

As already implied, the breakdown of tissue and organ proteins is an extensive, continuous and regulated process. In association with protein synthesis, the degradation or breakdown of proteins determines the qualitative and quantitative nature of the cellular protein profile.

In mammalian cells, there are separate lysosomal and non-lysosomal mechanisms that are involved in different aspects of protein degradation; proteins that enter the cell from the extracellular milieu (such as via receptor-mediated endocytosis and pinocytosis) are degraded in lysosomes. Lysosomal degradation of intracellular protein occurs mostly under stressed conditions, such as in starvation; this process is activated by glucocorticoids and suppressed by insulin or by a dietary protein deficiency.

Non-lysosomal mechanisms are responsible for the selective turnover of intracellular proteins that occurs under basal metabolic conditions and for many of the changes that occur in response to diet and hormones. The proteolytic system that degrades the bulk of cell proteins, including rapidly eliminated abnormal proteins and short-lived regulatory polypeptides, is non-lysosomal and ATP-dependent. It occurs in a large multiple-protein complex, the 26S

Figure 5.2 The ubiquitin–proteasome pathway of intracellular protein breakdown. (a) 20S core particle (white) and 19S cap complex (grey) of the 26S proteasome. (b) Ubiquitin is added to the target protein, the polyubiquinated target is fed into the 26S proteasome, where it is deubiquitinated and hydrolysed to peptides, which are released from the proteasome.

proteasome, consisting at a minimum of two copies each of 33 distinct subunits, which in total might account for as much as 1% of the total cell protein (Figure 5.2a). Proteins are degraded within the central core of the proteasome, the 20S particle, which contains different proteolytic activities (chymotrypsin-like, trypsin-like and caspase-like active sites). Proteasomes hydrolyse most peptide bonds and generate peptides that are typically 3–22 amino acids long. These peptides are then released from the 20S core and are hydrolysed to amino acids by peptidases in the cytoplasm.

An initial step in the hydrolysis of most such proteins is a 'marking' reaction involving their covalent conjugation by the 76-residue polypeptide ubiquitin, via a multistep process; the C-terminus of ubiquitin becomes attached by an isopeptide bond to ε-amino groups on lysine residues or in some cases to the free amino group on the N-terminal of the protein substrate. Much of the selectivity for proteolysis resides in this conjugation step, which requires ATP as well as ubiquitin activating enzyme (E1), ubiquitin carrier protein (E2) and ubiquitin-protein ligase (E3). Figure 5.2b shows a proposed sequence of events in the conjugation and degradation of protein via this system. The proteasome also recognises and degrades some non-ubiquitinylated proteins such as ornithine decarboxylase, which is presented to the proteasome by another protein (antizyme). In addition to lysosomal proteolysis and the proteasome, there are two

cytoplasmic proteolytic systems, neither of which requires ATP. The calpain system involves Ca^{2+}-activated cysteine proteases. It appears to be important as cellular calcium concentration varies, for example during the cell cycle, cell fusion, signal transduction and apoptosis. Caspases are also cysteine proteases but they specifically cleave proteins after aspartyl residues and they do not require calcium for activation; rather they are zymogens, which must be activated by limited proteolysis. They appear to be most important in the activation of proinflammatory cytokines and in promotion of apoptosis.

5.7 Selectivity of protein turnover

The proteins of a single tissue (e.g. skeletal muscle, liver and kidney) turn over at different rates. This general characteristic of protein metabolism is illustrated for the liver in Table 5.3. Not only do the cytoplasmic proteins in a liver cell turn over at vastly different rates, by as much as 2000-fold difference, but also the proteins of the mitochondrion have differential rates of turnover. Half-lives of some enzymes can vary markedly, depending on conditions in the cell. For example, cortisol causes a lengthening of the half-life for tyrosine aminotransferase in liver, befitting its role in gluconeogenesis.

Based on their turnover, as measured most often by tracer techniques, proteins have been classified as

Table 5.3 Half-lives of selected proteins in liver

Protein type	Name	EC number	Half-life (h)
Cytoplasmic	Ornithine decarboxylase	4.1.1.17	0.2
	Tyrosine aminotransferase	2.6.1.5	2.0
	HMG-CoA reductase	1.1.1.3 3.0	
	Arginase	3.5.3.1	96
	Lactate dehydrogenase (isoenzyme 5) 1.1.1.27	144	
Nuclear	RNA polymerase I	2.7.7.6	1.3
	RNA polymerase II	2.7.7.6	12
	Histone	432	
Mitochondrial	δ-Aminolevulinate synthetase (matrix) 2.3.1.37	1.1	
	Ornithine oxo-acid aminotransferase (matrix) 2.6.1.13		19
	Glutamate dehydrogenase (matrix) 1.4.1.3	24	
	Pyruvate carboxylase (matrix) 6.4.1.1	110	
	Pyruvate dehydrogenase (matrix) 1.2.4.1	194	

Data taken from Jennissen (1995). HMG-CoA, 3-hydroxy-3-methylglutaryl-coenzyme A.

short-lived proteins (half-life of minutes to a few hours) and long-lived proteins (half-life of many hours). Furthermore, the different subunits of a functional protein can turn over at different rates. For example, the light chain of myosin turns over about three times as rapidly as the myosin heavy chain. Finally, the mature collagen in skin does not reveal a turnover but is lost from the body by shedding of cells from the surface.

5.8 An integration of these processes of turnover with respect to amino acid metabolism

The metabolism of the amino acids that are released into the body pools during the process of protein breakdown, as well as those coming from the diet, is determined by, and also in turn affects, the status of protein synthesis and breakdown. The metabolism of amino acids differs from that of lipid and carbohydrate macromolecules in two important ways, both of which determine the overall pattern of amino acid metabolism. The first is that the body has no specific store for amino acids, in contrast to its ability, albeit limited, to store carbohydrate as glycogen and the considerable capacity to store fatty acids as triacylglycerol. It is true that, in certain circumstances, proteolysis in the liver and musculature can make amino acids available for particular purposes (e.g. acute-phase protein synthesis or gluconeogenesis), but

these liver and muscle proteins, together with all other body proteins (with the possible exception of some milk proteins), are primarily synthesised for their specific physiological function and not as a nutritional store of amino acids.

Protein synthesis requires that all amino acids must be available to tissues simultaneously; this is the basis for dietary protein complementation (see Chapter 5 in *Introduction to Human Nutrition* in this series). The corollary of this is that tissue amino acids in excess of the capacity and requirements for protein synthesis are very rapidly oxidised. The need for rapid metabolism of dietary protein can also be argued simply on osmotic grounds. A typical North American adult ingests about 100 g of protein per day. On digestion and absorption, this amounts to about 1000 mmoles of amino acids. This quantity of amino acids, if distributed evenly throughout body water (about 42 l in a 70 kg person), would increase the osmotic pressure by about 24 mOsm, hence the need to remove these amino acids rapidly by catabolising those that are not required for protein synthesis.

The second way in which the metabolism of amino acids differs from that of carbohydrate or of fat is in the nature of its end-products. In addition to carbon dioxide and water, amino acid catabolism produces nitrogen-containing end-products (principally urea and ammonia) and sulphur-containing end-products (principally sulphate). These, too, have important implications for shaping amino acid catabolism. Since ammonia is a potent neurotoxin, its blood concentration must be kept low (about 30 µmol/l in humans). Ammonia detoxification via urea synthesis is confined to the liver, therefore much of amino acid disposal occurs in the liver. When amino acid metabolism occurs in the periphery, mechanisms exist for transporting the nitrogen to the liver in a form that avoids elevation of the blood ammonia concentration. There are also important acid–base consequences to the catabolism of the sulphur amino acids as this involves the production of a strong metabolic acid. The elimination of this acid is also accomplished via amino acid metabolism.

5.9 Regulation of amino acid metabolism

As for the case of protein synthesis and breakdown, there is a fine regulation of amino acid metabolism, particularly in reference to the metabolism of the indispensable amino acids. Thus, a variety of mechanisms, both short and long term, come into play. These include enzyme induction and turnover, covalent modification of enzymes and control by K_m. For example, glucagon secretion is increased on ingestion of a high-protein meal. This response plays two roles. First, a high-protein intake also stimulates insulin secretion. Insulin promotes protein synthesis from the ingested amino acids, but will also increase glucose utilisation. This latter action, if unopposed, could result in hypoglycaemia after the ingestion of a high-protein, low-carbohydrate meal. The increased glucagon levels prevent this by increasing hepatic glucose production. The second action of glucagon is to stimulate amino acid catabolism. That glucagon plays a major role in the catabolism of many amino acids is evident from the generalised hypoamminoacidaemia in patients with a glucagonoma.

- Glucagon activates phenylalanine hydroxylase by an adenosine 3′5′-cyclic monophosphate (cAMP)-dependent mechanism.
- Glucagon activates glutaminase and the glycine cleavage enzyme, although the mechanism of these effects remains obscure.
- Glucagon and glucocorticoids induce the synthesis of a number of amino acid catabolising enzymes.

In addition to hormones that stimulate the catabolism of a variety of amino acids, there must be mechanisms specific to individual amino acids that can accommodate appropriate amino acid oxidation in the face of varying amounts of different amino acids. The most obvious of these is control by K_m. Many enzymes that initiate amino acid degradation have quite high K_m values for their amino acid substrates, relative to the tissue concentrations of the amino acids. Thus, these enzymes can automatically respond to increased postprandial tissue levels of amino acids with increased catabolism. The corollary of this is that as tissue concentrations of amino acids decrease, so will their catabolism. However, it is clear that control by K_m is not sufficient to protect indispensable amino acids from excessive catabolism, and a number of other mechanisms have evolved. A particularly effective mechanism is that of rapid enzyme induction and degradation. Many of the hepatic enzymes that initiate amino acid catabolism, particularly the catabolism of the indispensable amino acids, are highly inducible. Increased dietary protein brings about increased synthesis of these enzymes; these effects are often hormonally mediated. Furthermore, many of these enzymes have quite short half-lives, as already noted above. The combination of these factors means that there are quite large amplitude changes (as much as 10-fold) in the hepatic activities of enzymes such as tyrosine aminotransferase, ornithine aminotransferase, tryptophan dioxygenase, serine dehydratase and histidase. The physiological significance of these effects is clear. The induction of the enzymes can facilitate increased catabolism when the amino acid supply is high, while the virtual disappearance of some of these enzymes when the amino acid supply is low serves to conserve these indispensable amino acids.

Finally, some of the key enzymes of amino acid catabolism are regulated by covalent modification. The branched-chain α-ketoacid dehydrogenase (BCKADH) is the controlling enzyme in the catabolism of the three branched-chain amino acids (valine, leucine and isoleucine). Existing as a multienzyme complex, similar to that of pyruvate dehydrogenase, the BCKADH complex contains a protein kinase and a protein phosphatase that can regulate its activity by reversible phosphorylation (Figure 5.3). The enzyme is inhibited by phosphorylation. The BCKADH kinase is inhibited by the branched-chain α-ketoacids (most potently by α-ketoisocaproate, the α-ketoacid derived from leucine), which results in a dephosphorylation, and hence activation, of the BCKADH. Another

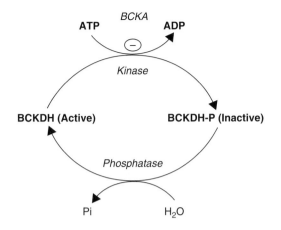

Figure 5.3 Regulation of the branched-chain α-keto acid (BCKA) dehydrogenase.

striking regulatory mechanism is found in the catabolism of phenylalanine. Phenylalanine hydroxylase, the controlling enzyme in the conversion of phenylalanine to tyrosine, is regulated by its amino acid substrate and by phosphorylation/dephosphorylation. Glucagon can activate the enzyme via a cAMP-dependent phosphorylation. However, the enzyme can also exist in two forms, dimeric and tetrameric, and can be converted to the more active tetrameric form in the presence of phenylalanine. These two forms of activation appear to be synergistic in that phenylalanine also increases the rate of phosphorylation by glucagon. Tyrosine, the product of phenylalanine hydroxylase, is generally considered to be dispensable since it can be synthesised by humans. If both phenylalanine and tyrosine are present in excess the limiting enzyme for their degradation, tyrosine aminotransferase, can be induced and the half-life can be lengthened (as mentioned previously) to markedly increase the amount of enzyme present. Thus, these enzymes are activated by increased substrate concentrations, providing elegant mechanisms whereby these amino acids are readily catabolised when their supply is high and conserved when supply is low.

5.10 Amino acid synthesis: the dispensable amino acids

Nutritionists pay great attention to the indispensable (essential) amino acids. It can be argued, however, that the retention, during evolution, of the synthetic pathways for the dispensable (non-essential) amino acids speaks of their importance in metabolism.

The synthesis of many of these amino acids is fairly simple, for example alanine is synthesised in a single transamination reaction, in which glutamate provides the amino group and the carbon skeleton, pyruvate, is readily available from glycolysis. However, for other amino acids the situation is more complex. Arginine (a conditionally indispensable amino acid) provides an excellent example of a complex synthetic pathway in which there are both developmental variations and important interspecies differences.

In many adult mammals, including humans, arginine is synthesised by a pathway that involves the small intestine and the kidney (Figure 5.4). In brief, citrulline produced in the enterocytes is added to the blood and removed by the kidneys, which convert it to arginine. This arginine is then released in the renal vein. Citrulline is produced, in the intestine, in two ways. A major portion arises from the metabolism of glutamine. A key enzyme in this pathway is pyrroline-5-carboxylate synthetase, which is found only in these cells. Proline can also be a source of citrulline (Figure 5.4). Citrulline is taken up by the kidneys, where it is converted to arginine, in cells of the proximal tubule, by the combined action of argininosuccinate synthetase and argininosuccinate lyase (Figure 5.4). The importance of this intestinal/renal axis for arginine synthesis is evident from the arginine deficiency that occurs when intestinal citrulline synthesis is inhibited or after massive surgical resection of the small intestine. A similar situation occurs in strict carnivores, such as cats and ferrets, whose intestines synthesise almost no citrulline owing to low activities of pyrroline-5-carboxylate synthetase and ornithine aminotransferase. In these animals, ingestion of a single arginine-free meal can result in hyperammonaemia, convulsions and even death. Finally, the entire pathway for arginine synthesis is expressed in enterocytes from newborn animals and newly synthesised arginine is released into the hepatic portal vein. However, such intestinal arginine synthesis is strictly a neonatal event, as it declines within a few days of birth (in piglets), and intestinal citrulline production is evident a few days after weaning.

The synthesis of dispensable amino acids such as arginine, as described above, glutamine, glycine and

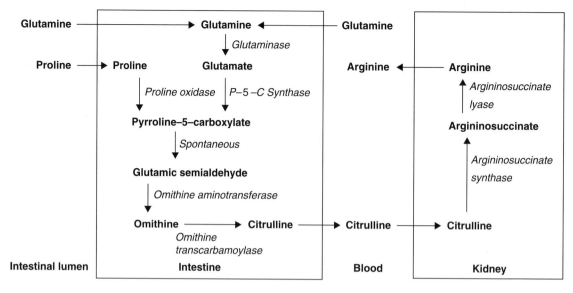

Figure 5.4 Intestinal–renal axis for endogenous arginine synthesis.

proline normally proceeds at rates commensurate with metabolic needs. However, under certain conditions, such as in prematurity or in catabolic stress, their synthesis may not proceed at rates sufficient to meet the metabolic requirement. In this case a dietary source of the amino acid is required and in this context these amino acids are classified as being 'conditionally indispensable' or 'conditionally essential'.

5.11 *In vivo* aspects of protein and amino acid turnover

Techniques for measurement of protein turnover

Various tracer techniques have been used to estimate amino acid fluxes and protein kinetics at the whole-body level and in individual tissues and organs (Table 5.4). The different whole-body approaches may be classified into one of two major categories:

- methods involving the use of ^{15}N and measurement of the label in end-products of nitrogen metabolism (end-product method)
- methods involving administration of specifically labelled amino acids and measurement of the tracer in body fluids, such as plasma or urine (plasma or precursor method).

Table 5.4 Methods of measuring protein turnover *in vivo*: whole-body, region and specific proteins

	Example of tracer
Whole body	
End-product (EP) methods	[^{15}N]glycine
Precursor methods	[^{13}C]leucine/[^{13}C]KIC
Specific proteins	
Bolus/constant infusion tracer protocols	[^{13}C]leucine, [^{2}H$_5$]phenylalanine
Region	
Constant infusion/biopsy	[^{2}H$_5$]phenylalanine
Arteriovenous difference tracer studies	[^{15}N-1–^{13}C]leucine
Multiple isotope (iv/ig-splanchnic)	[^{2}H$_3$]leucine (iv), [1–^{13}C]leucine (ig)

iv, intravenous; ig, intragastric.

^{15}N end-product methods

The principle behind ^{15}N end-product approaches for the measurement of protein (nitrogen) turnover in the whole body is depicted in Figure 5.5; it involves administration of a ^{15}N-labelled precursor (often [^{15}N]-glycine) as a continuous infusion or as a single bolus and measurement of the appearance of the isotope in urine, either as ammonia or total nitrogen. In its simplest form the metabolic nitrogen pool is depicted as a single homogeneous pool into which nitrogen enters from protein breakdown and from the diet. Nitrogen leaves via protein synthesis and by pathways of nitrogen excretion. This model, or modifications of it, has been used extensively by many investigators since it was first used more than 50 years ago by Schoenheimer at Columbia University in New York.

The isotopic data generated from ^{15}N-labelled tracer administration may be evaluated using a compartmental modelling approach or by applying a stochastic model in which the overall flow of nitrogen into and out of the metabolic pool is of interest, rather than the movement of nitrogen within and among the intermediate pools. The stochastic method gives less information than the compartmental modelling approach, but is obtained more easily; this might be an advantage in studies dealing with protein

and amino acid turnover that are conducted under demanding experimental conditions such as in various clinical settings or even in the field. Additional details, problems and limitations of this approach are to be found by consulting the further reading list.

Precursor, plasma or substrate-specific methods

Under this general category an isotopically-labelled amino acid is administered, most often by continuous intravenous infusion, often immediately preceded by a priming dose to help to achieve a rapid approach to a plateau of isotopic enrichment within the sampled compartment. In human studies, the latter is most often the venous blood circulation, although urine could be sampled as a basis for the non-invasive determination of the isotopic enrichment in the free amino acid pool. Alternative procedures within this class of methods include giving the isotope tracer(s) by bolus intravenous injection or by oral administration or by both, where simultaneous doses of different specific labelled tracers of an amino acid are given via these routes.

The basic features of the precursor procedure are depicted in Figure 5.6, where enrichment of the tracer is measured in the plasma and, if appropriate, the appearance of the label in expired carbon dioxide is also monitored. Using simple dilution principles, the flux of the amino acid in the sampled compartment can be determined. Under steady-state metabolic and isotopic conditions, when a nutritionally indispensable amino acid is used as a tracer, estimates can be made of the rate of disappearance of the tracer via non-oxidative metabolism, assumed to be a measure of protein synthesis, and of the rate of appearance of

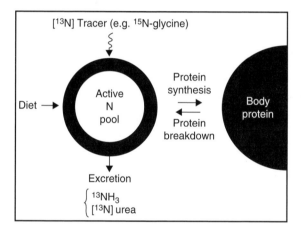

Figure 5.5 Schematic of the ^{15}N-end-product model for determination of whole-body protein turnover.

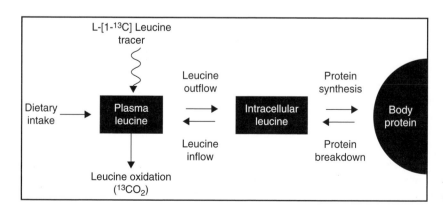

Figure 5.6 Schematic of the plasma precursor model, using ^{13}C-leucine as the example tracer, for determination of whole-body protein turnover.

Table 5.5 Some issues and questions related to precursor or 'plasma' approach for measurement of amino acid fluxes and whole-body and organ/tissue protein turnover

---

1. What model and why?
    (a) for whole-body protein turnover
    (b) for measurement of organ (regional) protein and amino acid metabolism
    (c) for study of specific amino acid metabolism; its conversions and interconversions and metabolic fate
    (d) for studying the carbon and/or nitrogen moiety and/or functional groups of the molecule
2. What is the isotopic enrichment of the 'precursor' amino acid pool(s) for accurate measurement of whole-body flux and oxidation rates?
3. What is the appropriate amount of tracer and length of infusion period, and is there a problem of recycling of label?
4. Are infusion and sampling sites important? Which are best?
5. For measurement of components of flux, what is the retention of $^{13}CO_2$?

---

the tracer into the compartment via protein breakdown. The most widely used tracer protocol in studies of human whole-body protein turnover has been L-[1–^{13}C] leucine, given as a primed continuous intravenous infusion. The isotopic enrichment of α-ketoisocaproate in plasma reflects its isotopic enrichment in cells and may be used as a surrogate for the intracellular isotopic enrichment of leucine.

Several technical and modelling issues need to be considered when using the plasma or precursor approach for measurement of amino acid fluxes and for estimation of whole-body protein dynamics. For summary purposes, Table 5.5 lists some of the questions that must be answered when attempting to estimate the whole-body amino acid flux and rate of protein synthesis in the body as a whole. A particularly important problem is that of determining isotopic enrichment of the precursor of interest in order to estimate whole-body amino acid fluxes, rates of protein synthesis or rates of synthesis of specific proteins. Since in most clinical investigations it would be difficult, or unethical, to sample the tissue or organ pools of interest, the problem might be overcome, at least in part, by measuring in blood the enrichment of a metabolite derived from the intracellular metabolism of the tracer and which is in rapid equilibrium with the extracellular compartment. In this context the transamination product of leucine, α-ketoisocaproate (KIC), is often used to predict intracellular leucine labelling and various studies have generally

supported the validity of this approach. However, other approaches have been used for specific purposes, and that of mass isotopomer distribution analysis (MIDA) is particularly powerful; this involves quantifying precursor–product events from the distribution of mass isotopomer patterns in the labelled precursor and product.

The flooding-dose technique

Finally, mention should be made of the flooding-dose method, which has been used in both experimental animals and humans to determine rates of synthesis of muscle proteins and of various blood proteins, such as albumin in humans. This approach involves giving the tracer (e.g. [1–^{13}C]-leucine or [^{2}H$_5$]-phenylalanine) together with a large amount of unlabelled amino acid to create a similar isotopic enrichment in the extracellular and intracellular compartments, including the pool supplying amino acids for tRNA charging and thus protein synthesis. The idea and approach is highly attractive, particularly since it involves a relatively brief study period for any one experimental subject and, therefore, is potentially applicable in complex clinical settings. Estimates of albumin synthesis obtained by this method are in general agreement with those derived from the constant tracer infusion approach, but concern has been raised about the appropriateness of the technique for estimating synthesis rates of muscle proteins. The flooding-dose approach is particularly suited to measurements made on tissues that can be taken during surgery.

5.12 *In vivo* rates of protein turnover

Whole body

The various methods summarised above have provided a picture of human protein metabolism where, for example, protein synthesis rates are high in the newborn and, per unit of body weight, these rates decline with progressive growth and development (Table 5.6). Three points emerge from the values shown in this table. Firstly, not only is the higher rate of protein synthesis in the young, compared with that for the adult, related to the net protein deposition that occurs during growth, but also there is a high rate of total protein turnover (synthesis and breakdown) related, in part, to tissue remodelling. Hence,

Table 5.6 Some representative estimates of whole-body protein synthesis rates, in humans at various ages compared with dietary protein allowances

Age group	Protein synthesis (g/kg per day)	Protein allowance (g/kg per day)
Infant (premature)	11.3, 14	~3.0
Child (15 months)	6.3	1.3
Child (2–8 years)	3.9	~1.1
Adolescent (~13 years)	~5	~1.0
Young adult (~20 years)	~4.6	0.75

Data compiled from Young *et al.* (1985), where references to the original studies are given.

Table 5.7 Some estimates of tissue protein synthesis in adult humans

Tissue/organ	Fractional synthesis rate (%/day)
Skeletal muscle	2
Stomach	43
Oesophagus	30
Colon	9
Liver	21
Heart	5
Lymphocytes	6

Data compiled from Garlick *et al.* (1994).

Table 5.8 Effects of various nutritional and pathological states on muscle and liver protein synthesis in young rats or mice

Treatment	Protein synthesis (% of control)	
	Liver	Muscle
Starvation (2 days)	71	47
Protein-free diet (9 days)	70	27
Diabetes	51	41
Malaria infection	66	49
Turpentine injection	116	66
Interleukin-1β	145	68
Cancer	126	56

Data compiled from Garlick and McNurlan (1994), where references to original sources of the data are given.

protein synthesis in the premature infant is about twice as high as in the preschool child and approximately three or four times as high as in the adult. Secondly, at all ages, the rates of whole-body protein synthesis and breakdown are considerably greater than the intakes of dietary protein apparently necessary to meet the needs for maintenance or for the support of growth. It follows, therefore, that there is an extensive reutilisation within the body of the amino acids entering tissue pools during the course of protein breakdown. Thirdly, there is a general relationship between the age- and developmental-associated changes in protein turnover and the dietary protein needs for each specific age group. This implies that when rates of synthesis and breakdown of body proteins change in response to various stimuli, such as infection and trauma, the dietary requirement for nitrogen and specific amino acids intakes will change. This prediction is consistent with the increased total protein (nitrogen) needs of patients following severe trauma.

Organs and tissues

Although whole-body rates of protein turnover change with different physiological and pathological states, these measurements do not provide information on the status of protein turnover in different tissues and organs. Hence, estimates of protein turnover by individual organs and tissues have also been made and a summary of some of these is presented in Table 5.7. The fractional rates of synthesis differ among the organs, with those for liver being about 10 times the value for skeletal muscle. However, because of the size of the musculature it

accounts for about 20% of whole-body protein synthesis or about the same as that for the liver.

It should now be clear that there are major differences among the various tissues and organs in their rates of protein turnover. As might be expected, therefore, the responses of different organs to nutritional and pathological stimuli also differ, and this can be with respect to the direction of change and the extent of change. To illustrate this point, Table 5.8 summarises the responses of the liver and muscle of young rats to a variety of nutritional and pathological treatments. As shown here, the rates of protein synthesis in these rat tissues change in the same direction during nutrient deprivation, but they respond differently to various disease states. Although the available data are more limited in humans, similar differences in the pattern of response appear to apply. Thus, the higher rate of whole-body protein turnover in severely traumatised patients is associated with

Figure 5.7 mTORC1 activation by nutrients and growth factors. (Reproduced with permission from Shaw, 2008).

higher rates of muscle protein breakdown and also higher rates of liver protein and immune cell protein synthesis. For example, in severely burned adult patients, rates of whole-body protein synthesis might be as much as double those for healthy subjects. It has been estimated that in response to infection acute-phase protein synthesis might account for an additional 1 g protein synthesis/kg body weight per day, which is six times the normal rate of albumin synthesis in adult humans.

5.13 Mechanisms and factors responsible for alterations in protein turnover

Protein synthesis

As is already evident, rates of protein synthesis and breakdown are not constant but change in response to different pathophysiological conditions. Among

the important factors responsible for alterations in protein synthesis rates is the availability of amino acids. They regulate the expression of a number of genes involved in growth, cellular function and amino acid metabolism. The finer details of the mechanisms involved are only now being revealed.

An increase in amino acid availability can up-regulate the translational phase of protein synthesis via an effect on translation initiation by activation of the kinase mTOR (Figure 5.7). Rag proteins (a subfamily of Ras small GTPases) interact with amino acids and mTORC1 (the mTOR complex with Raptor) to cause redistribution of mTORC1 to vesicles containing Rheb, which activates mTOR. Phosphorylated targets in response to mTOR include 4E-BP1, which is inhibited, permitting the cap complex to form (Figure 5.1) and S6 Kinase, which phosphorylates several targets to increase translation. Insulin and several growth factors also activate mTORC1 through the PI3 Kinase/PK-B pathway, which results in Rheb activation. Thus amino acids and insulin/growth factors work synergistically to activate translation. A second mechanism has been proposed to explain the down-regulation of translation as a result of amino acid starvation. In this case, free tRNA accumulates when amino acids are lacking and activates the kinase GCN2, which phosphorylates EIF2a, thus inhibiting formation of the preinitiation complex (Figure 5.1). There is still more to be learned about how the cell senses changes in amino acid availability, the basis for the specificity of the response to particular amino acids, and the nature and extent of the cooperativity between amino acids and growth-promoting hormones in the regulation of protein synthesis.

Protein breakdown

A profound loss of muscle mass may occur under various experimental conditions, such as following glucocorticoid treatment, denervation, immobilisation, microgravity and fasting. A similar loss also occurs in patients suffering from major trauma, including burn injury, sepsis and cancer. This erosion of muscle protein is due, in part, to enhanced rates of protein breakdown or proteolysis, and the contractile or myofibrillar proteins may be particularly affected. In models of muscle wasting there are various changes that indicate an activation of the proteasome–ubiquitin-dependent pathway. The increases in mRNA levels for ubiquitin, for certain proteasome subunits and for specific ubiquitination enzymes, suggest a coordinated series of biochemical adaptations in the atrophying muscle that enhance the activity and capacity of this pathway, leading to muscle wasting. It is now thought that activation of FoxO transcription factors leads to activation of both lysosomal proteolysis and the proteasomal system to result in a marked increase in proteolysis of muscle proteins (Figure 5.8).

In contrast to the stimulation of muscle breakdown, there are other conditions that favour conservation of muscle cell protein. Thus, after a meal, when insulin is increased, protein turnover in muscle is reduced. Insulin activates Akt, which inhibits FoxO3 (Figure 5.8), leading to a reduced capacity to degrade proteins, associated with a suppression of the ubiquitin-dependent proteasome pathway as well as a reduction in the activity of the lysosomal pathway.

Such adaptations to protein inadequacy are seen in humans in prolonged starvation or malnutrition, where physiological mechanisms have evolved that

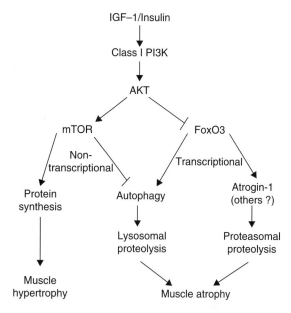

Figure 5.8 Schematic of FoxO3 regulation of lysosomal and proteasomal proteolysis leading to muscle atrophy. Insulin would oppose muscle atrophy by activating AKT which inhibits FoxO3 and activates mTOR, leading to increased muscle protein synthesis. (Reprinted from Cell Metabolism, Vol 6, FoxO3 Coordinately Activates Protein Degradation by the Autophagic/lysosomal and Proteasomal Pathways in Atrophying Muscle Cells. pp. 472–483, (2007) Copyright © Elsevier.)

permit survival to continue with little or no energy and protein intake for relatively long periods. However, a continued and sustained loss of cell proteins is lethal and so the capacity to mobilise protein from cells as a source of energy is limited. In the initial days of a fast or catabolic illness, muscle and skin proteins are mobilised and amino acids are metabolised for energy and/or used to meet the amino acid needs for protein synthesis in the splanchnic region and by the immune system. After several days of food deprivation, that catabolic response ceases and other mechanisms are activated to suppress muscle protein breakdown and amino acid oxidation. The conservation of muscle protein occurs concomitantly with a reduction in oxygen consumption and metabolic rate, and the overall rates of protein breakdown vary with changes in nutrient supply and endocrine factors. Thus, muscle proteolysis is controlled by several hormones, especially insulin and glucocorticoids.

The turnover of proteins and their response to changes in the internal and external environments occur in the context of the movement of amino acids among organs and within tissues. This aspect of the integration of protein and amino acid metabolism will be discussed in the following section.

5.14 Interorgan amino acid metabolism

Fed and fasted states

There is considerable amino acid traffic between the various organs of the body. The principal vehicles for this transport are the free amino acids themselves. However, distribution via proteins and peptides should also be considered. The liver is the site of synthesis of a number of plasma proteins, of which albumin is quantitatively the most important. In a well-nourished healthy adult, approximately 20 g of albumin is synthesised by the liver per day and catabolised in the periphery. Albumin synthesis is sensitive to nutritional and pathological conditions, increasing with the feeding of protein-rich meals and decreasing in kwashiorkor, for example. Albumin degradation occurs in many tissues of the body, including skin, muscle, kidneys and even in the liver itself; it seems that fibroblasts in these tissues are particularly active. In terms of amino acid traffic, it can be estimated that some 20 g of amino acids per day are normally made available to peripheral tissues as a result of albumin catabolism.

Peptides have also been suggested as a vehicle for interorgan amino acid traffic. Certainly, some peptides that arise physiologically, such as the C-peptide of proinsulin or peptide products of angiotensinogen proteolysis, are very rapidly catabolised. The kidney has a high capacity for such peptide catabolism. It has also been suggested that peptides can play a major role in interorgan amino acid metabolism. However, the situation is far from clear as the evidence for the existence of a significant circulating peptide pool is controversial.

The principal technique for the study of interorgan amino acid metabolism is that of arteriovenous (or A-V) difference. When combined with simultaneously measured rates of blood flow, such A-V differences provide quantitative data on the net uptake or output of amino acids across different organs. There are two important points to appreciate about this technique. First, it measures *net* metabolic exchanges. It is entirely possible that there may be simultaneous utilisation and production of an amino acid across an organ (e.g. glutamine utilisation in periportal hepatocytes and glutamine synthesis in perivenous hepatocytes). Delineation of these individual processes requires the application of isotopic techniques, in addition to that of the A-V difference approach. Secondly, A-V differences are, almost always, small differences between two large numbers. As such, they require great analytical precision and it can be assumed that many small, although physiologically important, differences escape detection.

Major A-V differences for amino acids have been found across many tissues. Across the fed intestine, there is a net outflow of amino acids into the hepatic portal vein as proteins are digested and amino acids are absorbed, but in addition there is an uptake of glutamine and an output of alanine and citrulline. The carbon skeleton of alanine arises from glycolytically derived pyruvate, while the nitrogen arises from glutamine metabolism. Kidneys remove citrulline and convert it to arginine, which is released (Figure 5.4). They also remove glycine and produce serine. Kidneys take up glutamine, for acid–base homeostasis, and this uptake increases dramatically in metabolic acidosis (e.g. diabetic ketoacidosis) or during ingestion of a high-protein diet when increased quantities of sulphuric acid are produced from methionine and cysteine oxidation. Skeletal muscle oxidises an important proportion of dietary branched-chain amino acids. It also releases substantial quantities of alanine and glutamine. Alanine is synthesised via alanine aminotransferase; its nitrogen comes from the branched-chain amino acids and its carbon from glucose by glycolysis. This alanine is taken up by the liver and converted to glucose (the glucose–alanine cycle). Thus, alanine serves as an innocuous means of transferring nitrogen to the liver without increasing blood ammonia concentrations. In the fed state, more glutamine than alanine is released by muscle. The nitrogen for glutamine synthesis is derived from all three of the branched chain amino acids, but the carbon skeleton can only be provided from isoleucine and valine.

During starvation there is marked muscle proteolysis to provide amino acids to the liver for gluconeogenesis. However, the pattern of amino acids released by the liver does not correspond to the amino acid composition of muscle protein, in that alanine and glutamine comprise at least 50% of the amino acids

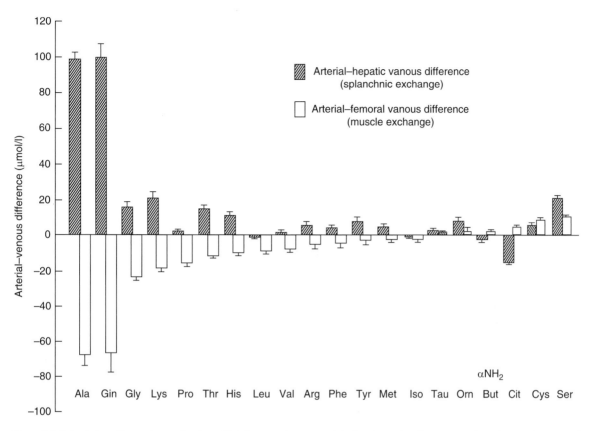

Figure 5.9 Splanchnic and leg exchange of amino acids in humans after an overnight fast. (Printed, with permission, from the Annual Review of Biochemistry, Vol.44 © 1975 by Annual Reviews http://www.annualreviews.org.)

released. Much of the alanine arises via the glucose–alanine cycle. The carbon skeletons for glutamine synthesis are derived from the intramuscular metabolism of glutamate, aspartate, asparagine, valine and isoleucine. The concordance is between the pattern of amino acids released from skeletal muscle after an overnight fast (shown in white in Figure 5.9) and the pattern of amino acids taken up by splanchnic tissues after an overnight fast (shown in grey in Figure 5.9).

5.15 Amino acid and peptide transport

Amino acid pools

Free amino acids comprise a very small portion of total body amino acids, whereas about 99% are found in proteins. However, the free amino acid pools are, metabolically, very dynamic. The extracellular pool is the major vehicle for interorgan amino acid exchange. Cellular amino acid pools are heterogeneous, both between cell types and within intracellular compartments. Thus, the brain contains particularly high concentrations of glutamate, an important neurotransmitter, while muscle contains the great bulk of the body's free glutamine. Cellular amino acid pools are crucial for the specific metabolic functions of individual cell types (e.g. the role of arginine, ornithine and citrulline in the liver's urea cycle) as well as, more generally, being the immediate pool of amino acids from which proteins are synthesised and to which amino acids are returned by intracellular proteolysis. Table 5.9 gives the concentrations of free amino acids in human plasma and within human muscle cells. It is apparent that there is considerable variability in the intracellular/extracellular gradients for different amino acids. These gradients are largely determined by amino acid transport mechanisms.

Table 5.9 Concentrations of free amino acids in human muscle and plasma

Amino acid	Plasma (mM)	Intracellular muscle (mM)
Citrulline	0.03	0.04
Phenylalanine	0.05	0.07
Tyrosine	0.05	0.10
Methionine	0.02	0.11
Isoleucine	0.06	0.11
Leucine	0.12	0.15
Cysteine	0.11	0.18
Valine	0.22	0.26
Ornithine	0.06	0.30
Histidine	0.08	0.37
Asparagine	0.05	0.47
Arginine	0.08	0.51
Proline	0.17	0.83
Serine	0.12	0.9
Threonine	0.15	1.03
Lysine	0.18	1.15
Glycine	0.21	1.33
Alanine	0.33	2.34
Glutamate	0.06	4.38
Glutamine	0.57	19.45
Taurine	0.07	15.44

Compiled from Bergstrom *et al.* (1974).

Amino acid transporters

Since the early 1990s enormous progress has been made in this field as many amino acid transporters have been identified, cloned and studied in detail. This new knowledge has complemented and expanded our earlier understanding, which was almost entirely derived from kinetic studies and genetic defects. Most cells contain systems A, ASC, L, y^+, N, y^+L and X_{AG}^- (Figure 5.10 and Table 5.10), as well as tissue-specific transport systems. From these new molecular studies it is now appreciated that there are many individual transporters within these different systems. Each transport protein is given a name, as is the gene that codes for the protein (Table 5.10). A common feature of these transporters is that, generally, they transport a number of amino acids that share common structural features.

Amino acid transporters differ in their preferred substrates and in the thermodynamic driving forces they use. Systems A, ASC and L transport neutral amino acids; systems A and ASC mediate transport of amino acids with small side-chains, whereas system L prefers amino acids with bulky side-chains (i.e.

branched and aromatic groups). Alanine, serine and glutamine are preferred substrates for system A, and alanine, serine and cysteine for system ASC. Transport via systems A and ASC is in symport with sodium ions and uses sodium entry down its electrochemical gradient as a driving force. System L is not sodium linked and may, in many circumstances, mediate amino acid efflux from cells. System y^+ mediates high-affinity sodium-independent transport of cationic amino acids as well as sodium-dependent transport of neutral amino acids. System X_{AG}^- transports glutamate or aspartate together with sodium into the cell and potassium out of the cell. For a more complete review, see Hyde *et al.* (2003).

In addition to these fairly ubiquitous transporters, mention should be made of system B° (ASCT2, SLC1A5) and related systems, which are found on the apical poles of epithelial cells, such as in the intestine and kidney. These effect the sodium-dependent accumulation of a broad range of neutral amino acids, including those transported, in other cells, by system L. Transport of glutamine, asparagine and histidine occurs via a sodium-dependent system N in hepatocytes and system N^m in skeletal muscle. It is thought that the massive loss of glutamine from skeletal muscle during catabolic illness occurs via system N^m. It should be emphasised that the amino acid transporters are described in general terms and represent only a fraction of those that have been identified. In addition, with the continuing application of molecular techniques many more of these transporters may be discovered. Chapter 8 of this volume deals in greater detail with amino acid transporters of importance to brain function.

Peptide transporters

Peptide transporters have been identified that transport dipeptides and tripeptides in intestinal and renal epithelia. PEPT1 is expressed in the intestine and, to a lesser degree, in the kidney. PEPT2 is found only in the kidney. These transporters have quite broad specificity with respect to the amino acid composition of the dipeptides and tripeptides transported, but they will not transport amino acids or tetrapeptides. The peptide transport occurs together with a hydrogen ion; the driving force for peptide accumulation is the transmembrane electrochemical H^+ gradient. These peptides are hydrolysed to amino acids within renal and intestinal cells. The peptide transporters are also

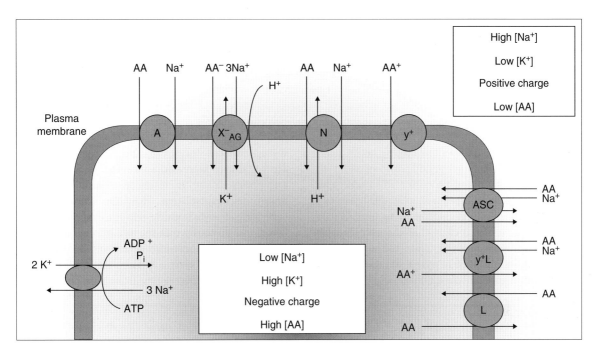

Figure 5.10 Transport mechanisms involved in the maintenance of transmembrane gradients of amino acids. The amino acid transport systems shown differ in terms of transport mechanism, regulatory properties and substrate specificity. The Na$^+$/K$^+$-ATP^{ase} (on the left) is a primary active transporter and helps to maintain transmembrane Na$^+$ and K$^+$ gradients. Secondary active transporters, such as systems A, N and ASC, couple amino acid transport to the sodium gradient. Facilitated transporters, such as system L, permit neutral amino acids to move down their concentration gradient. (Reproduced with permission from Hyde, Taylor & Hundal, 2003, Biochem J 373, 1–18. © The Biochemical Society. http://www.biochemj.org)

Table 5.10 Some major amino acid transport systems in mammalian cells

System	Protein	Gene	Substrate
A	SAT1–3	SLC38A1,2,4	Small neutral
ASC	ASCT1,2	SLC1A4,5	A S C
N	SN1,2	SLC38A3,5	Q N H
L	LAT1,2	SLC7A5,8	Large hydrophobic
Y$^+$	Cat1,2,3,4	SLC7A1–4	R K H
X$_{AG}^-$	EAAT1–5	SLC1A1–3,6,7	E D
Y$^+$L	Y$^+$LAT1,2	SLC7A6,7	K R Q H M L

of considerable pharmacological importance as they transport a number of drugs, including cephalosporins and penicillins, which contain peptide-like structures.

Physiological function and regulation of amino acid and peptide transport

The most obvious function of the amino acid and peptide transporters is in the absorption of amino acids from the intestine, the reabsorption of filtered amino acids in the kidney, and the cellular uptake and interorgan metabolism of amino acids. Amino acid transporters also play important roles in the maintenance of cell volume. Transepithelial amino acid transport (e.g. in the intestine and kidney) requires two amino acid transporters, one on the apical (brush-border) membrane and the other on the basolateral membrane. These two transporters are, invariably, distinct. In the intestine, the combination of amino acid and peptide transporters is responsible for the absorption of about 160 g of amino acids per day, comprising about 100 g of dietary protein and about 60 g from intestinal secretions and sloughed cells. In the intestine, the peptide transporters are quantitatively more important than the amino acid transporters.

The total plasma amino acid concentration is about 2.5 mmol/l, and the glomerular filtration rate, in humans, is about 180 l/day. Therefore, it can be calculated that the renal amino acid transporters reabsorb about 450 mmoles of amino acids per day (equivalent to the amino acids in about 45 g of protein). In the absence of reliable data on the plasma concentrations of dipeptides and tripeptides a similar calculation cannot be made for the amount of peptide transport in the kidney, but it is believed to be much less than amino acid transport. It should be noted that the brush-border membranes of the cells of the proximal tubule contain highly active peptidases that can attack larger peptides and small filtered proteins, and that these processes will make additional dipeptides and tripeptides available to the peptide transporters, but it is difficult to quantify this activity. However, it is clear that the renal peptide transport systems will play a major role in the hydrolysis of peptides provided in parenteral nutrition.

In addition to facilitating amino acid uptake and output by cells, amino acid transporters may exercise control on such amino acid traffic. It has already been indicated that the loss of glutamine from skeletal muscle during catabolic illness is attributable to the system N^m transporter. The hepatic uptake of alanine may be limited by its transport. Competition between large neutral amino acids limits their uptake into the brain (Chapter 8). The capacity of many of these transport systems is also controlled. Perhaps the best examples come from system A, whose activity, in a variety of tissues, can be made to vary markedly. For example, hepatic system A activity is up-regulated in diabetes and during starvation as well as by the administration of glucorticoids and interleukin-6 (IL-6), and by both glucagon and insulin. Its expression is decreased by growth hormone.

There are three well-described situations where system A is markedly up-regulated in almost all cells: adaptive regulation, hypertonicity and cell proliferation. In each of these situations the up-regulation requires protein synthesis. Adaptive regulation refers to the increase in system A activity that becomes apparent when cells are placed in a medium lacking system A substrates. (Conversely, system A activity is down-regulated when cells are transferred to an amino acid-rich medium.) This mechanism relates to the fundamental nutritional needs of cells as the up-regulation helps cells to cope with a limited extracellular availability of amino acids. System A also shows remarkable sensitivity to osmotic pressure. Cells shrink when placed in a hypertonic medium but, after some time, exhibit a regulatory volume increase in which up-regulation of system A and the expansion of the amino acid pool play a key role in the restoration of cell volume. System A can also regulate cell volume during isotonic conditions. In particular, increased system A activity has been implicated in the increased cell volume associated with cell proliferation. System A is up-regulated as cells leave the G_0 phase and enter the cell cycle, while the marked increase in cell volume in the G_1 and S phases is attributable to increased accumulation of potassium and amino acids. These effects expand the role of amino acid transporters, from the simplest one of supplying cells with amino acid substrates for metabolism and protein synthesis, to a more complex and fundamental role in osmoregulation. The signalling pathway whereby system A is enhanced in these conditions is, currently, a highly active research field.

Genetic diseases of plasma amino acid transport

Various amino acid transport disorders are known. These have provided valuable knowledge about the transport process as well as providing nutritional challenges for patient care. Cystinuria is an autosomal recessive disease, often associated with increased urinary loss of cationic amino acids that share a transporter with cystine. The intestinal transport mechanisms for the absorption of cystine and the cationic amino acids are also often defective in cystinuria; however, this appears to have no nutritional consequences owing to alternative uptake mechanisms. Hartnup disorder is an autosomal recessive impairment of neutral amino acid reabsorption in the kidney. Defective transport is also evident in the intestine. Lysinuric protein intolerance is an autosomal recessive disease associated with greatly increased urinary excretion of lysine, arginine and ornithine. These amino acids are also poorly absorbed in the intestine. The transport defect is localised in the basolateral membrane of these epithelia. The condition is associated with intolerance and rejection of high-protein food as well as hyper-ammonaemia, which has been attributed to impaired urea synthesis. Other amino acid transporter defects include aminoaciduria, characterised by increased urinary excretion of glycine, proline and hydroxyproline, and dicarboxylate aminoaciduria, characterised by massive urinary excretion of glutamate and aspartate. It is obvious that most of these genetic transporter diseases have been discovered as a result of increased urinary amino acid excretion. It may be assumed that comparable defects occur in which the lesion is exclusively expressed in internal organs but which have not yet been discovered because of the lack of so convenient a means for their identification.

5.16 Disposal of dietary amino acids and roles of specific organs

With the continuous turnover of proteins and movement of amino acids between organs there is an inevitable and irreversible loss of indispensable amino acids and of end-products of nitrogen metabolism. Hence, a dietary supply of indispensable amino acids in adequate amounts and proportions, together with suitable carbon and nitrogen sources that can be used to synthesise dispensable and conditionally indispensable amino acids, is needed to maintain this dynamic state of protein turnover and cell and organ function. It is necessary, therefore, to consider here the metabolism of amino acids entering from the diet.

Events in the intestine

The digestion and absorption of dietary protein is dealt with in detail in Chapter 10. In terms of quantitation, it is important to appreciate that, although an adult may ingest some 100 g of protein per day, the quantity digested and absorbed is much greater than this. It is estimated that approximately another 70 g arises in the intestine as a result of the sloughing of mucosal cells and the protein content of secreted juices. Since faecal nitrogen is equivalent to some 10 g of protein daily, it follows that about 160 g of protein might be available for digestion and absorption per day. However, it is not known at this time how the enteric microbiota would influence this calculation.

It is now apparent that the small intestine is a major site of amino acid catabolism and, in the fed state, can obtain a significant amount of its energy requirements from this process. As much as 90% of dietary glutamate and aspartate and much glutamine are catabolised within the small intestinal mucosa in the first pass. In addition, appreciable quantities of indispensable amino acids (isoleucine, leucine, valine, lysine, methionine and phenylalanine) are catabolised.

There is also substantial metabolism of threonine, but this may be due largely to mucin synthesis (a threonine-rich protein) rather than catabolism. In the case of many of these amino acids, as much as 30–50% does not enter the hepatic portal circulation, so that intestinal metabolism is a major determinant of whole-body amino acid requirements. In addition, this phenomenon has important implications for amino acid nutrition during parenteral feeding, as the elimination of first pass intestinal metabolism means that indispensable amino acid requirements will be decreased.

Finally, it should be noted that intestinal amino acid catabolism is often not complete, and products released into the hepatic portal vein include other amino acids such as alanine, citrulline and proline. It is clear that first-pass intestinal metabolism substantially modifies the pattern of amino acids that are available to the rest of the body.

Role of the liver

The liver has long been recognised as the principal organ that metabolises dietary amino acids. It is the only organ that contains the enzymic capacity to catabolise all of the amino acids, although its ability to metabolise branched-chain amino acids is limited. It also contains the urea cycle, so that ammonia arising from amino acid catabolism can be readily detoxified. Indeed, the ammonia concentration in the hepatic venous blood that exits the liver is much lower than in the blood that enters via the hepatic portal vein, which is enriched in ammonia partly as a result of bacterial activity in the intestine. However, ammonia detoxification cannot be entirely attributed to urea synthesis. It is now apparent that there are two hepatic processes that remove ammonia: urea synthesis and glutamine synthesis. Furthermore, these two processes do not occur in the same liver cells. The enzymes of the urea cycle are found in the periportal and central hepatocytes, whereas glutamine synthetase is restricted to the perivenous hepatocytes, where it can serve to scavenge ammonia that escapes detoxification in the earlier part of the hepatic acinus (Figure 5.11). As the K_m of glutamine synthetase for ammonia is much lower than that of carbamylphosphate synthetase 1, the hepatic ammonia detoxification system can be thought of as a low-affinity, high-capacity system (urea synthesis) in series with a high-affinity, low-capacity system (glutamine

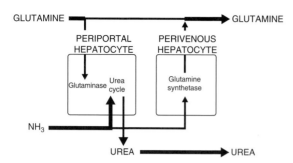

Figure 5.11 The intercellular hepatic glutamine cycle. Urea synthesis in periportal cells and glutamine synthesis in perivenous cells provide an in-series (fail-safe) system for ammonia removal by liver.

synthesis). These two systems, together, are responsible for the very low levels of ammonia that are normally found in the systemic circulation.

The capacity of the liver for urea synthesis is very high, so that it can readily respond to increased substrate supply. In addition, there are important acute and long-term controls that act on this process (see also Chapter 4 of *Introduction to Human Nutrition* in this series). The principal acute regulation occurs via changes in the concentration of *N*-acetylglutamate, an obligatory activator of carbamylphosphate synthetase-1, the first enzyme of urea synthesis. Levels of *N*-acetylglutamate can change very rapidly and are very responsive to protein intake. The mechanism by which *N*-acetylglutamate increases rapidly in response to a high-protein meal is not clear, but it is known that glucagon can rapidly increase the hepatic concentration of this regulator. Long-term regulation of the urea cycle occurs via alterations in the activities of its enzymes in response to changes in habitual protein intake or to endogenous protein catabolism. These enzymes are not known to be regulated by covalent modification and changes in their activities are due to corresponding changes in the amounts of the enzyme proteins. A variety of mechanisms underlies these alterations in enzyme activity. Certainly, altered rates of gene transcription (mediated by glucagon and glucocorticoids) play a major role, but other mechanisms, such as alterations in mRNA translation and protein stability, may also be important.

Traditionally, urea was thought of as a classical end-product. It is now apparent, however, that there is appreciable recycling of urea nitrogen. Urea diffuses into the intestinal lumen and is also a constituent of pancreatic and biliary secretions. This urea is hydrolysed by urease-containing gut bacteria and much of the ammonia is returned to the body in the hepatic portal vein. It is estimated that approximately 25% of total hepatic urea production is recycled in this way. As discussed in Chapter 4 of *Introduction to Human Nutrition*, the extent to which this recycled nitrogen contributes to nitrogen retention is still unclear.

Amino acid oxidation provides a substantial fraction of the body's energy. The oxidation of the amino acids in 100 g of protein requires the consumption of about 5 moles of oxygen. This compares with a consumption of approximately 3 moles of oxygen per day by the typical adult liver. Clearly, the traditional textbook description of amino acid oxidation, that dietary amino acids are almost completely oxidised in the liver, cannot be true. Even if the dietary amino acids were the liver's only fuel, their oxidation would require more oxygen than the liver actually consumes and would produce more ATP than the liver could use. The solution to this conundrum is two-fold. First, there is substantial extrahepatic amino acid oxidation and, secondly, many of the amino acids metabolised by the liver are only partially oxidised there; their carbon chains are converted to glucose or to the ketone bodies that are released and may be oxidised by other tissues. The principal extrahepatic tissues for amino acid catabolism are the small intestine (see above), skeletal muscle and kidney.

The liver removes about two-thirds of the absorbed amino acids. Of these, perhaps as much as two-thirds are metabolised and one-third is used for protein synthesis, of both plasma proteins and hepatic protein, which undergoes a temporary post-prandial increase. About one-third of the absorbed amino acids, enriched in the branched-chain amino acids, reach the peripheral tissues.

Skeletal muscle and kidney

Skeletal muscle plays a crucial role in branched-chain amino acid catabolism. The first two enzymes in their catabolism (the branched-chain aminotransferase and the branched-chain α-keto acid dehydrogenase) are common to the catabolism of each of the three branched-chain amino acids. The liver has very low activities of the aminotransferase, so that almost all dietary branched-chain amino acids are delivered to the systemic circulation. Skeletal muscle, which has substantial activities of both enzymes, is the major catabolic organ for these amino acids. The nitrogenous end-products are glutamine and alanine, which are released from muscle. In some animals (e.g. the rat) many of the branched-chain keto acids produced by transamination are released from the muscle and metabolised in the liver. However, it is evident that in humans the bulk of these α-keto acids are metabolised within the muscle.

The kidney uses amino acid metabolism to maintain acid–base status. The two sulphur-containing amino acids, methionine and cysteine, generate sulphuric acid on oxidation (equations 5.1 and 5.2).

$$2C_5O_2NH_{11}S \text{ (methionine)} + 15O_2 \rightarrow (NH_2)_2CO$$
$$\text{(urea)} + 9CO_2 + 7H_2O + 4H^+ + 2SO_4^{2-} \quad (5.1)$$

$$2C_3O_2NH_7S \text{ (cysteine)} + 9O_2 \rightarrow (NH_2)_2CO$$
$$\text{(urea)} + 5CO_2 + 3H_2O + 4H^+ + 2SO_4^{2-} \quad (5.2)$$

In an individual ingesting 100 g of protein a day these reactions can amount to some 60–70 mmoles of hydrogen ions per day. This production of acid cannot be considered in isolation, as it will be offset by any base produced from other dietary constituents, such as from the oxidation of alkali salts of carboxylic acids, which are abundant in fruits. Most individuals on a typical Western diet will have a net daily generation of about 30 mmoles of hydrogen ions. Significant concentrations of hydrogen ions are not allowed to accumulate; they are promptly neutralised by the blood bicarbonate buffer system (equation 5.3).

$$H^+ + HCO_3^- \leftrightarrow H_2CO_3 \leftrightarrow H_2O + CO_2 \quad (5.3)$$

However, the buffering of 30 mmoles of hydrogen ions amounts to a daily bicarbonate loss of similar magnitude. A process that can regenerate bicarbonate is necessary. Such a process, involving amino acid metabolism, is found in the kidney (Figure 5.12). The principle behind the process is simple. The kidney does not contain a urea cycle, so amino acid nitrogen gives rise to ammonium. Metabolism of a neutral amino acid to a neutral end-product (e.g. carbon dioxide or glucose) will produce, as end-products, NH_4^+ and HCO_3^-. Transport processes within the renal tubules effect the separation of NH_4^+ from HCO_3^- such that NH_4^+ is excreted in the urine while HCO_3^- is returned to the body via the renal vein (Figure 5.12). This regenerates the bicarbonate

Figure 5.12 Renal glutamine uptake, ammonium excretion and bicarbonate regeneration.

that was lost when hydrogen ions were buffered. In addition to glutamine, glycine is used as a source of NH_4^+ and HCO_3^-. However, glutamine is the predominant substrate in situations where there is massive acid production, such as diabetic ketoacidosis. In human kidneys, the carbon skeleton of glutamine is converted to glucose via renal gluconeogenesis.

5.17 Catabolic illnesses

As mentioned above, patients suffering from burn injuries, cancer, trauma or sepsis, or who have undergone major surgery frequently have greatly increased rates of protein turnover and catabolism. The origins of these catabolic states are complex and anorexia may play a role. However, if so, anorexia only plays a minor role since the provision of nutrients by way of intravenous nutrition does not arrest the catabolism. These pathological catabolic conditions are clearly different from the physiological response to starvation, where lipid oxidation provides the bulk of the energy and protein catabolism is somewhat restrained. The pathological catabolic states are characterised by massive loss of lean body mass (muscle protein catabolism) as well as high rates of lipolysis and fat oxidation. They are also often accompanied by hypermetabolism (increased resting energy expenditure). Circulating levels of cortisol, glucagon, epinephrine and tumour necrosis factor (TNFα) are invariably elevated and many of the features of the muscle protein catabolism can be reproduced by infusions of these hormones. Of these hormones, cortisol appears to be an important contributor to the catabolic state, with the protein imbalance being further increased by a decreased concentration or responsiveness to various anabolic hormones, such as growth hormone or insulin-like growth factor 1.

Thus, a high rate of protein and amino acid turnover in catabolic illness inevitably means a relatively high requirement for nitrogen and for specific amino acids. Indeed, rates of turnover (or flux) of nitrogen and indispensable amino acids as well as their oxidation rates in patients suffering from burn injury, for example, are generally much higher than in healthy adults. The turnover of protein amounts to about 7.3 g protein/kg per day in severely burned patients, in comparison with the healthy adult where turnover approximates 4 g protein/kg per day.

Another relationship of both metabolic and nutritional interest is that between energy metabolism and the rate of whole-body protein turnover. As mentioned earlier, protein synthesis, amino acid transport and protein breakdown are all energy-dependent processes. While their energy requirements differ, it can be estimated that in normal adults amino acid transport and protein synthesis alone appear to account for at least 20% of basal energy metabolism. It follows, once again, that major changes in body protein turnover due, for example, to severe infection or major trauma affect not only the protein and amino acid utilisation and requirements but also the status of body energy expenditure and requirements. In adult burn patients, the increased rate of protein turnover has also been estimated to account for about 20% of the increased metabolic rate characteristic of this stressful condition.

One of the most remarkable features of muscle metabolism in these conditions is the massive loss of free glutamine. Glutamine is the most abundant free amino acid in human skeletal muscle, being present at concentrations of about 20–25 µmol/l (Table 5.9). During these catabolic illnesses it can decrease to as little as 8–10 mmol. This is quite specific for glutamine; the other free amino acid pools of muscle are not comparably decreased. The importance of glutamine depletion relates to evidence, from *in vitro* studies with rat muscle, that intracellular glutamine may exert some control of protein synthesis and degradation. High glutamine concentrations favour net protein accretion and lower concentrations favour net proteolysis. The mechanism whereby glutamine may bring this about is uncertain, but it may be related to osmotically induced changes in cell volume.

The increased muscle protein catabolism and glutamine efflux seen in these catabolic conditions serve functions that are designed to improve the

organism's survival. Glutamine is directed to the liver where, with other amino acids, it serves as a gluconeogenic precursor, and to rapidly dividing cells, cells of the immune system and wounded tissue, where it is used as a metabolic fuel and a precursor for nucleotide synthesis. The increased gluconeogenesis seen in these situations often leads to hyperglycaemia, which may serve the physiological role of increasing the delivery of glucose to poorly perfused wounded tissue, since glucose is the preferred fuel of tissues with limiting oxygen delivery. The hyperglycaemia may also maintain glucose delivery to the brain in situations where its perfusion is decreased due to shock. Arginine delivery to macrophages will be used for the synthesis of nitric oxide, which is used by these cells as a bacteriocidal agent. In addition, these amino acids will be used for repair of damaged tissue and by the liver for increased synthesis of acute-phase proteins. Despite these beneficial functions of muscle protein catabolism, it is apparent that when the catabolism is excessive it can contribute to increased mortality and morbidity. For this reason, many studies have provided substantial amounts of glutamine (either as free glutamine or in peptide form) to such patients in attempts to replace muscle glutamine and to arrest or reverse the loss of lean body mass. Beneficial results, such as improved nitrogen balance and gut integrity and reduced rates of infection while in hospital, have been reported.

Another point to note, of particular interest in surgical metabolism and nutrition, relates to the post-translational modifications of protein mentioned earlier. Thus, there is a methylation of histidine residues within actin and myosin, the major fibrillar proteins in skeletal muscle. Since the 3-methylhistidine released during the degradation of myosin and actin is not further metabolised to any extent or reabsorbed by the renal tubule, it is largely excreted via the urine unchanged. Hence, its rate of output serves as an index of the approximate rate of muscle myofibrillar protein degradation. This technique offers a relatively simple *in vivo*, non-invasive index of protein breakdown that can be used to provide an understanding of the *in vivo* regulation of muscle protein degradation and its response to nutritional and pharmacological treatment. In addition, methylated derivatives of arginine occur in many proteins and they are also excreted in urine when the proteins are degraded. In particular, it has been shown that asymmetric

($N^G N^G$)-dimethyl-L-arginine (ADMA), another product of proteolysis, can be produced in quantities that inhibit nitric oxide synthase. Nitric oxide is one of the major endothelium-derived vasoactive mediators. Excess ADMA has been reported to occur in patients with hypertension and with chronic heart failure. Thus these two examples of modified amino acids further illustrate the intimate relationship between protein turnover, amino acid metabolism and function in chronic illness.

5.18 Non-proteinogenic metabolic functions of amino acids

In addition to their roles as substrates for protein synthesis and as regulators of protein turnover, amino acids display more functional diversity than any of the other major nutrients. They are extraordinarily important in the brain as neurotransmitters (glutamate, glycine) and as neurotransmitter precursors (tyrosine, tryptophan, histidine, glutamate, cysteine). These issues are discussed in Chapter 8 of this volume. In the other tissues of the body, amino acids also play crucial roles in metabolism and biosynthesis (Table 5.11).

Many of the dispensable amino acids are involved in high-capacity metabolic fluxes. For example, the malate–aspartate shuttle is the principal means of oxidising NADH generated in the cytoplasm during glycolysis and, therefore, is involved in the oxidation of some 200–400 g of carbohydrate per day, in most adults. Glutamate is involved in the transamination of almost all of the amino acids and, thus, in the metabolic disposal of about 100 g of protein per day (on a typical Western diet). Alanine is the major vehicle for shuttling nitrogen to the liver after amino acid catabolism in muscle or intestine. There is a very high rate of glutamine synthesis and degradation (40–80 g/day in adults), which is only partly explained by the fact that glutamine is a major fuel for intestinal cells and for cells of the immune system. Arginine is involved in the synthesis of some 30 g of urea per day (on a typical Western diet). Aspartate is the immediate source of half of the nitrogen in urea. It could be argued that the magnitude of the fluxes involved in these processes obliged the retention of pathways for the synthesis of these amino acids. However, both dispensable and indispensable amino acids play key

Table 5.11 Some biochemical functions of amino acids

Amino acid	Functions
Alanine	Nitrogen transport in blood
Arginine	Urea cycle intermediate
	Substrate for nitric oxide synthesis
	Substrate for creatine synthesis
	Substrate for polyamine synthesis
Aspartate	Nitrogen donor for urea synthesis
	Substrate for purine and pyrimidine synthesis
Cysteine	Substrate for glutathione synthesis
	Substrate for taurine synthesis
Glutamate	Partner in transamination reactions
	Neurotransmitter
	Substrate for glutathione synthesis
	Precursor for GABA synthesis
	Agonist for umami taste receptor
Glutamine	Nitrogen donor for purine, pyrimidine and amino sugar synthesis
	Acid–base balance: source of urinary ammonia
	Metabolic fuel for enterocytes and cells of the immune system
	Nitrogen transport in blood
	Substrate for citrulline and arginine synthesis in gut
Glycine	Bile salt synthesis
	Substrate for haem synthesis
	Neurotransmitter
	Source of methylene groups for one-carbon pool
	Substrate for creatine synthesis
Histidine	Precursor of histamine
Methionine	Major methyl donor via S-adenosylmethionine
	Substrate for polyamine synthesis via decarboxylated S-adenosylmethionine
Serine	Source of hydroxymethylene groups for the one-carbon pool
	Precursor in phospholipid and sphingosine biosynthesis
Tryptophan	Precursor for serotonin synthesis
Tyrosine	Precursor for epinephrine (adrenaline), norepinephrine (noradrenaline) and dopamine synthesis

roles in many lower flux pathways. Some of these are given in Table 5.11. Three aspects of amino acids that are of particular interest are selected here. These are the role of methionine as a methyl donor, the biosynthesis of creatine, and the synthesis and function of glutathione.

Methionine metabolism

The metabolism of methionine provides an excellent example of:

- a key amino acid function (methylation)
- the crucial involvement of vitamin-derived cofactors

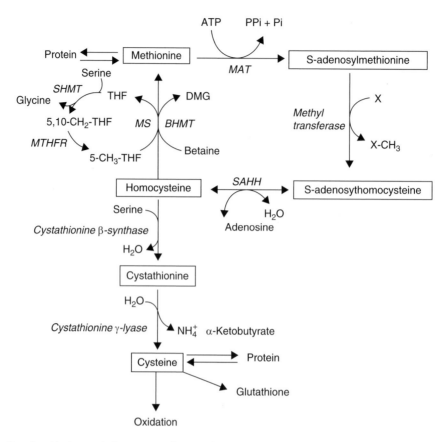

Figure 5.13 Outline of methionine metabolism. MAT: methionine adenosyltransferase; SHMT: serine hydroxymethyltransferase; MTHFR: 5,10-methylenetetrahydrofolate reductase; MS: methionine synthase; BHMT: betaine: homocysteine, methyltransferase; SAHH: *S*-adenosylhomocysteine hydrolase; THF: tetrahydrofolate reductase; DMG: dimethylglycine

- the adaptation of metabolic fluxes to nutritional conditions
- the influence of a common genetic polymorphism on metabolism.

It also provides insight into factors that affect the production of homocysteine, which has been identified as an important risk factor for cardiovascular disease. Figure 5.13 shows an outline of the major pathways of methionine metabolism. In fact, Figure 5.13 depicts two separate pathways: the catabolism of methionine via the transsulphuration pathway and the methionine cycle. Probably all cells have the methionine cycle, while the transsulphuration pathway, which converts homocysteine to cysteine, is most active in the liver but is also found in the kidney, intestine and pancreas.

The methionine cycle describes the reactions whereby the methyl group of methionine is used in methylation reactions and then regenerated, while preserving the carbon skeleton of this indispensable amino acid. The reactions involve the conversion of methionine to *S*-adenosylmethionine, which serves as a universal methylating agent in more than 50 different methyltransferases. Examples of such methyltransferases are found in the synthesis of epinephrine, creatine and phosphatidylcholine, and in the methylation of DNA, RNA and protein. *S*-adenosylhomocysteine, produced in these methylation reactions, is hydrolysed to adenosine and homocysteine. To complete the cycle, homocysteine is remethylated to methionine by one of two enzymes: either by the ubiquitously distributed methionine synthase, which uses 5-methyltetrahydrofolate (5-methyl THF) as the methyl donor, or by betaine methyltransferase, which is restricted to the liver and the kidney. Betaine arises from the catabolism of choline. The transsulphuration pathway affects the catabolism of methionine. Homocysteine is removed from the cycle and converted to cysteine by the successive actions of cystathionine β-synthase and cystathionine γ-lyase. An important feature of these pathways is the role of vitamin-derived cofactors. Methionine synthase has methylcobalamin as its cofactor; both cystathionine β-synthase and cystathionine γ-lyase contain pyridoxal phosphate. In addition, methionine synthase utilises a methyl group from the folic acid–one-carbon pool.

In Figure 5.13 it can be seen that homocysteine sits at a metabolic crossroads as it may be reconverted to methionine or catabolised to cysteine. Careful balance data and isotopic measurements of methionine's fate in both humans and rats show that the partitioning of homocysteine between remethylation and transsulphuration depends on the dietary supply of methyl groups. When methionine and choline intake is low, homocysteine is predominantly remethylated. However, when dietary methyl groups, in the form of methionine and choline, are abundant, remethylation is decreased and flux through the transsulphuration pathway is increased.

Since the early 1990s, convincing epidemiological evidence has accumulated to support the proposition that elevated plasma homocysteine is an important risk factor for cardiovascular disease. This has stimulated a great deal of interest in factors that affect the plasma level of homocysteine. Deficiencies in the B vitamins important in methionine metabolism (folic acid, vitamin B_{12} and pyridoxal) are all associated with elevated plasma homocysteine. Of these, it is apparent that folic acid deficiency is the most important contributor to hyperhomocystinaemia. Indeed, the US 'national' plasma homocysteine level has decreased by some 5–10% since the advent of folic acid fortification.

Finally, the metabolism of methionine and homocysteine provides a remarkable example of the influence of common genetic polymorphisms. Methylenetetrahydrofolate reductase (MTHFR) reduces 5,10-methylene THF to 5-methyl THF, which is used by methionine synthase to remethylate homocysteine to methionine (Figure 5.13). An MTHFR polymorphism (C677T), in which alanine-222 is replaced by valine, is remarkably common. Indeed, in most populations that have been examined, homozygosity for this polymorphism varies from 4 to 24%.

Individuals with this variant tend to have an increased folate requirement, as well as increased plasma homocysteine because of impaired provision of 5-methyl THF for methionine synthase. Whether or not this genetic polymorphism is a risk factor for cardiovascular disease is controversial, but there is no question that the C677T polymorphism predisposes to neural tube defects.

Creatine synthesis

Creatine synthesis provides an excellent example of amino acids as biosynthetic precursors. It is also a pathway that consumes substantial amounts of arginine and methyl groups. An adult human loses some 1–2 g of creatinine per day in the urine. This creatinine arises from the spontaneous breakdown of both creatine and phosphocreatine. Creatine synthesis (which replaces the loss) involves three different amino acids, but only two enzymes. The first step (equation 5.4) is catalysed by arginine, glycine amidinotransferase:

$$\text{glycine + arginine} \rightarrow \text{guanidinoacetate} \\ \text{+ ornithine} \qquad (5.4)$$

The second reaction is catalysed by guanidinoacetate methyltransferase (equation 4.5):

$$\text{guanidinoacetate} + S\text{-adenosylmethionine} \\ \rightarrow \text{creatine} + S\text{-adenosylhomocysteine} \quad (5.5)$$

These two enzymes occur in different tissues: the amidinotransferase is most abundant in the kidney and absent from the liver, while the methyltransferase is largely restricted to the liver. Thus, creatine synthesis is an interorgan process in which guanidinoacetate is released by the kidney and taken up by the liver. Creatine synthesis makes major demands on arginine and on methyl groups. It can be calculated that an 18–29-year-old male requires about 2.5 g of arginine per day for creatine synthesis. This is about 50% of dietary arginine if he ingests 100 g protein/day. Creatine synthesis is also a major consumer of methyl groups. Indeed, the methylation of guanidinoacetate uses approximately 40% of physiologically labile methyl groups.

Glutathione

Glutathione provides an excellent example of a key amino acid-derived molecule whose synthesis may be restricted, in certain nutritional and pathological conditions, by the availability of its amino acid constituents and whose function is determined by an inorganic micronutrient, selenium. Glutathione is a tripeptide (L-γ-glutamyl-L-cysteinylglycine) composed of three amino acids in which the glutamate is joined to cysteine by an unusual iso-peptide linkage. It plays a number of roles within cells in such diverse areas as:

• conjugation and elimination of xenobiotics
• covalent modification of protein via gluta-thionylation
• transfer of nitric oxide as *S*-nitrosoglutathione.

Glutathione is also the major low molecular weight thiol in animal cells and, as such, serves both as a redox buffer and as an agent for the detoxification of reactive oxygen species (ROS). The key to glutathione's function in these processes lies in its ability to undergo oxidation. Glutathione with a free thiol (GSH) can be oxidised to glutathione disulphide (GSSG). In cells most of the glutathione exists as GSH owing to the action of glutathione reductase (equation 5.6):

$$\text{NADPH} + \text{H}^+ + \text{GSSG} \rightarrow \text{NADP}^+ + 2\text{GSH} \quad (5.6)$$

The NADPH is provided by the pentose phosphate pathway. Glutathione plays a major role in the destruction of hydrogen peroxide (equation 5.7) and a variety of organic hydroperoxides (equation 5.8) via the action of glutathione peroxidase:

$$2\text{GSH} + \text{H}_2\text{O}_2 \rightarrow \text{GSSG} + 2\text{H}_2\text{O} \quad (5.7)$$

$$2\text{GSH} + \text{ROOH} \rightarrow \text{GSSG} + \text{H}_2\text{O} + \text{ROH} \quad (5.8)$$

Hydrogen peroxide arises from a variety of reactions, including the scavenging of superoxide radicals by superoxide dismutase. Organic hydroperoxides arise from lipid peroxidation of polyunsaturated fatty acids. Thus, glutathione can deal with a variety of ROS. It can also prevent lipid peroxidation because of its ability to scavenge free radicals, such as those that propagate lipid peroxidation. Glutathione, therefore, is part of the cell's defence against oxidative stress. Depletion of glutathione or excessive production of ROS is associated with peroxidative cell damage in a variety of pathological conditions.

Glutathione peroxidase contains selenium in the form of an unusual amino acid, selenocysteine. The

selenium replaces the sulphur atom of cysteine. Synthesis of selenocysteine occurs on its cognate tRNA and it is incorporated into selenoproteins during their synthesis. The activity of glutathione peroxidase is therefore greatly reduced in selenium deficiency, with a consequent increased susceptibility to an oxidative challenge. Recent work has examined red blood cell glutathione synthesis in humans. This is quite sensitive to sulphur amino acid availability. Patients infected with human immunodeficiency virus (HIV) have quite low erythrocyte GSH levels because of decreased erythrocyte cysteine concentrations: cysteine supplementation leads to an increased rate of GSH synthesis and an increase in the erythrocyte GSH concentration. Thus, precursor amino acid availability can determine the concentration of this key molecule.

5.19 Perspectives on the future

Protein synthesis, protein turnover and amino acid metabolism play major roles in the bodily economy. Isotopic and other techniques have revealed the magnitude of these fluxes. In a healthy adult human, some 300 g of new protein is synthesised each day and a comparable quantity of protein is catabolised. This compares with approximately 100 g of protein consumed per day on a typical Western diet. Protein synthesis and turnover are major components of resting energy expenditure. Such a high metabolic price underlies important functions, including adjusting to changes in the internal environment, tissue remodelling and the removal of mutant or damaged proteins. A crucial feature of these processes is their physiological selectivity, with regard to both individual proteins (rates of turnover of individual proteins vary by factors of over 1000) and individual tissues (e.g. catabolic illnesses are associated with a marked loss of muscle protein but with net increases in the rates of protein synthesis in cells of the immune system). Both protein synthesis and degradation are regulated, in complex ways, by amino acid availability and by hormones.

Amino acids serve as the building blocks of proteins and they also serve other functions. Thus, amino acid metabolism is an intimate component of the protein and nitrogen economy of the body. The catabolism of dietary amino acids is finely regulated by a variety of mechanisms. This is critical as the rate of amino acid catabolism is an important determinant of amino acid requirements. Gluconeogenesis, from muscle-derived amino acids, is a major component of the physiological response to starvation. Certain tissues have a specific requirement for certain amino acids. For example, intestinal cells and cells of the immune system require glutamine as an energy substrate; kidney requires glutamine for acid–base homeostasis; cells that produce nitric oxide, such as endothelial cells and macrophages, require arginine; the brain requires amino acids as neurotransmitter precursors; the kidney and liver combine to produce creatine from glycine, arginine and methionine; glutathione serves as a defence against ROS. Interorgan amino acid metabolism integrates these different tissue amino acid requirements. These interorgan amino acid fluxes are facilitated, and in some cases regulated, by specific amino acid transporters.

The study of proteins and amino acids continues to provide novel insights and stimulation for the nutritionist. Scarcely a year goes by without some major discovery that forces us to look at things in a new light. One of the most extraordinary of discoveries has been that of the production of nitric oxide from arginine and its many biological functions. It is now also understood that a retrovirus (the murine leukaemia virus) uses the y$^+$ amino acid transport system as its cell-surface receptor. Recently, it has been discovered that the brain contains a serine racemase that converts L-serine to D-serine, which may be used as a coagonist of the N-methyl-D-aspartate receptor. Hydrogen sulphide (H$_2$S), derived from the metabolism of the sulphur-containing amino acids, has recently been proposed to be a physiological cell regulator. It is a certainty that there will be more surprises. The sequencing of the human genome and that of other organisms has accelerated the pace of discovery and there can be no doubt that we will uncover spectacular new vistas in the field of amino acid and protein nutrition. There is also the possibility of genetic engineering. Will mammals or species of agricultural importance always require the same spectrum of indispensable amino acids? Genes that encode for threonine synthesis in bacteria have already been introduced into mouse cells such that these cells, in culture, no longer require exogenous

threonine. Could a similar approach be taken with intact animals, say with poultry, so that they could be fed a lower quality protein ration? Such approaches may be limited more by ethical and regulatory constraints than by technical ones.

Further reading

Bergstrom J *et al*. Intracellular free amino acid concentration in human muscle tissue. J Appl Physiol 1974; 36: 693–697.

Brosnan JT, Brosnan ME. Creatine: endogenous metabolite, dietary, and therapeutic supplement. Annu Rev Nutr 2007; 27: 241–261.

Carthew RW, Sontheimer EJ. Origins and mechanisms of miRNAs and siRNAs. Cell 2009; 136: 642–655.

Duggle SL, Waterlow JC. The end-product method of measuring whole-body protein turnover: a review of published results and a comparison with those obtained by leucine infusion. Brit J Nutr 2005; 94: 141–153.

Fafournoux P, Bruhat A, Jousse C. Amino acid regulation of gene expression. Biochem J 2000; 351: 1–12.

Felig P. Amino acid metabolism in man. Annu Rev Biochem 1975; 44: 933–955.

Garlick PJ, McNurlan MA. Isotopic methods for studying protein turnover. In: Protein Metabolism During Infancy (Railia NCR, ed.). Nestlé Nutrition Workshop Series Vol. 33, pp. 29–42. New York: Raven Press, 1994.

Garlick PJ, McNurlan MA, Essen P, Wernerman J. Measurement of tissue protein synthesis rates in vivo: a critical analysis of contrasting methods. Am J Physiol 1994; 266: E287–E297.

Hyde R, Taylor PM, Hundal HS. Amino acid transporters: roles in amino acid sensing and signaling in animal cells. Biochem J 2003; 373: 1–18.

Jennissen HP. Ubiquitin and the enigma of intracellular protein degradation. Eur J Biochem 1995; 231: 1–30.

Lecker SH, Goldberg AL, Mitch WE. Protein degradation by the ubiquitin-proteasome pathway in normal and disease states. J Am Soc Nephrol 2006; 17: 1807–1819.

Libao-Mercado AJ *et al*. Dietary and endogenous amino acids are the main contributors to microbial protein in the upper gut of normally nourished pigs. J Nutr 2009; 139: 1088–1094.

Seo J, Lee K-J. Post-translational modifications and their biological functions: proteomic analysis and systematic approaches. J Biochem Mol Biol 2004; 37: 35–44.

Shaw RJ. mTOR signaling: RAG GTPases transmit the amino acid signal. Trends Biochem Sci 2008; 33: 565–568.

Sonenberg N, Hinnebusch AG. Regulation of translation initiation in eukaryotes: mechanisms and biological targets. Cell 2009; 136: 731–745.

Watford M. Glutamine and glutamate metabolism across the liver sinusoid. J Nutr 2000; 130: 983S–987S.

Young VR *et al*. Amino acid kinetics in relation to protein and amino acid requirements: the primary importance of amino acid oxidation. In: Substrate and Energy Metabolism in Man (JS Garrow, D Halliday eds), pp. 119–133. London: John Libbey, 1985.

Zhao J *et al*. FoxO3 coordinately activates protein degradation by the autophagic/lysosomal and proteasomal pathways in atrophying muscle cells. Cell Metab 2007; 6: 472–483.

6
Pregnancy and Lactation

Joop MA van Raaij and Lisette CPGM de Groot

Key messages

Pregnancy
- There is growing evidence that foetus and young infants are protected from deficiencies in diets of their mothers.
- Critical periods during prenatal development have been identified in which specific nutrients, such as iodine, DHA, choline and folate, are required for optimal development. There are likely to be many more such critical nutrients
- Common genetic variations may influence nutrient requirements in pregnancy during critical periods. Single nucleotide polymorphisms (SNPs) have been shown to exist in pathways for the biosynthesis of DHA and of choline. Many more SNPs must influence metabolism and should be characterised.
- The approach to nutritional needs in pregnancy is mainly focused on the amount and composition of the pregnancy weight gain, on increased metabolism and on improved absorption rates.
- If the energy costs of pregnancy are to be covered solely by increased food intake, the mother should eat about 15% more than she did before her pregnancy. However, in observational studies, none or very small increments in food intake are observed. Whether this depends on the level of maternal nutritional status remains to be clarified.
- Since mothers have several options to meet the energy and nutrient needs of pregnancy, for example by increasing intakes, by decreasing physical activity or by limiting storage, there are good arguments against setting one specific recommendation for increased intake for all pregnant women.

Lactation
- Maintenance of milk production appears to be under feedback control by a substance called 'the feedback inhibitor of lactation', a polypeptide that is present in breast milk and enables women to adjust milk synthesis to the amount withdrawn by their infants.
- Breast milk changes in consistency during time. Initially, colostrum is produced, low in macronutrients but high in immunoglobulins. The concentrations of fat and lactose increase over time with transitional milk and mature breast milk.
- Breast-feeding confers several benefits on infants and is considered the perfect food for the normal infant, as long as the maternal system can sustain lactation and as long as there are no contraindications, such as the use of alcohol or certain medications by the mother.
- In well-nourished women, little relationship exists between maternal diet and milk production: Mothers appear to protect breast-feeding through the depletion of their own body stores.

6.1 Pregnancy

Introduction

Nutrition before and during pregnancy, and during lactation, can have significant effects on the short- and long-term health of mothers and their children. The potential impact of nutrition is greater at this time than during any other stage of life. Insufficient preconceptional energy stores may negatively affect ovulation and menses, and challenge the beginning of pregnancy. On the other hand, excessive fat stores may also make conceiving difficult by affecting ovulation

because of insensitivity to insulin, an excess of male sex hormones and the overproduction of leptin. A woman who enters pregnancy with an inadequate nutritional status risks having inadequate pregnancy performance, depleting her body's own stores of nutrients and of commencing lactation in a state of suboptimal nutrition, which may deteriorate further as lactation progresses. Similarly, women who enter pregnancy in an overweight or obese state have an increased risk of maternal complications during pregnancy, such as gestational hypertension, gestational diabetes, caesarean delivery, macrosomia and certain

Nutrition and Metabolism, Second Edition, edited by S. A. Lanham-New, I. A. Macdonald and H. M. Roche.   © 2011 The Nutrition Society.

birth defects. Infants who are undernourished in the womb are at risk of a variety of adverse outcomes, ranging from low birth weight to severe mental and physical retardation, and even death. Foetal undernourishment has also been linked to an increased prevalence of coronary heart disease, raised lipids, obesity and decreased glucose tolerance in adult life. Similarly, if the weight or fat mass increments of a foetus are too high, there may be short- and long-term adverse effects.

The effects of under- and overnutrition before and during pregnancy and lactation depend on the nutrient or nutrients involved and the stage at which under- or overnutrition occurs. Each stage of this part of the life cycle has specific tissue needs for nutrients, and shortcomings or surplus in the tissue supply of these nutrients may have undesirable consequences. The success of pregnancy and lactation involves other factors, such as the mother's age, the intake of substances such as alcohol, nicotine and drugs, the physical and emotional stresses to which she is subjected, and the presence of any infections or other diseases. This chapter, however, will concentrate mainly on aspects of nutrition.

Physiological stages of pregnancy and their nutritional demands

Pregnancy can be divided into three main physiological stages: implantation, organogenesis and growth.

Implantation

The implantation stage includes the first 2 weeks of gestation, when the fertilised ovum becomes embedded in the wall of the uterus. The nutrients provided by the secretions of the uterine gland pass directly into the fertilised ovum and developing embryo. Specific nutritional needs are undoubtedly required at this stage but, quantitatively speaking, these demands will be negligible.

Organogenesis

The next 6 weeks of pregnancy are known as the period of organogenesis or embryogenesis. During this stage, the cells of the embryo begin to differentiate into distinct tissues and functional units that later become organs, such as heart, lungs and liver. The development of the skeleton also begins at this time. During organogenesis, the foetus obtains nourishment mainly from the mother's blood. When organogenesis

is complete, the foetus weighs approximately 6 g and is less than 3 cm long.

Evidence from animal studies indicates that the presence of particular nutrients at specific times is crucial for the normal development of various tissues. There are critical periods of organogenesis during which the absence of certain nutrients can cause specific congenital abnormalities. For example, riboflavin deficiency during a critical period has been associated with poor skeletal formation, pyridoxine and manganese deficiencies with neuromotor problems, and vitamin B_{12}, vitamin A, niacin and folate deficiencies with defects in the central nervous system. Not surprisingly, little information is known on nutrient deficiencies and critical periods of organogenesis in humans. Recently, it has become clear that folate is important for the prevention of neural tube defects (NTD). NTDs occur when the brain and skull and/or the spinal cord and their protective spinal column do not develop properly within the first 4 weeks after conception. It has been shown that ample folate intake before and in early pregnancy may significantly reduce the risk of this form of foetal abnormality and so nowadays an extra folate intake as a supplement, or in the form of fortified foods at a level of 400 µg/day of folic acid, is recommended for at least 1 month before and 3 months after conception, in addition to consuming food folate from a varied diet.

Growth

The remaining 7 months of pregnancy are known as the growth period. Most of the nutrients for growth are delivered through the placenta. Blood does not flow directly from the mother's circulation to the foetal circulation. Altogether, about 10–11 m^2 of surface area are available for the transfer of materials between the placental and the foetal circulation. Free fatty acids and cholesterol can be transferred across the placenta by simple diffusion: carbohydrates (mainly glucose) cross by facilitated diffusion (diffusion assisted by the presence of a protein embedded in the membrane) and amino acids by active transport (transport against a concentration gradient powered by the release of cellular energy). Most water-soluble vitamins are present in the foetal circulation at higher concentrations than in the maternal circulation and so presumably enter the foetus by active transport. Fat-soluble vitamins are present at lower concentrations in the foetus than in the mother and probably enter the foetus by passive diffusion. Both calcium and iron cross the placenta by active transport, via mechanisms that are not well understood.

During the period of growth, the tissues and organs formed during organogenesis continue to grow and mature. Growth of the foetus occurs in three phases. During the first phase, known as hyperplasia, there is a rapid increase in the number of cells. The large numbers of cell divisions involved require sufficient supplies of folate and vitamin B_{12}. In the next phase, when cells are growing in size, cellular replication continues with hypertrophy. This requires sufficient supplies of amino acids and vitamin B_6. In the final phase of growth, hypertrophy or cellular growth predominates, whereas cellular division ceases.

Just as with the phase of organogenesis, little is known of the consequences of specific nutritional deficiencies in humans during the growth phase. What we do know is that inadequate nutrition during the growth phase may cause intra-uterine growth retardation (IuGR) and a low birth weight, but at this stage it will not cause the more serious abnormalities associated with deficiencies at earlier times. This is certainly not to say that IuGR can be considered to be a problem of minor importance. On the contrary, it should be clearly recognised that infants with low birth weights (i) show higher rates of morbidity and mortality, probably due to infectious diseases and impaired immunity, and (ii) are at increased risk of growth failure and abnormal cognitive development as infants. It should be noted, however, that a depression of growth during a temporary period of undernutrition is often compensated for by increased growth when nutrition becomes adequate again. This means that nutritional interventions in pregnancy during the growth phase of the foetus may still have beneficial effects on the growth performance of the foetus.

In summary, variations in the nutritional demands throughout pregnancy are evident. Inadequate food intakes in pregnancy, quantitatively and/or qualitatively, have obvious effects on pregnancy performance, in terms of weight gain and pregnancy outcome, but little is known of the consequences regarding deficiencies of individual nutrients.

Principles for estimating nutritional needs in pregnancy

Since little is known on the role of individual nutrients, it is not surprising that in the approach to nutri-

tional needs in pregnancy attention is focused on the amount and composition of pregnancy weight gain and altered metabolism. This so-called 'factorial approach' implies that due consideration must be made of the following fact: that the extra energy and nutrient needs imposed by pregnancy are over and above the baseline needs for non-pregnant, non-lactating women.

If recommendations are already in place, then a decision must be reached on what is considered an appropriate, or desirable, pregnancy weight gain. A desirable weight gain should result in a desirable pregnancy outcome, for example a full-term birth weight between 3 and 4 kg. However, the size of the desirable weight gain will also depend on the woman's weight before pregnancy. For a woman who is clearly underweight, a higher desirable weight gain should be projected than for an overweight woman of the same height.

In the remainder of this chapter, the energy content of the pregnancy weight gain and the increased energy metabolism in pregnancy will be discussed in this chapter.

Energy content of reference weight gain over pregnancy

In well-nourished women from affluent countries, with a pre-pregnant body weight between 60 and 65 kg, an average weight gain during pregnancy of 12.5 kg, and an average infant birth weight of 3.4 kg, is observed. The components of weight gain can be divided into three categories: (i) the products of conception, that is the foetus, amniotic fluid and placenta, (ii) the increased amounts of maternal tissues other than fat, that is extracellular fluid, uterus, breasts and blood, and (iii) the increased amount of fat stores. A representative proportion of the total weight gain during pregnancy that can be attributed to each of the components is shown in Table 6.1. The distribution of the total weight gain of 12 500 g over the four quarters of pregnancy is calculated on 650, 3350, 4500 and 4000 g, respectively.

This typical pregnancy weight gain, and composition of weight gain, was first described in the 1960s by Hytten and Leitch, who derived theoretical estimates of the extra nutritional needs from this outline. Since then, many national and international bodies have adopted this as a 'reference pregnancy' for developing recommended intakes in pregnancy.

Table 6.1 Components of weight gain over pregnancy

Products of conception	4850 g
Foetus	3400 g
Amniotic fluid	800 g
Placenta	650 g
Maternal tissues (excluding fat stores)	4305 g
Extracellular fluid	1680 g
Uterus and breasts	1375 g
Blood	1250 g
Maternal fat stores	3345 g
Fat stores	3345 g
Total weight gain	12 500 g

The energy equivalent of the reference weight gain is about 200 MJ for the 9-month period and is composed of two components: the energy deposited in fat stores, which is about 150 MJ (154 MJ based on 3345 g fat, at an energy cost of 46 kJ/g fat), and the energy deposited in other tissues such as foetus, placenta, uterus, breasts, amniotic fluid and blood, which is about 50 MJ (47 MJ based on 440 g fat and 925 g protein, at an energy cost of 46 kJ/g and 29 kJ/g).

Energy needs for maintaining the new metabolism

An increase in the maintenance of metabolism during pregnancy is approached by studying basal metabolic rate (BMR) throughout pregnancy. Measurements are made under standardised conditions (rest, post-absorption and thermoneutrality). Any increase in the maintenance of metabolism is calculated as the cumulative area under the curve, represented by the rise in a mother's BMR above the pre-pregnancy baseline metabolic rate.

Between populations, a wide variation was observed relating to accumulative increases in metabolic maintenance during pregnancy, for example +210 MJ in Swedish women to −45 MJ in unsupplemented Gambian women. When results from all available studies are combined, a good correlation appears between pregnancy weight gain and the cumulative increase of metabolic maintenance during pregnancy. For the reference weight gain of 12.5 kg, the increase in BMR is estimated to be about 160 MJ, which is very close to the estimate based on theoretical calculations by Hytten & Leitch (150 MJ), so for a reference pregnancy a total energy cost has been projected of approximately 360 MJ

(200 MJ energy content of weight gain plus 150 MJ for increased metabolism).

Physiological adjustments that may affect the energy and nutrient needs of pregnancy

Energy metabolism

Many studies have investigated whether basal metabolism, diet-induced thermogenesis (which refers to the increase in energy expenditure above basal metabolism after food ingestion) or the performance of physical exercise may be more efficient and energetic during pregnancy. There is, however, no convincing evidence for such 'energy-saving' mechanisms. Rather, it would appear that savings in energy expenditure are mainly realised by changes in the lowered pattern and pace of daily activity, and not by improvements in energy metabolism.

Protein metabolism

Shifts in protein metabolism are complex and change gradually throughout gestation so that nitrogen conservation for foetal growth achieves full potential during the last quarter of pregnancy. Studies of nitrogen balance in pregnant and non-pregnant women have revealed that there is no evidence to suggest that nitrogen deposit in early pregnancy will mobilised later. However, nitrogen retention is increased in late pregnancy and is due to a reduction in urinary nitrogen excretion. A decrease in urea synthesis seems to account for this reduction in urinary urea nitrogen and suggests that amino acids are conserved for tissue synthesis. As there is no evidence to suggest that pregnant women store protein in early pregnancy for later foetal demands, the increased requirements of late pregnancy might, at least in part, be met by physiological adjustments that enhance dietary protein utilisation. If the dietary supply is low, greater physiological adjustments are required to meet foetal needs than if the dietary intake is liberal. However, the extent to which low intakes of dietary protein may affect urea synthesis or circulating concentrations of amino acids is yet to be established in pregnant women. Presumably, maternal protein status at conception also influences the physiological adjustments made in nitrogen metabolism. Further research is needed into the study of nutrient metabolic adjustments in women who consume a marginal to adequate diet in order to fully understand the interactions between physiology of pregnancy, nutrient metabolism and maternal nutritional status.

Micronutrient metabolism

Although foetal demand for nutrients occurs primarily during the latter half of gestation when more than 90% of foetal growth occurs, adjustments in nutrient metabolism are apparent within the first weeks of pregnancy. There is an increase in the concentration of serum lipids during pregnancy, while circulating concentrations of most other nutrients have decreased by the end of the first 10 weeks of gestation, and remain lower than non-pregnant values until term. The decrease starts before there is an increase in plasma volume, and the reduction in later stages is less than the change in plasma volume. Thus, the total amount of vitamins and minerals in circulation increases during pregnancy.

For many nutrients, an increased absorption rate in pregnancy has been found, although the underlying mechanisms are yet to be clarified. These absorption rates will be taken into consideration when suggesting recommendations. Total plasma calcium levels fall very early in pregnancy, mediated by a fall in plasma albumin, as part of the process of haemodilution. However, ionised calcium and phosphate levels remain normal throughout. Plasma levels of 1,25-dihydroxy-D_3 are elevated early in pregnancy and remain elevated throughout. Intestinal calcium absorption doubles in pregnancy, probably owing to the changes in vitamin D status. The earliest study of calcium absorption was conducted at 12 weeks and even at this early stage the very dramatic rise in calcium absorption was noted. The observed elevation in 1,25-dihydroxy-D_3 is associated with an observed rise in calcium binding protein $_{9K}$-D. Given that foetal need for calcium does not arrive until later in pregnancy, it is possible that the increased calcium flow from the gut leads to storage in the skeletal pool. Indeed, increased bone density has been observed in animal models.

It is important that the fall in serum nutrient concentration caused by haemodilution should not be interpreted as a sign of nutritional deficiency. It is therefore essential that, in order to achieve a valid assessment of a pregnant woman's micronutrient status, appropriate pregnancy standards are used.

Ways in which mothers may deal with the energy and nutrient needs of pregnancy

Mothers have several behavioural options when dealing with the energy and nutrient needs of pregnancy: They may eat more and/or eat other types of food products, they may consume supplements or they may become less active.

Amount of food consumed

To cover the energy costs of pregnancy solely by increased food intake, the mother should eat 10–15% more than she did before her pregnancy. However, most studies in well-nourished women revealed either no change or only minor increases in the amount of energy and nutrients consumed in pregnancy; where an increased intake was found, hen the observed level of increment only partly covered the energy cost of pregnancy. An analysis of available data, from longitudinal studies in populations with average birth weights >3 kg, has revealed a cumulative intake of only 85 MJ during the whole pregnancy, or only 0.3 MJ/day, which equates to only 25% of the estimated needs.

Food choice

In addition to eating more, the diet of the pregnant mother should be well balanced and fully in line with dietary guidelines. Beliefs about pre-natal diets and food cravings (strong desires to eat particular foods) or food aversions (strong desires to avoid particular foods) may influence food choices in pregnant women. Food cravings and aversions do not necessarily have a deleterious effect on the quality of the diet. Cravings and aversions that arise during pregnancy are most likely due to hormone-induced changes in sensitivity to taste and smell, and do not seem to reflect real physiological needs.

Use of supplements

In general, pregnant women are encouraged to obtain their nutrients from a well-balanced, varied diet, rather than from vitamin or mineral supplements. In situations where a well-balanced, varied diet cannot be realised and for specific risk groups, dietary supplements might be an option. There is a paucity of data concerning the use of dietary supplements during pregnancy and lactation. Demographic, sociologic and economic factors seem to influence supplement use, and recent data suggest that individuals with possibly the greatest risk of having inadequate diets are the least likely to take a supplement. If we are going to supplement diets, we need to know much more about the risk of over-indulging a critical nutrient, which will then help to identify the proper balance of both benefits and risks (benefit–risk analysis).

Level of physical activity

The energy costs for a person's daily physical activity depend on (i) the time–activity pattern (amount of time spent on various activities), (ii) the pace or intensity of performing the various activities and (iii) the person's body weight.

Since body weight increases during pregnancy, an increase in energy costs might be expected, at least for weight-bearing activities. However, a mother may compensate for this by reducing the pace or intensity with which the activity is performed. A pregnant woman may also choose to change her activity pattern and, for example, reduce the amount of time spent on weight-bearing activities. However, this assumes that mothers will be more or less free to change their daily activities, or to change the pace or intensity of the work performed. This might be the case for many women from affluent societies, but is certainly not applicable to all societies. For example, low-income women from developing countries often have to continue their strenuous activity pattern until delivery, and so for them the option to save energy by reducing physical activity is not available. Also, for mothers who enter pregnancy with a light, daily activity pattern (not uncommon in affluent societies), the possibilities to save energy, by reducing physical activity, are limited. This is especially true for those mothers who already have the daily care of younger children. It should also be realised that, even if women voluntarily decrease their pace and consequently the energy expenditure per minute, the energy cost to complete a task may be unchanged, or even increased, since the performance of the task will take more time.

Women who had a high level of recreational exercise before pregnancy, and continued to do so during pregnancy, tended to gain less weight and to deliver smaller babies. There is little information from good-quality studies to suggest whether active women have better pregnancy outcomes than less active women.

Dietary recommendations for pregnancy

The increased demands of pregnancy may be met in a variety of ways. Some mothers will meet the demands by increasing intake, others by decreasing the level of physical activity or by limiting storage (e.g. fat storage), and still others by a combination of these options. It is not possible to advise women before pregnancy on the most appropriate strategies to balance intake and expenditure. With respect to the option of increasing food intake, it is clear that adequate and appropriate foods must be available to and accessible by women. With respect to the option of changing the physical activity level, it should be recognised that activity levels are sometimes already very low and that in situations where the levels might be high, women do not always have the social or economic freedom to reduce that level. Finally, the option of limiting storage clearly depends on the pre-pregnant nutritional status of the mother. Mothers with no low reserves or no reserves at all should be able to build up an appropriate reserve to enter lactation in an appropriate nutritional status, and mothers who already have ample reserves before pregnancy probably do not need to create an additional reserve.

Thus, there are good arguments against setting a specific recommendation regarding increased intake for all pregnant women. It may be good policy to permit considerable freedom regarding recommendations of food intake on the basis of individual preferences and to monitor weight gain carefully; adjustments in food intake can then be made only in response to deviations from the normal pattern of gain.

To estimate energy and nutrient needs during pregnancy the 'factorial approach' is commonly used. This means that the extra energy and nutrient needs imposed by pregnancy are added to the baseline estimates for non-pregnant, non-lactating women. Table 6.2 shows the dietary reference values on vitamins and minerals for pregnant as well as non-pregnant and non-lactating women.

Energy

The reference pregnancy, based on an increase in maternal fat stores of 2.0–2.5 kg and a protein deposition of 925 g, takes an extra 290–310 MJ approximately over the whole pregnancy. The average extra requirement is nil in the first trimester, 1.4 MJ/day in the second trimester and 1.9 MJ/day in the third trimester.

Table 6.2 Nutrient reference values of vitamins and minerals for pregnant women (from Nutrient Reference Values for Australia and New Zealand, 2006)

	Women, 19–50 years			
	Non-pregnant, non-lactating		Pregnant	
	EAR	RDI	EAR	RDI
Water-soluble vitamins				
Thiamin (mg/day)	0.9	1.1	1.2	1.4
Riboflavin (mg/day)	0.9	1.1	1.2	1.4
Niacin (mg/day)	11	14	14	18
Vitamin B_6 (mg/day)	1.1	1.3	1.6	1.9
Vitamin B_{12} (µg/day)	2	2.4	2.2	2.6
Folate (µg/day)	320	400	520	600
Pantothenic acid (mg/day)		4.0[a]		5.0[a]
Biotin (µg/day)		25[a]		30[a]
Vitamin C (mg/day)	30	45	40	60
Fat-soluble vitamins				
Vitamin A (µg/day)	500	700	550	800
Vitamin D (µg/day)		5[a]		5[a]
Vitamin E (mg/day)		7[a]		7[a]
Vitamin K (µg/day)		60[a]		60[a]
Choline (mg/day)		425[a]		440[a]
Minerals				
Calcium (mg/day)	840	1000	840	1000
Phosphorus (mg/day)	580	1000	580	1000
Zinc (mg/day)	6.5	8	9	11
Iron (mg/day)	8	18	22	27
Magnesium (mg/day)	255/265	310/320	290/350	300/360
Iodine (µg/day)	100	150	160	220
Selenium (µg/day)	50	60	55	65
Molybdenum (µg/day)	34	45	40	50
Copper (mg/day)		1.2[a]		1.3[a]
Chromium (µg/day)		25[a]		30[a]
Manganese (mg/day)		5.0[a]		5.0[a]
Fluoride (mg/day)		3.0[a]		3.0[a]
Sodium (mg/day)		460/920		460/920
Potassium (mg/day)		2800		2800

[a] AI in stead of RDI. EAR, estimated average requirement; RDI, recommended dietary intake.

Protein

No additional requirement is set for the first trimester, as there is little additional weight gain during this period. The recommendations are for the second and third trimesters, and are based on the estimated 925 g of protein deposited during pregnancy in the foetal, placental and maternal tissues, and on the observed efficiency of utilisation. The increase in body weight requires an additional 0.2 g of protein/kg/day. The estimated average requirement (EAR) for non-pregnant and non-lactating (NPNL) women of 19–50 years is 0.6 g/kg/day and for pregnant women is 0.8 g/kg/day. The recommended dietary intake (RDI; $RDI = EAR + 2SD_{EAR}$) is 0.25 g/kg/day higher in pregnancy: 0.75 g/kg/day for NPNL-women and 1.00 g/kg/day for pregnant women..

Essential fatty acids

Transplacental transfer of essential fatty acids is of crucial importance for foetal development, particularly membrane formation and cellular development in the brain. Demand for n-6 and n-3 fatty acids for placental and foetal tissue must be met from maternal stores or by increased dietary intake. The AIs (adequate intakes) for pregnancy are based on those for NPNL women, with an additional amount based on increased body weight (25% higher). For pregnant women the amounts are 10 g/day for linoleic acid, 1.0 g/day for α-linolenic acid and 115 mg/day for the total of long-chain n-3 fatty acids. Docosahexaenoic acid (DHA) is the major omega-3 fatty acid needed to build foetal brain and is therefore important in pregnancy. To make more DHA available for brain development, the maternal diet could include more fish. Where that is not possible, a supplement could be used.

For pregnant women, there are no other specific recommendations with respect to fat. This is also the case for *carbohydrates*. There is also no evidence for increased metabolic needs for *dietary fibre* in pregnancy, but the AI is increased in relation to the increased energy needs: 28 g/day versus 25 g/day for NPNL women. Pregnant women are recommended to abstain from alcohol.

Fat-soluble vitamins

Although it is well established that adaptive mechanisms improve the body's use of minerals during pregnancy, there is less evidence of similar mechanisms for adapting to vitamin requirements. Dietary reference values for pregnancy include a small increase for vitamin A, and no increments for vitamins D, E and K.

Little is known about the need for vitamin A during human pregnancy. However, if the mother is adequately nourished, her infant will be born with a reserve of vitamin A in the liver, even if the mother did not increase her vitamin A intake during pregnancy. The extra requirement is based on the desired accumulation of vitamin A in the liver of the foetus. It is important to note that high intakes of vitamin A can be damaging for the developing foetus and should be avoided.

Active forms of vitamin D readily cross the placenta to play an active role in the metabolism of calcium in the foetus. However, the amounts required are too small to affect the mother's vitamin D requirement, particularly since serum calcitriol is increased and there is an improvement in calcium resorption during late pregnancy. Mothers who consume enough milk to meet calcium requirements do not need an additional source of vitamin D. For women who have little access to sunlight, a supplement of 10 μg/day would not be excessive.

Water-soluble vitamins

The requirement for most B vitamins is increased by 10–50% in pregnancy, based on maternal and foetal growth, and increase in energy use. Folate requirements increase substantially in pregnancy (by 60–70%). This recommendation does not include consideration of additional needs to prevent neural tube defects, as the neural tube is formed before most women are aware of their pregnancy.

Choline

Choline also belongs to the nutrients for which there is limited capacity for endogenous biosynthesis and therefore it is conditionally required in the diet. Choline is required for membrane synthesis, methylation reactions and neurotransmitter synthesis, and is metabolically inter-related to folate. The AI for pregnancy is based on the foetal and placental accumulation of choline, plus turnover in the mother.

Minerals

Mineral requirements in pregnancy are estimated from the amounts transferred to the foetus. These amounts might come from the mother's stores, an increased consumption or an increased absorption rate. The extent to which these various options may contribute probably depends on maternal pre-pregnancy nutritional status and the mother's access to food. Calcium, iron, zinc and iodine are the main minerals of interest during pregnancy. Recommended dietary intakes for these minerals during pregnancy are given in Table 6.2.

The mother transfers about 30 g of calcium to her infant before birth, most of it during the last trimester of gestation. A well-nourished woman has more than 1000 g of stored calcium from which she might draw. However, recent findings suggest that the maternal skeleton is not used for the calcium needs of the foetus. Available data suggest that there is no need for additional dietary intake in pregnancy, as maternal adaptive mechanisms, including enhanced efficiency of absorption, more than meet additional requirements in the last trimester. This means that the normal calcium intake is sufficient to meet calcium requirements during pregnancy. Infants are born with a supply of iron stored in the liver, sufficient to last for 3–6 months. To achieve this storage, the mother must transfer about 200–400 mg of iron to the foetus during gestation. In addition, the pregnant woman requires additional iron for the formation of the placenta, for the haemoglobin (required by the expansion of blood volume) and to compensate for the loss of blood during delivery. Once this is taken into account, the total requirement for iron over the course of pregnancy amounts to 800–900 mg, therefore approximately 3 mg of iron must be supplied each day from the diet or maternal iron stores. However, many young women enter pregnancy with practically no reserves of iron. Fortunately, the efficiency of iron absorption may increase from 10 to 30% during the second half of pregnancy. Taking all this into consideration, the EAR for pregnancy is 22 mg/day, which is 14 mg/day more than for non-pregnant women.

As stated before, the amount of iron that must be absorbed by pregnant women, or supplied by maternal stores, amounts to 3 mg/day. This figure is substantially more than the amount of iron that must be absorbed by menstruating women. Menstrual iron losses vary greatly among women, but they usually amount to about 0.5–1 mg/day, when averaged over the whole menstrual cycle. Thus, the cessation of menstrual iron losses can contribute between one-sixth and one-third of the iron requirements in pregnancy.

The EAR for zinc is 2.5 mg/day, at an absorption rate of about 30%, and is based on the needs of the additional maternal and foetal tissues. As absorption is higher from animal foods than plant sources, vegetarians will need to increase their intake of the set value by 50% or more. This is also true for iron recommendations.

The EAR for iodine is based on the thyroid content of newborns, iodine balance studies and iodine supplementation studies in pregnancy, and is estimated as 160 μg/day, 60% more than for non-pregnant women.

Perspectives on the future

There is growing evidence that the foetus and the young infant are not protected from the inadequate diets of their mothers. Periods during perinatal development have been identified in which specific nutrients are required for optimal development, such as iodine, DHA, choline and folate. There are likely to be many more critical nutrients. However, a trend appears to emerge whereby the search is made for nutrients that have a wide range of dietary intake and

whose pathways for biosynthesis are either a marginal or non-existent, or they are needed to divide progenitor cells.

We also need to know more on how common genetic variations influence nutrient requirements during these periods. Single nucleotide polymorphisms (SNPs) have been shown to exist in pathways for the biosynthesis of DHA and of choline. Many more SNPs must influence metabolism and should be characterised. As soon as our knowledge of SNPs increases, we will be able to identify women who appear to be consuming enough of a nutrient, but who need to consume more because of a metabolic inefficiency.

DRVs might be used for designing appropriate intervention strategies in pregnancy. Further studies should be performed to establish whether such strategies indeed result in more optimal health outcomes for mother and baby. In general, pregnant women are encouraged to obtain their nutrients from a well-balanced, varied diet, rather than from vitamin and mineral supplements. In some situations, dietary supplements might be required. If supplements are used, we need to know much more about the risk of over-indulging the critical nutrients, and attention should be given to the benefit–risk-analyses of the supplements or fortified foods.

Different ethnic groups have been shown to vary widely in their energy requirements during pregnancy. Observational studies on the relationship between pregnancy, body mass index (BMI) and maternal energy needs, in a variety of ecological and ethnic settings, are necessary to explain this variability. In addition, further work would be valuable in assessing the causes and consequences of extremes of weight gain in pregnancy. Dietary studies would be useful in looking at the influences of diet on the prevalence of low birth weight. It is clear that many women gain excessive weight during pregnancy and yet there is still an occurrence of low infant birth weight in this group.

Many physiological adaptations occur during pregnancy to supply the growing foetus with its increasing demand for macro- and micronutrients. This increase in nutrient bioavailability, manifested by an increase in gastrointestinal absorption, has not been fully elucidated and work is required in this area.

Table 6.3 Concentrations of selected immunological factors in several human phases of lactation

	2–3 days	1 month	6 months	1 year
Lactoferrin (ng/ml)	5.3 ± 12.9	1.9 ± 0.3	1.4 ± 0.4	1.0 ± 0.2
Lysosyme (ng/ml)	0.09 ± 0.03	0.02 ± 0.03	0.25 ± 0.12	0.2 ± 0.1
Serum immunoglobulin A (ng/ml)	2 ± 2.5	1 ± 0.3	0.5 ± 0.1	1.0 ± 0.3
IgA (%)	90	87		
IgG (%)	2	3		
IgM (%)	8	10		

Data are shown as mean ± standard deviation.
Reproduced with kind permission from Springer Science+Business Media: J Mammary Gland Biolog Neoplasia, 12(4), Immune components of Colostrum and milk – A Historical Perspective, Wheeler T.T. et al, 237–247 (2007).

6.2 Lactation

Regulation of milk production

Lactation is an integral part of the reproductive cycle. During pregnancy, the alveolar system of the mammary gland develops (mammogenesis) under the combined action of oestrogen and progesterone, and is supplemented by greatly increased amounts of prolactin from the mother's anterior pituitary gland. Oestrogens and progesterone in the circulation during pregnancy inhibit prolactin from being effective. Following delivery of the infant and placenta, a sharp fall in the levels of maternal oestrogen and progesterone occurs, prolactin is released and the flow of breast milk begins. Suckling from the infant induces a variety of hormonal responses. In the mother, it stimulates the continued production of prolactin by the anterior lobe of the pituitary gland and induces the release of oxytocin from the posterior lobe. Oxytocin is essential for the milk letdown reflex. This reflex initiates the release of milk from the alveoli into the ducts and to the nipple. Milk is then withdrawn by the infant's suckling.

Following the birth of the infant, the prolactin level starts to return to the non-pregnant level, and it remains one of the two major hormones involved in initiating and sustaining milk secretion. Each time the mother nurses the infant, nerve impulses from the nipples to the hypothalamus increase the release of prolactin-releasing hormone, resulting in a 10-fold increase in prolactin secretion by the anterior pituitary, which lasts for about an hour. Concurrently, the oxytocin response is transient and intermittent, rather than sustained. Plasma levels often return to basal between milk ejections, even though suckling continues.

Maintenance of milk production appears to be under feedback control by a polypeptide substance called the feedback inhibitor of lactation (FIL), which is present in breast milk and enables women to adjust milk synthesis to the amount withdrawn by their infants. Key factors in the regulation of milk synthesis are the frequency and thorough removal of milk. Thus, it is essential for mothers to be adequately instructed on the art of breast-feeding. The most common causes of poor lactational performance are the infant's lack of access to the breast or inappropriate suckling behaviour.

Colostrum, transitional and mature milk

In the first 2–3 days after birth, the mammary glands secrete around 30–40 ml/day of fluid called colostrum. This volume increases following suckling-induced milk production, which also stimulates the synthesis of lactose and attracts water osmotically. Although colostrum contains relatively little water, lactose and fat, it contains a larger percentage of protein, minerals and fat-soluble vitamins than later milk. Moreover it is rich in constituents that enhance the neonate's immune system and protects the infant during the first few months of life (Table 6.3). During the colostral period, concentrations of fat and lactose increase, while those of protein and minerals decrease. Thus, colostrum serves adequately until the appearance of transitional milk (days 7–14 postpartum), which gradually changes to become mature over the first 2 weeks of breast-feeding.

Protective aspects of human milk

Breast milk contains a complex system of bioactive factors that augment the infant's immature systems and provide protection against infection. These include:

- antibodies such as secretory immunoglobulin A (IgA, and to some extent serum IgG), which prevent binding and proliferation of pathogens and may actively prime the newborn's immune system
- white blood cells, which can kill micro-organisms
- whey proteins, for example lactoferrin, an iron-binding protein that inhibits proliferation of iron-requiring bacteria, and lysosyme, an enzyme that attacks microbial pathogens
- oligosaccharides, which inhibit binding of certain bacterial pathogens to epithelial cells, and N-acetyl-D-glucosamine-containing oligosaccharides (bifidus factor), which promote growth of beneficial lacto-bacilli and bifidobacteria in the lower intestinal tract and create an environment of pH 5, which discourages growth of potential pathogens
- antioxidants, which are important for the integrity of epithelial surfaces
- epidermal growth factor, which stimulates maturation of the lining of the infant's intestine to receive the nutrients in milk
- anti-inflammatory agents, antiviral lipids and anti-protozoan factors.

Such protection is most valuable during the first year, when the infant's immune system is not fully prepared to mount a response to infection. The defending role of other components of breast milk, such as hormones, growth promoting factors, cytokines and prostaglandins, is not fully understood, but it may go beyond infection to protection against non-communicable diseases of later life.

Breast-feeding confers several benefits to the infant and is considered the perfect food for the normal infant, provided the maternal system can sustain lactation and as long as there are no contraindications, such as the use of certain drugs by the mother. Thus, for normal full-term infants, breast-feeding is generally considered the preferred method of feeding for the first 6 months of life, not only because human breast milk provides all of the nutrients needed by the infant, but also because of its short- and long-term benefits for the child. Evidence for these benefits has emerged in relation to reducing mortality, diarrhoea, pneumonia, acute infections, long-term diseases with an immunologi-

cal basis, obesity, risks to cardiovascular health and improved intelligence. In March 2001, a WHO expert consultation on the optimal duration for exclusive breast-feeding recommended a 6-month period, recognising that some mothers are unable to, or choose not to, follow this recommendation (*WHO*, 2001). These mothers should also be supported to optimise their infants' nutrition. Despite the numerous recognised advantages of breast-feeding, no more than an estimated 35% of the world's infant population are exclusively breast-fed between 0 and 4 months of age (WHO Global Data Bank on Breastfeeding, 2001). Between 1996 and 2006, there have been improvements in this situation, for example in Europe exclusive breast-feeding rates increased from 10 to 19%. As a substitute for breast milk, cow's milk is considered inadequate, owing to its high contents of protein, sodium, calcium, phosphate and chloride, and low concentrations of iron and copper Based on the current knowledge of infant requirements and the composition of breast milk, industries have modified the composition of cow's milk and put a variety of formula milks on the market. Recommendations on the compositional requirements for a standard infant formula have been developed by an international expert group, which concluded that infant formulae should specifically contain, in acceptable amounts, *only* those components that serve a nutritional purpose or provide another benefit, in order to maximise the support of the infant's normal growth and development. Thus, nutritional safety and adequacy should be scientifically underpinned (Koletzko *et al.,* 2005).

Maternal nutrition and lactational performance

Milk volume

In well-nourished women, little relationship exists between maternal diet and milk production. Longitudinal studies indicate that during exclusive breast-feeding, human milk production rates gradually increase from approximately 700 to 850 g/day at 6 months. Actual measurements of milk yield, from groups of women belonging to a wide range of nutritional and cultural conditions, revealed that breast-milk output was remarkably similar in early lactation (Figure 6.1). Thus, even underprivileged women

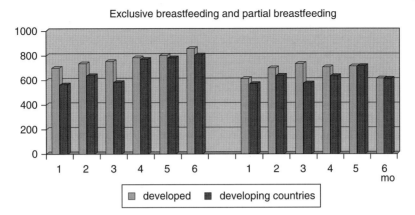

Figure 6.1 Average milk production rates (g/day) in developed and developing countries. (Source: Butte, Lopez-Alarcon and Garza. Nutrient adequacy of exclusive breast feeding for the term infant during the first six months of life. WHO, Geneva 2002.)

from developing countries are able to produce about 600 to 800 ml of breast milk/day early in lactation, provided they are not actually starving. Milk production for the partially breast-fed compares well to these latter values.

From the age of 6 months onwards, when infants are partially breast-fed, milk production tends to fall to approximately 550 g/day in full breast-feeders and to 50% of this amount in partial breast-feeders. Although the mother's milk yield appears to be relatively robust, the quality of the mother's diet can influence the secretion of specific components of breast milk.

Energy and macronutrient content of breast milk

As in the case of milk volume, the macronutrient content of human breast milk (Table 6.4) appears rather insensitive to differences in maternal nutrition. Estimates of the gross energy content of milk vary from 2.5 to 3.0 kJ/g, with 2.80 kJ/g as a compromise.

Protein

Compared with the milk of other mammals, human milk contains a very low concentration of protein. It declines from 20–30 g/l at 1–5 days of lactation to 8–9 g/l at 1 month and to about 7 g/l at 3.5–6.5 months of lactation. Human milk proteins consist mainly of whey proteins (60%, mostly α-lactalbumin) and caseins (40%). Proteins in human milk have multiple functions:

- they supply the essential amino acids
- they protect against infection (sIgA, lactoferrin and lysozyme)

Table 6.4 Estimates of the mean concentration of nutrients per litre of mature human milk

Nutrient	Amount	Unit
Lactose	67	g
Protein	9	g
Fat	37–40	g
Minerals		
Calcium	200–250	mg
Phosphorus	120–140	mg
Magnesium	30–35	mg
Iron	0.3–0.9	mg
Zinc	1–3	mg
Copper	0.2–04	mg
Vitamins		
A	0.3–0.6	mg
E	3–8	mg
D	0.33	μg
K	2–3	μg
C	100	mg
Thiamin	200	μg
Riboflavin	400–600	μg
Niacin	1.8–6.0	mg
B_6	0.9–1.1	mg
Folate	80–140	μg
B_{12}	0.5–1.0	μg

Reprinted from Pediatric Clinics of North America, volume 48, M. Picciano, Appendix: Representative values of constituents of human milk (2001) © with permission from Elsevier.

- they are components of lactose synthesis within the mammary gland
- they carry metals (calcium, zinc and magnesium).

The exact functions of non-protein nitrogen in human milk are mostly unknown. These compounds contribute about 25% to total nitrogen and include nitrogen-containing oligosaccharides ('bifidus factor'). Together with lactose, the principal carbohydrate (80%) in human milk, they enhance colonisation of the intestine with *Lactobacillus bifidus*. In established lactation, the concentrations of lactose (70–74 g/l) and oligosaccharides (about 12 g/l) are high.

Fat

By concentration, lipids are the second largest component of breast milk. The lipid fraction not only contributes to the energy content of human milk, but also serves as a carrier of fat-soluble vitamins and certain fat-soluble hormones. In well-nourished women, milk fat averages about 37–40 g/l. A positive correlation exists between the concentration of milk fat and the mother's measured body fat. More importantly, the nature of the fat consumed by the mother influences the fatty acid composition of milk, which provides the essential fatty acids linoleic acid (C18: 2n-6) and linolenic acid (C18: 3n-3). From these, long-chain (20- and 22-carbon) polyunsaturated metabolites (LCPUFAs, e.g. eicosapentaenoic acid (EPA: C20: 5n-3) and docosahexaenoic acid (DHA: C22: 6n-3)) can be derived. These LCPUFAs have profound biological activity and, as structural components of membranes, they may affect cognitive development and visual acuity. Although human milk contains small amounts of LCPUFAs, these may benefit the psychomotor and visual development of the infant (see Chapter 9), therefore the current consensus is that lactating women should aim to achieve an average daily intake of at least 200 mg DHA (Koletzko *et al.*, 2007).

Vitamins and minerals

The water-soluble vitamins in milk are all linked to the current dietary intake of the mother. Thus, they respond quickly to supplementation of the mother's diet. Fat-soluble vitamins are less responsive, since maternal stores and carrier proteins are able to buffer the effects of inadequate postpartum intakes. Also, breast-milk concentrations of iron, zinc, chromium, copper, sodium, calcium and magnesium do not appear to be related to dietary intake. In general, it seems that levels of milk nutrients are well protected, if necessary, through depletion of the mother's own body stores. Yet growing evidence places increased dietary importance on specific nutrients during pregnancy and lactation, for example for choline, folate and iodine, which are needed by dividing progenitor cells, there is a wide range of dietary intake, but marginal or no pathways for biosynthesis. Awaiting better understanding of how, for example, common genetic variations influence the mother's requirements, lactating women are encouraged to obtain their nutrients from a well-balanced, varied diet.

Recommended intakes during lactation

The total amount of nutrients secreted in milk is directly related to the extent and duration of lactation. Thus, nutrient needs during lactation depend primarily on the volume and composition of milk produced and on the mother's initial nutrient needs and nutritional status. There may be some variation in milk composition related to maternal nutrition, but the main factors that influence the needs of lactating women are the breast-feeding practices and the duration of exclusive breast-feeding. Micronutrient intakes that might be of concern to lactating women include vitamin A (in developing countries), calcium, iodine, zinc, folate, and vitamins E, D and B_6.

Energy

Ideally, women are well nourished throughout pregnancy and maintain adequate nutritional intakes with appropriate weight gain that may act as an energy substrate to cover part of the additional energy costs during lactation.

There is a wide range of variability in breast-milk volume among women. This may vary from about 550 g/day to over 1000 g/day. Accordingly, energy needs can vary considerably between women. The average energy costs of lactation can be calculated as the sum of:

- maternal requirements, including non-pregnant, non-lactating requirements ± changes in activity; any effects of possible changes in physical activity are thus included in the maternal requirements
- breast milk volume × energy density × conversion efficiency
- ± changes in body fat.

Table 6.5 summarises supplemental requirements, assuming:

- energy density of milk to be 2.8 kJ/g
- a dietary milk energy conversion efficiency of 80%

Table 6.5 Energy cost of human milk production by women who practice exclusive breastfeeding

Period: month	Milk volume (g/day)	Energy requirement (kJ/day)	
		Energy cost of milk production	Allowing for
1	699	2569	1849
2	731	2686	1966
3	751	2760	2040
4	780	2867	2147
5	796	2925	2205
6	854	3138	2418
Mean	769	2824	2104

With kind permission from the Food and Agriculture Organisation of the United Nations. Report on human energy requirements, 2004 © FAO.

- an allowance for fat loss of 0.8 kg/month up to 6 months postpartum
- no changes in maternal physical activity.

The average additional requirement may be taken as an extra 2824 kJ/day as full costs or as 2104 kJ/day allowing for fat loss. There is little evidence of energy-sparing adaptations in BMR, or dietary-induced thermogenesis, which have been suggested to compensate for part of the energy demand of lactation.

Lactating women predominantly meet the energy costs of lactation by increasing their energy intake. Some studies show that next to mobilisation of body fat, they tend to decrease their physical activity. The fat-loss allowance is not considered obligatory, depending on the initial stores of the mother. In overweight women, weight losses of approximately 2 kg/month do not seem to affect milk production or infant growth adversely. For undernourished, stressed women, the fat-loss allowance should probably not be assumed, particularly when pregnancy fat gain has been minimal. To their personal energy demands these women should add the full 2.8 MJ/day during the first semester of lactation.

Protein

Additional protein requirement during lactation amounts to 21.2 g/day (Food and Nutrition Board and Institute of Medicine, 2002). Taking the non-protein fraction of human milk into account, the additional requirement is about 17 g/day. As yet, there is no clear evidence that low maternal protein intake compro-

mises milk volume, although some short-term studies suggest an impact on the milk nitrogen fraction.

Vitamin A

Estimates of vitamin A requirements during lactation have been based on calculations of how much would be needed to replace that which is excreted daily in breast milk (Table 6.6). Consequently, the vitamin A content of human milk depends on maternal vitamin A status. There is a relatively wide range of recommended daily allowances, from 850 µg/day (WHO/FAO, 2004) to 1500 µg/day (German Nutrition society et al., 2000), related to the extent of inadequate vitamin A status, vitamin A availability and the socioeconomic constraints of the community. Useful specific guidelines for supplementation have been published by WHO (2009). In industrialised countries, there is no need for vitamin A supplementation. In areas of endemic vitamin A deficiency caution should be applied regarding vitamin A supplementation, given the potential risk of teratogenesis. The upper level of vitamin A intake has been set at 2800 µg/day (14–18 years) or 3000 µg/day (19–50 years). After the infant reaches the age of 6 months, or when solid foods are introduced, there is less maternal need for additional vitamin A.

Folate

The folate concentration of human milk remains relatively constant. The average daily amount secreted in human milk is estimated to be 85 µg/l. The additional dietary intake needed to provide this amount is 133 µg/day. Women who are only partially breast-feeding have less demand. There may be a profound effect on offspring if either a deficiency or an excess of methyl donors, such as folate, is experienced. It is therefore considered best to limit supplementation – if any – to levels that are within the range of population intakes.

Vitamin D and calcium

Available data indicate that vitamin D requirements are not increased during lactation. Concentrations of vitamin D in breast milk are low, between 12 and 60 IU/l. Although the milk 25-hydroxy-vitamin D (25(OH)D) concentration correlates with maternal 25(OH)D concentration and maternal vitamin D intake, infant 25(OH)D concentrations do not correlate with milk 25(OH)D unless the mother

Table 6.6 Recommended levels for micronutrient intake during lactation

| Micronutrient | Commonwealth of Australia (2006) National Health and Medical Research Council* | | WHO (2004) |
	EAR	RDA	RNI (or RDA)
Thiamin (mg/day)	1.2	1.4	1.5
Riboflavin (mg/day)	1.3	1.6	1.6
Niacin (mg/day)	13	17	17
Vitamin B$_6$ (mg/day)	1.7	2.0	2.0
Folate (µg/day)	450	500	500
Vitamin B$_{12}$ (µg/day)	2.4	2.8	2.8
Pantothenic acid (mg/day)[a]		6	7.0
Biotin (µg/day)[a]		35	35
Choline (mg/day)[a]		550	
Iron (mg/day)	7 (6.5) 14–18 years (19–50 years)	10 (9) 14–18 years (19–50 years)	10–30 (15–5% bioavailability)
Calcium (mg/day)	1050 (840) 14–18 years (19–50 years)	1300 (1000) 14–18 years (19–50 years)	1000
Phosphorus (mg/day)	1055 (580) 14–18 years (19–50 years)	1250 (1000) 14–18 years (19–50 years)	
Magnesium (mg/day)	300 (255, 265) 14–18 years (19–30 years, 31–50 years)	360 (310, 320) 14–18 years (19–30 years, 31–50 years)	270
Vitamin D (µg/day)[a]			5
Fluoride (mg/day)	3.0		
Vitamin A (µg/day)	780 (800) 14–18 years (19–50 years)	1100	850
Vitamin K (µg/day)[a]		60	55
Vitamin C (mg/day)	58 (60) up to 18 years (19–50 years)	80 (85) up to 18 years (19–50 years)	70
Vitamin E (α-tocopherol) (mg/day)[a]		11	–
Selenium (µg/day)	65	75	35 (42) 0–6 months (7–12 months)
Iodine (µg/day)	190	270	

Recommendations from the US/Canada, UK, Germany and the EU.

[a] AI, adequate intake; to replace RDA if sufficient scientific evidence is not available. EAR, estimated average requirement; RNI, reference nutrient intake, two standard deviations above EAR; RDA, recommended dietary allowance, two standard deviations above EAR. Safe level is the upper end of normal storage requirement.

receives high doses of supplemental vitamin D (e.g. 4000 IU/day). Within 8 weeks of delivery, vitamin D stores are depleted in vitamin D-replete mothers. When maternal vitamin D status is poor, vitamin D should be administered to newborns just after birth, as this can easily achieve vitamin D sufficiency. Dietary guidance for lactating women should ensure good nutrition and exposure to sunshine. Daily supplementation with 10 µg/day should be considered for mothers who avoid milk, eggs and fish, as well as for populations with limited sunshine exposure.

As is the case in pregnancy, lactation is a period of high calcium requirement. If milk products are not a major part of the diet, it is difficult for many lactating women to consume the recommended amount. During lactation, physiological adaptive processes ensure that calcium is provided for milk production. Thus, although there are wide differences among women, the concentration of calcium in breast milk is not influenced by the calcium intake of the mother during the breast-feeding period. Furthermore, calcium nutrition does not influence the changes in bone mineral status, calcium and bone metabolism, and these changes are not responsive to an increase in calcium intake by breast-feeding women. This evidence supports the view that calcium increments are no longer necessary in lactation, despite the current poor understanding of mechanisms involved in calcium regulation during lactation.

Iodine

Universal salt iodisation (USI) is recommended as a safe, cost-effective and sustainable strategy to ensure sufficient iodine intakes by all individuals worldwide. As universal implementation of salt iodisation appears not to be feasible, iodine supplementation has been proposed for pregnant and lactating women who have insufficient access to iodised salt (WHO, UNICEF 2007). Dosages amount to 250 µg/day or a single annual dose of an iodised oil supplement of 400 µg.

Energy and nutrient inadequacies

In general, lactating women are considered at high risk of energy and nutrient inadequacies. Selected groups of lactating women may need special nutritional attention, including:

- groups with restricted eating patterns
- complete vegetarians
- women who diet to lose weight
- women who avoid dairy products
- women on a low income
- women with HIV infections
- women using substances which penetrate into breastmilk, for example alcohol, nicotine.

Vegetarian mothers

In vegetarian women, vitamin D and calcium status may be low and vitamin B_{12} deficiency has been reported in their offspring. Given sufficient sunlight exposure, supplemental vitamin D does not appear to be necessary and the low calcium intake in vegetarian women does not result in a lower milk calcium content. One of the major nutritional concerns for vegetarian women is vitamin B_{12}, a lack of which leads to elevated methyl malonic acid levels in both mothers and infants.

Mothers with insulin-dependent diabetes mellitus

The goal for the treatment of insulin-dependent diabetes mellitus (IDDM) during lactation is to decrease infant mortality and morbidity, as well as the sequelae of the disease in the mother. The extra needs of lactation must be recognised, and both energy and insulin dose adjusted to meet those needs. To ensure adequate infant nutrition, mothers with IDDM should receive lactation counselling, addressing all factors that may influence the success of lactation:

hyperglycaemia, hypoglycaemia, method of delivery, feeding frequency, foetal condition, gestational age, incidence of mastitis, metabolic control and maternal dietary intake.

Maternal caloric restriction and exercise during lactation

Following lactation many women in affluent populations are eager to return to their pre-pregnancy weight. To achieve this goal, they may restrict energy intake or increase exercise. For women with adequate reserves, milk energy output is maintained, even if they are losing weight at a rate of up to 0.5 kg/week. Only when women with low energy reserves are in negative energy balance does milk energy output decrease. The threshold at which low energy reserves and negative energy balance affect milk energy output has, however, yet to be identified.

HIV infections

Mothers with HIV infections can transmit the virus to their infants through breast milk, especially during the early months of breast-feeding. To prevent the mother-to-child transmission of HIV, WHO and Unicef urge mothers in specific areas not to breast-feed and to find suitable feeding alternatives.

Alcohol and smoking

Both alcohol and smoking interfere with breast-feeding. They hinder milk production, enter breast milk and alter its flavour, so that the infants drink less. In this way, infant development may be impaired.

6.4 Perspectives on the future

Research is needed to identify the threshold of nutritional status at which mothers can no longer sustain lactation. Further clarification is required in cross-cultural comparisons, which suggest that lactational performance is remarkably unaffected by environmental factors, since many possible confounding differences may exist between cultures. More research is required to define whether low nutrient intakes before or during pregnancy can have deleterious effects on lactational performance.

To confirm the ecological studies in well- and undernourished mothers, additional studies are needed to explore the impact of supplementation practices on lactational performance and infant development.

Supplementation studies should also aim to examine growth, body composition and bone mineralisation, visual and cognitive development, and effects on immune outcomes and cardiovascular function.

Future research should consider the short- and long-term effects of LCPUFA status, prior to and during pregnancy, lactation and infancy, according to inter-individual differences, such as genetic variation in fatty acid desaturase activities or gender.

Studies addressing sub-groups with potential specific needs and benefits, such as women with at-risk pregnancies, restricted dietary intakes, or short-term intervals between pregnancies, are to be encouraged.

References

Food and Nutrition Board: Institute of Medicine. Dietary Reference Intakes for Energy, Carbohydrates, Fiber, Fat, Fatty Acids, Cholesterol, Protein and Amino Acids. Washington, DC: National Academy Press, 2002.

German Nutrition Society, Austrian Nutrition Society, Swiss Society for Nutrition Research, Swiss Nutrition Association: Reference Values for Nutrient Intake (D-A-CH), 1st edn. Frankfurt am Main: Umschau/Braus, 2000.

Koletzko B *et al.* Global standard for the composition of infant formula: recommendations of an ESPGHAN coordinated international expert group. Pediatr Gastroenterol Nutr. 2005; 41: 584–99.

Koletzko B *et al.* Dietary fat intakes for pregnant and lactating women. Br J Nutr 2007; 98: 873–7.

Nutrient Reference Values for Australia and New Zealand Including Recommended Dietary Intakes, 2060

WHO Guideline Development: Effects and Safety of Vitamin A Supplementation in Populations. Geneva: World Health Organization, 2009.

WHO/UNICEF. Reaching Optimal Iodine Nutrition in Pregnant and Lactating Women and Young Children. Joint Statement by the World Health Organization and the United Nations Children's Fund. Geneva: World Health Organization, 2007.

World Health Organization. Expert Consultation on the Optimal Duration of Exclusive Breastfeeding. Conclusions and Recommendations. Geneva: WHO, 2001. Available from: http://www.who.int/inf-pr-2001/en/note2001-07

World Health Organization. The WHO Global Data Bank on Breastfeeding and Complementary Feeding. Geneva: WHO, 2001. Available from: http://www.who.int/research/iycf/bfcf/bfcf.asp

World Health Organization/Food and Agriculture Organization. Human Vitamin and Mineral Requirements. Rome: FAO, 2004.

Further reading

Butte NF, Lopez-Alarcon MG, Garza C. Nutrient adequacy of exclusive breastfeeding for the term infant during the first six months of life. World Health Organization, Geneva, 2002.

Commonwealth Department of Health and Ageing Australia, Ministry of Health, New Zealand, National Health and Medical Research Council. Nutrient Reference Values for Australia and New Zealand including Recommended Dietary Intakes. Canberra: Commonwealth of Australia and New Zealand Government, 2006.

FAO Food And Nutrition Technical Report Series 1.Human energy requirements. Report of a Joint FAO/WHO/UNU Expert Consultation. Rome: United Nations University, World Health Organization, Food and Agriculture Organization of the United Nations, 2004

Joint FAO/WHO Expert Consultation on Human Vitamin and Mineral Requirements. Vitamin and Mineral Requirements in Human Nutrition. Rome: World Health Organization and Food and Agriculture Organization of the United Nations, 2004.

National Health and Medical Research Council of Australia. Nutrient Reference Values for Australia and New Zealand, 2006.

Picciano MF. Nutrient composition of human milk. Ped Clin North Am 2001; 48: 53–67.

Riediger ND *et al.* A systematic review of the roles of n-3 fatty acids in health and disease. J Am Diet Assoc 2009; 109: 668–679.

Wheeler TT, Hodgkinson AJ, Prosser CG, Davis SR. Immune components of colostrum and milk – a historical perspective. J Mamm Gland Biol Neoplasia 2007; 12: 237–47.

WHO. Vitamin and mineral requirements in human nutrition. World Health Organization and Food and Agriculture Organization of the United Nations, Rome, 2004.

World Health Organization. Infant and Young Child Feeding. Model chapter for textbooks for medical students and allied health professionals. Geneva: WHO, 2009. Available from: http://www.who.int/child_adolescent_health/documents/9789241597494/en/print.html

Zeisel SH. Is maternal diet supplementation beneficial? Optimal development of infant depends on mother's diet. Am J Clin Nutr 2009; 89(suppl): 685–7S.

7
Growth and Ageing

Mark L Wahlqvist and Prasong Tienboon

Key messages

- Growth provides an indication of nutritional status in pre-adult years.
- Changes in body composition and anthropometry reflect changes in growth and thus nutritional status.
- Nutritional needs change in accordance with the demands of growth throughout the different stages of life.
- The interplay of genetic and environmental factors determines growth outcomes and disease risk.
- Inadequate nutrition during the early years of life can drastically impair growth, and can affect stature and health outcomes in later life.
- 'Catch-up growth' is a phenomenon that compensates for deviations in growth from the genetic trajectory.
- Maximum height may not be equivalent to 'optimal' height with respect to positive health outcomes.

- Obesity and overweight in early life, and especially during adolescence, increase the likelihood of obesity and associated risk factors in adult life.
- Chronological and biological age do not necessarily correlate.
- Energy requirements generally decrease with age, but nutrient needs remain relatively high. Animal studies suggest that energy restriction promotes longevity, but human studies suggest that 'eating better not less' is desirable.
- Physical activity can improve health and well-being, and reduce morbidity risk at any stage of the lifespan.
- Many health problems commonly associated with older age are not necessarily products of 'ageing', instead they can be prevented or delayed by consuming a nutritionally adequate diet and engaging in regular physical activity.

7.1 Introduction

Nutrition plays an important role in human growth and development throughout life. Infancy and childhood are important times for nutrition and growth, as they strongly predict health outcomes later in life. Nutrition once again plays an important role in later life, when prevention of chronic disease and system degeneration becomes a major priority. All people require the same nutrients to maintain health and well-being, but these are required in differing amounts according to their stage of life. Optimal growth and healthy ageing will occur if nutritional requirements are met and environmental influences are conducive to health throughout life.

7.2 Growth and development

'Growth' may be defined as the acquisition of tissue with a concomitant increase in body size. 'Development' refers to changes in the body's capacity to function both physically and intellectually through increased tissue and organ complexity. Different individuals experience these processes at different rates.

There are five stages under which major growth and developmental changes occur in humans:

- infancy
- childhood
- adolescence
- adulthood
- late adulthood.

Nutrition and Metabolism, Second Edition, edited by S. A. Lanham-New, I. A. Macdonald and H. M. Roche. © 2011 The Nutrition Society.

These stages can be distinguished by changes in growth velocity and distinct biological and behavioural characteristics. Nutritional needs change in response to the demands that these stages of growth place on the body. If nutritional needs are met and adverse social circumstances or diseases are not encountered, optimal growth will occur.

Cellular aspects of growth and death

Cell division

Cells are subject to wear and tear, as well as to accidents and death, therefore we must create new cells at a rate as fast as that at which our cells die. As a result, cell division is central to the life of all organisms. Cell division or the M phase (M = mitotic) consists of two sequential processes: nuclear division (mitosis) and cytoplasmic division (cytokinesis). Before a cell can divide, it must double its mass and duplicate all of its contents to ensure that the new cell contains all of the components required to begin its own cycle of cell growth, followed by division. Preparation for division goes on invisibly during the growth phase of the cell cycle and is denoted the interphase. During interphase, cell components are continually being made. Interphase can last for up to 16–24 h, whereas the M phase lasts for only 1–2 h. Interphase starts with the G_1 phase (G = gap) in which the cells, whose biosynthetic activities have been slowed during the M phase, resume a high rate of biosynthesis. The S phase begins when DNA synthesis starts and ends when the DNA content of the nucleus has doubled and the chromosomes have replicated. When DNA synthesis is complete, the cell enters the G_2 phase, which ends when mitosis starts. Terminally differentiated and other non-replicating cells represent a quiescent stage, often referred to as the G_0 phase (Figure 7.1).

In multicellular animals, like humans, the survival of the organism is paramount rather than the survival of its individual cells. As a result, the 10^{13} cells of the human body divide at very different rates depending on their location, and are programmed and co-ordinated with their neighbours. Something in the order of 10^{16} cell divisions take place in a human body during the course of a lifetime. Different cell types sacrifice their potential for rapid division, so that their numbers are monitored at a level that is optimal for the organism as a whole. Some cells, such as red blood cells, do not divide again once they are

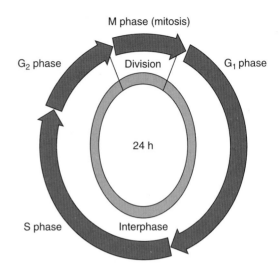

Figure 7.1 Cell growth and division: The four successive phases of a typical cell cycle.

mature. Other cells, such as epithelial cells, divide continually. The observed cell-cycle times, also called generation times, range from 8 h to 100 days or more. Cells that do not actively proliferate have a reduced rate of protein synthesis and are arrested in the G_1 phase. A cell that has become committed to division by passing through a special restriction point (R) in its G_1 cycle will then go on to make DNA in the S phase and proceed through to the following stages. Growth stops for those cells arrested at R, although biosynthesis continues. This specific restriction point of the growth-control mechanism may have evolved partly due to the need of a safe resting state (at R) for those cells whose growth conditions or interactions with other cells demand that they stop dividing. Cells that have been arrested at this stable resting state are said to have entered a G_0 phase of the cell cycle. Whether or not a cell will grow and divide is determined by a variety of feedback control mechanisms. These include the availability of space in which a cell can flatten (contact inhibition of cell division) and the secretion of specific stimulatory and inhibitory factors (peptides, steroids, hormones, short-range local chemical mediators and others still to be identified) by cells in the immediate environment.

Cancer cells have escaped from or respond abnormally to many of the control mechanisms that regulate cell division. Cancer cells require fewer protein growth factors than do normal cells in order to survive and divide in culture; in some cases this may be because they produce their own growth factors. A second fundamental difference between normal and cancer cells is that the latter can go on dividing indefinitely. For example, cells taken from older animals will divide fewer times in culture than the same cells taken from young animals, suggesting that older cells have used up many of their allotted divisions whilst in the animal. As cells differentiate they become programmed to die after a certain number of divisions. This programmed cell death is an additional safeguard against the unbridled growth of one particular cell. However, cancer involves something more than just abnormalities of proliferation and programmed senescence; it requires the coincidental occurrence of several specific mutations in a single cell, enabling it to proliferate in disregard to the usual constraints and to invade regions of the body from which it would normally be excluded.

Cell death

Apoptosis is an active process in which cells undergo genetically programmed death. Apoptosis occurs when a calcium-dependent enzyme (endonuclease) fragments the genome of the cell into approximately 180 base pairs. The dead cells are then removed by phagocytosis. It is still unclear how many mechanisms are involved in causing cell death, but it is known that alterations in intracellular calcium levels can trigger apoptosis. Cell death appears to be activated by special genes in dying cells. For cell death to occur genes identified as *ced-3* and *ced-4* must be expressed in a dying cell. A third gene, *ced-9*, is a major control factor, which negatively regulates the *ced-3* and *ced-4* genes. Animal studies have shown that mutations to *ced-9* inactivate the gene, causing the death of cells that were otherwise intended to survive and thereby killing the animal under study. Cell senescence occurs when the cell does not divide or proliferate and DNA synthesis is blocked. Cells are programmed to carry out a finite number of divisions, which is called the Hayflick limit. If cells do not reach senescence they continue to divide and in effect become immortal. Immortal cells eventually form tumours, and this is therefore an area where research into ageing and cancer is inter-related. It is thought that senescence may have evolved exactly because its action protects against cancer. Cells exhibiting evidence of DNA damage and oxidative stress may

recover from these stresses provided they are equipped with an adequate DNA repair system and an adequate level of stress-response proteins and/or antioxidant defences. Most theories that aim to explain the ageing process suggest that senescence results from the accumulation of unrepaired damage. Telomeres (the sections of DNA at the end of chromosomes) shorten with each division of the cell, resulting in a set lifetime for each normal cell. Inhibition of telomerase is thought to reduce cellular ageing. Although genes play an important role and can be an indicator of disease risk in later life, environmental factors also strongly influence the development of disease. The general degenerative properties of ageing are also a factor in disease development. Greater understanding of the molecular events regulating cell progression and apoptosis is rapidly emerging. The non-nutritional and nutritional factors affecting cell division and growth are outlined below.

Non-nutritional factors affecting growth

Growth is influenced by a number of important factors, including genetics and endocrine control, and also by the surrounding environment, such as nutritional factors, social factors (socioeconomic status and cultural practice) and psychological factors. For example, the physical growth of school children aged 6–9 years is the result of environmental and genetic factors, and the interaction between the two. It is too simplistic to think that these factors affect growth in isolation, as ultimately it is the interaction of all of these factors that will affect growth. It is often difficult to isolate the effects on growth of these individual factors, as they are often closely linked.

Genetic factors

Genetic factors arguably play the most important role in determining the outcome of growth and development. It is clear that the genetic make-up of the individual and what has been inherited from previous generations greatly influences how they advance through life. Studies of twins have shown that patterns of growth, age of menarche, body shape, composition and size, and deposition of fat are all closely linked to genetic factors. Many studies support a genetic component in obesity-related traits. Height is influenced strongly by genetic predisposition, whereas weight appears to be mostly influenced by environment. The effects of genetic control are often quite explicit and limited in terms of their action. Dental maturation, for example, appears to be independent of skeletal maturation, and some evidence suggests that genes regulating the growth of different sections of limbs are also independent. Evolution and genetic factors largely explain racial differences, but the role of socioeconomic and educational advantage and disadvantage, together with living conditions, including food, is likely to be underestimated. For example, skeletal maturation and growth rates differ between white American children and black African–Americans in the first few years of life. Whilst this is largely attributed to genetic factors, there is increasing evidence to show that the intra- and intergenerational effects of intrauterine nutrition and early childhood rearing are important qualifiers.

Gender differences are predominantly explained by genetic factors, such as differences in both the timing of the adolescent growth spurt and the sex-specific changes that occur during puberty. At the age of 10 years, males and females are of a similar height, weight and body fatness. However, after puberty, major differences are evident. Although the timing of the growth spurt is controlled largely genetically, hormonal factors are thought to control its intensity and duration, while environmental factors also play an important role. Females typically achieve skeletal maturation at an earlier age than males. Genes on the Y chromosome, which are found only in males, are thought to retard skeletal maturation relative to females. A disturbance in the expression of a single gene, or group of genes, can have widespread and drastic effects, leading to compromised growth and development. Insults to gene expression during intrauterine life in particular can have important consequences in later life in terms of growth and development, and even in the formation of degenerative diseases. Inborn errors of metabolism such as phenylketonuria, galactosaemia and hereditary fructose intolerance are all genetic conditions that require vigilant dietary management to avoid deficiencies of essential nutrients.

Hormones and growth factors

Hormones are responsible for coordinating much of the appropriate timing and rates of growth. There are many hormones that have recognised effects on growth. Generally, there are three distinct endocrine phases of linear growth: infancy (including foetal growth), childhood and puberty. Each of these phases is regulated by different endocrine growth-promoting systems. Thyroid and parathyroid hormones, through thyroxine and triiodothyronine, stimulate general metabolism. Other hormones and growth factors include epidermal growth factor (important for actions in the epidermis), platelet-derived growth factor (involved in blood clots and possibly cell division) and melatonin (plays a role in regulating puberty and possibly growth velocity). Hormones are largely responsible for many changes in body composition and the development of secondary sexual characteristics, which occur as individuals grow older. The effects of hormones are often influenced and regulated by other hormones and growth factors.

One of the most important hormones that regulates growth is the human growth hormone (GH). GH exerts a powerful effect on growth, at least in part, through somatomedins or insulin-like growth factors (IGF-I, IGF-2). IGF acts by stimulating muscle cell differentiation and is therefore important in foetal and postnatal growth and development. GH is important in regulating protein synthesis and cellular division, and is thus thought to be the major regulator of the rate of human growth and development from the latter few months of the first year of life. Synthetic forms of GH are regularly used in a clinical setting to encourage growth in children of a small stature. It is thought that sex steroids, which are active around puberty, may trigger significant secretions of GH and thus IGF. Hormones such as thyroxine and cortisol may also influence IGF plasma levels. Disturbances to genetic programming *in utero* during critical phases of foetal development may result in the impairment of the endocrine factors, responsible for growth in later life. Studies have reported associations between growth retardation and abnormalities in levels of hormones such as GH and hormone-mediated factors, such as IGF.

Neural control

It has been proposed that within the brain there is a 'growth centre', which is responsible for regulating growth. The hypothalamus has been implicated as a possible growth centre, owing to its close association with the anterior pituitary, a hormonal gland closely involved in growth. By this action, any deviation of growth from its pre-determined genetic pathway will be identified by the hypothalamus and will then be compensated for by the subsequent release of growth-specific hormones from the anterior pituitary gland, thereby inhibiting the potential for damage to any growth or development. The peripheral nervous system may also play an important role in growth. This effect is thought to be achieved through the secretion of neural chemicals, which have the ability to influence growth.

Local biochemical control

To attain optimal growth, areas of localised growth rely on complex regional influences, whether they are mechanical or chemical stimuli. These can be paracrine factors, such as neighbouring proteins, which act as local signalling and growth factors. Alternatively they may be autocrine factors, such as hormones or growth factors that influence the growth of quite localised areas, despite being secreted from a more distant position. These mechanisms appear to be responsible for the growth of specific tissue. Furthermore, the age of groups of cells, or a specific tissue, can determine the amount of cell replication and division that is possible. This is the case where cells undergo a finite number of mitotic divisions.

Social and cultural factors

The major social factors affecting growth are culture, age, family, gender and socioeconomic status. Emotional disorders have also been related to growth abnormalities. Different countries or regions may exhibit their own cultures and cuisines, which reflect a mixture of geographical, agricultural, historical, religious and economic factors, among others. These factors may either directly or indirectly affect growth through their influence on a number of factors, such as health, nutrition, food selection and cooking methods. Infants and children who emigrate to other areas may often experience changes to growth patterns. Generational differences in stature, for example, often reflect changing environments. Many adolescents eagerly seek independence, and factors associated with this have an effect on nutritional status. Levels of physical activity, peer pressure, self- esteem and distorted body image, chronic dieting and disordered eating, together with substance abuse, are all factors that can affect nutritional status and, consequently, growth. Chronic dieting, in particular, can also place an individual at risk of many micronutrient deficiencies, infertility, long-term degenerative diseases, such as osteoporosis and a compromised immune system, which can negatively affect growth and health outcomes.

Family factors that have been associated with compromised growth and development include single-parent families, family conflict and disturbance to the family unit, such as divorce and separation. Growth retardation in conflict situations may partly be a result of stress, which is thought to affect GH levels. The amount of care and attention that an infant receives will also have an important impact on growth. This can be related to the number of children and birth position in the family. Various cultures may practice a gender bias and favour one gender over the other. This can be seen to a larger degree in developing countries, where boys may be more favoured and thus receive more care and nourishment. In both developing and industrialised countries, socioeconomic status is associated with many behavioural, nutritional and health outcomes, which can influence growth. Usually children of a higher socioeconomic class are taller, display faster growth rates and become taller adults. Children of lower classes are typically smaller at birth, shorter and, particularly in industrialised countries, have higher levels of body fat. Socioeconomic status is also a strong predictor of certain micronutrient deficiencies, such as vitamin A and iron deficiencies.

Independently, educational attainment and income have been positively associated with growth and development, mainly through the alleviation of poverty. Females, in particular, benefit from schooling, as they are able to exert greater control over their environment and show improved growth and pregnancy outcomes. Typically, as income increases, a larger amount of money will be spent on animal products, such as meat, owing to the prestige factor associated with such foods. The inclusion of greater amounts of animal protein in the diet can influence growth and development. Infant feeding practices, such as breastfeeding and weaning, may also follow the culturally or socially acceptable patterns of a region. Women of a higher socioeconomic status are known to breastfeed for longer periods than women of lower classes. This can have important growth and development outcomes on the infant. Dental caries are common in both developing and industrialised countries, where dental hygiene is inadequate and in areas where water fluoridation is absent. Under such conditions, dietary factors associated with increased dental caries include the regular consumption of foods high in sucrose, particularly sticky sweet forms.

7.3 Nutritional factors affecting growth

In order for growth to proceed at its pre-determined genetic rate, adequate nutrition is essential. Food supplies the individual with the required energy, nutrients and food components to influence growth. The strong link between food intake and growth is supported from studies of food intake patterns during famines, encountered at the time of the two world wars. Children of Dutch and German families living in these areas exhibited impaired growth, while in Japan a reduction in the mean height of adults was observed between 1945 and 1949. Nutrition affects all body systems and factors influencing growth. For example, a compromised nutrient intake can influence gene replication and expression, hormonal control and neural control; as stated earlier, other environmental factors are also important for growth.

Inadequate nutrition is the predominant factor leading to malnutrition, which can be expressed as either undernutrition or overnutrition. Undernutrition occurs when there is not only inadequate energy, but also a lack or imbalance of specific food components and nutrients. Chronic energy deficiency, commonly referred to as protein–energy malnutrition (PEM), occurs in both developing and industrialised countries, but it is more prevalent in the former. Characteristic features of PEM include stunted growth, delayed maturation, reduced muscle mass and decreased physical working capacity.

In addition to sufficient energy, adequate supplies of macronutrients and micronutrients are required to promote optimum growth. The proportions and amounts of these nutrients may change according to the various stages of growth. For example, protein is a prerequisite for optimal growth at all life stages, while fat may arguably have its most important role during infancy and childhood, as a major supplier of energy and long-chain polyunsaturated (n-3) fatty acids, which are important in neural development. Components of certain foods, called growth factors, may have powerful effects on growth. For example,

Table 7.1 Micronutrients affecting growth

Children	Adolescents
Iodide	Calcium
Zinc	Folate
Iron	
Vitamin A	
Vitamin K	
Riboflavin	
Vitamin C	
Vitamin D	

some of the proteins present in milk are thought to promote growth. Population groups that consume large amounts of milk also exhibit typically taller statures.

Nutritional status is found to greatly affect hormonal status. GH, for example, will not stimulate linear growth, unless there is adequate nutrition. IGF plasma levels appear to respond closely to acute directional changes in the body's nitrogen balance. This suggests that the ingestion of several dietary components, such as essential amino acids, adequate energy and an optimal nitrogen balance may be critical for optimal hormonal control: When this is not the case, there may be negative effects on growth and development. Food and its components, such as metabolites of vitamins A and D, fatty acids, together with some sterols and zinc, can directly influence gene expression and thus growth. Components of dietary fibre are thought to influence gene expression indirectly by a number of pathways, including altering hormonal signalling, mechanical stimulation and through metabolites, which are produced by flora of the intestine. The specific micronutrients that are frequently held responsible for much of the functional impairment and growth retardation experienced globally are shown in Table 7.1.

Iodide

Iodide deficiency at different life stages produces differing health outcomes. Its intake is of most critical importance *in utero* and during the first 2 years of life, when neural cells in the brain undergo major cellular division. Adequate iodide intakes during these times are therefore essential for mental and cognitive growth and development. The extent of mental dysfunction may be lessened, if sufficient dietary iodide levels are administered in the early years of life. Complications associated with iodide deficiency in childhood and adolescence may appear as goitre, hypothyroidism, mental dysfunction, retarded mental and physical growth, and reduced school performance.

Vitamin A

Severe deficiency in vitamin A is commonly associated with impaired vision, retarded growth and development, poor bone health, compromised immune functioning, and complications with reproductive health and outcomes. In industrialised countries, vitamin A deficiency is rare. Too much vitamin A in the diet can also slow growth. Subclinical vitamin A deficiency greatly increases the risk of morbidity and mortality in vulnerable population groups. Reductions in mortality rates of around 20–25% can be achieved by improving the vitamin A status in young children in populations where deficiency has been identified.

Zinc

Zinc is of crucial importance in over 200 enzyme reactions. It is of structural and functional importance in biomembranes, DNA, RNA and ribosomal structures. Zinc deficiency has been linked with disturbed gene expression, protein synthesis, immunity, skeletal growth and maturation, gonad development, pregnancy outcomes, behaviour, skin integrity, eyesight, appetite and taste perception. Zinc deficiency can cause major intrauterine growth retardation (IUGR) if the maternal diet provides inadequate sources of zinc. It is therefore of great importance for linear growth, as well as the development of lean body mass.

Iron

In industrialised countries, iron represents the major micronutrient deficiency, but in developing countries iron deficiency occurs on a much larger scale. Although iron is important at all life stages, iron deficiency commonly affects preschool and school-aged children, who, as a consequence, face compromised growth if dietary intake is inadequate. Iron is very important in pregnant women, as low intakes can have wide implications for the newborn infant with limited iron stores. The effects of iron deficiency are varied, but a major effect is its impairment of cognitive development in children. Other consequences of iron deficiency include a reduced work capacity and a decreased resistance to fatigue.

Other nutrients

Other nutrients of importance to growth include vitamin B_2, which affects general growth, vitamin C, which is important in bone structure, and vitamin D, which is involved in calcium absorption from the intestines. Chronically low dietary intakes of these vitamins can greatly impair growth and bone health. Calcium and folate appear to be micronutrients of importance for growth during adolescence. Vitamin K has also emerged as a factor in bone health and growth through osteocalcin.

Phytochemicals

There is emerging evidence that certain phytochemicals, such as the isoflavones genistein and daidzein (found in legumes, especially soy), may help to inhibit tumour formation by regulating cell-cycle progression and by promoting cell differentiation and apoptosis (cell death). Formation of new vasculature is required for a cancer to grow and metastasize; isoflavones have also been identified as antiangiogenic agents that inhibit the formation of new vasculature and thus the development and dissemination of tumours.

7.4 Nutrition and the life cycle

Energy and nutrient needs differ according to the different stages in life and it is therefore important for food intake to reflect these changing demands. Inadequate nutrition exerts its most detrimental impact on pre-pubertal growth. Supplementation programmes and interventions that are provided before this time will have the most beneficial growth and development outcomes. Nutrient needs during infancy are influenced by length of gestation, the newborn's nutrient reserves, body composition, growth rate, activity levels, and the length and duration of breast-feeding. An infant is wholly dependent on a carer for some or all nourishment, ideally via breast milk.

The essential long-chain fatty acids (LCPUFA), such as the n-3 fatty acids docosahexaenoic acid

(DHA) and arachidonic acid (AA), are structurally important in cell membranes, particularly in the central nervous system. Most infant formulae contain only the precursor essential fatty acids, α-linolenic acid (ALA, the n-3 precursor) and linoleic acid (LA, the n-6 precursor), from which infants must assemble their own DHA and AA, respectively. Studies have suggested that such formulae may not be effective in fully meeting the essential fatty acid requirements that are needed by most infants. Reduced cognitive, motor and visual acuity outcomes have been reported in formula-fed infants, compared with their breast-fed counterparts, but not all studies have reported such findings. From 6 to 24 months of infant life breast-feeding alone cannot provide all of the nutrients and energy needed to promote and sustain adequate growth, therefore complementary feeding is necessary. If complementary feeding is introduced too late, there is a risk of impaired growth, macronutrient deficiency, impaired cognitive and physical development, and stunting as a result of PEM.

Early weaning (4 months or earlier) has been associated with negative health outcomes, such as the formation of allergies, diarrhoea and even death. Chronic or episodic diarrhoea may affect the absorption of nutrients which, if not addressed, may lead to growth impairment. Common reasons for introducing complementary feeding with formula milk or solids include a perceived inferior quality of milk, poor weight gain, difficulties or pain with feeding, mother's employment, refusal by the infant to feed and lack of mother's confidence. Many people perceive formula to be of a higher quality than breast milk, particularly as a result of aggressive marketing strategies from infant formula manufacturers. This may cause the mother to abandon exclusive breast-feeding from an early age. In 2001, the World Health Organization (WHO) released a systematic review on the optimal duration of exclusive breast-feeding. These results indicate that breast-feeding should be exclusive for the first 6 months of life (http://www.who.int/inf-pr-2001/en/note2001-07.html).

Some individuals experience erratic growth during childhood, largely reflecting changes in appetite and food intake, or even an underlying illness. Nutrient needs increase throughout childhood, reflecting the continuing growth of all body systems. Children can exhibit good growth and thrive on most lacto–ovo vegetarian and vegan diets, provided they are well planned and supplemented. Growth delays have occasionally been reported in children fed severely restricted diets (primarily macrobiotic, Rastafarian and fruitarian forms). However, by school age, the growth of vegetarians and non-vegetarians becomes more alike. Few differences have been found in the timing of puberty or completed adult growth. Little effect is evident on intelligence quotient (IQ), assuming a reasonably adequate vegetarian diet. Typically, girls tend to consume less than boys at all ages. However, it is during adolescence that males begin to increase their intake to levels well above that of most females. Adolescence is a time that requires the greatest total energy intake of all of the life stages, as a result of the body being in a highly metabolically active state. Inadequate intakes of nutrients and energy during this time can potentially impede growth and delay sexual maturation. Pregnancy during adolescence has many increased risks for both the mother and the child, as the foetus and the mother must compete for nutrients to maintain and promote their respective growth. This is of even greater concern if the adolescent is malnourished. Calcium is of particular concern as it is needed for continuing bone development in the mother while also being required in large quantities by the developing foetus. Birth and maternal complications during adolescent pregnancy are greater than those for older women of similar nutritional status. For example, adolescent mothers face increased risks of infant and maternal mortality, pre-term delivery and giving birth to babies prematurely and of a low birth weight. The Australian dietary guidelines for children and adolescents and the American dietary guidelines for healthy people over 2 years old are shown in Tables 7.2 and 7.3.

7.5 Effects of undernutrition

Identifying the cause of undernourishment is not always an easy task. Inadequate dietary intake may not be the sole cause. Social, cultural, genetic, hormonal, economic and political factors may also be important. Underlying health problems and inadequate care and hygiene may also be contributing factors to undernourishment. The outcomes of undernutrition are largely determined by its severity and duration. Consequences of undernutrition include death, disability, and stunted mental and physical growth. Poor

Table 7.2 Dietary guidelines for children and adolescents in Australia 2003

Encourage and support breast-feeding
Children and adolescents need sufficient nutritious foods to grow and develop normally:
- growth should be checked regularly for young children
- physical activity is important for all children and adolescents

Enjoy a wide variety of nutritious foods
Children and adolescents should be encouraged to:
- eat plenty of vegetables, legumes and fruits
- eat plenty of cereals (including breads, rice, pasta and noodles), preferably wholegrain
- include lean meat, fish, poultry and/or alternatives
- include milks, yoghurts, cheese and/or alternatives (reduced-fat milks are not suitable for young children under 2 years because of their high energy needs, but reduced-fat varieties should be encouraged for older children and adolescents)
- choose water as a drink (alcohol is not recommended for children)

Care should be taken to:
- limit saturated fat and moderate total fat intake (low-fat diets are not suitable for infants)
- choose foods low in salt
- consume only moderate amounts of sugars and foods containing added sugars

Care for your child's food: prepare and store it safely
These guidelines are not in order of importance.
Each one deals with an issue that is key to optimal health.
Two relate to the quantity and quality of the food we eat – getting the right types of foods in the right amounts to meet the body's nutrient needs and to reduce the risk of chronic disease. Given the epidemic of obesity we are currently experiencing in Australia, one of these guidelines specifically relates to the need to be active and to avoid overeating. Another guideline stresses the need to be vigilant about food safety, and, in view of the increasing awareness of the importance of early nutrition, there is a further guideline that encourages everyone to support and promote

Dietary Guidelines for Children and Adolescents in Australia incorporating the Infant Feeding Guidelines for Health Workers, National Health & Medical Research Council, 2003, Copyright Commonwealth of Australia, reproduced by permission http://www.nhmrc.gov.au/publications/synopses/dietsyn.htm

Table 7.3 American dietary guidelines for healthy people over 2 years old, 2000, modified in 2005 with greater emphasis on weight and physical activity because of childhood and community-wide obesity epidemic

Aim for fitness
Aim for a healthy weight
Be physically active each day
Build a healthy base
Let the pyramid ('My Pyramid') guide your food choices
Choose a variety of grains daily, especially whole grains
Choose a variety of fruits and vegetables daily
Keep food safe to eat
Choose sensibly
Choose a diet that is low in saturated fat and cholesterol and moderate in total fat
Choose beverages and foods to moderate your intake of sugars
Choose and prepare foods with less salt
If you drink alcoholic beverages, do so in moderation

Reproduced from American dietary guidelines for healthy people over 2 years old, 2000, USDA (2000 and 2005) and http: //www.mypyramid.gov/

nutrition often commences *in utero* and in many cases extends into adolescence and adult life. Females in particular are affected by life-long poor nutrition. Evidence from epidemiological studies from both developing and industrialised countries now suggests a causal relationship between foetal undernutrition and increased risks of impaired growth and various adult chronic diseases. This forms the basis of the hypothesis that disease originates at the foetal stage. Wasting is often one of the earliest signs of acute undernutrition. Wasting can be detected by reduced measures of weight-for-age and skinfold thickness, reflecting a loss of weight or a failure to gain weight. In severe cases of undernourishment individuals may exhibit other clinical symptoms such as hair loss, skin discolouration or pigmentation (in marasmus) and oedema (in kwashiorkor), and evidence of deficiencies that are characteristic when lacking specific nutrients. Stunting reflects chronic undernutrition and is detected as impaired linear growth. However, where stunting and wasting are both present, as in chronic cases of undernourishment, growth charts may not detect abnormal weights-(or heights)-for-length owing to proportional growth retardation of both weight and height (or length). A stunted infant is likely to remain stunted throughout childhood and adolescence and is likely to become a stunted adult, particularly if the individual continues to live in the same environment that instigated the stunting. Adult stunting and underweight have direct effects not only on a woman's health and productivity, but also by increasing the risks of pregnancy complications, such as gestational diabetes, and the likelihood that her off-spring will be born of a low birth weight (LBW); thus, stunting commonly spans generations.

Most growth impairment, of which underweight and stunting are outcomes, occurs within a relatively short period, from before birth until about 2 years of age. Severe undernutrition during infancy can be particularly damaging to the growth of the brain. This can result in major retardation of cognitive growth and functioning. Delayed intellectual development is a risk factor for absenteeism from school and poor school performance. Infants born of LBW and who have suffered IUGR are born undernourished and face a greatly increased risk of mortality in the neonatal period or later infancy. Suboptimal intakes of energy, protein, vitamin A, zinc and iron during the early years of life may exacerbate the effects of foetal growth retardation. There is a cumulative negative impact on the growth and development of an LBW infant if undernutrition continues during childhood, adolescence and pregnancy. The LBW infant is thus more likely to be underweight or stunted in early life. Undernourished girls tend to have a delayed menarche and grow at lower velocities, but for longer periods, compared with their better nourished counterparts. This means that they may attain similar heights to better nourished girls if undernutrition is limited to adolescence. However, if childhood stunting was also experienced, undernourished adolescent females are unlikely to reach similar heights to well-nourished girls. Optimal development during adolescence is reliant on both the present and past nutritional intake. Malnourishment and impaired growth during infancy and early childhood can greatly affect an individual's attainment of height.

Catch-up growth

'Catch-up' or 'catch-down' growth is a phenomenon that appears to compensate for retarded or accelerated intrauterine growth, whereby children return to their genetic trajectory. Many studies have suggested that the potential for catch-up growth and reversal of cognitive impairment among children who have

suffered growth retardation during infancy and/or early childhood is thought to be limited after the age of 2 years, particularly when children remain in poor environments. However, other studies have shown that undernourished children in poor environments can display spontaneous catch-up, even without environmental change. As adolescence is a time of rapid growth, this provides an opportunity for further catch-up growth. It is thought, however, that the potential for significant catch-up during this time is limited. Reversed stunting in women may reduce the risk of pregnancy outcomes that are commonly associated with women of small stature. However, in most cases, regardless of whether growth catch-up has occurred, problems associated with reduced cognitive function remain. Females appear to display greater catch-up than males. Zinc deficiency, of which growth retardation is an outcome, is a commonly reported reason why males may be less able to catch up. At all ages, zinc requirements are very much higher for males than females and therefore a zinc limitation may explain restricted growth in males to a much greater extent than females, and clarify why males are unable to catch up to the same extent as females. Catch-up growth has been associated with a number of adverse outcomes in later life. It is not known why catch-up growth is detrimental, but one theory suggests that IUGR restricts cell numbers, therefore ensuing catch-up growth is achieved by the overgrowth of a restricted cell mass.

Short stature and plant food environments

Many populations in developing countries exist on diets that are predominantly plant based. Such diets are commonly associated with micronutrient deficiencies, chronic energy deficiency and poor growth outcomes. Thus, populations who consume a predominantly plant-based diet are often seen to exhibit short stature. In addition to containing fewer kilojoules, plant-based diets are thought to contain large amounts of protective phytochemicals, which may act to limit the amount of 'metabolic dysregulation', leading to the development of degenerative diseases; the antinutrients may also act to limit growth. It has been suggested that short stature and micronutrient deficiencies may represent adaptations for group survival in adverse environmental conditions. For example, slow growth rates associated with zinc deficiency may represent an adaptation to situations where this is a survival advantage.

Maximal versus optimal height

As undernutrition and stunting during infancy and early childhood have been consistently found to detrimentally affect both the short- and long-term health of an individual, the common health focus of the general public has been on either encouraging secular growth or following the trend towards quicker growth and bigger size. Secular growth is apparent in many cultures. There is evidence, however, that secular growth in many developed countries, such as North America, Western Europe and Australia, is slowing and reaching a plateau. Current nutrition theory holds that an individual should achieve their maximal height potential in order to achieve the best health outcomes. Recent studies, however, have questioned this theory and have introduced the concept of 'optimal' rather than 'maximal' stature. It has been suggested that smaller stature confers many health benefits and represents an adaptive response to an individual's environment. Although small stature carries with it an increased risk of abdominal obesity and heart disease, tall stature increases the risk of developing cancer and degenerative diseases.

7.6 Effects of overnutrition

Obesity is of global epidemic proportions, affecting children, adolescents and adults in growing numbers. In some countries over half of the adult population is affected, thus leading to increasing death rates from heart disease, hypertension, stroke and diabetes. It is the growing prevalence of obesity in younger age groups that has raised alarm. Obesity is multifactorial and a problem of both nutrient imbalance and insufficient physical activity levels. Declining physical activity levels have been associated with television viewing and other modern technological advances. Children who watch large amounts of television are particularly at risk of becoming overweight or obese.

Effects of overweight and obesity

Being overweight or obese as a child and adolescent has many associated health, social and psychological implications. Overweight and obese children may suffer from impaired social interaction and self-esteem.

They are often taller than their non-overweight peers and are often viewed as more mature. This inappropriate expectation may result in adverse effects on their socialisation. Obese individuals at all ages often do less well academically, leading to higher rates of poverty and lower job prospects in later life. Being overweight or obese can negatively affect mobility and physical fitness. Serious physical complications associated with high weights in children are rare, but include cardiomyopathy, pancreatitis, orthopaedic disorders and respiratory disorders such as upper airway obstruction and chest wall restriction. These are largely restricted to the severely obese and are of low prevalence. In adolescents, obesity confers significant cardiovascular risks, abnormal glucose tolerance, hypertension and lipid profile abnormalities. Furthermore, a greater percentage of abdominal fat in children of both genders is associated with early maturity. Few studies have investigated the long-term effects of childhood obesity on adult health outcomes, but obesity experienced during childhood or adolescence seems to increase the risk of adult morbidity and mortality.

Age of onset and obesity in later life

Differences exist in the prevalence of obesity between boys and girls, men and women, and between social classes. Social factors are a predominant determinant of body fatness and thus obesity. Obesity is, however, also a familial condition. It has been reported that less than 10% of obese children have both parents of a normal weight, with 50 and 80% of obese children having one and two obese parents, respectively. Obese children are more likely to remain obese as adolescents and as adults. The age of the onset of obesity strongly influences this risk. The older the obese child, the more probable it is that he or she will become an obese adult. The correlation between adult and childhood obesity rises with age and with the severity of childhood obesity, while the rate of spontaneous weight reduction decreases with age. The proportion of overweight or obese adults, who had been overweight or obese in adolescence, ranges from 20 to 45%, while from 25 to 50% of overweight or obese adolescents had been overweight or obese in early childhood. Obese adolescents have significantly more abdominal fat than the non-obese. Obesity that begins during, or close, to adolescence is often characterised by the abdominal type of fat distribution. In the 1960s it was reported that both hypermasculine and hyperfeminine types of body fat distribution in women often began prior to adulthood, with the hyperfeminine variety tending to originate pre-pubertally and the hypermasculine type tending to originate during adolescence. Adolescence may thus be a sensitive period for the development of android or abdominal obesity, in both males and females.

Predictors of body size and fatness in adolescence

The interaction of both genetic and environmental factors appears to determine human body fatness. Measures that predict body size and fatness in adolescence have been identified. Predictors in early life of body size and fatness in adolescence include birth weight, anthropometric measures at 12, 50 and 80 months, weight and height velocities during the first year, the presence of a major illness and parental socioeconomic status in early life. Tienboon *et al.* (1992) found that the consumption of fish liver oil [high in vitamins A and D and in eicosapentaenoic acid (EPA) and DHA] in early life, lowered the risk of developing obesity, particularly abdominal obesity. Self-reported measures of exercise, appetite and consumption of some specific food items correlated more closely with contemporary predictors of adolescent body size and fatness when measured at adolescence.

Factors affecting weight status in children and adolescence

Many factors, including season, geographical region, population density, ethnicity, socioeconomic status, family size, gender, parental education, levels of physical activity, maternal age and maternal preference for a chubby baby, have been reported to affect the development of obesity in children and adolescents. Weight status may differ between children and adolescents living in rural and urban areas. Adolescents from urban areas may be significantly taller and heavier, and have more superficial fat and longer legs, than adolescents from rural areas.

Rate of weight gain and mode of feeding in early life

Early feeding experience is related to the development of excess weight in infancy. Both breast-feeding and the delayed introduction of solid foods appear to exert a protective effect against adiposity up to 2 years of age, and probably in later life. However, not all studies have shown this effect. The ages where most obesity arises before adulthood are between 0 and 4 years, 7 and 11 years and during adolescence. During infancy, rapid increases in weight have been associated with obesity at adolescence in boys. Early catch-up growth, between the ages of 0 and 2 years, has been frequently reported as a predictor of childhood obesity, particularly for central or abdominal obesity.

Familial aggregation of weight status

In the 1920s one of the first and more detailed of the early genetic studies was conducted. It was found that alleles for obesity tended to be dominant, and thus more likely to be expressed, compared with non-obese alleles. Slender individuals tended to be homozygous, whereas obese persons were often heterozygous for these alleles. Overweight or obese individuals generally have at least one overweight or obese parent, with current statistics between 49 and 69%; of these, a fat mother (26–43%) is more common than a fat father (12–16%). When all other family members are obese, the likelihood of children being obese is very high (24–28%).

Many studies have investigated the relationship between body fatness and fat distribution among families. The effects of environmental factors, with respect to weight status, have been demonstrated in studies of twins and siblings. Both genetic and environmental factors appear to play a role in total body fat levels and distribution patterns. Measures of body mass index (BMI) for immediate family members are often highly correlated. In addition, it appears that people living together can have similar degrees of fatness. Under shared environmental conditions, both genetically related and unrelated household members show similar amounts of total body fatness. In this sense, genetically unrelated subjects are generally as similar, fat-wise, as genetically related individuals. However, studies have found that genetic, rather than environmental, factors may be more influential in determining the fat distribution pattern. Spouses who do not share genetic make-up often show little relationship in fat distribution, even after 20 years of co-habitation. However, family members of shared genetic origin show similarities in fat distribution patterns and the degree of correlation is gender specific.

(a)

(b)

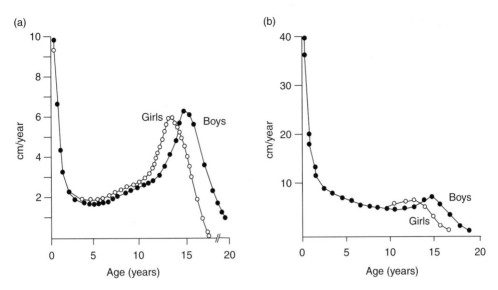

Figure 7.2 Growth velocities throughout childhood and adolescence: (a) 50th centile weight velocities; (b) 50th centile height velocities. (Reproduced with permission from Gracey M, Hetzel B and Smallwood R, Responsibility for Nutritional Diagnosis: A Report by the Nutrition Working Party of the Social Issues Committee of the Royal Australasian College of Physicians. London: Smith-Gordon, 1989.)

7.7 Growth during childhood and adolescence

The most rapid periods of growth take place during the first few months of life and during adolescence. Growth velocity slows significantly after the first year of life. The growth rate accelerates again as an individual enters puberty in adolescence over a period of 1–3 years. After the peak velocity of growth in puberty has been attained, the growth rate slows considerably until growth in height ceases at around 16 years of age in girls and 18 years in boys (Figure 7.2).

During the first year of life, a well-nourished infant will ideally increase in length by 50% and in weight by 300%. Rapid and essentially linear growth occurs in well-nourished infants, with rates of weight and height keeping pace with each other. Infants have a high surface area to body weight, which means that their energy and nutritional needs are much higher than adults on a per kilogram of body weight basis. As a result of this, infants are prone to heat stress and dehydration, but the ratio of surface area to body weight decreases with age. The period of infancy ends when the child is weaned from the breast (or bottle), which in pre-industrialised societies occurs at a median age of 36 months, and less in more developed countries. During early childhood, height and weight increase in an essentially linear fashion. Steady growth necessitates a gradual increase in the intake of most nutrients to support growth and development. It is thought that the age of 6–7 years is a critical period for determining future weight and height status. During childhood, an individual is still largely dependent on the caregiver for providing nourishment, but this begins to change during late childhood, when a child begins to develop increased control over his or her food intake and relies less on caregivers.

During adolescence, the body undergoes a large number of changes as a result of puberty. Once puberty is reached, an individual is capable of sexual reproduction. The onset of puberty is characteristically earlier in females than in males (10.5–11 years and 12.5–13 years, respectively). As males reach puberty later than females, they experience on average 2 more years of pre-pubertal growth than females, resulting in typically higher statures at the onset of puberty for males.

Before puberty there are no significant height differences between girls and boys. It is during the adolescent growth spurt that major skeletal differences between males and females become apparent. In males, there is a widening of the shoulders with respect to the pelvis, while the opposite is seen in females. Typically, height gains of approximately 20 and 15 cm are realised in males and females, respectively.

In both genders, a sequential pattern of growth is observed: the feet and hands, the calves and forearms, the hips and chest, and the shoulders, followed by the trunk. Skeletal growth ceases once the epiphyses, the active areas of bone at the end of long bones, have closed. Once this occurs, bones cannot become any longer and are largely unresponsive to exogenous GH administration. In males, puberty is marked by growth of the sexual organs, followed by changes in the larynx, skin and hair distribution. The growth of the ovaries signifies the beginning of puberty in females. Fat is deposited in the breasts and around the hips, dramatically changing the female body shape. Menarche coincides with the peak growth spurt of adolescence, after which growth decelerates.

Body composition changes during childhood and adolescence

Growth and development in children and adolescents are associated with changes in body composition, which affects body fatness and leanness. Body composition is therefore used as one of the measures of growth. It also provides an indication of both nutritional status and physical fitness.

Changes in fat-free mass and body water content

Lean body mass (LBM) includes all non-lipid body constituents, as well as essential fats and phospholipids. In adolescence, LBM increases to a much greater extent in males than in females, with muscle and bone representing the largest gains in growth. Fat-free mass (FFM) is similar to LBM, but it excludes all essential fats and phospholipids. FFM density (effectively lean mass) increases from the first year of life through to 10 years of age, and then again dramatically during puberty. Both males and females show a linear increase in FFM mineral content from the age of 8–15 years. The body's water content, measured as FFM–water content, decreases from 81 to 72% during the period of birth to adulthood. This drop in water content coincides with the abrupt rise in the mean FFM density seen between these ages.

Changes in body fat

Full-term infants have 10–15% body fat. In infancy, the amount of fat is correlated with body weight. Body fat shows a remarkable increase during the first year of life. By the end of this year, it is estimated that body fat represents 20–25% of total body weight. Thereafter, there is a decline in the percentage of body fat to its lowest level in the mid-childhood years, and then an increase in adolescence. Girls experience a much larger increase in body fat than boys during adolescence. Adolescent boys typically have significantly less superficial fat, less total body fat and less percentage body fat than adolescent girls. Furthermore, adolescent boys have a significantly higher abdominal or central fat distribution than girls, as shown by waist–hip ratio and the ratio of subscapular–triceps skinfold thickness.

Fat patterning in children and adolescents

The waist-to-hip circumference ratio (WHR) measures the predominance of fat storage in the abdominal region, relative to the gluteal region. A high WHR is indicative of excess abdominal fat; that is, a central fat distribution. In adults, the WHR has been related to a number of metabolic diseases and is a strong predictor of mortality, but the implications of a high WHR in children are not clear. WHR is significantly influenced by age and gender. Boys generally have higher measures of WHR than girls. The WHR decreases with age from approximately 1.1 in the youngest children to approximately 0.8 in pubertal children. From puberty onwards, the WHR approaches the values reported for adults. In children, WHR is more or less independent of the total body fatness. In adults, however, the WHR is positively correlated with body fatness, as measured by BMI. In general, subcutaneous adipose tissue is distributed peripherally for most children up until puberty. For the majority of boys, but only a few girls, fat begins to be stored more centrally. The rate of change towards a more central fat distribution decreases in girls after about 13–14 years of age, but continues in boys. In adults, a central fat pattern is common in men, but not in women. However, a central fat pattern is more prevalent in elderly women than in younger, adult women.

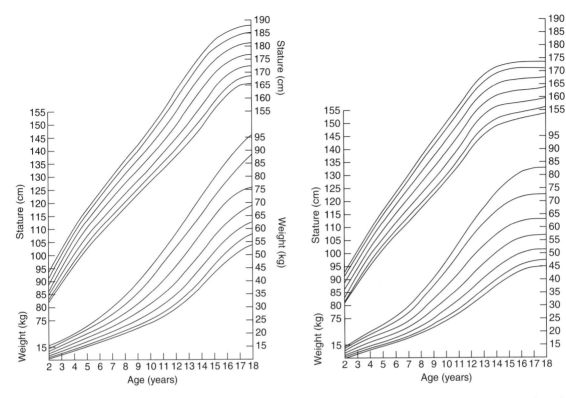

Figure 7.3 Growth chart (attained): boys 2–18 years. (Reproduced with kind permission from World Health Organization, http://www. who.int/growthref/en 2009 © WHO.)

Figure 7.4 Growth chart (attained): girls 2–18 years. (Reproduced with kind permission from World Health Organization, http://www. who.int/growthref/en 2009 © WHO.)

Assessment of growth

Growth charts are routinely used to assess growth and are used in the diagnosis and management of diseases, and in monitoring the efficacy of therapy. Chronic undernutrition or overnutrition is typically reflected in growth rates and therefore the monitoring of growth is used as an integral part of nutritional assessment. Common growth charts include weight-for-age, length-for-age (for children below 2 years of age) and height-for-age (for children 2 years and over) (Figures 7.3 and 7.4). Those to 60 months of age, based on breast-fed infants in various cultural settings, are now provided by WHO (http://www.who.int/childgrowth/standards/technical_report/en/index.html).

Although growth charts that show attained growth may show a steady progressive increase in anthropometric body measures with age, growth velocity charts reveal the changing rates of growth more visibly (see Figure 7.2). The growth charts may suggest that an infant or child who is above the 97th centile, or below the third centile, is unusually large or small. However,

such a conclusion is not always appropriate. A well-nourished individual will follow a typical growth curve and it is therefore possible that a misinterpretation may occur for an individual whose growth is considered to be small or large from their chart, but is simply a reflection of individual variation. A greater cause for alarm is when an individual crosses centiles, particularly if this happens over a short period. This may indicate inappropriate weight gain or acute growth failure or retardation, such as wasting or stunting, as a result of chronic undernutrition due to either chronic malnourishment or an underlying disease condition. Wasting is detectable on weight-for-age growth charts and by reduced skinfold measures, while stunting is seen as impairment of linear growth, as detected by length- or height-for-age growth charts. It should be noted, however, that there are large variations between individuals in rates and patterns of growth, and these variations must be taken into consideration when determining whether or not a child's growth is abnormal.

Appropriate measures must be used for specific population groups. Growth charts based on Caucasian bottle-fed babies are unlikely to be appropriate for use in certain developing countries, as using such charts may misclassify an individual or population group as underweight. New international growth references are being developed by WHO based on pooled data from seven countries, combining measurements from over 13 000 breast-fed healthy infants and children. They are now available to 60 months of age, as indicated above. This will provide a more scientifically reliable tool for use in all countries to monitor growth and nutritional status. Other anthropometric measures that are routinely used to monitor growth and nutritional status include head circumference, which is used in young infants, mid–upper arm circumference, which is widely used in developing countries as a measure of muscle and fat in both children and adults, and skinfold thickness, which measures subcutaneous fat. BMI centiles (Table 7.4), using Quetelet's ratio (weight in kilograms divided by the square of height in metres) have been developed to detect overweight and obesity in children.

Tienboon P (2003) has developed cut-off levels for BMI for children, both boys and girls aged 1–7 years, to screen for under and over-nutrition. The healthy cut-off levels are 14.5–18.0 kg/m². They have utility in the evaluation of service delivery in out patient departments (OPD) or in field work in developing countries. These BMI values have been evaluated in apparently healthy children and in patients with various degrees of undernutrition, (Table 7.5). They correspond closely to current WHO criteria.

Both GH and IGFs can be measured in the plasma and their levels are thought to reflect changes in growth and cellular activity. IGF plasma levels are considerably more stable and do not display such large fluctuations as displayed by GH. As a result of this greater stability, plasma levels of IGF can provide a sensitive measure of growth. Growth is a process that is multifactorial. The relative contributions of genetic and environmental factors, to growth and development outcomes, of an individual are still under investigation. Both overnutrition and undernutrition exert negative and often irreversible impacts on growth at all life stages and unless addressed in the early years of life, long deficits may result.

Table 7.4 International cut-off points for body mass index (BMI) for overweight and obesity by gender between the ages of 2 and 18 years

Age (years)	Overweight		Obese	
	Males	Females	Males	Females
2	18.41	18.02	20.09	19.81
2.5	18.13	17.76	19.80	19.55
3	17.89	17.56	19.57	19.36
3.5	17.69	17.40	19.39	19.23
4	17.55	17.28	19.29	19.15
4.5	17.47	17.19	19.26	19.12
5	17.42	17.15	19.30	19.17
5.5	17.45	17.20	19.47	19.34
6	17.55	17.34	19.78	19.65
6.5	17.71	17.53	20.23	20.08
7	17.92	17.75	20.63	20.51
7.5	18.16	18.03	21.09	21.01
8	18.44	18.35	21.60	21.57
8.5	18.76	18.69	22.17	22.18
9	19.10	19.07	22.77	22.81
9.5	19.46	19.45	23.39	23.46
10	19.84	19.86	24.00	24.11
10.5	20.20	20.29	24.57	24.77
11	20.55	20.74	25.10	25.42
11.5	20.89	21.20	25.58	26.05
12	21.22	21.68	26.02	26.67
12.5	21.56	22.14	26.43	27.24
13	21.91	22.58	26.84	27.76
13.5	22.27	22.98	27.25	28.20
14	22.62	23.34	27.63	28.57
14.5	22.96	23.66	27.98	28.87
15	23.29	23.94	28.30	29.11
15.5	23.60	24.17	28.60	29.29
16	23.90	24.37	28.88	29.43
16.5	24.19	24.54	29.14	29.56
17	24.46	24.70	29.41	29.69
17.5	24.73	24.85	29.70	29.84
18	25	25	30	30

7.8 Ageing

Ageing is not a disease, nor are the so-called diseases of ageing – cancer, heart disease, arthritis and senility – the inevitable consequences of advancing years. If we live long enough, changes in body composition, physical function and performance will occur in all of us. Many of these changes, as well as health problems which become more common in old age, have long been attributed to the 'normal ageing process'. This section will highlight that these health problems can be delayed to the last few years of life (i.e. compression of morbidity).

Table 7.5 Body mass index as an indicator for nutritional status of children aged 1-7 years

Nutritional status	Body mass index (kg/m²)
Underweight	
Mild degree	<14.5–13.0
Moderate degree	<13.0–11.5
Severe degree	<11.5
Normal weight	14.5–18.0
Overweight	>18.0–19.5
Obesity	
Mild degree	>19.5–21.0
Moderate degree	>21.0–22.5
Severe degree	>22.5

Using body mass index to assess undernutrition and overnutrition of preschool children, Tienboon P., Thai Journal of Parenteral and Enteral Nutrtion, 14(2)Copyright © (2003) Reproduced by permission of Thai Journal of Parenteral and Enteral Nutrition.

Table 7.6 Proportion of the population aged 65 years and over, selected countries 1985 and 2005

	Population aged 65+ (%)	
	1985	2005
Europe		
France	12.4	14.8
Germany (FRG)	14.5	18.9
Greece	13.1	16.9
Hungary	12.5	15.0
Italy	13.0	16.9
Poland	9.4	12.3
Sweden	16.9	17.2
UK	15.1	15.3
North America		
Canada	10.4	12.5
USA	12.0	13.1
Other developed countries		
Australia	10.1	11.4
Japan	10.0	16.5
Less-developed countries		
Brazil	4.3	5.8
China	5.1	7.4
India	4.3	6.1
Kenya	2.1[a]	2.1
Mexico	3.5	4.6

Reprinted from Textbook of Geriatic Medicine and Gerontology, 4th edn (JC Brocklehurst, RC Tallis, HM Filit, eds) pp 3–20 copyright © 1992.

Sociodemography

Humans are living longer than ever before, with several population life expectancies at birth now exceeding 80 years. Since the early 1970s life expectancies have increased globally by approximately 1 year every 3 years. The elderly today are living almost 20 years longer than their ancestors at the beginning of the twentieth century. At present, the proportion of centenarians is also increasing (upwards of 1 in 1000 of the population in economically advantaged countries), but individuals do not appear to exceed a maximal lifespan of about 120 years. Maximal lifespan may yet increase as biotechnology, lifestyle and health care develop in favour of greater longevity.

Adults are reaching older age in better health and the majority will live independently. Life expectancy is increasing for men and women alike. Between 1981 and 2001 the number of older people in the population increased by 50%, with an even greater increase in those aged over 70. Although maximum life expectancy has not increased over the past century, average life expectancy has changed substantially. Men born in 2020 can expect to live to 79, and women to 87. Our ability to live longer is, in part, attributable to better nutrition and to other lifestyle changes (e.g. reduced substance abuse, greater recreational opportunities), to improved health care (e.g. reduced infant and maternal mortality, earlier diagnosis and management of cancers and heart disease), to educational

and economic improvements, and to better housing (especially less crowding) and social support systems. But as we live longer, our nutritional needs may change, either with 'healthy' ageing or because of the advent of disease. Keeping an elderly population well is of great importance for the individuals themselves and the well-being of society in general, that is the transfer of knowledge and skills to younger people, especially descendants and a reduced burden on others, and for reasons of available resources to care for the aged. Remarkably, the numbers of elderly people in developing countries now approach and will exceed those in developed countries (Table 7.6), so that the problem is global.

Biological and chronological age and compression of morbidity

Biological and chronological age

Ageing may be defined as chronological age (a person's age in years since birth) or biological age (the decline in function that occurs in every human being with time). Some elderly people look and function as though they were older and others as though they were younger, even though they are at the same 'chronological age'. Prospective studies, where some assessment of biological age has been made during the twentieth century in Sweden, indicate that people are less biologically old at the same chronological age than they used to be, and that this difference may be as much as 10 years of biological age. This is a rather remarkable change and some of it is likely to be attributable to improved lifelong nutrition. It may well be that much of what we currently regard as ageing is preventable by nutritional means. In other words, even though genes have a strong influence on biological age, it is now believed that lifestyle factors also have a strong influence. You may be able to remain biologically younger if you look after yourself in your younger adult years. The question is, what aspects of ageing are biologically inevitable, having to do, for example, with the programmed death of cells (apopotosis), and how much is age related? While the clock cannot be turned back in terms of chronological age, the search for prolonged youth continues to invoke much interest and research. The older people are, the more dissimilar they become from others of the same chronological age. Some of this variability may reflect heterogeneity in true rates of ageing, but other factors that accompany ageing also seem to be of major importance. These include lifestyle factors, such as poor eating habits, a sedentary lifestyle and smoking, and the development of disease. Each of these factors can contribute to deterioration in cardiovascular, lung or endocrine functions, thereby accelerating one's apparent rate of ageing. For example, declining cardiovascular function was observed in the Baltimore Longitudinal Study of Aging. However, after careful exclusion of those with heart disease, no consistent declines in function with age remained. Thus, the apparent declines in the study group members as they aged were due to inclusion of people with defined disease, rather than to the ageing process per se. As discussed later in this chapter, the accumulating effects of years of poor eating habits can increase the risk of many health conditions as one grows older; yet it is never too late to change!

Compression of morbidity

The accumulating effects of years of poor eating habits can increase the risk of many health conditions as one grows older. The good news is, however, that food habits may be amenable to modification. In other words, we can adopt lifestyle habits, such as regular exercise and healthy eating, that will slow functional decline and compositional changes, within the limits set by genetics. It is possible to compress morbidity into the last few years of life (i.e. increase health span potential) if we take care of lifestyle and environmental factors throughout life, even once we reach old age. For example, an exercise intervention study in mid-life has been shown to compress morbidity (measured with disability score) towards the end of life. Several of the health problems and bodily changes experienced by older adults that have been attributed to the normal ageing process are increasingly recognised as being linked to lifestyle or environmental factors. For example, decline in LBM and increases in body fat, which tend to occur as people grow older, cannot be entirely attributed to the ageing process per se. A major contributor to these changes is the increasingly sedentary nature of people's lifestyles as they grow older in Western countries. Social and physical inactivity and inadequate nutrient and phytochemical intakes are now thought to be instrumental in trying to compress morbidity towards the end of life, and in maintaining or increasing physiological and nutritional reserves.

Physiological reserves, frailty and prevention strategies

Many bodily functions remain relatively unaffected until about 75 years of age when, on average, they start to decrease more noticeably. Nutritionally related health problems are often compounded in later life by reduced physiological reserves of many organs and functions. This applies to both reduced metabolic tissues (e.g. insulin resistance or reduced insulin response to a meal load, or a greater glycaemic response to the same food) and organ tissues (e.g. reduced cardiac reserve means that an added salt load may tip someone into heart failure, whereas otherwise it would not). While a younger person will be able to consume an inadequate diet with no foreseeable consequences, an elderly person is more likely to experience problems because of diminished physiological function. Many studies have shown significant reductions in different body functions with age. These may not be inevitable, however. For example, what used to be regarded as a decline in brain function at about the age of 70 may not be seen until much later, raising the possibility that biological age in some body functions may be occurring at a later and later chronological age. Measures of physiological and nutritional reserves may be important indicators of health in older adults. Prevention of associated health problems may be possible, if physiological and nutritional reserve levels are known.

Frailty

Avoidance of frailty is one of the major challenges facing older people and their carers. Frailty among older people has been defined as 'a condition or syndrome which results from a multi-system reduction in reserve capacity, to the extent that a number of physiological systems are close to, or past, the threshold of symptomatic clinical failure. As a consequence, the frail person is at an increased risk of disability and death from minor external stresses' (Campbell and Buchner, 1997). As the number of chronic conditions increases with age, they contribute to disability and frailty which, in turn, reduce a person's level of independence, sometimes resulting in institutionalisation. Falls, incontinence and confusion are regarded as clinical consequences of frailty, and a number of risk factors are associated with each of these conditions. The risk of falling is increased as muscle strength and flexibility decline, and if balance and reaction time are impaired. Urinary incontinence is also a risk factor for falls among elderly people. Dehydration and PEM are two nutritional factors that can contribute to the confusion often experienced by elderly adults. Urinary incontinence often results in elderly people restricting their fluid intake in an effort to control their incontinence or reduce their frequency of urination. Studies are underway in relation to its prevention and management, and there is great interest in the extent to which it is reversible.

Prevention strategies

The major prevention strategies that elderly individuals can take to increase their physiological and nutritional reserves include:

- consuming a wide variety of foods
- engaging in physical activity, as this maintains lean muscle and bone mass, thus increasing nutritional and physiological reserves to prevent major health problems

- engaging in social activity
- avoiding substance abuse (including alcohol, tobacco, excessive caffeine intake and unnecessary intake of medications).

By focusing on the complete lifestyle rather than on just one component, such as nutrition, elderly people can enjoy life without experiencing major consequences of nutritional error.

Food variety

Research has shown that food variety has an important role to play in preventing the onset of diseases such as diabetes, cancer and cardiovascular disease. A varied diet, ideally containing 20–30 biologically distinct foods a week, is seen to be beneficial in the prevention of certain disease states. Specifically, an association between increased food variety and lower glycaemic response, in both insulin-dependent and non-insulin-dependent diabetes mellitus (IDDM and NIDDM), has been found. Greater dietary diversity has also been found to be predictive of less morbidity and greater longevity in people aged over 70 years. Mortality follow-up studies of elderly people aged 70 and over in Australia, Greece, Spain and Denmark have found that more varied food patterns, even as late as 70 years and onwards, could reduce the risk of death by more than 50%. To obtain this mortality advantage, it was necessary for the elderly in these studies to have their old patterns consistent with the following food groups, giving a score ranging from 0 to 8: (1) high in vegetables (>300 g/day), (2) high in legumes (>50 g/day), (3) high in fruits (>200 g/day), (4) high in cereals (>250 g/day), (5) moderate in dairy products (<300 g of milk/day or equivalent in cheese/yogurt), (6) moderate in meat and meat products (<100 g/day), (7) moderate in alcohol (<10 g/day), (8) high in monounsaturated fat (mainly from olive oil) and low in saturated fat (i.e. high monounsaturated: saturated fat ratio). This food pattern is consistent with food patterns prevalent in Greece in the 1960s, when Greeks enjoyed the longest life expectancy in the world. The subjects achieved greater mortality advantage if they followed the entire food pattern (i.e. had high dietary variety scores ≥4), as opposed to just achieving the required amount for one or two of the food groups (Figure 7.5).

This suggests that there may be synergy between the food groups and we need to follow dietary recommendations as a whole, rather than focusing on just one food group or nutrient.

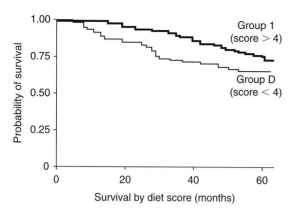

Figure 7.5 Kaplan–Meier survival curves for individual subjects with diet score up to 3 and 4 or more. (Reproduced from Diet and overall survival in elderly people, Trichopoulou A, Kouris-Blazos A, Wahlqvist M, 311: 1457–1460 (1995) Copyright © with permission from BMJ Publishing Group Ltd.)

Physical activity

Ageing as we know it in modern society is, in many ways, an exercise deficiency syndrome, implying that we may have far more control over the rate and extent of the ageing process than we previou sly thought. (Fiatarone, 1996)

Some of the most dramatic changes that we see with age are changes in body composition. A decline in muscle mass and increases in body fat tend to occur as people grow older. What is often not appreciated, however, is that these too cannot be blamed on the ageing process per se. A major contributor to these changes is the increasingly sedentary nature of people's lifestyles as they grow older. Reduced physical activity leads to loss of muscle and, as a direct consequence, basal metabolic rate (BMR) falls. A lower metabolic rate means that we need to eat less in order to maintain the same body weight. If one does indeed eat less to avoid weight gain, rather than remaining (or becoming) active, it becomes increasingly difficult to meet the needs for essential nutrients. Without doubt, it is preferable to keep physically active, maintain muscle mass and continue to enjoy eating.

Physical activity has been associated with greater energy intakes and subsequently nutrient intakes and quality of life in the aged. This results in a higher plane of energy nutrition and runs counter to the disturbing advocacy that energy restriction prolongs life. These studies were conducted on rats and have no direct application to humans. To suggest that elderly people restrict their food intake to prolong life is absurd, when this may contribute to frailty and loss of lean mass. The evidence is, however, that any extra energy intake must be from nutrient (and phytochemical)-dense foods, without excessive abdominal fatness. Many studies have shown that energy intake declines with age, making a nutritionally adequate diet more difficult to achieve. Older men consume about 800 kcal less than younger men, and older women consume about 400 kcal less than younger women. A reduction in BMR is partly responsible for this decline in energy intake, but physical inactivity appears to be the major cause. Prospective studies show that increased energy intakes in the order of 300–500 kcal/day, which is balanced with increased physical activity to avoid fat gain, confer either decreased cardiovascular or total mortality and improve life expectancy. Physical activity also seems to protect against osteoporosis and fractures, diabetes, and breast and colon cancers, to improve mental health and cognitive function, reduce symptoms of anxiety and depression and enhance feelings of well-being in older people. An exercise intervention study in mid-life has been shown to compress morbidity (measured with disability score) towards the end of life. The subjects who belonged to a 'runner's club' in mid-life had significantly less disability in their 80s, compared with control subjects. While the evidence points to the value of early and lifelong regular physical activity, recent evidence underlines just how much survivors can gain from the combination of endurance and strength training well into later life, with studies available on people well into their 80s. In other words, physical activity in old age can defer morbidity and mortality, and compress the morbidity period before death.

Social activity

Social activity is now thought to be one of the most important determinants of longevity. Participation in fewer social activities outside the home and limited social networks have been linked with higher mortality in old age. The impact of social activity on longevity could be through its impact on psychological well-being and nutrition. For example, elderly people who are socially isolated, lonely, institutionalised, recently bereaved and socially inactive have been found to have inadequate food intakes. Glass *et al.* (1999) examined associations between social (e.g. church), productive (e.g. shopping) and physical/fitness activities (e.g. walking) at baseline and 13-year survival in 3000 older people. Social and productive activities were found to be as effective as fitness activities in lowering the risk of death. Further studies of this kind indicate the importance of social activity to the health and mortality of older people, and perhaps younger people as well.

Effects of ageing on physiological function

Physiological changes that occur with ageing contribute to the body's declining function which, in turn, influences nutritional status, just as growth and development do in the earlier stages of the life cycle. Some physiological changes are:

- hormone activity alters body composition
- changes in the immune system raise the risk of infections and some chronic diseases
- atrophic gastritis interferes with nutrient digestion and absorption
- tooth loss and depression can adversely influence food choice.

Animal studies suggest that energy restriction promotes longevity, but human studies suggest that 'eating better, not less' is desirable.

Theories of ageing and energy restriction

There are three main theories of ageing which predict the role that genes play in the ageing process:

- programmed ageing
- error theory
- free radical theory.

The theory of programmed ageing suggests that the body has a built-in clock that begins ticking at birth. This theory is supported by the discovery that normal cells have a limited capacity to divide because telomeres (the sections of DNA at the end of chromosomes) shorten at each division, resulting in a fixed lifespan for each normal cell. Furthermore, the ageing process accelerates so rapidly in some individuals that they become biologically 'old' in their teens. The error theory attributes ageing to increasing damage to DNA and the progressive decline in the function of specialised enzymes that repair DNA. It is thought that diseases such as cancer, heart disease, osteoporosis and diabetes may be the result of an accumulation of errors. The free radical theory proposes that free radicals (highly reactive oxygen molecules) are produced by oxygen-consuming biological reactions in the body. Free radicals damage cells and have been implicated in the development of cancer and heart disease. There is no evidence that taking antioxidants will improve longevity, but antioxidants consumed from food may have an indirect effect by reducing the damage produced by free radicals. A free radical is a molecule with an unpaired, highly reactive electron, which is often associated with the development of cancer, arteriosclerosis, autoimmune diseases and ageing. Antioxidants include phytochemicals (flavonoids) and nutrients (vitamins C and E and β-carotene), as well as enzymes such as superoxide dismutase (SOD), catalase and glutathione peroxidase. These prevent most, but not all, oxidative damage. Bit by bit, the damage mounts and contributes, so the theory goes, to deteriorating tissues and organs. Antioxidants may reduce the risk of cancer by protecting cellular DNA from free radical damage.

There has been a popularised view, derived mainly from rodent experiments, which has argued that energy restriction may decrease the risk of cancer and increase longevity. Most of these studies are flawed insofar as extrapolation to humans is concerned because either they are conducted from early life with excessive early mortality or they do not account for energy expenditure, and therefore energy balance, reflected in body fatness and/or its distribution. Where the full energy equation is available, increased energy throughput (e.g. higher energy intakes with no increase in body fatness) has been associated with decreased cancer risk and/or increased life expectancy. Increased energy intake (and possibly its frequency) has, in its own right, been associated with increased cancer risk at several sites. Again, the quality of extra food intake seems important. The Zutphen prospective study in The Netherlands showed that increased energy intake, which included relatively more plant-derived food and fish, was associated with lower cancer and total mortality over a period of 10 years.

Body composition

Some of the most dramatic changes seen with age are changes in body composition. A decline in muscle, bone mass and increases in body fat tend to occur as people grow older, and subcutaneous fat is redistributed from limbs to the trunk. Some of these changes occur because some hormonal activity that regulates metabolism decreases with age (e.g. insulin, GH, androgens), while the activity of others increases (e.g. prolactin): the former contribute to a decrease in lean mass and the latter to an increase in fat mass. However, what is often not appreciated is that these cannot be blamed entirely on the ageing process per se. A major contributor to these changes is the increasingly sedentary nature of people's lives as they grow older. Reduced physical activity leads to loss of muscle and, as a direct consequence, BMR falls. A lower metabolic rate means that older people need to eat less energy in order to maintain the same body weight, but should ensure that this does not lead to a decrease in micronutrient intake. The incidence of people becoming underweight has been shown to increase with age. A lower body weight has been more strongly linked with morbidity in the elderly than mild to moderate excess weight, and the problem is often insidious. Survival rates in elderly Finnish people, (85 years and over) during a 5-year period, showed the highest mortality to be in those with a BMI less than $20\,kg/m^2$ and the lowest mortality to be in the group with a BMI of 30 or more. Other studies have shown that elderly people with BMIs below $27\,kg/m^2$ lived shorter lives than those with higher BMIs. Weight changes, and especially weight loss, are of greater concern in the elderly than too much fat. In developed countries, 30–50% of older adults have been reported to be at high risk of developing health problems as a result of an inadequate food and nutrient intake.

Immune system

Both physical stressors (e.g. alcohol abuse, other drug abuse, smoking, pain, heat and illness) and psychological stressors (e.g. divorces, exams, migration and loss of a loved one) elicit the body's stress response: the classic fight-or-flight response. Stress that is prolonged or severe can drain the body of its reserves and leave it weakened, aged and vulnerable to illness. As people age, their ability to adapt to both external and internal stressors, especially via the immune system, is diminished owing to physiological changes that occur with ageing. The immune system can also be compromised by nutrient deficiencies (see below), and so a combination of age and sub-

clinical nutrient deficiencies makes older adults vulnerable to infectious diseases, including chronic diseases where the immune system is involved, such as arthritis and cancer.

Gastrointestinal tract

The intestine loses strength and elasticity with age; this slows motility and increases the risk of developing constipation (which is four to eight times more common in the elderly than in younger adults). Atrophic gastritis is also more common among older adults; about 30% of adults aged over 60 have this condition. It is a condition characterised by chronic inflammation of the stomach, accompanied by a diminished size and functioning of the mucosa and glands, resulting in less hydrochloric acid being secreted and increased levels of bacteria. These changes in the stomach can impair digestion and the absorption of nutrients, especially vitamin B_{12}, biotin, calcium and iron.

Tooth loss

Chewing can be painful or difficult in old age as a result of tooth loss, gum disease and ill-fitting dentures. This can result in a reduced variety of foods consumed and an increased risk of developing nutrient deficiencies.

Sensory loss

Changes in taste and smell are variable and are often associated with lifelong cigarette smoking, poor dental hygiene and disease. Nevertheless, this phenomenon may make eating less enjoyable and may partly explain why older people tend to increase salt intake and use caffeinated beverages (caffeine may briefly suppress, but then increase their appetite). Ageing is associated with a decrease in the opioid (dynorphin) feeding drive and an increase in the satiety effect of cholecystokinin. Recent studies suggest that early satiety in older people may be caused by a nitric oxide deficiency, which decreases the adaptive relaxation of the fundus of the stomach in response to food.

Psychological changes

Depression is common among older adults, but is not an inevitable component of ageing. It is frequently accompanied by loss of appetite and the motivation to cook.

Nutritionally vulnerable older adults

Contrary to the popular 'tea 'n' toast' myth, it appears that many older adults outside institutions eat reasonably well. The dietary patterns of older adults have generally been found to be similar to, or healthier than, those of their younger counterparts. Nevertheless, their intakes of cereals, fruit, vegetables and milk products are still below the recommended amounts. Some older people may consume a higher calorie diet without adverse health effects, which may be attributed to higher levels of physical activity or intake of protective nutrients, such as phytochemicals. Ageing is often associated with less efficient processing of some essential nutrients, so older people may require higher intakes of particular nutrients, while requiring lower intakes of others.

As a general guide, adult energy requirements decline by an estimated 5% per decade. In developed countries, energy intakes fall with advancing age (from 2800 to 2000 kcal for men and from 1900 to 1500 kcal for women), but average intakes of protein, total fat, polyunsaturated n-6 linoleic acid, vitamin A, thiamin, riboflavin, niacin, vitamin C, iron and phosphorus remain adequate in the 65-plus age group. Saturated fat and refined carbohydrates (high sugar content) continue to be consumed in excess of the recommended levels, and intakes of monounsaturated fats, n-3 fatty acids (from plants and fish), unrefined carbohydrates, fibre, folate, vitamin B_6, calcium, magnesium and zinc tend to be below the recommended intakes. These intakes may not result in the appearance of any diagnostic features or symptoms of true deficiency, but may result in subtle or sub-clinical nutrient deficiencies. In developed countries, mild vitamin and mineral deficiencies are very common in older people, particularly those in institutions; 30–50% of older adults have been reported to be at high risk of developing health problems as a result of an inadequate food and nutrient intake, including cognitive impairment, poor wound healing, anaemia, bruising, an increased propensity for developing infections, neurological disorders, stroke and some cancers (e.g. vitamin A deficiency is associated with lung cancer).

Nutritionally vulnerable 'at-risk' groups

Some sub-groups within older populations appear more likely to be consuming inadequate diets (e.g. less regular consumption of cooked meals). In Australia in 1998, 50% of older people lived with their partner and 63% lived with at least one relative; 28% lived alone and 6% in cared-for accommodation. Providing nutritious food via a Meals-on-Wheels programme may not overcome the associated problem of social isolation, a risk factor for poor nutrition. This may be overcome by encouraging the individual to eat with family or friends, as this has been shown to increase food intake. An elderly person may eat less food for several reasons.

Nutritionally vulnerable 'at-risk' groups within older populations, who are more likely to be consuming inadequate diets (e.g. less regular consumption of cooked meals) and to be at risk of protein–energy malnutrition, include those who are:

- institutionalised
- older men living alone
- from low socioeconomic status groups
- socially isolated and lonely
- recently bereaved
- depressed or cognitively impaired
- physically and socially inactive.

and those with:

- physical handicaps, impaired motor performance and mobility
- presence of chronic diseases (e.g. arthritis, diabetes, hypertension, heart disease, cancer)
- polypharmacy (unnecessary intake of medications, drug–nutrient interactions; some drugs affect appetite/mood and cause nausea)
- sensory impairment: taste/smell (reduction in taste), eyesight (cataracts)
- reduced sense of thirst (hypodypsia)
- problems with chewing (loss of teeth and poorly fitting dentures)
- limited food storage, shopping difficulties and inadequate cooking skills
- erroneous beliefs and food fadism, food preferences.

Medications, depression, dementia, chronic illness, disability, loneliness and diminished senses of smell and taste may decrease the pleasure of eating. Food beliefs, in relation to health, can be strongly held among elderly people and lead to both food fads and undesirable food avoidance. There may be a significant association between food beliefs and food habits, as evidenced in studies of various elderly communities around the world. Nutrients at greatest risk of inadequate intake in 'at-risk' elderly groups are:

- protein
- folate
- vitamin B6
- vitamin B12
- vitamin D
- zinc
- calcium
- magnesium
- phytonutrients
- water.

Low intakes of these nutrients have important implications for bone health (calcium), wound healing (zinc, protein, energy), impaired immune response (zinc, vitamin B_6, protein, energy) and vascular disease via elevated homocysteine levels (folate, vitamin B_6).

Risky food patterns

When older people are physically active, marginal food patterns are less likely to lead to problems of the aged, such as:

- frailty
- protein energy dysnutrition
- micronutrient and phytochemical deficiency, because greater amounts of nutritious food can be eaten without positive energy balance
- chronic metabolic disease (NIDDM, cardiovascular disease, osteoporosis) and certain cancers (breast, colonic, prostate)
- depression (there is growing evidence that n-3 fatty acid deficiency can contribute to depression in some individuals, and that exercise can alleviate it)
- cognitive impairment with the apoE4 genotype; excess dietary saturated fat is likely to increase the risk of Alzheimer's disease and some antioxidants such as vitamin E and glutathione may reduce the risk.

Specific risky food patterns in later life include:

- large rather than smaller, frequent meals or snacks because of the inability of insulin reserve to match the carbohydrate load in those proven to have impaired glucose tolerance (IGT) or in those with

NIDDM, or because, where appetite is impaired, nutritious snacks can help to avoid chronic energy undernutrition

- alcohol excess, no alcohol-free days and/or alcohol without food (since food reduces the impact of alcohol ingestion on blood, alcohol concentration and its consequences)
- eating alone most of the time (since social activity encourages interest in food and, usually, healthy food preferences)
- use of salt or salty food rather than intrinsic food flavour (especially as taste and smell tend to decline with age), as excess sodium contributes to hypertension through an increased Na/K molar ratio, and to salt and water retention in cardiac decompensation, and promotes the loss of urinary calcium.

Nutrients at risk of inadequate intake

Protein–energy dysnutrition

It is usual to speak about protein–energy malnutrition (PEM), otherwise known as protein–calorie malnutrition (PCM), but in the aged, the body's compositional disorder may be rather more complex. The most common nutritional scenario in the aged is for there to be a decrease in lean mass (comprising water and protein-dominant tissues such as muscle, organs such as liver and also bone) and an increase in abdominal fat. This disorder could not be described as PEM, but can be described as protein–energy dysnutrition (PED). Illness or inadequate food intake may result in PED, a condition more common among elderly adults, especially in institutionalised care. It is associated with impaired immune responses, infections, poor wound healing, osteoporosis/hip fracture and decreased muscle strength (frailty), and is a risk factor for falls in the elderly. About 16% of elderly people living in the community consume <1000 kcal/day, an amount that cannot maintain adequate nutrition. Undernutrition also occurs in 3–12% of older outpatients, 17–65% of older people in acute-care hospitals and 26–59% of older people living in long-term care institutions. Studies show that being underweight in middle age and later places a person at greater risk of death than being overweight. Marasmus is a condition of borderline nutritional compensation in which there is marked depletion of muscle mass and fat stores, but normal visceral protein and organ function. As there is a depletion of nutritional reserves, any additional metabolic stress (e.g. surgery, infection, burns) may rapidly lead to kwashiorkor (hypoalbuminemic PEM). Characteristically, elderly people deteriorate to this state more rapidly than younger people, and even relatively minor stress may be the cause. Usually, susceptible elderly people are underweight, but even those who appear to have ample fat and muscle mass are susceptible if they have a recent history of rapid weight loss. The protein requirements of older people seem to be similar to, or higher than, those of younger people. The current dietary recommendation of protein for adults is 0.75–0.8 g/kg, whereas the recommendation for the elderly is slightly higher at 0.91 g/kg. In elderly people with PEM, oedema is usually absent; serum albumin and haemoglobin levels, total iron-binding capacity and tests of cell-mediated immune function are usually normal. When hypoalbuminemic PEM occurs, the serum albumin level is <3.5 g/dl and anaemia, hypotransferrinaemia and lymphocytopaenia (evidenced by a total iron-binding capacity <250 µg/dl) are likely. Often, anergy and oedema are present. Albumin has a 21-day half-life, and is an excellent measure of protein status, except in people suffering from illness or trauma and after surgery. Normal, able-bodied elderly people should have serum albumin levels >4 g/dl; only when a person is recumbent do fluid shifts result in a normal albumin level of 3.5 g/dl. Albumin levels <3.2 g/dl in hospitalised, older people are highly predictive of subsequent mortality. Cholesterol levels <160 mg/dl in nursing-home residents predict mortality, presumably because such levels reflect malnutrition. Acute illness associated with cytokine release can also lower cholesterol levels. Anergy (failure to respond to common antigens, such as mumps, injected into the skin) can occur in healthy, as well as malnourished, older people. The combination of anergy and signs of malnutrition correlate more strongly, resulting in a poorer outcome, than either one alone.

Folate

Before mandatory folate fortification of cereals in several developed countries, such as America and Australia, many older adults did not consume enough folate. This was compounded by the fact that folate absorption appears to be affected by atrophic gastritis, which is common in older adults. Elevated homocysteine levels have recently been defined as a marker of poor folate status in older people, and elevated levels of the former have been linked with an increased risk of heart disease and strokes. Folate metabolism may also be altered by the ingestion of antacids, anti-inflammatory drugs and diuretics commonly used by older adults. Several governments have legislated for the fortification of grain products with artificial folate since about 1998. The aim of this fortification exercise was to reduce birth defects of the spine, called spina bifida. Pregnant women need enough folate early in pregnancy to prevent most cases of spina bifida. A study in Framingham, Massachusetts, USA, studied folate levels in over 1100 people before and after fortification was mandated. The folate levels in blood more than doubled, and the percentage of people, including older adults, with low folate levels dropped by more than 90%. This is partly explained by the greater bioavailability of artificial folate in fortified foods. For example, only about half of the folate found naturally in food is available for use in the body; in contrast, the folate found in fortified foods is nearly all absorbed.

Can folate fortification have any adverse effects on elderly people? Vitamin B_{12} deficiency is quite common in older adults owing to inadequate absorption (see below). Vitamin B_{12} is needed to convert folate to its active form, therefore one of the most obvious vitamin B_{12} deficiency symptoms is the anaemia of folate deficiency (megaloblastic anaemia). Vitamin B_{12}, but not folate, is also needed to maintain the sheath that surrounds and protects nerve fibres. Either B_{12} or folate will clear up the anaemia, but if folate is consumed via fortified foods when a B_{12} supplement is needed instead, the result is devastating owing to permanent nerve damage and paralysis. In other words, folate 'cures' the blood symptoms of a vitamin B_{12} deficiency, but allows the nerve symptoms to progress and this means that folate can mask a vitamin B_{12} deficiency. With sufficient folate in the diet, the neurological symptoms of vitamin B_{12} deficiency can develop in older adults without evidence of anaemia. This highlights some of the safety issues surrounding the fortification of the food supply.

Vitamin B_6

During the course of life, plasma vitamin B_6 falls by approximately 3.6 µmol/l per decade. A number of studies suggest that age-related changes occur in both the absorption and metabolism of this vitamin and as a consequence aged adults may have a higher requirement. Studies also show that vitamin B_6 deficiency results in decreased immune response. Vitamin B_6 deficiencies (as well as vitamin B_{12} and folate) also result in higher concentrations of homocysteine. Supplementation of vitamin B_6 in healthy elderly people has been found to improve immune function and long-term memory.

Vitamin B_{12}

The prevalence of pernicious anaemia increases with age, as does atrophic gastritis; the absorption of vitamin B_{12} is reduced in individuals with either condition. The prevalence of *Helicobacter pylori* also increases with age and has been shown to be associated with vitamin B_{12} malabsorption, possibly because it contributes to gastric atrophy. As the likelihood of vitamin B_{12} deficiency is more common among older adults, this not only increases the risk of irreversible neurological damage, but is likely also to contribute to megaloblastic anaemia and homocysteine concentrations associated with vascular disease (see section on folate).

Vitamin D

Older adults are at greater risk of vitamin D deficiency than younger people and therefore at greater risk of exacerbated bone health decline (and resulting osteopenia and osteoporosis).

Risk factors for vitamin D deficiency include:

- lack of exposure to sunlight (may be due to less physical activity or sunscreen use)
- decline in renal function
- impaired skin synthesis (may be due to ageing skin)
- low fish intake (especially fatty fish)
- low intake of egg yolks, butter, vitamin D-fortified margarine and cheese.

The diet becomes an important source of vitamin D in people who do not receive enough sunlight. The diets of elderly people are often deficient in vitamin D-rich foods such as oily fish, and so fat-soluble vitamin absorption may be impaired. This is thought to contribute to the high incidence of vitamin D deficiency in older people. It appears that in the USA and the UK some 30–40% of older patients with hip fractures are vitamin D deficient. However, even during old age improving vitamin D status can provide profound benefits for bone health. In a Finnish study of outpatients over the age of 85 years and municipal home residents aged 75–84 years, those randomly assigned to receiving an annual vitamin D injection had significantly fewer fractures over a 5-year follow-up period. Probably the most striking and impressive study is one by Chapuy *et al.* (1992) of a nursing-home population of 3270 women, with an average age of 84 years. In a randomised, controlled trial of vitamin D (20 µg/day) and calcium (1200 mg/day), those receiving the supplement experienced 43% fewer hip fractures and 32% fewer non-vertebral fractures over an 18-month period. If blood levels of vitamin D are not reduced, vitamin D resistance may occur. Vitamin D resistance is relatively common because of impaired renal function in later life and the best indicator of this is an elevated parathyroid hormone (PTH) concentration in blood, a phenomenon referred to as secondary hyperparathyroidism. Vitamin D is important not only for bone, but also for immune function and muscle strength, and as a cell differentiator to reduce the risk of neoplastic disease.

Zinc

Zinc plays an important role in wound healing, taste acuity and normal immune function, and may affect albumin status in older adults. It is a crucial element in numerous metalloenzymes, and its intake is dependent on foods such as meat, with limited intake from plant foods, in which it is bound to phytic acid, oxalate and dietary fibre. It is more bioavailable in cereals that are leavened because of the presence of phytase in yeast, which breaks down phytic acid. Low zinc intakes are associated with low energy and a diet low in meat. Older adults may absorb zinc less effectively than younger people and so a diet including zinc-rich foods is important in later life. Zinc deficiency in older people is likely to compromise immune function with greater risk of infection, particularly respiratory, such as pneumonia. Some of the symptoms of zinc deficiency are similar to symptoms associated with normal ageing, such as diminished taste and dermatitis; the difficulty is in determining whether to attribute these symptoms to zinc deficiency or simply to the ageing process.

Calcium

Ageing is associated with a decrease in calcium absorption, which is probably due to alterations in the metabolism of vitamin D. However, calcium is a very important nutrient in older age as osteoporosis becomes a problem. Postmenopausal women not on hormone replacement therapy (HRT) have higher calcium needs. Many women do not meet the current Australian recommended calcium intake for postmenopausal women (1000 mg/day). Recent studies suggest that postmenopausal women need 1500 mg calcium per day. It is recommended that elderly people who suffer from a milk allergy or are lactose intolerant seek calcium from non-milk sources or supplements to help them meet their daily requirements.

Phytonutrients

Phytochemicals (from the Greek *phyto*, meaning plant) are unlike vitamins and minerals in that they have no known nutritional value. Phytochemicals are naturally occurring plant secondary metabolites which plants produce to protect themselves against bacteria, viruses and fungi. Many phytochemicals function as antioxidants, which protect cells from the effects of oxidation and free radicals within the body. Only recently have they been recognised as potentially powerful agents that may offer protection from diseases and conditions such as heart disease, diabetes, some cancers, arthritis, osteoporosis and ageing. They are present in a number of frequently consumed foods, especially fruits, vegetables, grains, legumes and seeds, and in a number of less frequently consumed foods, such as liquorice, soy and green tea. Phytonutrients may play a protective role in cardiovascular disease, certain cancers and menopausal symptoms. They are likely to lend protection against many of the diseases associated with ageing. A diet rich in phytoestrogens (isoflavones, lignans) may lessen the symptoms and impact of the menopause by improving vaginal health, reducing the incidence of hot flushes and improving bone mineral content (BMC). Food sources of phytoestrogens include soy, chickpeas, sesame seeds, flax seed (linseed) and olives.

One study in particular has shown that ingestion of soy may be more effective than HRT in improving BMC and therefore reducing the risks of osteopenia and osteoporosis.

In studies looking at the effect of HRT on BMC, it took 36 months to achieve an increase of just under 4%. In another study, however, an increase of 5.2% in BMC was detected after just 12 weeks of soy consumption.

Water

Total body water declines with age. As a result, an adequate intake of fluids, especially water, becomes increasingly important in later life, as thirst regulation is impaired and renal function declines. Dehydration is a particular risk for those who may not notice or pay attention to thirst, or who may find it hard to get up to make a drink or reach the bathroom. Older people who have decreased bladder control may also be at risk because they may be afraid to drink too much water.

Dehydrated elderly people appear to be more susceptible to urinary tract infections, pressure ulcers, pneumonia and confusion. Recommended intakes for the elderly are approximately 6–8 glasses of fluid a day, preferably water.

Nutrition-related health problems in the aged

There is growing awareness that the major health problems in the aged, and even mortality, have nutritional contributors and can be (in part) prevented by food intake. These health problems do not necessarily need to occur with ageing and death can be delayed. As the number of chronic conditions increases with age, they contribute to disability and frailty, which in turn reduces a person's level of independence, sometimes resulting in institutionalisation. The primary nutritional problems affecting the elderly are:

- protein–energy dysnutrition
- sub-clinical/mild vitamin deficiencies and trace mineral deficiencies
- obesity

all of which can contribute to the development of chronic conditions seen with ageing. Some common nutrition-related problems in the aged are outlined below.

Sarcopenia

The condition or state of sarcopenia is the specific involuntary loss of flesh or muscle that occurs with age, and is more marked in women. It has been demonstrated that reduced muscle mass and body cell mass is associated with a loss of muscle strength, and impaired immune and pulmonary function. Furthermore, this decline in muscle strength is responsible for much of the disability observed in older adults and in the advanced elderly, as muscle strength is a crucial component of walking ability. It is thought that human life cannot be sustained if levels of body cell mass fall below 60% of the normal levels of young adults. The prevalence, incidence and aetiology of sarcopenia are currently unknown, and therefore require further study. Decreasing physical activity and GH levels are two likely contributing factors to the advancement of sarcopenia, along with poor nutrition (especially inadequate energy and protein intakes, which may be due to poor food intake or disease), disease and the ageing process.

Obesity

Overweight and obesity are common problems in the aged, not because they are an inevitable part of growing older, but because of the associated sedentary lifestyle. Although a less serious problem in older people than PEM, obesity can impair functional status, increase the risk of pulmonary embolus and pressure sores, and aggravate chronic diseases such as diabetes mellitus and hypertension. Greater body fatness, especially if centrally distributed, increases the risk of insulin resistance, hypertension and hypercholesterolemia in the aged. In contrast, heavier women have a lower risk of hip fracture. This is partly due to 'padding' and better muscle development, but may also be due to maintenance of higher oestrogen levels from the conversion of precursor steroids to oestrogen in adipose tissue. Abdominal obesity is defined as an abdominal circumference of greater than 102 cm for men and 88 cm for women. However, abdominal obesity can be reduced in old age by engaging in some form of daily physical activity. An appropriate body weight is a protective factor in older people with advancing age. Body weight maintenance, at a suitable level, is desirable to maintain physical strength and activity, resistance to infection and skin breakdown, and quality of life.

Immune function

Infections are a common cause of illness and death among the aged. Ageing adults are more susceptible to infection and this is probably due, in part, to the age-associated decline in immune function, but this decline may be preventable with good nutrition and physical activity. A decline in immunity may also increase the risk of cancer and arthritis. The observed decline in immune function with ageing may be prevented with nutrient intakes greater than those currently recommended for 'normal' health. Nutrients important in immune function include protein, zinc, vitamin A, vitamin C, pyridoxine, riboflavin and tocopherols. Other food components not considered to be essential for health in earlier life may become more important with age.

The non-essential amino acid glutamine has an important role in DNA and RNA synthesis. It is stored primarily in skeletal muscle and is utilised by intestinal cells, lymphocytes and macrophages. As the contribution of skeletal muscle to whole-body protein metabolism declines with age, the rate of glutamine formation and availability may be impaired. As such, it may compromise immune function, resulting in a sub-optimal response to infection or trauma. Glutamine can be synthesised from glutamic acid, which is found in wheat, soybeans, lean meat and eggs. Glutathione (a tripeptide) and phytochemicals, such as flavonoids and carotenoids, also appear to play a role in the immune function. Meat is a good source of glutathione, with moderate amounts being found in fruits and vegetables. Whey proteins, although low in glutathione, are capable of stimulating endogenous glutathione production.

Osteoporosis and fractures

Old age is associated with decreased bone mass, and osteoporosis is one of the most prevalent diseases of ageing. Amongst the ageing population, there is an increase in the incidence of osteoporosis, with females most affected. It has been estimated that about 25% of the female population over 60 years is affected by osteoporosis, and 70% of the fractures that occur annually in Australia can be attributed to osteoporosis. In 1986, 10 000 hip fractures were recorded in Australia, and this rate is expected to rise to 18 000 per year by 2011. Hip fractures result in both mortality and morbidity. Two types of osteoporosis have been identified. Type I involves the loss of trabecular bone (calcium-containing crystals that fill the interior of the bone). Women are more affected by this type of osteoporosis, with the most effective preventive measure being the administration of oestrogen for at least 7 years after the menopause. Type II osteoporosis progresses more slowly than type I and involves the loss of both the cortical (exterior shell of the bone) and the trabecular bone. As the person ages, the disease becomes evident with compressed vertebrae forming wedge shapes into what is commonly referred to as 'dowager's hump'. Once again, women are more affected by this disease than men. Women are more prone to osteoporosis than men for two reasons: bone loss is accelerated after the menopause and women have a lower bone mineral density than men. A large study of elderly men and women conducted in Australia found that after the age of 60 years approximately 60% of women and 30% of men would sustain an osteoporotic fracture. A high intake of calcium appears to prevent or reduce bone loss in postmenopausal women. While adequate intakes of calcium appear to be protective against osteoporosis, other potentially protective factors include vitamins C, D and K, protein, boron, copper and possibly phytoestrogens. Recent evidence indicates that soy consumption may also provide benefits to bone health. A vitamin D supplement from fish liver oil has also been shown to reduce fracture rates in later life. While nutrition and physical activity can maximise peak bone mass during growth, other factors such as excess sodium, caffeine, smoking and alcohol can accelerate bone loss in later life.

Cardiovascular disease

Cardiovascular disease is the most common cause of death and disability in the developed world. Dietary habits may contribute to, or provide protection against, risk factors associated with cardiovascular disease. In a longitudinal health survey of elderly people living in The Netherlands, an inverse relationship was found between fish consumption and coronary heart disease mortality. Elevated serum homocystine concentrations have been identified as an independent risk factor for cardiovascular disease. In the Framingham study, elderly adults with better folate status had lower homocystine concentrations. Inadequate intake of folate, together with vitamins B_6 and B_{12}, can lead to homocystinaemia then to vascular damage and proneness to thrombosis.

Cancer

Specific dietary patterns that protect against cancer remain unclear. However, certain food groups are associated with a reduced risk of cancer, for instance a high intake of fruit and vegetables appears to be associated with a reduced risk of cancer at many sites. Fruit and vegetables are excellent sources of antioxidants, phytochemicals and dietary fibre. Particular foods that may protect against prostate cancer include soy products, tomatoes and pumpkin seeds. Foods high in resistant starch, dietary fibre and salicylates may protect against colorectal cancer. Foods that appear to increase the risk of cancer at specific sites include salt, smoked/cured foods (stomach cancer) and alcohol (oesophageal cancer). Factors that occur early in life may affect the risk of breast cancer in later life. For instance, rapid early growth, greater adult height and starting menstruation at a younger age, are associated with an increased risk of breast cancer. Although it is unlikely that appropriate interventions could be undertaken to avoid these, other nutritional and lifestyle factors are amenable to change and may reduce the risk of breast cancer. These include consuming diets high in vegetables and fruits, avoiding alcohol, maintaining a healthy body weight and remaining physically active throughout life. There is some evidence that phytoestrogens (compounds found in plants that possess mild Oestrogenic properties) may reduce the risk of breast cancer. Soy and linseed are two excellent sources of phytoestrogens and recently Australian food manufacturers have been adding soy and linseed to a variety of breads and cereals. Increased prevalence of nutritionally related immunodeficiency with ageing is likely to contribute to the development of neoplastic disease.

Diabetes

Ageing is associated with an increased prevalence of NIDDM and glucose intolerance. Two risk factors associated with the development of both these conditions include obesity and physical inactivity. In older adults, modest weight reductions can contribute to improvements in diabetic control. This is important, as retrospective studies indicate that good blood glucose control reduces the likelihood and severity of stroke, cardiovascular disease, visual impairment, nephropathy, infections and cognitive dysfunction. Dietary modification can reduce cardiovascular disease risk; even a relatively small reduction in salt and saturated fat intake can have a substantial effect on cardiovascular disease.

Endocrine function

Ageing sees a decline in hormone secretion throughout the body. The decline in the level of human GH seems to play a role in the ageing process, at least in some individuals. GH also plays a role in body composition and bone strength. Oestrogen levels also drop with age. Low levels of oestrogen are associated with bone thinning, frailty and disability. Low testosterone levels in the body may weaken muscles and promote frailty and disability. Melatonin responds to light and seems to regulate seasonal changes in the body. As melatonin levels decline with age, other changes in the endocrine system may be triggered. Dehydroepiandrosterone (DHEA) is currently being studied to establish its effects on immune system decline and its potential to prevent certain chronic diseases, such as cancer and multiple sclerosis.

Cognitive function

Prevention of cognitive loss, or dementia, poses a particular challenge in older people. Some deterioration can be attributed to atherosclerotic disease and thus interventions such as aspirin, or particular dietary patterns that reduce cardiovascular risk, may also prevent dementia. High educational status early in life and continued mental stimulation may also be protective. Living alone has recently been reported to increase the risk of dementia. It is generally accepted that dementing illnesses and depression have a strong genetic background. However, the genetic susceptibility to a certain disease is strongly influenced by environmental factors. Thus, it may be possible to delay the onset of poor cognitive function in old age if food intake is adequate. For example, cognitive status assessed in a group of older adults from Madrid, using Folstein's Mini-Mental State Examination and Pfeiffer's Mental Status Questionnaire, was found to be better in those who consumed a more satisfactory global diet. This diet was characterised by a greater intake of total food, fruit and vegetables. Dementia can result in forgetting to eat, indifference to food, failure to see the need to eat and behavioural abnormalities, such as holding food in the mouth. Changes in smell and taste may also lead to weight loss, which is common in older adults with dementia, or even anorexia in older adults. Long-term moderate (sub-clinical) nutrient deficiencies are now

believed to produce memory impairments and declining immunity in older adults. Certain nutrients or toxic substances may directly affect brain development (e.g. alcohol and folic acid deficiency) or brain function (e.g. alcohol, vitamins B_1, B_2, B_6, B_{12}, C and E, and zinc deficiencies). Brain ageing is associated with oxidative stress, thus antioxidants and pro-oxidants (such as iron) are of particular interest. There is some epidemiological evidence that the antioxidants, carotene and carotenoids, ascorbic acid and α-tocopherol may delay brain ageing and iron may accelerate it. Vitamin K may also be protective against cognitive decline and Alzheimer's dementia. Depression in the elderly is a very common symptom. There is a growing body of evidence to suggest that n-3 polyunsaturated fatty acids may play an important role in the aetiology of depression. Caffeine ingested as either tea or coffee has also been shown to improve mood and reduce anxiety.

Nutritional assessment of the aged

One of the greatest difficulties in making any assessment of the aged is the biological heterogeneity ('biological age'). There are clearly many health problems seen in the aged in some communities that are not seen in others, making them more age-related than ageing; nutritional assessment of the aged needs to pay attention to a number of sociodemographic variables and the food culture in which the elderly person has lived. Another challenge for nutritional assessment in the aged is the question of 'timing', that is when nutritional factors will have operated during the lifespan and the resulting consequences on health in later life. With these considerations taken into account, the areas of nutritional assessment to consider are:

- food and nutrient intake
- anthropometry and body composition
- laboratory investigations by way of biochemistry, haematology and immunology
- nutritionally related risk factors for various health problems in the aged.

In Australia a tool has been developed that identifies older adults at risk of poor nutritional health by giving warning signs (Figure 7.6).

Food and nutrient intake

Assessment of food and nutrient intake is an important tool in the health assessment of the aged. As a

---

DETERMINE YOUR NUTRITIONAL HEALTH

The warning signs of poor nutritional health in the older person are often overlooked. Use this checklist to find out if you, or someone you know, is at nutritional risk.

Read the statements below. Circle the number in the column that applies to you or the person you know. For each answer, score the number in the box. Total your nutritional score.

	YES	NO
I have an illness or condition that made me change the kind and/or amount of food I eat	2	0
I eat at least three meals per day	0	3
I eat fruit or vegetables most days	0	2
I eat dairy products most days	0	2
I have three or more glasses of beer, wine or spirits almost every day	3	0
I have six to eight cups of fluids (e.g. water, juice, tea or coffee) most days	0	1
I have teeth, mouth or swallowing problems that make it hard for me to eat	4	0
I always have enough money to buy food	0	3
I eat alone most of the time	2	0
I take three or more differently prescribed or over-the-counter medicines every day	3	0
Without wanting to, I have lost or gained 5 kg in the last 6 months	2	0
I am always able to shop, cook and/or feed myself	0	2
TOTAL		

Add up all the numbers you have circled. If your nutritional score is ...

0–3	**Good!** Recheck your nutritional score in 6 months
4–5	**You are at moderate nutritional risk.** See what can be done to improve your eating habits and lifestyle. Your Council on Ageing or healthcare professional can help. Recheck your nutritional score in 3 months.
6 or more	**You are at high nutritional risk.** Bring this checklist the next time you see your doctor, dietician or other qualified health or social service professional. Talk with them about any problems you may have. Ask for help to improve your nutritional health.

Reproduced from the Australian Nutrition Screening Initiative, a project of RACGP, Council on the Ageing, Dietitians Association of Australia, and Self Care Pharmacy, a joint program of the Pharmaceutical Society of Pharmacy Guild of Australia.

Figure 7.6 Example of a checklist to identify older persons at risk of poor nutritional health.

result of the positive decline in memory, instruments used for food intake assessment should be as simple and practical as possible, and should involve corroboration from other observers, such as family or friends. Knowledge of appetite, the special senses for smell and taste, and the overall food patterns facilitates an understanding of the various factors that may affect food intake. Food and nutrient intake can alert the healthcare worker to possible nutritionally related disease, for example osteoporosis, by asking 'What do you have in the way of dairy products, fish, sesame based foods?' (sources of calcium). A systematic inquiry about food intake usually requires asking about each episode of eating during the day, that is main meals and snacks.

Anthropometry and body composition

Anthropometry is a simple, non-invasive, quick and reliable form of obtaining objective information about a person's nutritional status.

Weight

Ambulatory elderly persons are weighed on an upright balance beam scale or microprocessor-controlled digital scale. A movable wheelchair balance beam scale can also be used for those elderly who can only sit. A bed scale should be available in geriatric hospitals for measuring the weight of bed-ridden elderly patients. Weights less than 20% of the ideal body weight indicate a significant loss of total body protein, requiring immediate investigation and action. They are associated with reduced tolerance to trauma and an increased risk of morbidity, infection and mortality. Low body weight and/or unintended weight loss are significant risk factors as the ageing process progresses and require careful intervention and monitoring. General guidelines requiring action would be:

- a 2% decrease in body weight in 1 week
- a 5% decrease in body weight in 1 month (3.5 kg in a 70 kg man)
- a 7% decrease in body weight in 3 months
- a 10% decrease in body weight in 6 months.

Interpretation of the weight of elderly people should be done with circumspection. Increases in body weight may indicate overweight/obesity or oedema. Decreases in body weight can signify the correction of oedema, development of dehydration or emergence of a nutritional disorder.

Height

For the elderly who are agile and without stooped posture, height should be measured in an upright position. When this cannot be measured, knee height (using a knee-height calliper) in a recumbent position can be used to estimate stature. The following formulae are used to compute stature from knee height:

$$\text{stature for men} = (2.02 \times \text{knee height})$$
$$- (0.04 \times \text{age}) + 64.19$$
$$\text{stature for women} = (1.83 \times \text{knee height})$$
$$- (0.24 \times \text{age}) + 84.88$$

The knee-height measurement in these equations is in centimetres, and the age is rounded to the nearest whole year. The estimated stature derived from the equation is in centimetres. These equations are derived from observations which presume that elderly people will have lost some height, an inevitability that may not always continue as healthcare improves.

Arm span

Arm span is another substitute for height and happens to be the same as maximal height achieved. It is sometimes necessary to ask for maximum adult height to be recalled by the subject or by a carer. Gradual reduction in height may be an indicator of vertebral crush fractures due to osteoporosis or it may be due to loss of vertebral disk space.

Mid-arm circumference

Combined with triceps skinfold (TSF), mid-arm circumference (MAC; taken at the mid-point between the acromion and olecranon) can be used to calculate mid-arm muscle area (MAMA), which is an index of total body protein mass. The equation to estimate MAMA is:

$$\text{MAMA} = [\text{MAC} - (3.14 \times \text{TSF}/10)]^2 / 12.56$$

The MAC measurement in this equation is in centimetres and the TSF is in millimetres. The calculated MAMA derived from the equation is in centimetres squared. MAMA of less than 44 cm^2 for men and less than 30 cm^2 for women may indicate protein malnutrition.

Calf circumference

Calf circumference (taken at the largest circumference using non-elastic flexible measuring tape) in the absence of lower limb oedema can be used to calculate weight in a bed-ridden patient. Several anthropometric measurements, apart from calf circumference itself (calf C), are required to compute weight. They are knee height (knee H), MAC and subscapular skinfold thickness (subsc SF) (taken at posterior, in a line from the inferior angle of the left scapula to the left elbow). There are separate equations for men and women:

body weight for men
$$= (0.98 \times \text{calf C}) + (1.16 \times \text{knee H})$$
$$+ (1.73 \times \text{MAC}) + (0.36 \times \text{subsc SF})$$

body weight for women
$$= (1.27 \times \text{calf C}) + (0.87 \times \text{knee H})$$
$$+ (0.98 \times \text{MAC}) + (0.4 \times \text{subsc SF})$$
$$- 62.35$$

All measurements should be in centimetres and the resulting computed weight is in kilograms. Calf circumference is expected to have increasing application for assessment of lean mass. It can also be used as a measure of physical activity in the aged.

Anthropometric indices
BMI has been used widely to estimate total body fatness. BMI can be obtained by using the formula BMI = weight (kg)/height (m²). BMI can be calculated to help classify whether or not the subject is in the reference range. Inter-observer errors are possible. Height and weight having coefficient of variations in the order of less than 1% may be altered by kyphosis in the aged and make interpretation of BMI invalid. Circumferences ratio (AHR) measured at the abdominal (taken at the midpoint between lower ribcage and iliac crest) and hip (taken at the maximal gluteal protrusion) is another anthropometric index to estimate fat distribution and the one now recommended by the WHO. It is fat distribution reflected in abdominal fatness, which may account for a number of chronic non-communicable diseases in the elderly if the ratio is above 0.9 for men and 0.8 for women. Several studies are now showing that umbilical measurements alone can be used to safely decide whether weight loss is necessary to reduce the risk from diseases such as heart disease and diabetes. Statistical analyses of umbilical circumferences of Caucasian men and women aged 25–74 years indicated that the ideal circumference for men is less than 102 cm and for women is less than 88 cm. These conclusions are drawn from Caucasian subjects and thus may not apply in ethnic groups where the build is slight, such as in many Asian countries, and where a lesser degree of abdominal fatness may still put the person at risk of developing chronic diseases.

Laboratory investigations: biochemistry, haematology and immunology
Biochemical, haematological and immunological assessments are useful to confirm nutritional disorders and to identify specific complications that accompany them in the elderly (see also the chapter on metabolic and nutritional assessment in *Clinical Nutrition* in this series).

Various nutritionally related risk factors for health problems in the aged
Elderly people tend to have different degrees of risk factors (see section on nutritionally vulnerable 'at-risk' groups).

7.9 Guidelines for healthy ageing

Sometimes the assumption is made that, after reaching the age of 65 or 70 years, lifestyle changes will no longer confer significant health benefits. Are the remaining years sufficient to reap the benefits of modifications to food choice or exercise patterns? Several recent intervention and survival studies reveal that improvements in nutrition and regular exercise can benefit health, even in advanced old age. For example, older muscles are just as responsive to strength-training exercises as are young muscles. Non-agenarians have shown impressive increases in muscle mass, muscle strength and walking speed with weight-training programmes. Chronological age is, in itself, clearly no justification for deciding whether it is worthwhile to pursue lifestyle change. Behavioural risk factors (e.g. regularly not eating breakfast, lack of regular physical activity, being overweight and smoking) have been shown to remain predictors of 17-year mortality, even in people aged over 70. If elderly people pay attention to aspects of their lifestyle (physical and social activity) other than eating, they may be able to make nutritional errors with less consequence.

Physical activity
The type of physical activity undertaken can play an important role in the health of older people. The two principal forms of physical activity or exercise that are important in promoting health and well-being are endurance/aerobic exercise and strength training.

Endurance activities improve heart and lung fitness and psychological functioning, while strength training enhances muscle size and strength, thus preventing muscle atrophy. The level of physical activity required for older adults to achieve optimal health benefits has not yet been established. Resistance (or strength) training prevents lean muscle atrophy more effectively than aerobic activity, especially during weight loss, whereas aerobic exercise may be more involved in improving psychological functioning in older people (although group membership may also be a factor). Strength training in older adults seems particularly promising in reducing, or preventing, the decline in muscle mass observed with ageing. It can improve walking ability and balance and its associated risk for falls. Strength training also contributes to improved tendon and ligament strength, bone health and improvements in blood sugar levels. The benefits of physical activity, such as strength training, should make activities of daily living easier for older people. Such activities might include climbing stairs, getting out of a chair, pushing a vacuum cleaner, carrying groceries and crossing a road with sufficient speed. Research suggests that endurance activities should be performed daily (e.g. a walk of 30 min duration or three bouts of 8–10 min), along with some strength training. Endurance activities do not have to be continuous, but can be accrued throughout the day through short bursts of activity.

Protective foods and food variety

The first consideration when it comes to nutritional matters is that enough food is available for basic energy and nutritional needs. Food variety is another important consideration in terms of nutritional adequacy and health outcomes. Food variety has been demonstrated to be an accurate predictor of the nutritional adequacy of the diet and is invariably linked to food availability. Consuming a wide variety of foods (especially plant foods) has been associated with longevity. It is suggested that an ideal way to increase variety in the diet is to choose foods from across all five food groups and a wide selection within each of these groups. Several studies have shown that energy and total food intakes decline with age, making a nutritionally adequate diet more difficult to achieve. Older men consume about 800 kcal less than younger men, and older women about 400 kcal less than younger women. A reduction in BMR is partly responsible for this decline, but physical inactivity appears to be the major cause for reduced food intake. Compared with younger

adults, older adults need to reach at least the same levels of intake (and in some cases higher levels) of most vitamins, minerals and protein. As these usually need to be obtained from substantially lower overall food intakes, however, a nutrient and phytochemically dense diet becomes a high priority in later life. In other words, given the tendency for activity levels to decline and total food intakes to fall with advancing years, there is less room for energy-dense foods (e.g. indulgences, treats) which supply few of the essential nutrients that our bodies continue to need, therefore older adults need be selective about what they eat, in order to avoid excessive fat gain, and to develop a preference for foods that are nutrient dense and high in protein (e.g. nuts, lean red meat, low-fat dairy products, legumes, seeds). This principle also applies to younger adults who are sedentary. Eating in a traditional food culture context can provide a measure of food security for the aged. This is one of the arguments for food-based dietary guidelines (FBDGs) for the aged. The consumption of nutrient-dense foods reduces the risk of essential nutrient deficiencies. These foods include:

- eggs (little, if any, effect on serum cholesterol if not eaten with saturated fat)
- liver
- lean meat
- meat alternatives such as legumes (especially traditional soy products, e.g. tofu and tempeh) and nuts
- fish
- low-fat milk and dairy products
- fruits, vegetables and plant shoots
- wholegrain cereals
- wheat germ
- yeast
- unrefined fat from whole foods (nuts, seeds, beans, olives, avocado, fish)
- refined fat from liquid oils (cold pressed, from a variety of sources, predominant in n-3 and/or n-9 fatty acids).

The protective nutritional value of fruits and vegetables is derived particularly from their content of phytochemicals, which are multifunctional compounds, usually of benefit to health, (i.e. antioxidants, antimutagenics, antiangiogenics, immunomodulatory, phytoestrogens). In late 1999, the Australian government, based on the National Health and Medical Research Council report, released a set of dietary guidelines for older Australians (Table 7.7).

Table 7.7 Dietary guidelines for older Australians, 1999

1. Enjoy a wide variety of nutritious foods
2. Keep active to maintain muscle strength and a healthy body weight
3. Eat at least three meals every day
4. Care for your food: prepare and store it correctly
5. Eat plenty of vegetables (including legumes) and fruit
6. Eat plenty of cereals, breads and pastas
7. Eat a diet low in saturated fat
8. Drink adequate amounts of water and/or other fluids
9. If you drink alcohol, limit your intake
10. Choose foods low in salt and use salt sparingly
11. Include foods high in calcium
12. Use added sugars in moderation

Dietary Guidelines for Older Australians, National Health & Medical Research Council, 1999, copyright Commonwealth of Australia, reproduced by permission. http://www.nhmrc.gov.au/publications/synopses/n23syn.htm

The FBDGs were also recently published in conjunction with the WHO. They address traditional foods, dishes and, most importantly, cuisine, making such guidelines more practical and user-friendly on an individual level. These principles will need to be addressed by the various countries around the world when developing their own country/culture-specific FBDGs.

To summarise, the nutritional factors involved in healthy ageing include food variety, and nutrient and phytochemical density. A 'Mediterranean' food pattern may also reduce the risk of death in older adults. In the frail elderly, there should be more emphasis on the need for support and increased nourishment, together with the prevention of malnutrition. The best and main message for an older person at home is to be well nourished, to be as active as possible without overdoing it, to eat better, not less, to keep a proportionate weight and to drink plenty of fluids every day.

7.10 Perspectives on the future

While maximal lifespan is probably genetically determined, the probability of reaching that lifespan in good health seems largely determined by environmental and lifestyle factors. Thus, for humans to have the continued ability to increase their lifespan and associated quality of life, they will most likely need to make alterations, albeit very small, in the way they live their day-to-day lives. This may take the form of consuming more fruit and vegetables, reading or taking a daily walk. Owing to decreased energy requirements in old

age, diet plays an integral part in maintaining health and vitality. The quality of the diet is critical in ensuring that nutritional needs are met. The diet should consist of nutrient-rich, low-energy dense foods that are generally low in fat. There is not much room for indulgences in an elderly person's diet, especially if their lifestyle is mostly sedentary. Even though energy requirements are lower, nutrient needs are the same as, or higher than, those in younger adults. To reduce abdominal obesity and the development of sub-clinical deficiencies, older adults must choose foods wisely and maintain appropriate levels of physical activity.

Of increasing importance is the cost-effectiveness of health care, especially for older people. Much of this cost arises through disability, which improved nutrition could mitigate, and the use of multiple and costly pharmaceuticals, which could be reduced by nutritious diets. Better nutrition throughout the average lifespan could make health systems more affordable and sustainable.

References

Growth

Tienboon P, Rutishauser IHE, Wahlqvist ML. Early life factors affecting body mass index and waist-hip ratio in adolescence. Asia Pacific J Clin Nutr 1992; 1: 21–26.

Ageing

Campbell AJ, Buchner DM. Unstable disability and the fluctuations of frailty. Age and Aging 1997; 26: 315–318.

Chapuy MC et al. Vitamin D3 and calcium to prevent hip fractures in the elderly women. N Engl J Med. 1992 Dec 3; 327 (23): 1637–1642.

Fiatarone MA et al. Exercise training and nutritional supplementation for physical frailty in very elderly people. New Engl J Med 1995; 330 (25): 1769–1775.

Glass TA et al. Population based study of social and productive activities as predictors of survival among elderly Americans. BMJ 1999; 319 (21): 478–483.

Tienboon P. Using body mass index to assess under nutrition and over nutrition of preschool children. Thai J Paren and Enter 2003; 14(2): 122–129.

Further reading

Growth

Cole TJ, Bellizzi MC, Flegal KM, Dietz WH. Establishing a standard definition for child overweight and obesity worldwide: international survey. BMJ 2000; 320: 1240. http://www.bmj.com/cgi/content/full/320/7244/1240

Gracey M, Hetzel B, Smallwood R et al. Responsibility for Nutritional Diagnosis: A Report by the Nutrition Working Party of the Social Issues Committee of the Royal Australasian College of Physicians. London: Smith-Gordon, 1989.

Lee RD, Nieman DC. Nutritional Assessment, 2nd edn. Sydney: McGraw-Hill, 1996.

National Health and Medical Research Council. Dietary guidelines for children and adolescents in Australia incorporating the infant feeding guidelines for health workers. Canberra: Australian Government Publishing Service, 2003. On-line scientific background papers for each guideline. http://www.nhmrc.gov.au/publications/synopses/_files/n34.pdf

US Department of Health and Human Services and US Department of Agriculture. Dietary guidelines for Americans, 2005. On-line scientific background papers for each guideline. http://www.healthierus.gov/dietaryguidelines

US Department of Health Services. My Pyramid.gov, 2005. On-line scientific background papers for each guideline. http://www.mypyramid.gov/

World Health Organization. The WHO child growth standards, 2006. On-line scientific background papers for each guideline. http://www.who.int/childgrowth/standards/en/

Ageing

Committee on Nutrition Services for Medicare Beneficiaries, Food and Nutrition Board. The Role of Nutrition in Maintaining Health in the Nation's Elderly: Evaluating Coverage of Nutrition Services for the Medicare Population. Washington, DC: National Academy Press, 2000.

Grundy E. The epidemiology of aging. In: Textbook of Geriatric Medicine and Gerontology, 4th edn (Brocklehurst JC *et al.*, eds), pp. 3–20. New York: Churchill Livingstone, 1992.

Khaw K-T. Healthy ageing. BMJ 1997; 315: 1090–1096. On-line full text: http://www.bmj.com/cgi/content/full/315/7115/1090

Lee MS, Wahlqvist ML. Population-based studies of nutrition and health in Asia Pacific elderly. Asia Pac J Clin Nutr 2005; 14(4): 294–297. On-line full text: http://apjcn.nhri.org.tw/server/MarkWpapers/Papers/Papers%202005/P339.pdf

National Health and Medical Research Council. The Australian Dietary Guidelines for Older Adults. Canberra: Australian Government Publishing Service, 1999. On-line scientific background papers for each guideline. http://www.nhmrc.gov.au/filesnhmrc/file/publications/synopses/withdrawn/n23.pdf

National Policy and Research Center on Nutrition and Aging. Dietary Reference Intakes (DRIs)/Recommended Dietary Allowances (RDAs), 2003. On-line scientific background papers for each guideline. http://www.fiu.edu/~nutreldr/SubjectList/D/DRI_RDA.htm

Trichopoulou A. *et al.* Diet and overall survival in elderly people. BMJ 1995; 311: 1457–1460. On-line full text: http://www.bmj.com/cgi/content/full/311/7018/1457

Wahlqvist ML, Kouris-Blazos A. Requirements in maturity and aging. In: Food and Nutrition: Australia and New Zealand (ML Wahlqvist, ed.). Sydney: Allen & Unwin, 2002. http://www.healthyeatingclub.com/bookstore/

Wahlqvist ML *et al.* Does diet matter for survival in long-lived cultures? Asia Pac J Clin Nutr 2005; 14 (1): 2–6. On-line full text: http://apjcn.nhri.org.tw/server/APJCN/Volume14/vol14.1/fullArticles/Darmadi.pdf

8
Nutrition and the Brain

John D Fernstrom and Madelyn H Fernstrom

Key messages

- Brain chemistry and function are influenced by short-term and long-term changes in the diet.
- The blood–brain barrier is an important focal point for the nutrition of the brain: it is a selectively permeable barrier that promotes the uptake of water-soluble molecules via specific transporters (e.g. glucose, ketone bodies, amino acids, vitamins), excludes the uptake of other molecules, and allows the free diffusion of gases (e.g. oxygen, carbon dioxide) and other lipid-soluble molecules.
- Glucose is the principal energy substrate of the brain, although ketone bodies become major energy substrates during starvation.
- The dietary intake of carbohydrates, per se, does not influence the supply of hexoses to the brain.
- The dietary intake of protein and amino acids can influence the uptake of some amino acids into the brain, depending on the properties of amino acid transporters located at the blood–brain barrier.
- In the brain, amino acids are incorporated into proteins and functionally important small molecules, such as neurotransmitters. The production of these amino acid-derived small molecules is often surprisingly sensitive to the supply of amino acid precursors from the circulation and thus the diet.
- The brain does not use fatty acids directly as energy substrates, but does use them to construct a variety of complex lipid molecules that are incorporated into neuronal and glial cell membranes.
- Two fatty acids of functional importance to the brain are not synthesised in the brain or body of mammals (the essential fatty acids); certain brain functions thus depend on their adequate intake via the diet.
- Water-soluble vitamins gain access to the brain via blood–brain barrier (or blood–cerebrospinal fluid barrier) embedded transporters. Fat-soluble vitamins may also gain access to the brain by specialised transfer mechanisms that involve the macromolecules with which they circulate in the blood.
- Dietary deficiencies in certain water- and fat-soluble vitamins can produce functional deficits in the brain and retina of varying severity.
- The access of minerals to the brain, where studied, appears to involve the blood–brain barrier and special transport mechanisms; only prolonged deficiencies (for certain minerals) produce deficits in brain function.

8.1 Introduction

Until the 1960s, the brain was viewed as being 'protected' from both sudden and prolonged nutritional changes. This idea changed first with the realisation that severe nutritional insults, such as malnutrition, could seriously retard normal brain development in the foetus and newborn. During the 1970s, a number of experimental findings emerged suggesting that, in addition, fairly modest changes in the composition of the diet could directly influence the production of key signalling molecules in the brain (the neurotransmitters), and thus brain functions.

A further factor that helped to change this early viewpoint of the brain's metabolic invulnerability was the elucidation by scientists of the true nature of the blood–brain barrier (BBB), a very old concept. Originally, the BBB was thought of as a 'barrier' between the blood and the brain, preventing environmental insults and metabolic changes in the body from disturbing the brain's chemistry and function. New work revealed that the BBB is not really a barrier at all, but instead an extensive set of transport carriers, located on the membranes of the cells that make up the capillaries of the brain, promoting or restricting the entry of an endless number of molecules into

Nutrition and Metabolism, Second Edition, edited by S. A. Lanham-New, I. A. Macdonald and H. M. Roche. © 2011 The Nutrition Society.

brain, as well as their removal. Furthermore, in many cases transport carriers have been found to be 'plastic', that is, the properties of specific carriers can change in relation to current demands for the nutrients they transport. A contemporary appreciation of how nutrition influences the brain thus requires an understanding of the nutrient transporters on capillary cells that modulate the flow of these molecules into and out of the brain.

This chapter will begin by providing an overview of the structure of the nervous system and of the BBB. It will then consider how each of the nutrients in the diet finds its way into the brain and whether vagaries in the diet can influence the uptake of nutrients into and ultimately their function within the brain.

8.2 General organisation of the mammalian nervous system

The nervous system has two principal cell types, neurons and glia (Figure 8.1). Neurons are the cellular elements that provide information flow in the nervous system. They are organised into circuits that perform the various functions attributed to the nervous system. Neurons conduct electrical signals over short or long distances, depending on the circuit, and their anatomy bespeaks this function. Their cellular features are (i) one or more cellular extensions of variable length known as dendrites, which receive chemical and sometimes electrical signals from other neurons, (ii) a cell body, which provides the normal housekeeping functions of cells and passes electrical information received through dendrites across its surface membrane to (iii) the axon, which conducts electrical signals away from the cell body to specialised endings, the nerve terminals. The nerve terminal contains special molecules, neurotransmitters, which are released by electrical signals arriving via the axon, which serve to modify the electrical activity of adjacent neurons. The nerve terminal, together with the adjacent neuron and the intracellular space between the two, is termed a synapse. The axon is the long conducting portion of the neuron and, depending on the circuit, can be short or extremely long. For example, a neuron in the cerebral cortex that controls a motor neuron that innervates a muscle in the toe must project an axon from an upper portion of the brain down into the lower

reaches of the spinal cord, where it makes contact with the appropriate motor neuron. In a tall person, this axon could be 1 m in length; the axon of the motor neuron innervating the toe muscle could also be 1 m or more in length. This unusual cellular anatomy and function (maintenance and conduction of electrical impulses) suggests that neurons can have extraordinary metabolic needs.

Glial cells make up about 60% of the cellular mass of the brain and provide (i) insulation and physical support and packing around neurons, (ii) membranes (myelin sheaths) to insulate axons, which ensure privacy in the conduction of electrical impulses, and (iii) metabolic support for dendrites, axons, nerve terminals and synapses. The glial cells found in peripheral nerve bundles serve the same functions.

At the organ level, the nervous system is divided into two parts: the central nervous system (CNS) and the peripheral nervous system (PNS) (Figure 8.2). The CNS consists of the brain (including the retina) and the spinal cord, and contains networks of neurons organised into circuits of functional importance (e.g. the regulation of blood pressure, the control of appetite, or the initiation and control of movement). The PNS consists of neurons that either provide sensory information to the CNS (afferent neurons) or convey commands from the CNS to effector cells, such as muscle and gland cells (efferent neurons). The cell bodies of many sensory neurons lie outside the brain and spinal cord, while those of neurons conveying commands from the CNS lie within the brain or spinal cord. Hence, whilst the CNS provides a degree of metabolic organisation and protection to the neurons and glia within it, this is not provided to peripheral neurons and/or their cellular processes. The structural organisation of nerves and nerve bundles in the PNS and their attendant glial cells, however, appears to provide some of the metabolic features enjoyed by neurons and glia within the CNS.

The following nutritional and metabolic discussion therefore focuses on the CNS, primarily the brain (since it has been easier to study). The presumption is, however, that what is found to be true for the brain will also be true for the spinal cord. Where evidence is available, relevant comments will also be made regarding nutrient and metabolic effects on peripheral nerves.

Figure 8.1 (a) Typical neuron. (b) Glial cells and their relationships with brain neurons. Astroglia cells extend thin processes to surround regions where axon terminals make contact with neuronal surfaces (forming synapses) and separately to surround capillaries ('perivascular foot' in figure). Oligodendroglia cells can have relatively few processes and provide physical packing and metabolic support around neurons; they can also have extensive processes and form elaborate membranes around axons (myelin sheaths), as shown in (c). (c) Oligodendroglia wrapping axons with myelin. The three unmyelinated axons on the left lack myelin sheaths. The two axons on the right are myelinated by the same oligodendroglia cell (such cells can myelinate up to 50 axons). The myelin sheaths are connected by small cellular processes to the glial cell body. Outside the brain, the myelination of axons appears similar; glial cells performing this task are termed Schwann cells.

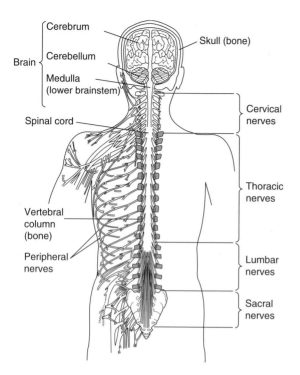

Figure 8.2 Gross structure of the human nervous system: brain, spinal cord and peripheral nerves.

8.3 The blood–brain barrier

A discussion of the BBB is central to any consideration of how food affects the brain (and other parts of the nervous system). This is because any solutes in blood that derive from food must pass through this barrier to gain access to the brain extracellular fluid. Hence, the way in which the barrier handles blood-borne nutrients affects their availability to brain cells.

What do we mean by a BBB? Historically, the concept arose a century ago with the observation that the intravenous administration to animals of certain dyes caused all tissues in the body, except for the brain, to be permeated by the dye. The brain, too, could become coloured, but only when the dye was injected directly into the brain. Hence, the absence of colour in the brain when the dye was administered into the blood did not result from some inability of brain cells to accumulate it when they were exposed to it directly. Rather, some mechanism, a 'barrier', prevented the dye from penetrating from the blood into the brain.

Figure 8.3 The physical nature of the blood–brain barrier. (a) The endothelial cells that form brain capillaries make tight junctions with each other, thereby preventing diffusion; capillary endothelial cells in other organs do not make tight junctions. (b) and (c) Capillaries that supply cerebral ventricles and choroid plexus are made up of endothelial cells *lacking* tight junctions. However, here the 'barrier' is provided by tight junctions made by special epithelial and arachnoid cells, which prevent non-lipid molecules from entering the cerebrospinal fluid by simple diffusion. (Reprinted with permission from Spector R, Vitamin homeostasis in the central nervous system. New Engl J Med 1977; 296: 1393–1398 Copyright © [1977] Massachusetts Medical Society. All Rights Reserved.)

With time, and much further experimentation, the BBB was found to be a selective barrier to the penetration of solutes that are present in the circulation. It is now known to be located in the endothelial cells that make up the capillaries of the brain. Unlike capillaries elsewhere in the body, the endothelial cells of brain capillaries form tight junctions with each other, such that no fluid or solutes can pass into (or out of) the brain without passing through these cells (Figure 8.3). Since this feature presents a continuous lipid barrier to solutes, as a first approximation, solutes in blood gain access to brain as a function of their lipid solubility. In fact, the ease of penetration of molecules into brain plots very reliably against their organic:aqueous partition coefficients: the greater the distribution into the organic phase, the greater the accessibility to brain by simple diffusion across cell membranes. However, many important exceptions exist since most molecules of biological importance are water soluble and thus do not readily diffuse into the brain. For example, the brain could not generate energy without a special, rapid means of acquiring glucose from the blood, since glucose is a water-soluble molecule. The same problem arises for other carbohydrates, as well as for amino acids, ketone bodies, vitamins and minerals. They are needed in the brain in amounts that could not be acquired rapidly enough if diffusion governed their rate of uptake into brain. The solution is that capillary endothelial cells have transport carriers for each of these (and other) nutrients that greatly accelerate their uptake into the brain (relative to diffusion).

It should also be noted that the brain does not have transport carriers for many water-soluble, biologically important compounds, for what seem to be very good reasons. Such molecules, when present in the blood, do not gain access to the brain. For example, certain neurotransmitters used by brain neurons are also used by peripheral neurons for the same purpose (e.g. norepinephrine, a neurotransmitter of the sympathetic nervous system). Significant concentrations of these molecules can sometimes occur in the blood, but they do not get into the brain, where they might indiscriminately modify brain functions. This protection occurs because they are water-soluble and brain capillary endothelial cells do not have transporters for them. Hence, viewed from this perspective, the BBB is a selectively permeable barrier, excluding some water-soluble molecules, promoting the uptake of other water-soluble molecules through carrier-mediated mechanisms, and further allowing the free penetration of gases (oxygen, carbon dioxide) and other lipid-soluble molecules. In addition, the BBB (capillary endothelial cells) appears to have transport carriers designed specifically to move molecules from the brain into the blood.

For completeness, it should be noted that not all parts of the CNS are protected by a BBB. Several small brain regions, known collectively as the circumventricular organs, receive their blood supplies from capillaries that do not have tight junctions. In such regions, neurons, nerve terminals and glial cells are exposed directly to all constituents of the blood. Compounds released by neurons and glia that would normally not penetrate the BBB are freely accessible to the blood in these areas. The absence of a BBB in these areas is presumably no accident. Indeed, it is thought that such areas lack a BBB because either they contain sensors for blood constituents that do not freely cross the barrier (e.g. the area postrema) or some of their neurons or glia release biologically important molecules into the circulation (e.g. nerve terminals in the median eminence, which release neurohormones into the blood that control the functions of the anterior pituitary gland). These areas have been of some interest from a dietary perspective, as they have been argued to be gateways into the brain of amino acids that act as excitatory neurotransmitters. When consumed in excessive amounts in pure form, such amino acids (glutamic acid, aspartic acid, cysteine) have been reported to gain entry into brain via these areas, cause over-excitation of neurons and lead to their death. This issue is discussed further below.

A barrier known as the blood–cerebrospinal fluid (CSF) barrier is also found in a special region termed the choroid plexus. This special collection of blood vessels and brain ependymal cells lines a portion of the brain's ventricular system. It is the site of transport into (and out of) the brain of some nutritionally important molecules and is also responsible for generating CSF. The blood–CSF barrier operates much like the BBB (Figure 8.3). It should also be noted that the retina (a portion of the CNS) is endowed with a blood–retinal barrier, the properties of which appear to be essentially identical to those of the BBB. Hence, as a first approximation, comments made in this chapter about the BBB also apply to the blood–retinal barrier.

Finally, the peripheral nerves lie outside the brain and thus do not have a BBB to protect them. However, they do appear to have protection in the form of a blood–nerve barrier. Nerves running through the body are supplied by capillaries that have endothelial cells like those found in brain. That is, they have tight junctions between cells, restricting the passage of solutes. The properties of transport between blood and nerve, to the extent that they have been studied, have been found to be quite similar to those between blood and brain. The blood–nerve barrier does not appear to extend all the way to peripheral nerve terminals, however, which suggests that nerve endings are exposed to the circulation. This is most clearly evidenced by the occurrence in blood of neurotransmitters such as norepinephrine, which escape from peripheral nerve terminals located in the heart and other parts of the body because no barrier surrounds terminal areas. It is also evident in the observation that when drugs such as 6-hydroxydopamine, which destroy norepinephrine nerve terminals in part by becoming concentrated in them, are given intravenously, they destroy peripheral, but not brain, norepinephrine terminals. The peripheral norepinephrine nerve terminal lacks a barrier to circulating 6-hydroxydopamine; the brain norepinephrine terminal is protected by the BBB.

The BBB is discussed here because it figures prominently in the discussion that follows. The access of dietary nutrients to the brain occurs by way of the circulation. The BBB sits between the blood and the brain. The access of any nutrient to brain therefore depends to a considerable extent on the properties of the BBB (and blood–CSF barrier) and its transport systems for that nutrient.

8.4 Energy substrates

The brain uses glucose as its primary energy substrate. Because glucose is hydrophilic, and thus does not easily penetrate lipid membranes, its uptake into brain requires a transporter, which is located at the BBB. The properties of the transporter for glucose (actually, there are a number of glucose transporters [GLUT] in the body – the one located at the BBB is termed GLUT1) can be described using simple Michelis–Menton kinetics. It is non-energy-requiring, saturable and competitive, non-concentrative and not insulin responsive. It has a K_m for glucose of about 10 mM, somewhat higher than normal blood glucose levels (4–6 mM). This means that the carrier is about half-saturated at normal blood glucose concentrations. The V_{max} of the transporter for glucose is 1.4 μmol/min per gram of brain, or about 1200 g/day for the entire brain (a human brain weighs about 1400 g). The human brain normally consumes 15–20% of the body's oxygen consumption, which allows an estimation of glucose utilisation by brain to be about 100 g/day. The carrier thus has a capacity for transporting glucose that is well in excess of that demanded daily by the brain. This fact presumably reflects the importance of glucose as the brain's primary fuel.

Once glucose has been transported across the BBB into the extracellular fluid, it is rapidly taken up into neurons primarily by GLUT3, a glucose transporter

located on the neuronal cell membrane. This transporter has a glucose affinity several times that of the BBB transporter (GLUT1). Within the cell, the glucose can then enter the glycolytic pathway. The initial enzyme, hexokinase, also has a very high affinity for glucose and is therefore fully saturated at normal brain glucose concentrations (3–4 mM). Overall, then, each step in the glucose pipeline from the circulation to brain neurons is tuned to maximise glucose supply for energy production. It only fails when the blood glucose supply is abruptly curtailed (e.g. the rapid hypoglycaemia that follows the accidental administration of too high a dose of insulin to a diabetic patient).

Blood glucose levels are normally regulated within bounds, except under unusual circumstances, such as starvation and diabetes. Hence, variations in the intake of carbohydrates, per se, are not thought to influence the uptake of glucose into the brain or cerebral function. For example, consuming more or less sugar on any given day does not influence brain glucose uptake. The brain, however, monitors blood glucose concentrations, presumably to insure adequacy of supply, and uses behaviour (food intake) as one mechanism for regulating blood glucose levels.

Blood glucose levels do not normally become low, but fall only under one extreme environmental circumstance, starvation. In starvation, when glucose supplies fall, the brain adds an additional energy source, ketone bodies. Ketone bodies are synthesised by the liver and are by-products of the breakdown of stored fat, providing an extended supply of energy in the absence of food-derived energy. The brain will use ketone bodies whenever provided with them (i.e. whenever blood ketone body levels rise), and blood ketone body concentrations rise in starvation. Indeed, the brain participates in the mobilisation of the body's fat stores by increasing the firing rate of the sympathetic nerves that innervate adipose tissue. This causes the fat stores to break down and release fatty acids, which is the initial event in a cascade leading to increased blood ketone body concentrations. The BBB transporter for ketone bodies, required because ketone bodies are hydrophilic compounds that do not readily cross cell membranes, is induced during starvation, further promoting the flow of ketone bodies into brain. This transporter, like the glucose transporter, has a K_m that exceeds the concentrations of circulating ketone bodies that occur during starvation, and a V_{max} well in excess of energy demands. Ketone body delivery to the brain will therefore never be limited by this transporter. During prolonged starvation, more than half of the energy used by the brain is derived from ketone bodies. Continued use of some glucose appears obligatory and is supplied by way of hepatic gluconeogenesis.

The ingestion of certain foods can also induce the brain to use ketone bodies as an energy source. The chronic ingestion of very-high-fat diets elevates blood ketone body concentrations, promoting their use by brain as an energy substrate. However, extremely high levels of fat intake are required to produce this effect and such diets are found by most to be unpalatable. Hence, in practice, ketogenic diets are not sought after and are hard to follow for extended periods. Diet is therefore not normally thought to influence cerebral energy production via dietary fat manipulation of ketone body supply to the brain (although it can).

High-fat diets are occasionally used clinically with success to treat intractable seizures, and the effect is linked to elevations in circulating ketone bodies. Although the mechanism of this effect is not understood, one hypothesis is that such diets somehow modify neuronal excitability to reduce seizure occurrence through the provision of this energy source to brain neurons.

As indicated earlier, blood glucose concentrations can fall abruptly, although not under physiological circumstances. An overdose of insulin administered by accident to a diabetic subject can cause a rapid, precipitous decline in blood glucose levels. The importance of maintaining blood glucose levels for the benefit of brain energy production quickly becomes evident, since confusion, delirium, seizures, coma and death occur as blood glucose concentrations drop below 50 mg/100 ml (2.5–3.0 mmoles/l), about half normal. That such effects occur, and are most effectively and rapidly reversed by the infusion of glucose, suggests that there is no other compound normally present in the blood that can readily substitute for glucose as the primary energy source for the brain. When gradual, long-term declines in blood glucose are produced experimentally, the brain adapts by increasing the functioning of BBB transport carriers for glucose. The BBB hexose transporter is thus somewhat 'plastic'. Indeed, faced with chronic hyperglycaemia, this hexose carrier can also reduce its ability to transport glucose into the brain.

The high rate of energy utilisation by the brain is thought to reflect in part the fact that 10 billion or so neurons must generate and maintain electrochemical gradients across their cell membranes, and then regenerate them whenever they are depolarised to produce impulses. This notion is supported by several types of evidence and leads to the obvious prediction that when neuronal sub-populations in brain conduct more business, as they often do, local glucose consumption rises. Conversely, when they conduct less, consumption falls. The mechanism for providing more glucose under conditions of increased neuronal firing involves increased blood flow to areas of enhanced neuronal activity. How is this increase in blood flow initiated? When local neuronal and synaptic activity increases, a variety of molecules is released into the local brain extracellular fluid by both neurons and adjacent glial cells (see Figure 8.4). Many of these molecules cause the smooth muscle cells that surround the capillaries to relax. Such molecules include metabolites like lactate (from increased glycolysis) and adenosine (from ATP utilisation), potassium (from membrane depolarisation), and local signalling molecules such as nitric oxide and prostaglandins (which are produced and released by neurons). The activated neuron in Figure 8.4 uses glutamate as a neurotransmitter (most of the synapses in brain use glutamate as a neurotransmitter). When it is released into synapses, in addition to depolarising adjacent neurons, glutamate interacts with specific receptors located on the membranes of surrounding glial cells (astrocytes), causing them to release many of the same molecules (such as prostaglandins [PG], as shown in Figure 8.4). Furthermore, the activation of nerve terminals that impinge directly on capillaries releases a variety of vasodilatory molecules. The barrage of such molecules, by causing capillary smooth muscle cells to relax, dilates local capillaries, resulting in increased blood flow.

With increased blood flow comes more glucose and greater glucose extraction to supply the energy needs of both neurons and glia. One route of glucose supply from the capillary to the neuron, as noted earlier, is simply via the transport of glucose by the capillary endothelial cell (GLUT1 transporter) into the extracellular space, and then the transport of this glucose into the neuron by the neuronal glucose transporter (primarily GLUT3). A more important route, at least for glutamate synapses in the cerebral

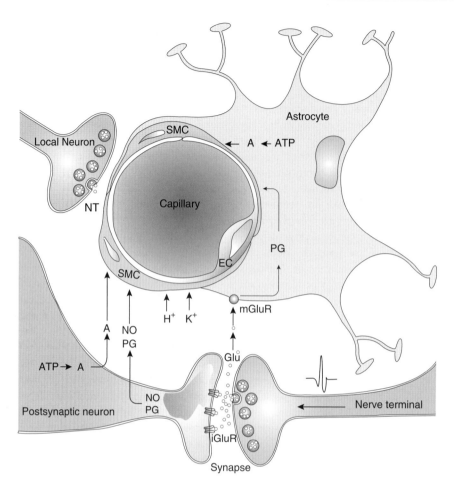

Figure 8.4 Chemicals released by neurons and glial cells during neural activity that cause vasodilatation of local capillaries by relaxing smooth muscle cells. In this figure, a local glutamate neuron has depolarised (lower right of figure), releasing glutamate into the synaptic space. The glutamate interacts with ionotropic GLU receptors (iGluR; such receptors activate ion channels, which are shown) on adjacent neurons (lower left), and metabotropic GLU receptors (mGluR; such receptors lead to intracellular second messenger production) on glial cells (astrocyte, which envelops the capillary), leading to the synthesis of nitric oxide (NO) and prostaglandins (PG) in these cells. The NO and PG are released into the extracellular space, by both cell types, where they can act on smooth muscle cells (SMCs) surrounding the capillary, causing them to relax and the capillary to dilate. The increase in the metabolic activity in neurons and glia that accompany the neuronal depolarisation elicits changes in the concentrations of extracellular ions, such as H^+ and K^+, and metabolic breakdown products, such as adenosine (A) from adenosine triphosphate (ATP), which also lead to the relaxation of capillary smooth muscle cells. Local neurons (upper left) that terminate on or around the capillary can release any of several neurotransmitters (NT) that lead to smooth muscle relaxation and capillary vasodilation. (Reprinted by permission from Macmillan Publishers Ltd: [Nature Review Neuroscience] Neurovascular regulation in normal brain and in Alzheimer's disease, Copyright © (2004).)

cortex, may be through glucose uptake into the astrocyte (via a membrane GLUT1 transporter), its partial metabolism to lactate and the release of the lactate for immediate use by adjacent glutamate neurons. Interestingly, this mechanism seeks to couple glutamate neurotransmission directly to the supply of an energy substrate needed to drive neurotransmission (lactate) and astrocytic glutamate recycling to the neuron. When glutamate is released by neurons, it interacts with receptors on adjacent neurons and is then rapidly cleared, so that the synapse can be reset for the next depolarisation event (see Figure 8.5). Glutamate is removed from the synapse primarily by surrounding astrocytes through a specific glutamate transporter located on the cell membrane. Once inside the astrocyte, the glutamate is quickly converted to glutamine, which has no activity as a neurotransmitter. The glutamine is then released by the

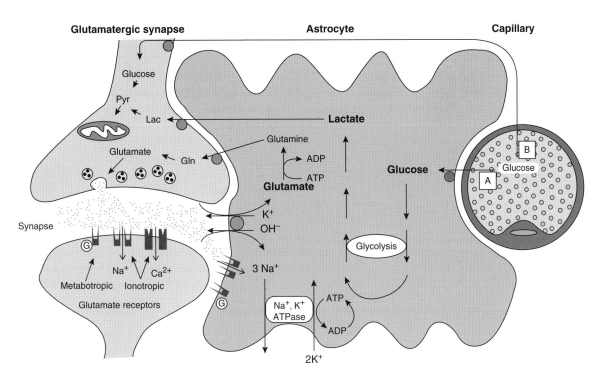

Figure 8.5 Model of the mechanism for glutamate-induced glycolysis in astrocytes during physiological activation. Glutamate release into synapses depolarises postsynaptic neurons by acting at specific receptor subtypes (ionotropic and metabotropic glutamate receptors). The action of glutamate is terminated by an efficient uptake system located primarily in astrocytes. Glutamate is co-transported with sodium ions, resulting in an increase in the sodium concentration in the astrocytes, which activates Na^+,K^+-ATPase. Activation of this enzyme stimulates glycolysis (glucose utilisation and lactate production). The stoichiometry of this process is such that for one glutamate molecule taken up with three Na^+ ions, one glucose molecule enters the astrocytes, two ATP molecules are produced by glycolysis and two lactate molecules are released. Within the astrocytes, one ATP molecule fuels the extrusion of the Na^+ ions taken up with the glutamate molecule and the other provides the energy required to convert glutamate to glutamine by glutamine synthase. Lactate, once released by astrocytes, can be taken up by neurons and serve as an energy substrate. This model, which summarises *in vitro* experimental evidence indicating glutamate-induced glycolysis, is taken to show cellular and molecular events occurring during activation of a given cortical area (arrow labelled A, activation). Direct glucose uptake into neurons under basal conditions is also shown (arrow labelled B, basal conditions). Pyr, pyruvate; lac, lactate; Gln, glutamine; G, G-protein. (Reproduced with permission Pellerin L, Magistretti J, Glutamate uptake into astrocytes stimulates aerobic glycolysis: A mechanism coupling neuronal activity to glucose utilization. Copyright © (1994) National Academy of Sciences, USA.)

astrocyte and is taken up by the nerve terminal, reconverted to glutamate and reused as a transmitter. The transport of one glutamate molecule into the astrocyte immediately stimulates the uptake of one glucose molecule into these cells from local capillaries (the same astrocyte can both surround a portion of an adjacent capillary and enclose a glutamate synapse). The glucose is rapidly converted to lactate, generating for each glucose molecule two ATP molecules to drive (i) the synthesis of one glutamine molecule (requiring 1 ATP) and (ii) the transport out of the cell of the sodium ions that accompanied the uptake of the glutamate molecule (requiring 1 ATP; see Figure 8.5). The lactate is released by the astrocytes

and taken up by adjacent glutamate neurons via a membrane transporter specific for monocarboxylic acids (lactate, ketone bodies), where it is converted to pyruvate and used to generate energy in the Krebs cycle. It should be noted that the key elements of this model are supported by experimental evidence, although its overall design (like that of other models) is presently the subject of active debate. Nonetheless, the feature of the model that makes it intriguing is that it offers a specific biochemical cascade that links an increase in the firing of a glutamate neuron to an increase in the supply of an energy substrate to that specific neuron. It will be interesting to follow the evolution and refinement of this and other metabolic models as the science progresses. For example, even if some version of this model is ultimately found to be correct, many brain synapses (30–40%) do *not* use glutamate as a neurotransmitter. Hence, this particular model cannot explain how increased signalling through such non-glutamate synapses supplies an increased flow of energy substrates to these neurons.

As a further note, although neurons can certainly take up and use lactate as an important source of energy, the lactate derives from other cells *within* the brain (e.g. astrocytes). While lactate can cross the BBB, and a transporter for it (a monocarboxylic acid transporter) is found on capillary endothelial cells, the capacity of the uptake process is not sufficient to supply biologically meaningful amounts to brain neurons from the circulation. Simply put, this means that changes in blood lactate levels are thought to have minimal effects on brain lactate levels or on the use of lactate by brain neurons. Hence, any changes in blood lactate that might be produced by food ingestion would not be expected to impact on the brain (at least as relates to energy supplies).

A final issue regarding brain energy substrates is ethanol, which supplies about 7 kcal/g when metabolised by the body (mainly in the liver and intestines). Is ethanol metabolised by the brain, and in the process does it contribute to the brain's energy supply? Ethanol is lipid soluble and thus readily penetrates the brain as blood ethanol concentrations rise. However, the brain contains very little alcohol dehydrogenase (it may possibly be found in very small amounts in some neurons) and thus does not metabolise ethanol in appreciable amounts. Hence, the brain does not derive energy directly from local ethanol metabolism. This is probably not an accident, since the immediate product of ethanol metabolism, acetaldehyde, is toxic to the brain (indeed, acetaldehyde is not taken up into the brain from the circulation). Ethanol consumption reduces glucose transport into and/or phosphorylation within the brain and thus may actually limit the brain's energy supply. This action may contribute to its behavioural effects (CNS depression).

In summary, the dietary intake of carbohydrates does not appear to influence the availability of glucose or other hexoses to the brain. Instead, blood glucose concentrations and cerebral blood flow are regulated, presumably to ensure the required supply to the brain. In starvation, when glucose supply becomes severely limited, the body accelerates ketone body production, and the brain switches to these molecules as its primary energy source. While diets very high in fat can also lead to ketone body formation, and thus use by the brain, such diets are not typically consumed. Ethanol, an energy source in some parts of the body, is not an energy substrate in the brain.

8.5 Amino acids and protein

Neuronal and glial cells in the brain use amino acids to produce proteins. In addition, they use certain amino acids for neurotransmission. The issue in relation to nutrition and the brain is the extent to which diet can influence the flow of amino acids into this organ and thus their individual uses. Like other needed substrates, the path from diet to brain proceeds from their absorption by the gastrointestinal tract, through their insertion into the circulation, to their extraction by the brain. As might be anticipated, this extraction process involves the BBB. The brain capillary endothelial cells that constitute the BBB contain on their cell surfaces a number of different transporters for amino acids. These transporters occur on both the luminal (facing into the capillary) and abluminal (facing into the brain extracellular fluid) cell membranes. The properties of these transporters dictate how much of each amino acid enters and exits the brain.

Amino acids enter and exit the brain by one of several transport carriers. The choice of carrier relates to the size and charge of the amino acid side-chain. Currently, six carriers have been identified (Figure 8.6). The first is the large neutral amino acid carrier (L in the figure), which is a non-energy requiring, bidirectional transporter that is saturable and stereospecific. This carrier is shared by several amino acids (Table 8.1), including some that are precursors for neurotransmitters (phenylalanine, tyrosine, tryptophan, histidine). Because the carrier is almost saturated at normal plasma concentrations of these amino acids, it is competitive. Hence, changes in the plasma concentration of any one large, neutral amino acid will affect not only that amino acid's transport into the brain, but also that of each of its transport competitors. Because glutamine is present in the brain in extremely large concentrations (it is produced there for a variety of uses), this large neutral amino acid is thought to drive the uptake into the brain of the other large neutral amino acids by serving as the principal amino acid that is counter-

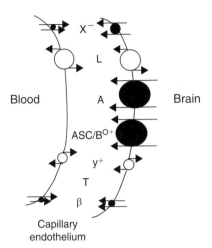

Blood

Brain

Figure 8.6 Blood–brain barrier amino acid transport carriers. Shaded systems, sodium dependent; unshaded systems, sodium independent. (Smith QR, Transport of glutamate and other amino acids at the blood–brain barrier, Journal of Nutrition, 2000. 130: 10165–225. Copyright © American Society for Nutrition.)

transported from brain to blood each time a large neutral amino acid is taken up into the brain.

The second transporter is the basic amino acid carrier (y^+ in Figure 8.6), which is also non-energy requiring, bidirectional, saturable and stereospecific. It is responsible for transporting arginine, lysine and ornithine, and is competitive. The third transporter is the acidic amino acid carrier (X^- in Figure 8.6), transporting glutamic and aspartic acids. This carrier is energy requiring, although little uptake occurs from blood to brain. Instead, the major activity of this carrier is seen on the abluminal membrane (i.e. the membrane on the brain side) of capillary endothelial cells, such that most of the glutamate and aspartate transport is *from* the brain *to* the circulation. Indeed, balance studies of glutamate indicate that the brain is a net exporter of this amino acid, synthesising much more than it needs. The fourth transporter is the small neutral amino acid carrier (A in Figure 8.6), preferring amino acids with small polar side-chains, also energy dependent, which transports primarily alanine, glycine, methionine and proline. This carrier is also located on the abluminal side of the capillary endothelial cell and, like the X^- transporter, is thought to move amino acids primarily *from* brain

Table 8.1 Blood–brain barrier transport constants for brain uptake of neutral and basic amino acids, as measured by the *in situ* rat brain perfusion technique

Amino acid	Plasma concentration (μM)	κ_m (μM)	V_{max} (nmol/min/g)	κ_m (app) (μM)	Influx (nmol/min/g)
Neutral amino acids (system L)					
Phe	81	11	41	170	13.2
Trp	82	15	55	330	8.2[a]
Leu	175	29	59	500	14.5
Met	64	40	25	860	1.7
Ile	87	56	60	1210	4.0
Tyr	63	64	96	1420	4.1
His	95	100	61	2220	2.5
Val	181	210	49	4690	1.8
Thr	237	220	17	4860	0.8
Gln	485	880	43	19900	1.0
Basic amino acids (system y⁺)					
Arg	117	56	24	302	6.7
Lys	245	70	22	279	10.3
Orn	98	109	26	718	3.1

[a] Estimated assuming ~70% of albumin-bound Trp contributes to brain uptake.
V_{max}, maximal saturable transport capacity; κ_m, half-saturation concentration in the absence of competitors; κ_m(app), 'apparent' κ_m under normal physiological conditions (i.e. in the presence of normal concentrations of plasma amino acids, κ_m(app) = κ_m(1 + $\Sigma(Ci/\kappa_m i)$)); influx, unidirectional amino acid flux rate from plasma to brain. Apparent κ_m values *in vivo* are much greater than true κ_m because of transport saturation and competition. (Reproduced with permission from Smith and Stoll, 1998.)

into blood. The fifth carrier (ASC/B°+ in Figure 8.6) is also abluminal and is specific to the small neutral amino acids alanine, serine and cysteine. Finally, the sixth carrier (β in Figure 8.6) is selective for taurine and is energy requiring.

It is evident from the above discussion that the carriers orientated to move amino acids into the brain are those that transport mostly essential amino acids (the large, neutral and basic amino acids), while those orientated to move amino acids out of brain are those transporting non-essential amino acids (the acidic and small neutral amino acids). A small net influx into the brain of the essential amino acids, notably tryptophan, tyrosine, phenylalanine, histidine and arginine, is no doubt required for the synthesis of the neurotransmitters that are derived from them (and are ultimately metabolised). The net efflux of the non-essential amino acids, notably aspartate, glutamate, glycine and cysteine, may serve as a means of removing amino acids that act *directly* as excitatory transmitters or cotransmitters in the brain. The brain carefully compartmentalises these amino acids metabolically, as discussed below, because they excite (i.e. depolarise) neurons. A mechanism to remove these amino acids from the brain may be a component of this compartmentalisation design.

A better understanding of the fundamentally different manner in which the brain uses transport carriers to handle the essential amino acids that are neurotransmitter precursors, and the non-essential amino acids that are neurotransmitters, can be gained by studying an example of each. These examples also reveal important distinctions regarding the impact of diet on amino acid transport into the brain. The examples are tryptophan, a large neutral amino acid, and glutamate, an acidic amino acid.

Tryptophan, a large neutral amino acid

Tryptophan is the precursor for the neurotransmitter serotonin (5-hydroxytryptamine). Serotonin neurons have their cell bodies in small regions (termed raphe nuclei) of the brainstem and midbrain (roughly at the level labelled 'medulla' in Figure 8.2), and project their axons extensively throughout the spinal cord and brain. This relatively small population of neurons (less than 1% of the total brain population) thus appears to communicate with most of the neurons in the CNS and

functions in neuronal circuitry that controls, for example, blood pressure, pituitary hormone secretion, sensory information processing (touch, pain, sound) and sleep.

Interest in this neurotransmitter in the present context derives from the fact that the concentration of tryptophan in the brain rapidly influences the rate of serotonin synthesis in and release from neurons. This relationship holds because the enzyme that catalyses the initial and rate-limiting step in serotonin synthesis (tryptophan hydroxylase; Figure 8.7) is relatively unsaturated with substrate at normal brain tryptophan concentrations. Hence, a rise in tryptophan concentration leads to an increase in serotonin synthesis as tryptophan hydroxylase becomes more saturated with substrate (causing the rate-limiting reaction to proceed more quickly). A fall in tryptophan concentration causes a reduction in serotonin synthesis as enzyme saturation declines (and the reaction proceeds more slowly).

Tryptophan concentrations in the brain are directly influenced by tryptophan concentrations in blood (serum). Hence, a change in serum tryptophan concentration can directly influence serotonin synthesis in brain neurons. However, because tryptophan is transported into the brain by the competitive carrier for large neutral amino acids, tryptophan uptake and concentrations in the brain, and thus serotonin synthesis, can *also* be modified by changing the serum concentrations of *any* of its transport competitors. The serum concentrations of most amino acids, including the large neutral amino acids, are readily influenced by food intake, thereby forming the final link between diet and serotonin synthesis in the brain. It is the competitive nature of the large neutral amino acid transporter, however, that explains a seemingly confusing feature of how food intake modifies brain tryptophan concentrations and serotonin synthesis. When fasting animals ingest a meal of carbohydrates, serum tryptophan increases within 1–2 h. This effect is paralleled by a similar increase in brain tryptophan concentrations and a rise in serotonin synthesis (and neuronal release). When animals ingest a meal of carbohydrates to which protein has been added, however, although serum tryptophan rises even more than when carbohydrates are consumed alone, no rise in brain tryptophan concentration or serotonin synthesis occurs. The explanation

Figure 8.7 Pathway of serotonin synthesis from L-tryptophan. Serotonin is synthesised in two steps catalysed by the enzymes tryptophan hydroxylase and aromatic L-amino acid decarboxylase. The cofactor for each reaction is also shown.

of this effect involves tryptophan's competitors for transport at the BBB, that is, when carbohydrates alone are consumed, not only does serum tryptophan rise, but the serum levels of most of its transport competitors fall, giving tryptophan a great advantage in competing for available transport sites into the brain. Brain tryptophan uptake and concentrations therefore increase. However, when a protein-containing meal is consumed, even though serum tryptophan rises considerably, the serum concentrations of its competitors not only fail to decline, but rise and by a proportionally *similar* amount to tryptophan (because they are present in the dietary protein). As a consequence, tryptophan experiences no change in its competitive standing for access to available transporters into the brain and brain tryptophan concentrations do not change. These effects of food on the serum concentrations of tryptophan and the other large neutral amino acids, in relation to competitive tryptophan transport at the BBB, can be summarised with a single expression of this competition, the serum tryptophan ratio (the serum concentration of tryptophan divided by the summed concentrations of its transport competitors). Following carbohydrate ingestion, the serum tryptophan ratio rises; after a protein meal, it does not.

A key assumption of this simple model is that it applies to all dietary proteins. Recent evidence indicates that this notion is no longer tenable. The original formulation was based on the testing of only a single dietary protein (casein, a milk protein). Surprisingly, no-one thought to examine other proteins. It now turns out that the protein ingested with carbohydrates has a tremendous effect on the post-meal changes in the serum levels of tryptophan and its transport competitors, and thus on post-meal brain tryptophan levels and serotonin synthesis. An experimental example is presented in Figure 8.8. In this study, groups of rats were fed a single meal containing carbohydrates and a protein at levels appropriate for a typical rat meal (about 18% as a percentage of total energy). Serum amino acids, brain tryptophan levels and serotonin synthesis were examined 2 h later. When rats ingested carbohydrate, the serum tryptophan ratio increased over fasting values, as expected, and brain tryptophan levels and serotonin synthesis also increased (compare inverted triangle symbol to X symbol in Figure 8.8). If a meal containing carbohydrates and casein was ingested, also as expected, no notable change occurred in the serum tryptophan ratio, brain tryptophan or serotonin synthesis (diamond symbol) compared to fasting values. If the

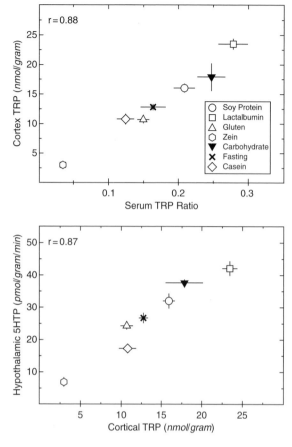

Figure 8.8 Brain tryptophan concentrations and serotonin synthesis in rats ingesting a single meal containing one of several dietary proteins. Food was not available during the daily light period (when rats normally eat little) and was supplied at the onset of the daily dark period (when rats normally begin to eat). Blood and brain samples were obtained 2 h into the dark period, after they had consumed a meal. Tryptophan was measured in the cerebral cortex (y-axis of the upper panel) and is representative of all brain regions. Serotonin synthesis (5HTP in the y-axis of the lower panel) was measured in hypothalamus, a brain region important in appetite and food intake control. The symbols represent group means; the lines are standard error bars. The dietary protein represented by each symbol is indicated in the upper panel. The correlation coefficient (r value in each panel) was very high, both for the relationship of the serum tryptophan (TRP) ratio to cortex tryptophan (upper panel), and the relationship of cortex TRP to hypothalamic serotonin synthesis (5HTP; lower panel). The serum TRP ratio is the serum concentration of TRP divided by the sum of the serum concentrations of its amino acid transport competitors (the other large, neutral amino acids) and is a reliable predictor of TRP uptake into brain. (Reprinted from Physiology & Behaviour, 98(1–2), Choi S, DiSilvio B, Fernstrom MH, Fernstrom JD, Meal ingestion, amino acids and brain neurotransmitters: effects of dietary protein in source serotonin and catecholamine, pp. 156–162, Copyright (2009), with permission from Elsevier.)

protein was lactalbumin (a milk protein), however, increases in the serum tryptophan ratio, brain tryptophan and serotonin synthesis occurred (square symbols) that were considerably larger than those observed when carbohydrates alone were consumed. If the protein added to the carbohydrates was zein (a corn protein), the opposite occurred, namely a marked reduction in the serum tryptophan ratio and in brain tryptophan level and serotonin synthesis (hexagonal symbols). Soy protein (circles) produced increases similar to those seen with carbohydrates alone, and wheat gluten (triangles) had effects like those seen with casein. Figure 8.8 shows that the correlations between the serum tryptophan ratio and brain tryptophan, and between brain tryptophan and serotonin synthesis, were remarkably good, supporting the idea that the impact of the meal on brain tryptophan and serotonin depends on how it changes the serum concentrations of tryptophan relative to those of its competitors. It is worth noting that since the amount of serotonin released by neurons tracks the rate of serotonin synthesis closely, the findings suggest that the ingestion of different proteins in a meal may produce different functional effects in the brain.

Altogether, such findings indicate that dietary proteins influence brain tryptophan and serotonin more than dietary carbohydrates, with some proteins causing increases that exceed those seen with carbohydrates. Indeed, carbohydrate effects seem modest in comparison. What might be the utility to the brain of having the function of a neurotransmitter so readily manipulated by the dietary protein in a meal? Changes of the magnitude observed are not seen with any other transmitter (as far as is presently known). One possibility is that the effect provides a signal to the brain regarding dietary protein quality (e.g. zein is a poor-quality protein, while lactalbumin is a high-quality protein, in relation to growth), which might be used to help the brain direct behaviour to insure the intake of sufficient high-quality protein by an animal to maximise growth rate. The only problem with this idea is that the rise in brain tryopthan and serotonin following the ingestion of carbohydrates alone might fool the brain into thinking that a protein of reasonably high quality had been ingested. However, this is not likely to be the only signal informing the brain about the quality or quantity of ingested protein. For example, glutamate is the dominant amino acid in almost all dietary proteins (about 10% by weight). When proteins are hydrolysed during digestion, glutamate receptors in the gut, which are linked to sensory nerves, are stimulated. These nerves run into the central nervous system and may provide the brain with an assessment of the total amount of protein ingested (independent of its quality). If this is the case, the tryptophan and serotonin increases produced by a carbohydrate meal would not fool the brain into thinking that a high-quality protein had been ingested: the absence of a glutamate signal would indicate that no protein had been consumed. Such ideas suggest interesting hypotheses for future experimentation. The broader question is: does the brain, and if so how does it, assess the nutritional adequacy of ingested matter in order to optimise growth and maintain optimal body function?

The above example considers the rapid effects of food on tryptophan and serotonin. Longer-term changes are also observed. For example, if rats ingest the above diets on a chronic basis (weeks), the same biochemical effects are present. Generally speaking, growth rate follows the diet's effects on brain tryptophan and serotonin. Given this fact, one might imagine that the brain of a rat containing low tryptophan and serotonin due to the ingestion of a protein such as zein (for example) would influence food-seeking behaviour to identify and consume foods containing better quality proteins. In addition, when animals consume diets low in protein (any protein) for extended periods, the plasma concentrations of all essential amino acids decline, including those of tryptophan and the other large neutral amino acids. In this case, even though the decline in plasma tryptophan may be proportionally similar to that of its transport competitors (i.e. competition for the brain transporters does not change), brain tryptophan and serotonin decline. The most likely explanation for this effect is that the transport carriers, which are about 95% saturated when normal amounts of protein are being consumed, become much less saturated at low levels of protein intake because of the decline in the plasma concentrations of all large neutral amino acids. At low carrier saturation competition ceases and simple changes in plasma tryptophan concentrations suffice to predict brain tryptophan uptake and concentrations. In such cases, tryptophan–serotonin signalling would not accurately communicate the quality of the dietary

protein being ingested (if indeed, that is what it does). Presumably, in such a case, other signals would indicate that protein intake is low (e.g. if the glutamate signal considered above is active) and direct protein-seeking behaviour.

Other large neutral amino acids serve as neurotransmitter precursors in substrate-driven pathways in the brain. Phenylalanine and tyrosine are substrates for the synthesis of the catecholamines (dopamine, norepinephrine, epinephrine), and histidine is the precursor of histamine. Like tryptophan, the brain concentrations of these amino acids are directly influenced by their uptakes from the circulation, which in turn reflect the plasma concentrations of all of the large neutral amino acids. For these transmitter precursors as well, the influence of diet on their brain concentrations reflects the impact the diet has on the plasma concentration of each amino acid in relation to those of its competitors. Presently, too little experimental information is available for these transmitters to conjecture how they might be linked to dietary protein or carbohydrate intake or the possible sensing of the intake of these macronutrients.

Glutamate, an acidic amino acid

As noted in Section 8.4, the non-essential amino acid glutamate is used as a transmitter by more than half of all nerve terminals in the brain. It is not known why there is such extensive use in neuronal transmission of a molecule of such great metabolic ubiquity. Glutamate is an excitatory neurotransmitter, which means that when it is applied to neurons with appropriate glutamate receptors on their surface, the neurons depolarise (become electrically active). Within nerve terminals, glutamate is packaged in small vesicles, where it resides until it is released. Once released into the synapse, it stimulates glutamate receptors on adjacent neurons and is then quickly cleared from the synapse (see Figure 8.5). Glutamate receptors fall into two broad categories, ionotropic and metabotropic. Ionotropic receptors are linked to ion channels and, when stimulated, directly alter transmembrane ion fluxes, thereby initiating depolarisation. Metabotropic receptors are linked to intracellular second messengers and, when stimulated, modify signalling pathways (such as those initiated by adenylate cyclase or protein kinases) that ultimately precipitate changes in neuronal function. Because glutamate is ubiquitous as a transmitter in the brain, it has been difficult to discern clearly the properties of the neuronal circuits in which it operates and the roles they play in brain function. Nonetheless, glutamate neurons are now actively studied, for example for their involvement in learning and memory, in the control of pituitary hormone secretion and in blood pressure control.

Because glutamate is an excitatory amino acid, neurons with excitatory glutamate receptors on their surface can become overexcited when exposed to high concentrations of the amino acid and die. The term 'excitotoxicity' was coined many years ago to describe this effect. It led to the concern that perhaps because glutamate is a major constituent of dietary proteins (up to 10% of the amino acid content of a typical protein, not including glutamine), and also added to many foods as a flavouring agent, the ingestion of food might cause the brain to become flooded with glutamate, leading to widespread neurotoxicity. However, this possibility turns out not to be the case. The principal reason relates to the function of the acidic amino acid transporter at the BBB (X^- transporter in Figure 8.6). As noted earlier, this transporter occurs primarily on the abluminal membrane of capillary endothelial cells. As a consequence, glutamate is transported out of the brain, not into it. Consequently, the BBB can be thought to function as a 'barrier' to glutamate penetration. This conclusion accords well with observations that extremely large increases in plasma glutamate concentrations are required before signs of excitotoxicity are evident in the brain (10–15-fold greater than would ever be produced by food ingestion), increases that can only be produced by administering extremely large doses of free glutamate.

There is a second mechanism that protects brain neurons from excessive exposure to glutamate, once released by other neurons. It can also protect them from glutamate that might accidentally penetrate into the brain from the blood. This mechanism was introduced in Section 8.4 and involves the role of glial cells in intracellular glutamate trafficking in the brain (see Figure 8.5). In order for information flow in neuronal circuits to be rapid and accurate, neurotransmitters, once released by nerve terminals, must quickly interact with receptors on adjacent neurons and then just as rapidly be removed from the synapse (to reset it for the next depolarisation). For glutamate synapses, this process of neurotransmitter removal is accomplished primarily by local glial cells, which have energy-requiring, high-affinity glutamate transporters on their surface. Once inside the glial cell, the glutamate is quickly converted to glutamine (by glutamine synthetase) and released into the intercellular spaces, from which it is taken back up into neurons, reconverted to glutamate (by glutaminase) and stored for reuse (Figure 8.5). While the efficient removal of synaptic glutamate by glial cells functions primarily in glutamate–glutamine recycling between neurons and glia, it can also serve to remove from the brain extracellular fluid glutamate molecules that may penetrate the BBB.

Hence, overall, the BBB transporter for glutamate (and brain glial cell glutamate transporters as a backup system) prevents the glutamate ingested in food from entering the brain or influencing brain glutamate neurotransmission.

There are exceptions to this rule. One relates to the existence of several small portions of the brain, termed the circumventricular organs, which lack a BBB. Presumably, this is not an accident of evolution, but serves to allow neurons in these regions to have access to blood constituents not permitted elsewhere in the brain (perhaps to allow sensing of particular molecules in blood) and their terminals to release molecules (e.g. neurohormones) into the circulation. It is possible that these areas are exposed to circulating glutamate, for reasons not presently understood. However, the glial elements in these areas function as they do elsewhere in the brain and rapidly accumulate the glutamate that penetrates in from the circulation. As a consequence, the glial cells in these areas protect neural processes with glutamate receptors on their surfaces.

Protein

Amino acids are also used to synthesise protein in the brain, by mechanisms common to all cells in the body. Does dietary protein intake influence this process (as it does in liver, for example)? In adult animals, variations in dietary protein intake have no effects on brain protein synthesis. This includes the chronic ingestion of very low levels of dietary protein, and probably means that brain cells are quite efficient in reusing amino acids liberated during intracellular protein breakdown. Low levels of protein intake by neonatal and infant animals, however, are associated with below-normal rates of protein synthesis in the brain. To date, one putative mechanism of this association, namely reduced uptake of essential amino acids into the brain and abnormally low brain concentrations of these amino acids, has not been proven.

Fatty acids and choline

Fatty acids

Unlike other tissues in the body, the brain does not appear to use fatty acids directly as energy substrates. However, fatty acids are required by the brain on a continuing basis for the synthesis of the complex fat molecules that are used to construct neuronal and glial cell membranes, and of cellular signalling molecules (e.g. prostaglandins). Membrane construction is particularly active in infant and growing animals, although it is also active in adults (due to membrane turnover). The brain is thought to synthesise some fatty acids from smaller molecules, but uptake from the circulation is also considered to be an important, possibly the major, source of most fatty acids found in the brain. (Indeed, the circulation is the ultimate source of all essential fatty acids in the brain.) In the blood, fatty acids circulate either as components of fat molecules or as non-esterified fatty acids. Some evidence suggests that lysophatidylcholine can be taken up into the brain, but non-esterified fatty acids presumably are the primary form in which fatty acids gain access to the brain. Indeed, uptake into the brain of both essential and non-essential fatty acids has repeatedly been demonstrated. The details of the uptake process are not presently understood, however, and fatty acid uptake presents certain conceptual problems. For example, the fact that fatty acids bind tightly to serum albumin suggests they might not be readily available for exchange with a transport carrier located at the BBB, and diffusion across capillary endothelial cell membranes may be limited, since fatty acids are almost completely ionised at physiological pH. At present, there is no generally accepted model of fatty acid transport to explain the available data for uptake into the brain and retina. Current hypotheses include multiple variants of the possibilities that fatty acids or albumin–fatty acid complexes bind to receptor/transporter sites on endothelial cells and are moved across the membrane into the cell interior, either as the free fatty acid or as the complex, or that fatty acids diffuse in the non-ionised form across cell membranes.

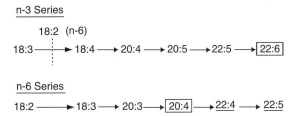

Figure 8.9 Pathways of conversion of essential fatty acids to polyunsaturated fatty acids. The major pathways for synthesis of longer chain n-3 and n-6 fatty acids from linolenic (18: 3) and linoleic (18: 2) acids are shown. As indicated by the dotted line, high levels of linoleic acid block the desaturation of linolenic acid. In tissues, docosahexaenoic acid is the major n-3 fatty acid and arachidonic acid (20:4) is the major n-6 fatty acid. (Reprinted from Connor WE, Neuringer M, Reisbick S, Essential fatty acids: The importance of N-3 fatty acids in the retina, Nutr Rev 1992; 50: 21–29 Copyright © Wiley-Blackwell.)

Whatever the ultimate mechanism of transport proves to be, from the nutritional perspective diet does influence essential fatty acid availability to brain, with potentially important functional consequences. In almost all mammals (cats are an exception), there are two long-chain fatty acids that cannot be synthesised and thus are essential in the diet. These are the polyunsaturated fatty acids linoleic acid and α-linolenic acid. In the body (including the nervous system), linoleic acid is converted into arachadonic acid, a key precursor in the synthesis of prostaglandins and leukotrienes, families of important second messenger molecules. α-Linolenic acid is converted into docosahexaenoic acid, a molecule found in very large amounts in the outer segments of rods and cones in retina, and in nerve terminal membranes in the brain (Figure 8.9). Docosahexaenoic acid is thought to be a key component of phototransduction cells and thus may be important in vision. The brain takes up both linoleic acid and α-linolenic acid, as well as arachidonic acid and docosahexaenoic acid. The calculation has been made that 3–5% of the arachadonic acid and 2–8% of the docosahexaenoic acid in adult (rat) brain turns over daily, which must be resupplied from the blood. Since both the essential fatty acids (linoleic acid and α-linolenic acid) and their products (arachidonic acid and docosahexaenoic acid) readily enter the brain from the blood, all may contribute to the resupply effort. However, the relative contribution of each is not presently known, although studies in the developing brain suggest that, from the *dietary* perspective, dietary docosahexaenoic acid may be more important as a source for brain docosahexaenoic acid pools than dietary α-linolenic acid (see below), particularly when linoleic acid intake is high enough to retard the conversion of α-linolenic acid to docosahexaenoic acid.

Inside the nervous system, linoleic and α-linolenic acid are incorporated into phospholipid molecules and inserted into cellular membranes. Typical phospholipids, which contain two fatty acid molecules, contain one saturated and one unsaturated fatty acid. In retinal rods and cones, where the docosahexaenoic acid content is extremely high, both of the fatty acids in phospholipids can be unsaturated. Because they contain double bonds, essential fatty acids influence membrane fluidity and membrane-associated functions (e.g. the functionality of receptors, transporters and other membrane-embedded molecules). Arachidonic acid is a constituent of lipids in all cells, including those in the nervous system. It is released into the cytoplasm by phospholipase molecules that are activated by the occupancy of membrane receptors (of a variety of types). Once released, arachidonic acid is converted into prostaglandins and leukotrienes. These molecules influence cellular responses to second messenger molecules, such as cyclic adenosine monophosphate (cAMP), and are also released into the extracellular fluid, where they influence the functions of other cells (see Figure 8.4). A dietary modification in essential fatty acid intake might therefore be expected to influence membrane functions in the brain (and elsewhere), leading to alterations in brain function.

Thus far, the most unambiguous studies linking the ingestion of an essential fatty acid to specific CNS functions have been those involving α-linolenic acid and docosahexaenoic acid. The outcome measure is vision. Unlike dietary amino acids, which can produce rapid changes in nervous system function (i.e. in hours), changes in the intake of α-linolenic acid require weeks to produce clearly observable functional effects. In addition, such effects are produced by restricting intake (producing a deficiency) or by restoring the essential fatty acid to the diet of deficient animals (i.e. correcting a deficiency; no effects are seen by increasing intake in normal animals). The functional effects of restricting α-linolenic acid intake are typically seen when applied to animals during the late gestational and early postnatal periods, times when neurons are developing axonal and dendritic extensions, and forming nerve terminals and synapses, and glial cells are proliferating and developing their variety of membrane structures. This also corresponds to the period when docosahexaenoic acid is most actively accumulating in the CNS. While it may ultimately be shown that vagaries in essential fatty acid intake influence brain functions at other times of life, present evidence most strongly links essential fatty acid deficiency to the developmental period of the life cycle.

Studies of α-linolenic acid deficiency have been conducted in both rodents and primates, but the primate results are of greatest interest because of the species proximity to humans. Female rhesus monkeys were fed a diet deficient in α-linolenic acid (but adequate in linoleic acid) throughout gestation, and the infants were fed an α-linolenic acid-deficient liquid diet from birth. Control animals were given diets containing adequate amounts of both α-linolenic and linoleic acids. At birth, biochemical determinations of blood and tissue samples affirmed that α-linolenic acid levels were greatly reduced in the offspring of the mothers fed the deficient diet, compared with those fed the adequate diet, and that this difference widened as the infants began to grow on their own. Moreover, brain and retinal docosahexaenoic acid levels were low at birth; this difference also widened as the infants aged. Measures of retinal function (non-invasive electrical recordings of retina activity, termed electroretinograms) in deficient animals were quite abnormal, and visual acuity was also found to be significantly below normal in α-linolenic acid-deficient infants (Figure 8.10). This effect persisted for at least 12 weeks postnatally. When animals were subsequently provided with diets containing adequate levels of α-linolenic acid, tissue levels of docosahexaenoic acid rose rapidly (4–12 weeks), but abnormalities in the electroretinograms persisted. Hence, while the biochemical deficit was corrected by restoring α-linolenic acid adequacy, features of the functional effects persisted. The persistence of the functional deficit could indicate that a biochemical inadequacy during a critical period of development produced permanent effects on CNS function. Alternatively, it might simply mean that the functional deficit took longer to recover, once adequate α-linolenic acid levels were restored, than was examined in the study.

Figure 8.10 Visual acuity in infant monkeys fed either a normal diet or a diet deficient in α-linolenic acid. (Reprinted from Connor WE, Neuringer M, Reisbick S, Essential fatty acids: The importance of N-3 fatty acids in the retina, Nutr Rev 1992; 50: 21–29 Copyright © Wiley–Blackwell.)

In humans, the development of the visual region of the cerebral cortex and the photoreceptors of the retina, as well as the accumulation of docosahexaenoic acid in the CNS, occur during the last trimester of pregnancy (gestation) and the early postnatal period. Some infants are born premature, however, removing them from the uterine environment during a significant portion of this important developmental period. For this reason, they may be deprived of the normal supply of α-linolenic and docosahexaenoic acids. In this case, visual development might be impaired, as it is in infant monkeys deprived of these fatty acids. Studies in premature infants, born at 7–8 months of gestation, suggest that this might be the case. The supplementation of a standard premature infant formula with α-linolenic acid, or α-linolenic acid and docosahexaenoic acids, was found to improve greatly the functional indices of visual acuity at about 6 months after birth, suggesting effects at both the retinal and visual cortex levels. The formula containing both α-linolenic acid and docosahexaenoic acid produced the greatest benefit. Red blood cell membranes in premature infants fed the unsupplemented infant formula had very low levels of docosahexaenoic acid, compared with those in infants fed breast milk, considered the gold standard infant diet. These levels were notably increased by the addition of α-linolenic acid to the formula, although they remained below those in breast-fed infants. They rose even further

with the additional inclusion of docosahexaenoic acid, to the point that they were no longer below those in breast-fed infants. (The red blood cell membrane is easily obtained in infants, and its fatty acid profile is used as an index of essential fatty acid adequacy in the diet.) Since it is known from animal studies that the addition of essential fatty acids to the diet of normal animals is without effect, but that such an addition to the diets of animals deficient in an essential fatty acid improves function, it may well be that the premature infants did indeed have a deficiency of α-linolenic acid and docosahexaenoic acid, since vision improved with supplementation of the infant formula. Another interesting feature of this work was that the infants supplemented with docosahexaenoic acid and α-linolenic acid showed a greater visual response that did those supplemented with α-linolenic acid alone. Breast milk contains docosahexaenoic acid, while infant formulas do not. The finding may indicate that, like breast milk, infant formulas might be improved by the inclusion of this long-chain polyunsaturated fatty acid, and several manufacturers have recently made this addition.

Choline

Choline occurs in the body as:

- a constituent of lipid molecules (phosphatidylcholine, lysophophatidylcholine, sphingomyelin, choline plasmalogen) that are building blocks of cell membranes
- a source of methyl groups
- a precursor for the neurotransmitter acetylcholine.

Choline is not considered to be an essential nutrient, at least in humans, since the body can synthesise it. Moreover, deficiencies are rarely seen, since it is ubiquitous in the diet.

However, in recent decades dietary choline has been a focus of interest in relation to brain function because of the possibility that changes in choline intake could influence neuronal acetylcholine synthesis. Acetylcholine is a neurotransmitter in neurons in the brain and in the PNS. Indeed, ample evidence indicates that acetylcholine synthesis in and release by brain cholinergic neurons is influenced by neuronal choline availability, and that neuronal choline concentrations can be altered by dietary choline intake, in the form of either free choline or phosphatidylcholine. In addition, oral choline and phosphatidylcholine have found some application in human disease and brain functions thought to involve cholinergic neurons. For example, they have been used successfully to treat movement disorders such as tardive dyskinesia. Tardive dyskinesia is a drug-induced muscular disorder seen in schizophrenic patients. Cholinesterase inhibitors, which raise acetylcholine levels by inhibiting the transmitter's metabolism, have been used with success to reduce the uncontrollable muscle movements associated with antipsychotic treatment in these patients, and choline ingestion has also been found to produce some beneficial effect. Choline and phosphatidylcholine, however, have proved to be of little value in controlling the muscle movements associated with Huntington's disease. Dietary choline and phosphatidylcholine supplements have also been studied as potential memory enhancers, based on the notion that acetylcholine neurons in the hippocampus have an important role in memory and that enhancing acetylcholine levels might improve memory. (Memory is sometimes improved when acetylcholine levels are raised by administering a cholinesterase inhibitor.) Patients with Alzheimer's disease have been most studied and, in general, the disappointing outcome has been that neither choline nor phosphatidylcholine has offered much improvement in memory.

The production of choline deficiency in experimental animals (dietary choline deficiency in humans is rare) has been reported sometimes to reduce the brain content of choline, choline-containing lipids and acetylcholine. Since this has not been a uniform finding, it is not possible at present to state whether or not occasional occurrences of choline deficiency in humans would be expected to diminish the brain's content of choline-containing and/or choline-derived molecules.

8.6 Vitamins and minerals

Vitamins

Neurons and glia have the same functional demands for vitamins as do other cells in the body. Their access to the brain is thus an important consideration, particularly given the existence of the BBB. *Water-soluble vitamins* appear to be transported across the BBB and, in some cases, the blood–CSF barrier, usually (though not always) by non-energy-requiring carriers.

After they are taken up into neurons and glial cells, most are rapidly converted into their biologically active derivatives, namely cofactors in enzyme-mediated reactions. Since cofactors are recycled, dietary deficiencies in one or another vitamin do not immediately lead to brain dysfunction, inasmuch as cofactor pools may take extended periods to become functionally compromised. *Fat-soluble vitamins* are hydrophobic (lipophilic), suggesting that their uptake into the CNS may involve simple diffusion across barrier endothelial cell membranes. The reality, however, is not so simple. The transport into and functions within the brain of micronutrients have not yet been studied to the same extent as has been the case for the macronutrients. However, available data do begin to provide some definition of these processes.

Water-soluble vitamins

Folic acid is transported into brain as methylenetetrahydrofolic acid, the major form of folic acid in the circulation. The transport site is located in the choroid plexus, at the blood–CSF barrier, and is about half-saturated at normal plasma concentrations of methylenetetrahydrofolate; little transport appears to occur at the BBB. CSF concentrations of methylenetetrahydrofolic acid are maintained at several times the circulating concentration, suggesting that transport is active (energy-requiring). The mechanism of transport of methylenetetrahydrofolate into neurons and glia from the CSF/extracellular fluid is not known, but is rapid. Once inside cells, folates are polyglutamated.

The brain appears to take up reduced folic acid, rather than folic acid itself, since it lacks the enzyme to reduce it (dihydrofolate reductase). Reduced folic acid (i.e. methylenetetrahydrofolate) is used by neurons and glia in transferring one-carbon groups, such as in the conversion of serine to glycine or homocysteine to methionine. As methylenetetrahydrofolate is consumed in these reactions, folic acid is transported out of the brain into the circulation.

Considerable interest has been generated in the past decade regarding the consequences of folate deficiency to CNS development. The incidence of neural tube defects (NTDs, e.g. spina bifida, an abnormality in the formation of the spinal cord) has been found to be increased above the population mean in the children of women who are folate deficient during pregnancy. Moreover, the occurrence of this abnormality can be reduced by folic acid supplementation during pregnancy, beginning before conception. Initiating supplementation before conception is essential, since the basic design of the CNS is laid down during the first trimester. At present, the mechanisms by which folic acid deficiency leads to the improper formation of the spinal cord are unknown. Folate is important in single-carbon metabolism, contributing carbon atoms to purines, thymidine and amino acids. Methylation reactions involving folate may also be important in the formation and maintenance of neuronal and glial membrane lipids. A folate deficiency, by impeding DNA, protein and/or lipid synthesis, could also conceivably influence neuronal and glial growth during critical points in neural tube development, leading to effects severe enough to induce NTDs. However, it is presently unknown which, if any, of these biochemical actions of folate might be involved in the production of NTDs.

Folate deficiency may also be linked to depression in adults. The clearest data supporting this connection come from findings in patients with megaloblastic anaemia (i.e. non-psychiatric patients). Patients having a clear folate deficiency in the absence of vitamin B_{12} deficiency showed a very high incidence of depression. Other findings then indicated that depressed patients (who do not have anaemia) have low plasma and red blood cell folate concentrations. Moreover, folate supplementation was found to improve mood in depressed patients. The mechanism(s) by which folate modifies mood might be related to the role of methylene tetrahydrofolate in methionine synthesis from homocysteine. It may thus help to maintain adequate methionine pools for S-adenosylmethionine synthesis. S-adenosylmethionine is a cofactor in methylation reactions in catecholamine synthesis and metabolism: catecholamines (dopamine, norepinephrine [or noradrenaline], epinephrine [or adrenaline]) are known to be important in maintaining mood, and S-adenosylmethionine ingestion is reputed to elevate mood. Folate has also been linked to the maintenance of adequate brain levels of tetrahydropterin, a cofactor in the synthesis of serotonin and catecholamines. It should be noted that although the above evidence suggests that a connection may exist between folate deficiency and abnormal mood, the connection is not widely accepted. Moreover, no mechanism for the effect has yet been convincingly demonstrated.

Ascorbic acid (vitamin C) is actively transported into the brain via the choroid plexus and the blood–CSF barrier, maintaining a concentration in the CSF that is four times circulating concentrations. Transport through the BBB does not occur; the absence of such transporters suggests that the BBB might retard the efflux of ascorbate from brain. The choroid plexus transporter is about half-saturated at normal blood ascorbate concentrations, such that increases in blood ascorbate do not produce large increments in brain concentrations. Moreover, the active transport mechanism ensures that when plasma ascorbate falls, brain levels do not decline appreciably. Consequently, brain ascorbate concentrations show minimal fluctuations over a wide range of plasma ascorbate concentrations (indeed, brain ascorbate concentrations have been shown to vary only two-fold when plasma ascorbate concentrations were varied over a 100-fold range). Inside the CNS, ascorbate is actively transported into cells, although it is not known whether this uptake process is confined to neurons or glial cells, or occurs in both. Ascorbate is lost into the circulation at a rate of about 2% of the brain pool each hour, a loss thought to be caused by diffusion into the circulation and by bulk flow of CSF returning to the circulation. The active transport mechanism readily compensates for this loss. Presumably because ascorbate is actively transported by the choroid plexus, and brain concentrations decline minimally at very low plasma concentrations, CNS signs are not notable in ascorbic acid deficiency states. To date, the only defined biochemical function of ascorbic acid in the brain is to serve as a cofactor for dopamine β-hydroxylase, the enzyme that converts dopamine to norepinephrine (although ascorbate is thought by some to function as an antioxidant).

Thiamin (vitamin B_1) is taken up into the brain by a transporter located at the BBB. It is non-energy requiring, and is about half-saturated at normal plasma thiamin concentrations. Small amounts of thiamin also gain entry via transport through the choroid plexus (blood–CSF barrier). Thiamin is then transported into neurons and glia, and phosphorylation effectively traps the molecule within the cell. In nervous tissue, thiamin functions as a cofactor for the pyruvate dehydrogenase complex, the α-ketoglutarate dehydrogenase complex, α-ketoacid decarboxylase and transketolase. It may also participate in nerve conduction. Severe thiamin deficiency in animals reduces thiamin pyrophosphate levels and the activities of thiamin-dependent reactions. It also produces difficulties in the coordinated control of muscle movement, suggestive of a compromise of vestibular function (e.g. unsteady gait, poor postural control and equilibrium). However, despite these biochemical–functional associations, the exact biochemical mechanism precipitating the functional deficits is unclear. The functional deficits are rapidly corrected with thiamin treatment, suggesting that neurons have not been damaged or destroyed. Thiamin deficiency in humans (Wernicke's disease) produces similar deficits in the control of complex muscle movements and also mental confusion. Korsakoff's syndrome, which occurs in almost all patients with Wernicke's disease, involves a loss of short-term memory as well as mental confusion. Severe thiamin deficiency in humans does appear to produce neuronal degeneration in certain brain regions. While the motor abnormalities can be corrected with thiamin treatment, the memory dysfunction is not improved.

Riboflavin enters the brain via a saturable transport carrier, by a mechanism that has not been well described. It is probably located on capillary endothelial cells, although some transport appears to occur at the choroid plexus (blood–CSF barrier), and is about half-saturated at normal plasma riboflavin concentrations. The vitamin is readily transported into neurons and glia from the extracellular fluid, and trapped intracellularly by phosphorylation and subsequent conversion to flavin adenine dinucleotide and covalent linkage to functionally-active proteins (flavoproteins). In nervous tissue, these functional forms of riboflavin participate in numerous oxidation–reduction reactions that are key components of metabolic pathways for carbohydrates, amino acids and fats. A key enzyme in neurotransmitter metabolism, monoamine oxidase, is a flavoprotein. The brain content of riboflavin and its derivatives is not notably altered in states of riboflavin deficiency or excess.

Pantothenic acid is transported into the brain by a saturable transport carrier located at the BBB. The carrier is almost completely unsaturated at normal plasma pantothenate concentrations, hence increases in plasma levels would never be likely to saturate the transporter completely and thereby limit transport. Neurons and glial cells take up pantothenic acid

slowly by a mechanism of facilitated diffusion. Inside the cell, the vitamin becomes a component of coenzyme A, the coenzyme of acyl group transfer reactions. Relative to other tissues, the brain contains a high concentration of pantothenate, mostly in the form of coenzyme A. Brain coenzyme A concentrations do not become depleted in pantothenate deficiency states, indicating that the supply to the brain of this vitamin is not the key factor governing coenzyme A concentrations in this organ.

Niacin (vitamin B$_3$) is transported into the brain as niacinamide, primarily via the BBB (capillary endothelial cells), but possibly also to a small extent via the choroid plexus (blood–CSF barrier). Most niacin in the brain is derived from the circulation, although the brain may be able to synthesise small amounts. Niacin is taken up into neurons and glia and rapidly converted to nicotinamide adenine dinucleotide (NAD). The half-life of NAD in the brain is considerably longer than in other tissues (e.g. seven to nine times that of liver). NAD and nicotinamide adenine dinucleotide phosphate (NADP) are involved in numerous oxidation–reduction reactions. Dietary niacin deficiency in the presence of a low intake of tryptophan causes pellagra in humans, a deficiency disease that includes changes in brain function such as mental depression and dementia, loss of motor coordination and tremor. The mechanisms for these effects have not been identified.

Pyridoxine (vitamin B$_6$) is taken up into the brain via a transport carrier that appears to be saturable; the details of the mechanism have not been well described. The carrier is probably located on capillary endothelial cells, although some transport appears to occur at the blood–CSF barrier. The vitamin can be transported in any of its non-phosphorylated forms (pyridoxine, pyridoxal, pyridoxamine). Once within the brain extracellular fluid compartment, the vitamin is readily transported into neurons and glia, and phosphorylated (primarily to pyridoxal phosphate or pyridoxine phosphate). In neurons and glia, pyridoxal phosphate serves as a cofactor in a variety of reactions, including decarboxylation reactions, such as those mediated by aromatic L-amino acid decarboxylase (which converts dihydroxyphenylalanine to dopamine, and 5-hydroxytryptophan to serotonin) and glutamic acid decarboxylase (which converts glutamate to γ-amino butyric acid [GABA]), and transamination reactions, such as that mediated by GABA transaminase (which catabolises GABA to glutamate and succinic semialdehyde). Dopamine, serotonin and GABA are neurotransmitters. In humans, pyridoxine deficiency is rare because of its widespread occurrence in foodstuffs. However, where it has been identified, it has been associated with increased seizure activity, an effect that is dissipated with pyridoxine treatment. Production of pyridoxine deficiency in laboratory animals leads to reductions in pyridoxal phosphate levels in the brain and in GABA concentrations. Reductions in GABA, an inhibitory transmitter, are known to be associated with increased seizure susceptibility, and electroencephalographic abnormalities have been recorded in deficient animals. Pyridoxine deficiency in rats also reduces serotonin concentrations in the brain, almost certainly the result of diminished 5-hydroxytryptophan decarboxylation (a pyridoxal phosphate-dependent reaction).

Biotin is transported into the brain by a saturable, sodium-dependent (energy-requiring), carrier-mediated mechanism located at the BBB. Essentially no transport occurs at the blood–CSF barrier. The affinity of the transporter for biotin is such that the carrier would never become saturated. The biotin carrier shows sufficient transport activity to compensate for normal daily turnover of the vitamin. Biotin is a coenzyme for a variety of carboxylation reactions (e.g. pyruvate carboxylase).

Cobalamin (vitamin B_{12}) is thought to be transported into the brain by a carrier-mediated mechanism. Relatively little is known about this process or about the function of vitamin B_{12} in the nervous system. However, vitamin B_{12} deficiency has been known for over a century to be associated with neurological abnormalities. The neurological deficits are presumed to derive from the demyelinisation of axons in spinal cord and brain that are seen in advanced deficiency cases. Left untreated, axonal degeneration eventually occurs. These effects can be reversed if vitamin B_{12} treatment is provided early enough. Vitamin B_{12} has been found to protect neurons from neurotoxin-induced damage, suggesting that it may be important in neuronal repair mechanisms, which may become compromised in deficiency states. Nervous system damage associated with vitamin B_{12} deficiency can occur at any age.

Fat-soluble vitamins

Of the fat-soluble vitamins, *vitamin A* (retinol) has been the most studied in relation to CNS availability and function. The others have been much less well examined, although vitamin E is currently a compound of some interest because of its function as an antioxidant. Vitamins D and K are not typically thought of as having the brain as a major focus of action and thus little information is available regarding their involvement in brain function. Vitamin A therefore presently provides the best candidate to illustrate some of the complexities of fat-soluble vitamin flux and function in the CNS. Some of vitamin E's putative brain actions will also be mentioned.

The most noted role of vitamin A in the CNS is as a component of the photoreceptive pigment of the eye, rhodopsin. Rhodopsin is contained in the outer segments of the photoreceptor cells of the retina, which are in intimate proximity to retinal pigmented epithelium (RPE) cells. The RPE cells serve several functions. One is as the cellular analogue to the ependymal cells of the brain that constitute the blood–CSF barrier. Another is as a participant in the maintenance of the rhodopsin pool in photoreceptor cells. The blood–retinal barrier function is served by the portion of the RPE cell membrane exposed to retinal capillaries. The photoreceptor functions are handled by another portion of the RPE cell membrane, which lies on the opposite side of the tight junctions that are formed between RPE cells (Figure 8.11).

As the physical representation of the blood–retinal barrier, the RPE cells, joined by tight junctions, serve the same functions as the capillary endothelial cells of the BBB and the ependymal cells of the blood–CSF barriers, regarding the flow of nutrients and other molecules between blood and tissue. In this capacity, the RPE cells are also the passageway for vitamin A entry into the retina. In the blood, vitamin A (retinol, in the all-*trans* form) circulates bound to a protein complex consisting of retinol binding protein and transthyretin (prealbumin). This binding enables the blood to carry much more retinol than would otherwise be possible, since the vitamin is very hydrophobic. Protein binding also protects retinol from oxidation. Because retinal capillary endothelial cells do not have tight junctions, the retinol–carrier protein complex can readily penetrate the immediate interstitial space. Here, it makes contact with the RPE

(a)

(b)

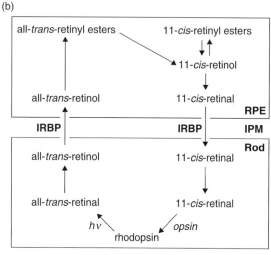

cells, which have specific receptors for retinol binding protein. In a process that has not been completely characterised, once the receptor is occupied retinol is released into the RPE cell. The retinol binding protein and transthyretin molecules are released back into the circulation. Inside the RPE cell, retinol is bound to a specific intracellular protein (cellular retinol binding protein [CRBP]) and ultimately esterified to a fatty acid. This latter molecule serves as the substrate for the conversion of retinol into the visually active form of the molecule 11-*cis*-retinaldehyde, which will ultimately find its way into the photoreceptor and rhodopsin.

The RPE cell also participates in the maintenance of the rhodopsin pool in the photoreceptor cells through its close proximity to these cells. RPE cells produce the active pigment molecule 11-*cis*-retinaldehyde (11-*cis*-retinal in Figure 8.11b) and export it to photoreceptor cells. The 11-*cis*-retinaldehyde is produced from retinol entering the cell from the circulation and from a very efficient mechanism for recycling the retinoid taken up from photoreceptor elements. This recycling process is not completely understood at the molecular level, but the general format is well described. Inside the photoreceptor, 11-*cis*-retinaldehyde is covalently bound to a protein, opsin, which resides in photoreceptor membranes. The 11-*cis*-retinaldehyde-opsin molecule is termed rhodopsin and is the light-responsive pigment of the eye. When light strikes rhodopsin, the phototransduction process occurs as an isomerisation of 11-*cis*-retinaldehyde to all-*trans*-retinaldehyde (all-*trans*-retinal in Figure 8.11b). Once this reaction has taken place, all-*trans*-retinaldehyde is hydrolysed enzymically from opsin as all-*trans* retinol, and released from the photoreceptor into the extracellular space between the photoreceptor and the RPE cell. The opsin is retained in the photoreceptor and reactivated by binding with a new 11-*cis*-retinaldehyde molecule. In the interstitial space, the released all-*trans* retinol is bound to a

Figure 8.11 (a) Schematic drawing of the relationship between the retinal pigment epithelial (RPE) cells and a rod (R) and a cone (C) in the retina. Villous processes containing pigment granules extend from the pigment epithelial cells and lie along the outer segments of both kinds of receptors. Adjacent RPE cells form close tight junctions, which serve to seal the extracellular space around the receptors from that found in the rest of the back of the eye. Some infoldings are found along the distal margin of the cell and above those infoldings is a basement membrane (BM) and the interstitial space of the capillaries. (Reprinted by permission of the publisher from The Retina: An Approachable Part of the Brain by John E Dowling. P. 179, Cambridge, Mass.: The Belknap Press of Harvard University Press Copyright ©1987 by John E Dowling.) (b) Retinoid cycle in the retina. IRBP, interstitial binding protein; IPM, interphotoreceptor matrix (Retinal Pigment Epithelium Fig. 7–8 p. 144 by Michael F Marnor and Thomas J Wolfenburger. By permission of Oxford University Press.)

carrier protein (IRBP in Figure 8.11b), which delivers it to the RPE cell membrane, from which it is transferred into the cell (this process has not yet been described at the molecular level). Inside the RPE cell, the all-*trans* retinol associates with CRBP and then is esterified to a fatty acid (all-*trans*-retinyl esters in Figure 8.11b).

The fatty acid-esterified form of all-*trans* retinol is enzymically converted to the 11-*cis*-retinaldehyde form, which is then exported into the interstitial space adjacent to the photoreceptors, where it again associates with a specific binding protein (IRBP in Figure 8.11b). It is delivered to the photoreceptor in this protein-bound form; the complex is presumed to bind to a receptor and release the 11-*cis*-retinaldehyde to the photoreceptor, where it can be covalently linked to opsin, thereby completing the cycle (Figure 8.11).

From the nutritional perspective, retinal cells clearly have a very refined system for managing and maintaining vitamin A pools. The molecule gains access to retina by a receptor specific for its transporter in blood and is immediately sequestered within the RPE cell. Photoreceptor and RPE cells carefully recycle and conserve the vitamin. Hence, depletion of retinal vitamin A pools in relation to a dietary deficiency only occurs over an extended period. The ultimate appearance of a retinal deficiency develops functionally as 'night-blindness', resulting from the loss of rhodopsin. Extended vitamin A deficiency leads to a loss of photoreceptor elements and eventually of the photoreceptor cells themselves. The cause of this cellular degeneration is not well understood.

Vitamin E is an antioxidant and free radical scavenger that (among other functions) protects fatty acids in cellular membranes. It is transported in blood associated with lipoproteins. The mechanism of its transfer into nervous tissue is presently unknown, but the vitamin generally transfers rapidly between lipoproteins and cellular membranes. Dietary vitamin E deficiency is extremely rare in humans. It occurs in association with certain abnormalities of vitamin E transport and fat absorption, and sometimes in individuals with protein–calorie malnutrition. The neurological manifestations are peripheral nerve degeneration, spinocerebellar ataxia and retinopathy.

Vitamin E has been proposed to play a role in a number of diseases of the CNS that have been linked to oxidative damage. One example is Parkinson's disease, a disorder of movement control induced by the degeneration of certain populations of brain neurons. Evidence of oxidative damage is present in the brains of Parkinsonian patients, although controlled clinical trials of vitamin E supplementation have proved to be of no benefit in retarding the disease's progression. Such negative findings question the likelihood of a vitamin E link to the aetiology of the degenerative changes. A second example is Alzheimer's disease (a form of senile dementia), which is associated with a progressive, generalised, ultimately catastrophic degeneration of the brain. Several types of oxidative damage have been found in the brains of Alzheimer's patients, although it is unclear whether this damage is cause or effect. Unfortunately, clinical trials of the ability of vitamin E to slow the development and progression of Alzheimer's disease have produced conflicting results. Moreover, the prolonged administration of high doses of vitamin E, such as are typical of such trials, has been associated with an increased risk of mortality.

Minerals

All of the essential minerals are important for cellular functions in the brain, as they are elsewhere in the body. These are sodium, potassium, calcium, magnesium, iron, copper, zinc, manganese, cobalt and molybdenum. While most function as cofactors in enzymic reactions, sodium and potassium are key ions in electrical conduction in neuronal membranes, calcium functions as a second messenger within neurons and magnesium functions at certain ligand-gated ion channels on neurons (e.g. the *N*-methyl-D-aspartate [NMDA] glutamate receptor). The diet normally provides more than adequate amounts of almost all minerals, except possibly for calcium, iron, magnesium and zinc. The permeability of the BBB to most metals is quite low, generally much lower than in other organs. Indeed, as a point of reference, the brain extracts 20–30% of the glucose in blood in a single capillary transit, but less than 0.3% of any metal is normally extracted. The mechanisms of transport into the brain for most metals are unknown. However, some details regarding the transport and or functions of iron, calcium and copper are available.

Iron (ferric) circulates bound to a protein, transferrin. More than 90% of plasma iron is bound to

Figure 8.12 Iron transport through the capillary endothelial cell. The left panel shows a cross- section of a brain capillary, indicating the capillary endothelial cells (EC), pericytes (P) and astrocytic feet (A). The small box in this panel is blown up in the right panel, which shows a possible route of iron–transferrin passage from the capillary lumen through the capillary endothelial cell into the brain extracellular space and ultimately into astrocytes. The transferrin–ferric iron complex circulating in blood binds to the transferrin receptor on the capillary endothelial cell (1), which internalises it to an endosome (2) that is moved to the abluminal membrane. The endosome joins with the membrane (3), releases only the ferric iron and then reforms to deliver the apotransferrin to the luminal membrane for release into the circulation (4). The ferric iron released into the brain extracellular fluid binds primarily to transferrin (5) or complexes with citrate or ATP (6). (Reprinted from Moos T, Nielsen TR, Skjørringe T, Morgan EH, Iron trafficking inside the brain. J Neurochem (2007) Copyright © Wiley–Blackwell.)

transferrin. Iron uptake into brain occurs primarily at the BBB. The process involves the uptake of the transferrin–iron complex by capillary endothelial cells, which express transferrin receptors on the luminal membrane (see Figure 8.12). Circulating transferrin–iron complexes bind to transferrin receptors and are internalised in endosomes. For most cells, the typical mechanism of iron transport and secretion into the extracellular fluid involves the release of iron (in the ferrous form) from transferrin in the endosomes and its transport out into the cytoplasma by a divalent metal transporter, located on the endosomal membrane. Cytoplasmic ferrous iron is then transported out of the cell by a cellular membrane protein, transportin, and then converted back to ferric iron by a membrane ferroxidase. However, curiously, brain capillary endothelial cells do *not* appear to express the divalent metal transporter or transportin. Consequently, the current hypothesis for iron movement across the capillary endothelial cell posits that the endosomes carry the iron–transferrin complex to the abluminal membrane and release ferric iron (but not transferrin) into brain extracellular fluid. The endosome then recycles to the luminal membrane and releases apotransferrin back into the circulation (Figure 8.12).

Transferrin is found in brain extracellular fluid and the ferric iron released from capillary endothelial cells associates with it. Transferrin-bound iron is the main form in which iron is found in brain extracellular fluid. *Neurons* express both the transferrin receptor and the divalent metal transporter. Hence, iron enters neurons by the endosomal process, as described above, and is released from the endosome into the cytoplasm. The importance of the uptake process to neuronal iron homeostasis is suggested by the fact that transferrin receptor expression by neurons (but not other brain cells) is markedly increased in iron-deficient animals. Neurons also express ferroportin and thus have the capacity to release iron into the extracellular fluid. Ferroportin is found on all parts of the neuron (dendrites, soma, axons), and the neuron is thought to use it to maintain intraneuronal iron levels at values appropriate for metabolic needs. However, it should be noted that certain neuron groups in the brain store large amounts of iron intracellularly as ferretin, for reasons that are presently unknown.

Curiously, *astrocytes* lack transferrin receptors. A current hypothesis therefore posits that astrocytes absorb iron from the extracellular fluid complexed with ATP or citrate (Figure 8.12). The process of iron release from astrocytes is not presently understood, although astrocyte cell membranes express a ferroxidase (ceruloplasmin), which is presumed to be involved. *Oligodendrocytes*, the glial cells that insulate axons (Figure 8.1c), also lack transferrin receptors, and thus are also thought to take up iron directly as an ATP or citrate complex. These cells, however, express ferroportin and thus can actively export iron.

Numerous, enzymes in brain are iron requiring, including several hydroxylases in neurons that mediate rate-limiting reactions in the production of neurotransmitters (tryptophan hydroxylase, phenylalanine hydroxylase, tyrosine hydroxylase) and monoamine oxidase, a key enzyme in the metabolism of the monoamine neurotransmitters (serotonin, dopamine, norepinephrine, epinephrine).

Iron deficiency can cause impairments in attention and cognition in children. Similar effects are seen in animals. In rats made iron deficient, despite increases in the efficiency of iron uptake by the brain, brain iron concentrations decline, with newborn and infant animals showing more rapid declines than older animals. Iron repletion in the brain occurs (slowly) in infant and adult rats with iron supplementation, but not in animals depleted at birth. While outside the brain the activities of many iron-dependent enzymes are depressed by iron deficiency, inside the brain their activities are unaffected. The activities of the hydroxylase enzymes are not reduced by severe iron restriction, nor are the rates of production of the neurotransmitters derived from them (serotonin for tryptophan hydroxylase; dopamine, norepinephrine and epinephrine from phenylalanine and tyrosine hydroxylases). However, a reduction in dopamine receptors (D_2 subtype) does occur, and coincides with aberrations in dopamine-dependent behaviours in rats. The inability of brain iron stores to recover in rats made iron deficient as newborns coincides with a persistence of dopamine receptor-linked behavioural deficits, despite normal repletion of iron stores elsewhere in the body. Restoration of normal behaviour with iron supplementation, along with brain iron stores, is seen in animals made iron deficient at other ages.

Iron deficiency also interferes with myelinisation. Since marked glial proliferation and myelin formation occur early in infancy, iron deficiency during this period could compromise the optimal development of neuronal communications (e.g. glial cells provide insulation for axons and synapses). This effect could account for some of the behavioural deficits associated with neonatal iron deficiency. If brain function is permanently affected by the occurrence of iron deficiency shortly after birth, this vulnerability should be an issue of great concern in those parts of the world where iron deficiency in infancy is an endemic problem.

Calcium is transported into the CNS via a saturable, probably active, transport mechanism located in the choroid plexus (the blood–CSF barrier). At normal plasma calcium concentrations (calcium circulates mostly in the free form, i.e. unbound to a blood protein), it operates at near saturation, presumably enabling brain calcium levels to remain relatively constant in the face of increases in plasma calcium. Unlike intestinal calcium transport, transport into the brain is not vitamin D sensitive. Some calcium is taken up into the brain via the brain capillary system (i.e. across the BBB), but this fraction is less than 40% of total calcium uptake each day. This transport mechanism has not been defined. The active transport of calcium at the blood–CSF barrier would presumably enable brain calcium levels to be maintained at or near normal levels in the face of dietary calcium deficits. Since calcium concentrations in the circulation are also regulated, under most circumstances, this process would also be expected to help maintain brain calcium uptake and levels in the face of vagaries in calcium intake. Deficiencies in brain calcium should thus be a relatively rare occurrence.

Copper functions as a cofactor for numerous enzymes, including dopamine β-hydroxylase, which mediates the reaction converting dopamine to norepinephrine. Dietary copper deficiency in humans is fairly rare, but when experimentally induced in animals lowers copper concentrations throughout the body, including the brain, and blocks the conversion of dopamine to norepinephrine in brain neurons. This enzyme block also occurs in peripheral sympathetic nerves and the adrenal gland, which synthesise norepinephrine and epinephrine. The mechanism of copper uptake into the brain is unknown, but recent evidence suggests that while copper circulates bound to serum proteins (notably ceruloplasmin), free (non-protein bound) copper is the form taken up into the brain, primarily across capillary endothelial cells (the BBB). One hypothesis is that copper transported into the endothelial cells is then directly transferred into astrocytes (through the 'end-feet' that surround brain capillaries) and subsequently provided to neurons through astrocytic processes that impinge on neurons. In this manner, copper availability to neurons could be metered, since excess copper is neurotoxic. Copper deficiency occurs as an X-linked genetic disease of copper transport in Menkes disease, in which tissue and brain copper levels become extremely low and produce neurodegeneration. Children with Menkes' disease die at a very young age.

8.7 Perspectives on the future

The brain is influenced by the availability to it of many of the nutrients it needs, and not simply in relation to chronic, dietary deficiencies. Indeed, the brain depends from minute to minute on its supply of glucose and this nutrient is therefore carefully regulated in blood (i.e. not directly dependent on the vagaries of dietary supply). Moreover, in the absence of an adequate glucose supply, the body turns to an alternative energy source, ketone bodies, which are supplied through mobilisation and metabolism of body fat deposits. Variations in amino acid supply to the brain do not influence protein synthesis, but hour-to-hour variations in the plasma concentrations of certain amino acids, such as those that follow a meal, can directly influence their conversion to neurotransmitter derivatives and thus presumably brain functions. Variations in the dietary intake of essential fatty acids also impact on brain and retinal composition, and on function (vision). These effects, however, take weeks to develop, and developing animals are most susceptible. Variations in micronutrient intake tend not to influence brain uptake and functions on a short-term basis. The manner in which they are supplied to, sequestered in and used by the brain indicates that considerable buffering exists between brain pools and dietary supply. Such seems to be the case for water-soluble and fat-soluble vitamins, and for minerals.

It is clear why glucose supply to the brain needs to occur without interruption (cutting off the glucose supply has an immediate, drastically negative impact on the brain) and why so many nutrient pools should be buffered from metabolic and dietary vagaries. It is thus somewhat surprising that the transmitter products of some amino acids are so vulnerable to diet-induced variations. Perhaps some function is served by this rapid diet–brain link, such as the monitoring of protein intake, but no real answer has yet been identified.

In contrast to the impact on brain chemistry and function of dietary vagaries in nutrient intake in relation to normal food sources, relatively little is known about the effects on the nervous system of consuming excessive amounts of most nutrients. The issue of potential toxicities of excessive nutrient intake gains importance with the current and growing practice of ingesting 'megadose' amounts of individual nutrients for perceived medical and physiological benefits, but this discussion remains for the future when, hopefully, the knowledge base will have expanded.

Further reading

Chader GJ *et al.* Retinoids and the retinal pigment epithelium. In: The Retinal Pigment Epithelium: Function and Disease (Marmor MF, Wolfensberger TJ, eds), New York: Oxford University Press, 1998, pp. 135–151.

Connor WE, Neuringer M, Reisbick S. Essential fatty acids: The importance of n-3 fatty acids in the retina and brain. Nutr Rev 1992; 50: 21–29.

Davson H *et al.*, eds. An Introduction to the Blood–Brain Barrier. Boca Raton, FL: CRC Press, 1993.

De Dominico I, Ward DM, Kaplan J. Regulation of iron acquisition and storage: consequences for iron-linked disorders. Nature Rev Mol Cell Biol 2008; 9: 72–81.

Deutsch AY, Roth RH. Neurotransmitters. In: Fundamental Neuroscience, 3rd edn. (Squire LR *et al.*, eds) Burlington: Academic Press, 2008, pp. 133–155.

Dowling JE. The Retina: An Approachable Part of the Brain, Cambridge, MA: Belknap, 1987.

Choi S *et al.* Meal ingestion, amino acids and brain neurotransmitters: Effects of dietary protein source on serotonin and catecholamine synthesis rates. Physiol Behav 2009; 98: 156–162.

Fernstrom JD, Fernstrom MH. Diet, monoamine neurotransmitters and appetite control. In: Nutrition and Brain, Nestlé Nutrition Workshop Series Clinical and Performance Program, Vol 5 (Fernstrom JD, Uauy R, Arroyo P, eds). Basel: Karger, 2001, pp. 117–134.

Fernstrom JD, Garattini S, eds. International Symposium on Glutamate. J Nutr 2000; 130 (4S): 891S–1079S.

Fernstrom JD *et al.*, eds. 100th Anniversary Symposium of Umami Discovery: The Roles of Glutamate in Taste, Gastrointestinal Function, Metabolism and Physiology. Am J Clin Nutr 2009; 90 (3S): 705S–885S.

Hamilton JA *et al.* Brain uptake and utilization of fatty acids, lipids and lipoproteins: Application to neurological disorders. J Mol Neurosci 2007; 33: 2–11.

Iadecola C. Neurovascular regulation in the normal brain and in Alzheimer's disease. Nature Rev Neurosci 2004; 5: 347–360.

Innis SM. Dietary omega 3 fatty acids and the developing brain. Brain Res 2008; 1237: 35–43.

Kamat CD *et al.* Antioxidants in central nervous system diseases: preclinical promise and translational challenges. J Alzheimers Dis 2008; 15: 473–493.

Magistretti PJ. Brain Energy Metabolism. In: Fundamental Neuroscience, 3rd edn. (Squire LR *et al.*, eds). Burlington MA: Academic Press, 2008, pp. 271–293.

Moos T *et al.* Iron trafficking inside the brain. J Neurochem 2007; 103: 1730–1740.

Pellerin L *et al.* Activity-dependent regulation of energy metabolism by astrocytes: an update. Glia 2007; 55: 1251–1262.

Rapaport SI, Chang MCJ, Spector AA. Delivery and turnover of plasma-derived essential PUFAs in mammalian brain. J Lipid Res 2001; 42: 678–685.

Simpson IA, Carruthers A, Vannucci S. Supply and demand in cerebral energy metabolism: The role of nutrient transporters. J Cereb Blood Flow Metab 2007; 27: 1766–1791.

Smith QR. Regulation of metal uptake and distribution within brain, in: Nutrition and the Brain, Volume 8 (Wurtman RJ, Wurtman JJ, eds). New York: Raven Press, 1990, pp. 25–74.

Smith QR, Stoll J. Blood–brain barrier amino acid transport, in: Introduction to the Blood–Brain Barrier (Partridge WM, ed.). New York: Cambridge University Press, 1998, pp. 188–197.

Spector R. Vitamin homeostasis in the central nervous system. New Engl J Med 1977; 296: 1393–1398.

Spector R. Micronutrient homeostasis in the mammalian brain and cerebrospinal fluid. J Neurochem 1989; 53: 1667–1774.

Squire LR *et al.*, eds. Fundamental Neuroscience, 3rd edn. Burlington MA: Academic Press, 2008.

9
The Sensory Systems and Food Palatability

Conor M Delahunty

Key messages

- Taste, smell, chemesthesis, somesthesis and vision are the human sensory systems that contribute to food perception and food palatability.
- Vision guides food selection, providing predictive signals for the other senses. Somesthesis evaluates texture during oral processing, preparing the food bolus for swallow and digestion. The chemical senses (taste, smell and chemesthesis) detect the flavour of foods, which is indicative of nutritional value, spoilage and potential toxicity.
- Each sense has distinct physiology and anatomy, but the psychophysical principles by which the senses detect and respond to stimuli are common to all.

- Cross-modal sensory interactions are observed when two or more perceptible components of a food system are studied together. The halo effect refers to how learning places greater reliance on one sensory modality over another. Flavour perception is influenced by the dominant visual sense and by changing food composition.
- Palatability can be defined as the hedonic reward provided by foods that are agreeable to the palate and is based on the integrated response to stimulation of all the human food senses. The performance of senses alters significantly across the lifespan; this in turn may change perceptions and palatability, and influence nutritional status.

9.1 Introduction to the sensory systems

The human senses play a very important role in the type and quantity of food consumed. The senses collectively function as 'gatekeepers', distinguish the foods that are acceptable for consumption from those that should be rejected and provide an early cue to cease consumption or to switch the type of food consumed.

The visual sense guides selection or choice, using overall appearance and colour as cues. The somesthetic sense detects and evaluates the rheology and structure of foods, enabling texture perception and the identification of food parts that should not be ingested, checking for texture that is unfamiliar, and preparing and evaluating the food (bolus) for digestion. Somesthesis is also used to perceive food temperature in the mouth. The chemical senses of taste, olfaction and chemesthesis (the common chemical sense) detect and evaluate chemical stimuli, in effect the flavour of foods, checking flavour against what is

familiar, screening for flavour associated with spoilage and confirming the presence of nutrients. The chemical senses are fundamental to food intake behaviour, as flavour is the primary signal of nutritional value and potential harm.

All food enters the body through the mouth. From the time of birth, we select what is beneficial to eat and reject that which will cause ill-health. The food senses have evolved to aid this decision-making process. In our modern world, the protective role of sensation is primarily to detect spoiled or tainted foods, as few now roam the countryside hunting, gathering and sampling unusual 'food'. However, we retain the psychological foundations upon which a 'safe and nutritious' diet from initially unknown foods is built, where we observe others, are encouraged to taste by information, sample by tasting and await the post-ingestion physiology consequences (without intention). This learning, often by association, results in a dietary habit of consuming foods with familiar sensory properties, but which may

Nutrition and Metabolism, Second Edition, edited by S. A. Lanham-New, I. A. Macdonald and H. M. Roche. © 2011 The Nutrition Society.

evolve slowly as we age. Within the range of palatable foods in the marketplace, subtle differences in taste, smell or texture can therefore have dramatic influence on individual preferences, ultimately determining quantity consumed, repeated intake and potential nutrition. Individual preferences are underpinned by genetics and determined by the impact of environment and experiences from early life.

The food senses have independent physiology and will be considered separately in this chapter. However, during consumption, these distinct sensory modalities interact to determine palatability and few consumers make any distinction. In fact, palatability is determined by a combination of all sensations relevant to food acceptability, including taste, smell, warmth or cold, touch, texture, pain and even visual sensations. In this chapter it will therefore be necessary to consider the perception of the senses together, particularly with regard to the understanding of sensory preferences.

9.2 The taste system

Unlike vision or olfaction, taste is a proximal sense, meaning that the primary stimulus for taste must make contact with the taste receptors, therefore the process of tasting begins in the oral cavity, primarily on the tongue. Taste receptors are stimulated by contact with liquid compounds, creating perceptions that endow distinctive taste qualities such as sweet, salty, sour, bitter and umami to these compounds.

Anatomy and physiology of the taste system

Taste receptors, located primarily on the tongue and soft palate, are termed taste buds (Figure 9.1). Each taste bud is a cluster of between 30 and 50 specialised epithelial cells. Taste bud cells end in hair-like cilia called microvilli, which make contact with the fluid environment in the mouth through a taste pore at the top of the taste bud. Taste receptors are primarily found on the microvilli, and stimulating compounds are believed to bind to these microvilli, initiating taste transduction. Taste buds, of which there are about 6000 in total, are located within small, but visible, structures known as papillae. There are four types: fungiform papillae (located at the tip and sides of the tongue), foliate papillae (appear as a series of folds

along the sides of the tongue), circumvallate papillae (found at the back of the tongue) and filliform papillae (cover the entire tongue surface and give the tongue a rough appearance). All papillae, apart from the filliform type, contain taste buds. Filliform papillae grip food on the tongue and play a role in mouthfeel. Stimulation of the back or sides of the tongue produces a broad range of taste sensations. The soft palate, root of the tongue and upper part of the throat are also sensitive to tastes. Taste papillae are supplied by a number of nerves. The chorda tympani nerve conducts signals from the front and sides of the tongue, and from the fungiform papillae in particular. The glossopharangeal nerve conducts signals from the back of the tongue. The vagus nerve conducts signals from taste receptors in the mouth and larynx. The sense of taste is robust by comparison with other sensory modalities, and this may be partly explained by the fact that different nerves innervate the tongue. It would therefore be difficult to knock out all taste areas through trauma.

As a large range of different compound types can stimulate taste, it is not surprising that taste transduction involves a variety of mechanisms, dependent on the chemical stimulus type. In general, sweet, bitter and umami tastants signal G-protein coupled receptors that initiate a cascade of events leading to changes in calcium deposits and membrane permeability to various ions such as K^+ and Ca^{2+}. On the other hand, salt and sour taste transduction involves the movement of the taste active Na^+ or H^+ through ion channels. The movement of ions into taste cells produces depolarising potentials that lead to transmission of the nerve signal at synaptic terminals via release packets of chemical neurotransmitters, which stimulate the next cell in the sequence.

Each taste cell has a lifespan of about 1 week. New cells differentiate from the surrounding epithelium and during their lifetime migrate towards the centre of the bud, where they eventually die. Differences in cell type within the taste bud represent differences in age and development. As a person ages, taste cell replacement may slow, and this may have adverse effects on taste function.

Taste coding

The taste neurons branch before entering the taste papillae, and branch again inside the taste

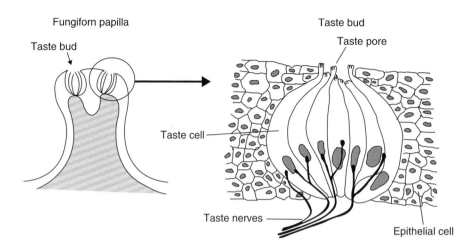

Figure 9.1 Cross section of a fungiform papilla showing the location of taste buds. Cross section of a taste bud, showing the taste pore where the taste enters, the taste cells, and the taste nerve fibres.

bud, therefore a single nerve fibre may innervate more than one papilla and a large number of taste buds. Two theories have been proposed to explain taste coding or how we can distinguish different taste qualities. The first is across-fibre pattern coding. The principle of this is that a taste compound stimulates many nerve fibres (groups of neurons), but not all to the same extent, and the pattern of stimulation across fibres is used to recognise, or code, the stimulus quality. The alternative theory is that of specificity coding, which assumes that some neurons respond best to specific compounds. However, results show that both mechanisms operate together. In general, individual taste cells respond to several types of chemical stimuli. However, it is also the case that taste cells can display selectivity, in particular with low threshold concentration compounds. The firing of specific neurons may identify, for example, compound group, or type, and then more subtle qualities of a compound can be determined by the pattern of firing across large groups of neurons.

Taste quality

It is widely recognised that there are five basic taste qualities, referred to as sweet, salty, sour, bitter and umami. Umami is a recognised 'fifth taste' that has been accepted more recently, particularly in Japan and other cultures where it is most familiar. There is also evidence of additional 'tastes', including metallic taste, ability to detect calcium and a 'fat taste'.

There have been attempts to define, or classify, the stimuli for specific taste qualities. Such a definition might explain an evolutionary basis for quality discrimination that is linked to the nutritional value of foods. Sweet taste is typical of sugars and other carbohydrates, although many artificial sweeteners are not carbohydrate. Salt taste is typical of salts of alkali metals and halogens, although again not without exception. Sour taste is very closely linked to the pH of a substance. Most bitter substances are organic compounds having biological activity, and many of them are poisonous. Thus bitter taste seems to be a poison detector. Umami is used to describe the taste of monosodium glutamate (MSG) and ribosides, such as salts of 5'-ionosine monophosphate (IMP) and 5'-guanine monophosphate (GMP). Europeans or Americans generally describe the umami taste as 'brothy', 'savoury' or 'meaty'. Umami taste guides the intake of peptides and proteins. A 'fat taste', which is thought to detect free fatty acids, may have evolved to select high-energy foods, foods containing fat-soluble vitamins and foods containing essential fatty acids.

Some compounds have a predominant taste: sodium chloride (NaCl) is predominantly salty, hydrochloric acid (HCl) is predominantly sour, sucrose is predominantly sweet and quinine predominantly bitter. However, most compounds have more than one taste quality. For example, potassium chloride (KCl) has substantial salty and bitter tastes, and sodium nitrate ($NaNO_3$) tastes of salty, sour and bitter.

Taste thresholds

Two types of taste threshold measurements can be considered. Absolute thresholds refer to the minimum concentration of a substance or compound that can be detected. Table 9.1 presents absolute thresholds for common compounds. Differential thresholds refer to the just noticeable difference between two levels of concentration above the absolute threshold (i.e. suprathreshold). At absolute threshold, a taste sensation may not have any discernable quality, but as its concentration in solution increases, quality becomes more defined. The taste quality of a compound may also change as concentration continues to increase. For example, NaCl tastes sweet at very low concentrations, and salt solutions below the concentration of saliva may give rise to bitter tastes. In general, intensity of perception increases with increases in the physical concentration of a compound. Psychometric taste functions relating concentration to response are sigmoidally shaped, with an initial flat portion where response at levels below threshold hover around a baseline or background noise level, an accelerating function as threshold is surpassed, and a decelerating function that eventually becomes flat as receptor sites are filled, or as the maximum number of sensitive nerves respond at or near their maximum frequency (Figure 9.2). Sigmoidal-shaped psychometric functions can also represent olfactory, chemesthesis, somesthesis and visual stimuli, and will be referred to again later in this chapter. The duration of taste sensation is also an important quality consideration and could be considered as a type of threshold. Long-lasting tastes are generally referred to as aftertastes and most often have negative association with preference, but recent evidence suggests a contribution to sensory specific satiety.

It was believed that different taste sensations were located exclusively on different areas of the tongue. This 'map' of the tongue was not accurate as a range of tastes can be detected on all parts. However, it is true that not all regions of the tongue are equally sensitive to all chemical stimuli: for sweet taste, threshold is lowest at the front; for sour taste, the rear sides are most sensitive; for salt taste, the front and sides are most sensitive; and for bitter taste, the front of the tongue and the soft palate are most sensitive. This localisation of taste sensitivity may aid in identification of food, manipulation of the food bolus or in

Table 9.1 Absolute taste thresholds for common taste compounds

Compounds	Threshold[a] (molar concentration)[b]
Bitter	
Urea	0.015
Caffeine	0.0005
Quinine HCl	0.000014
Sour	
HCl	0.00016
Acetic acid	0.00011
Citric acid	0.00007
Salt	
NaCl	0.001
KCl	0.0064
Sweet	
Glucose	0.0073
Sucrose	0.00065
Aspartame	0.00002
Umami	
Monosodium glutamate	0.0005

[a] Thresholds are based on compounds major taste quality, although several have additional tastes.
[b] Molar concentration represents the number of grams of solute divided by its molecular weight, per litre of solution.

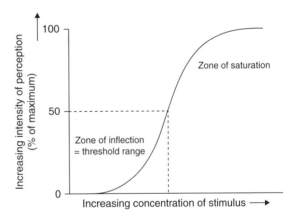

Figure 9.2 Psychometric function of increasing intensity of perception of a taste stimulus with increasing concentration of the stimulus in solution.

removal of selected portions of the bolus that have an unacceptable taste quality. However, this spatial ability also creates an obstacle for the development of substitute sweeteners and salts, as these generally have more than one taste quality and differ in the part of the tongue that they stimulate from the pure tastes of sucrose and NaCl, which they seek to replace.

Widespread individual differences in taste sensitivity are observed for most compounds, especially for bitter compounds, intensive sweeteners and multi-quality salts. For some compounds, the range in sensitivity across population can be several orders of magnitude. There is a genetically inherited difference in sensitivity to the bitter compound 6-n-propylthiouracil (PROP). Individuals may be classified into one of three PROP sensitivity statuses: non-tasters, medium tasters and super tasters. Anatomical differences have also been observed between groups with different PROP taste status, as papillae and taste bud numbers are correlated with taster status. PROP status has also been related to sensitivity to other taste compounds, and to chemical irritant and somesthesis sensitivity. However, these relationships are tentative and a high threshold for one compound does not predict high thresholds for all compounds.

Taste mixtures

The taste qualities of mixed compounds are perceived separately and no taste quality results from a mixture that is not present in the individual constituents of the mixture. Sapid compounds in the mixture cannot mutually suppress one another to produce a tasteless mixture. Consumers often assume that sweet and sour are opposite in taste quality. In fact, when acetic acid and sucrose are mixed, the resultant solution tastes both sweet and sour. Mutual suppression can raise the threshold of each mixed compound and if one compound is stronger than the other it will dominate, and may mask the weaker taste entirely. A solution of quinine and sucrose is less sweet than an equimolar concentration of sucrose tasted alone. Similarly, the mixture is less bitter than equimolar quinine. In general, this inhibitory criterion applies to mixtures of all four basic taste qualities and is referred to as mixture suppression. Since the majority of foods contain more than one taste compound, mixture suppression is important for determining a balanced sensation and providing overall appeal. For example, in fruit juices the unpleasant sourness of acids can be partially masked by the pleasant sweetness from sugars. Salt may be added in processed foods to suppress bitterness. However, it is difficult to characterise taste mixture interactions without also considering the sequential effects of adaptation, a concept that will be dealt with later in this chapter.

PROP taste status can also manifest itself in taste mixture sensitivity, as people who are not sensitive to PROP will not show some mixture suppression effects on other flavours, particularly when bitterness is present in the mixture. The relative intensity of other flavours may therefore be enhanced.

The sense of taste also demonstrates integrative, or additive, effects across the taste qualities. Solutions of taste compounds, regardless of quality, cannot be perceived when diluted below threshold. However, when two solutions of different taste quality that are diluted to 50% below absolute threshold are mixed, the mixture can be perceived. This additive effect has been demonstrated for up to 24 solutions of varied quality diluted to 1/24th of their absolute threshold.

9.3 The olfactory system

Like taste, the primary stimuli for smell must also make contact with the olfactory receptors. However, the stimuli for smell are airborne compounds of volatile substances. The odour-stimulating compounds create perceptions that are endowed with distinctive smells. The olfactory system responds to odour (sensed orthonasally) and aroma (sensed retronasally from volatile compounds released in the oral cavity during consumption). The largest contribution to the diversity of food flavours comes from volatile compounds sensed by the olfactory system, and much of what we commonly refer to as 'taste' is incorrectly localised smell detection. The significant contribution of smell to flavour can easily be demonstrated if you pinch your nose shut whilst eating, effectively blocking air circulation through the nasal passages. Familiar foods will not be recognised as themselves and it is even possible to confuse apples with onions if tasting blind.

Anatomy and physiology of the olfactory system

The receptors for odour are olfactory cells (Figure 9.3). These cells are long, narrow, column-shaped cells, each less than 1 micron in diameter. Olfactory cells are true nerve cells. There are between 6 and 10 million olfactory cells in the human nose. These are located within the olfactory epithelium, a region of tissue of around 5 cm^2 in area, located high in the upper part of each of two nasal cavities. A layer of

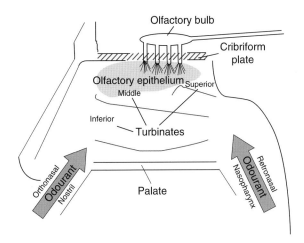

Figure 9.3 The human nasal cavity, illustrating the olfactory receptors, the olfactory epithelium and the different means of entry for volatile compounds.

mucus coats the olfactory epithelium. This mucus provides protection for the sensitive olfactory cells and also regulates transport of olfactory stimuli to the receptors, aiding in smell quality determination. The olfactory receptors have very fine fibres (cilia), which project into the mucous layer, where they contact the stimulus. The cilia serve to enlarge the surface area of the cell enormously so that it is about the same size as the total skin area for humans. Extending from the other end of the olfactory cells are nerve fibres, which pass through the cribriform plate of the skull into the olfactory bulb and connect at a junction called the glomerulus, then further connect with other parts of the brain by olfactory tracts. Therefore, olfactory receptors both receive and conduct stimulus.

During inspiration, or when air refluxes retronasally from the mouth carrying aroma during eating, air is directed into the nasal cavity below the level of the olfactory epithelium. At the interface of the air with the mucus layer covering the olfactory receptors there is an opportunity for chemically selective processes to take place. Compounds first partition from the air into the mucus medium and therefore for any compound to have smell potential it must be soluble in the olfactory mucosa. These compounds may then bind to other compounds, called olfactory receptor proteins, of which there are many hundreds of different types. Compounds eventually stimulate the cilia and, by some poorly understood biochemical process,

provoke the olfactory neural activity. The more vigorous the inhalation, the more of the olfactory epithelium is bathed by the odorant and the greater the stimulation. Olfactory receptors transmit signals directly to the olfactory bulb in the brain, where signals are then processed before being sent to the olfactory cortex and to the orbitofrontal cortex. In addition, olfactory nerves project to many different sites in the brain, some of them closely associated with emotion and memory.

Smell coding

Olfactory receptors respond to many hundreds of different odour-active compounds, giving rise to thousands of different odour qualities. To account for this incredible discriminative ability it is likely that smell is coded by a pattern of response across many receptors. The ability of the system to form a pattern is facilitated by differential movement of potential odorants through the olfactory mucosa. Some volatile compounds are strongly attracted to the mucosa, so they flow slowly through it and are potentially deposited close to its surface. Others are more weakly attracted to the mucosa and so flow more rapidly and stimulate receptors more uniformly throughout the mucosa. Each compound creates a different pattern of receptor stimulation because of differences in how each is deposited on the receptor surface, termed a regional sensitivity effect. In addition, the stimulus causes fairly widespread and diffuse activity in the olfactory bulb. Areas of the nervous system, higher than the olfactory bulb, may be important to interpret the complex neural activity, and the orbitofrontal cortex has been implicated. The amount of neural activity increases with increases in the concentration of a given odorant and it is also possible that different odorants, owing to specific differences in molecular properties, produce specific and distinctive spatial and temporal patterns of activity.

Smell quality

The sense of smell is capable of distinguishing and recognising a wide range of qualities. However, researchers have yet to identify a relationship between a compound's smell and a physical property that causes that smell. Compounds that are structurally very different from one another can smell the same, whereas compounds almost identical in structure can have very different smell qualities. In addition, many smells that we perceive as unitary are in fact complex mixtures of many volatile compounds. For example, the smell of coffee contains over 800 volatile compounds, although only 20 or 30 of these are above absolute threshold. Adding to the complexity, different individuals may describe the same sensation in different ways, although fixed terminologies and objective descriptive analysis techniques are now used to overcome this problem. However, terminology systems work better on a product-by-product basis (e.g. there are agreed terminologies for wine, beer and other product categories) than across product categories.

There have been many attempts to classify odour quality and researchers have searched for primary odours believing that their discovery will elucidate odour quality as did the discovery of the primary colours (see section on Vision). The stereochemical theory proposes seven primary odours (camphoraceous, musky, floral, minty, ethereal, pungent, putrid). This theory proposes that all compounds with similar odour quality have similar geometric structures that fit specific olfactory receptor sites. However, this theory is not widely accepted as there is no evidence of clear and distinct receptor sites and some compounds of similar quality have different structures. Odorants can be classified according to common structural features, such as aldehydes, alcohols, esters or ketones. Odours can also be classified according to physico-chemical features such as carbon chain length or the number and polarity of side groups. These properties determine the volatility and the mucus solubility of the odorant. In addition, the three-dimensional structure of the compound may determine what olfactory receptor protein the compound is capable of interacting with and thus the nature of the neuron activity it will elicit.

Smell thresholds

There are several million olfactory receptor cells on each side of the nose and these are highly ciliated, with 6 to 12 cilia per cell. The cilia greatly increase the surface area of exposure. In the olfactory bulb, a relatively large number of olfactory cells converge on a single glomerular cell, which in turn proceeds directly to the higher cortical regions. There is therefore neu-

Table 9.2 Absolute odour thresholds for common odour compounds

Compound	Smell quality	Threshold[a]
Methyl salicylate	Wintergreen	0.100
Amyl acetate	Banana	0.039
Butyric acid	Rancid butter	0.009
Pyridine	Burnt, smokey	0.0074
Safrol	Sassafras (woody-floral)	0.005
Ethyl acetate	Pineapple	0.0036
Benzaldehyde	Almond	0.003
Hydrogen sulphide	Rotten eggs	0.00018
Courmarin	Haylike, nutlike	0.00002
Citral	Lemon	0.000003
Methyl mercaptan	Rotten cabbage	0.0000002

[a] Milligrams per litre of air.

ral convergence from the cilia to the olfactory cells, and again from the olfactory cells to the olfactory bulb. This general funnelling of olfactory information makes the olfactory system extremely sensitive. As for taste, absolute and differential thresholds can be determined for smell. Olfaction has far lower absolute thresholds to concentration than does taste and may be 10 000 times more sensitive. On the other hand, the sense of smell has a poor ability to discriminate intensity levels and differential thresholds are high relative to other sensory modalities (in the region of 15–25% concentration change is required before a difference can be detected). Odour thresholds are not related only to the concentration of compound. Odour activity is also related to the physical and chemical properties described earlier. The absolute odour thresholds for some common odour compounds are presented in Table 9.2. Methyl mercaptan, which has the objectionable smell of rotten cabbage, can be detected at extremely low concentrations. Methyl salicylate, the smell of wintergreen, has a relatively high threshold, whereas water, which is also volatile, is odourless.

Odour thresholds can vary significantly, both within and between people, and some people with an otherwise normal sense of smell are unable to detect families of similar-smelling compounds. This condition is termed specific anosmia, and can be defined as a smell threshold more than two standard deviations above the population mean. Specific anosmias identified include that to androstenone, a component of boar taint, cineole, a terpene found in many herbs, diacetyl, which is a butter-like smell important for dairy flavour, and trimethyl amine, a fish spoilage taint. Thresholds for odour may also be affected by an interaction of gender and hormonal variation in an individual. It has been reported that the absolute threshold for exaltolide (cyclopentadecanolide), a musk-like synthetic lactone odorant used as a fixative in perfume, varies significantly in the human female according to the stage of her reproductive or menstrual cycle. Similar differences might be expected for food odours.

9.4 Smell mixtures

Like taste, the sense of smell also shows mixture interactions. In fact, it is smell mixtures and not single odorants that are encountered in almost every instance of everyday life. It may be for this reason that the sense of smell is limited in identifying individual odours even in the simplest of mixtures and in deciding whether a stimulus is a single odorant or a mixture. There are a number of basic principles that hold in general: odours of different quality tend to mask or suppress one another, or may remain distinct, whereas odours of similar quality tend to blend to produce a third unitary odour quality. The extent to which these interactions occur depends on the compounds that are mixed and can be influenced by chemical interaction between compounds, or by interaction or filtering at the olfactory receptor sites. The perception of the mixture is also determined by the odour thresholds of the compounds that are mixed, their concentration response functions and their potential to cause adaptation (adaptation will be discussed in more detail later in this chapter). In general, odour mixtures bear a strong resemblance in character to the quality characteristics of the individual components, and obtaining a wholly new odour as a function of mixing is rare. However, in very complex mixtures, such as those that are typical of cheese or wine, often odours of dissimilar quality can be found. In cheese, for example Cheddar, subtle fruity character is provided by fatty acid esters. However, this character complements the dairy characteristics of the cheese because of the inherent complexity of a blend of up to 30 compounds that are above threshold. In fact, the majority of natural odours are mixtures of many chemical components and none of the individual components of the mixture can produce the complexity of mixed odour on its own. It is this complexity and fine balance of natural odours that has made it difficult for flavour companies to reproduce accurately the character of natural flavours in manufactured foods.

9.5 Chemesthesis

Chemesthesis is the term used to describe the sensory system responsible for detecting chemical irritants. Detection is more general than that of taste and smell, and takes place primarily in the eyes, nose and mouth. The perception is closely related to the somatosensory characteristics of texture, pain and temperature change, and provokes a strong behavioural response. The primary function of chemesthesis is to protect the body from noxious chemical stimuli, but this high-influence sense has also been exploited to great effect commercially. The fizzy tingle of carbon dioxide (CO_2) so desired in soft drinks, the cooling sensation of menthol in mint sweets or toothpastes, and the burning sensation of chilli in curry or salsa are perhaps the best examples of how chemical irritation can provide additional character that is very much desired.

Anatomy and physiology of chemesthesis

The general chemical responsiveness to irritation is mediated by nerve fibres in the trigeminal (5th cranial) nerve, which innervate the mucosae and skin of the mouth, nose and eyes, as illustrated in Figure 9.4. The trigeminal nerve has three main branches: the ophthalmic, the maxillary and the mandibular. The chorda tympani and glossopharyngeal nerves, which serve taste reception, may also convey information about chemical irritation. All of the areas served by the trigeminal nerve are sensitive to chemical irritants. Tears caused when cutting onions readily demonstrate sensitivity in the eye, whereas the pungency of mustard readily demonstrates sensitivity in the nose. Chemical irritant sensitivity is by no means of less importance than that of taste or odour, and as already mentioned can have a strong influence on food acceptability.

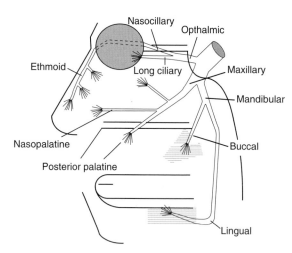

Figure 9.4 Diagram of the branches of the trigeminal nerves that innervate the nasal and oral cavities. A person is bilaterally symmetric with two of each of the branches illustrated.

Chemesthesis quality

The anatomical requirement to enable perception of different irritant qualities appears to be present, and there appears to be variety in the quality of irritative experiences. However, these differences could arise from intensity differences or additional taste or odour qualities. Examples of sensations arising from chemesthesis include the fizzy tingle of CO_2, the burn of hot peppers, the cooling of menthol, the nasal pungency of mustard and horseradish, the oral pungency of spices such as ginger, cumin and black pepper, and the bite of raw onions and garlic. However, each of these substances has additional qualities that stimulate other parts of the chemesthesis anatomy or stimulate olfaction and taste. Mustard, onions and garlic also have lachrymatory effects (tearing), not to mention strong odour. Menthol has a number of sensory properties, including cooling, warming, odour and other sensory effects depending on isomeric conformation, concentration and temporal parameters of exposure.

On the other hand, a majority of compounds, including those that stimulate common odours and tastes, have some degree of irritation. For example, completely anosmic individuals can detect many odour compounds, presumably from the ability of odorants to stimulate the trigeminal nerve branches in the nasal cavity. The trigeminal nerve also signals somesthetic sensations (i.e. tactile, thermal and pain)

and therefore the distinction between a true chemical sense and a somesthetic sense becomes blurred (see section on texture).

Chemesthesis thresholds

Psychophysical principles (absolute thresholds, differential thresholds, sigmoidal shaped concentration response functions) can again be applied to understanding the relationship between concentration and perception of chemical irritant stimuli. However, such relationships are often difficult to study as irritant stimuli can cause desensitisation following stimulation, which can be long lasting. On first stimulation with capsaicin, the irritant compound of chilli pepper, a warm, burning and painful sensation is perceived. This is termed sensitisation. However, repeated stimulation with the same concentration of capsaicin can be without effect as the receptors become desensitised. The quantity of irritant compound consumed is also important. Irritation from capsaicin continues to build to higher levels if stimulation proceeds in rapid sequences without allowing sufficient time for the senses to recover. The absolute threshold of capsaicin has been measured at below 1 ppm. In pure form, capsaicin causes a warm or burning sensation, with little or no apparent taste or smell. Piperine, black pepper, is around 100 times less potent. The rate of increase in perceived intensity as a function of concentration for common chemical irritants is often high relative to those for tastants and odorants. The relationship between the concentration of CO_2, which provides the fizziness in soft drinks, and perceived fizziness is greater than 1:2. This response to stimulus is much greater than that typical of other sensory modalities, apart from electric shock. The long-lasting nature of irritant stimulus is an important aspect of both quality and threshold of perception. Stimulation with capsaicin or piperine with concentrations above threshold may last 10 min or longer.

In addition, individual thresholds may change depending on regularity of exposure. People who regularly consume chilli peppers, or spices derived from chilli pepper, show chronic desensitisation. Interestingly, often reported 'addiction' to spicy food may have a physiological basis, as desensitisation by capsaicin is thought to be due to depletion of substance P, a neurotransmitter in the somatic pain system. Substance P has been linked to the functioning of endorphins, which have the effect of improving mood or giving a feeling of high. Irritant stimulation also has a strong cognitive component as it results in strong defensive mechanisms in the body, including sweating, tearing and salivary flow.

9.6 Texture

The International Organisation for Standardisation defines the texture of a food product as all the rheological and structural (geometric and surface) attributes of the product perceptible by means of mechanical, tactile and, where appropriate, visual and auditory receptors. In this section only the texture perception in-mouth will be considered, as visual perception will be described later. With this in mind, it is most likely that the primary role for texture perception is to determine progress in oral processing towards food bolus preparation for swallow, ensuring that the bolus is prepared adequately for passage to the stomach and for digestion. However, texture perception also contributes significantly to the palatability of foods (think soggy biscuits or hard bread) and texture contrast, both within and across foods (e.g. during a meal), is considered important for palatability of the food and of the meal. A meal would not be very appetising if all of its foods were blended so that texture was removed. Texture is important for food recognition when texture is removed by blending it is very difficult to recognise the food. Texture perception can also serve to determine if the food is homogeneous in texture or has the texture that is expected based on what is familiar.

Anatomy and physiology of somesthesis

Texture is not perceived by a single sense (or receptor type), as are taste or odour. As texture is a less specific construct of many variables, it requires multi-receptor integration for perception, including exteroception (e.g. the touch of food structures) and interoception (i.e. the proprioception of muscle movement). In broad terms, the somesthetic sense is responsible for the detection of food texture during oral processing. Somesthetic receptors are found in all regions of the oral cavity, including the lips, tongue, teeth and mucosa. Table 9.3 presents the sensory basis of texture perception in mouth.

Table 9.3 Somesthetic sense receptors and role in texture perception

Mechanoreceptors	Detect mechanical pressure or distortion and therefore perceive tactile stimuli or the physical structure of food.
Proprioceptors	Sense the static position and movements of the tongue and jaws during mastication, and the resistance to jaw movements during biting and chewing. Proprioception and kinesthesis are sometimes used interchangeably.
Periodontal receptors	Detect forces applied to the teeth.
Nociceptors	Detect potentially damaging stimuli, resulting in the perception of pain.
Thermoreceptors	Detect absolute and relative changes in temperature. There are cold receptors and warmth receptors that work together.

Sensations of the food attributes are gathered during each phase of the mastication process. As referred to earlier, the somesthetic sense is innervated by the trigeminal nerve (5th cranial nerve), and therefore somesthetic sense receptors perceive both chemical stimuli by chemesthesis and structure, rheology, pain and temperature stimuli. The auditory sense also plays a role in texture perception as sounds perceived during oral processing are related to texture attributes such as crispness and crunchiness.

Texture quality

Texture perception is dynamic in that it is continuously changing (dramatically when compared with flavour perception) as the food is manipulated and deformed, and by its very nature often requires movement of the food over the somesthetic sense receptors. Sensations of the food attributes are gathered during each phase of the mastication process. Sounds perceived during oral processing are related to crispness and crunchiness, and may give cues to differences in hardness, denseness and fracturability. In addition, the duration of sound may indicate differences in freshness (e.g. crisp apple) or toughness.

The most widely accepted classification of texture qualities contains three categories of terms: geometrical characteristics, mechanical characteristics and moisture-/fat-related characteristics. Geometrical characteristics relate to the size, shape and orientation of food particles, and are perceived mainly by the tongue and on the hard palate. Common quality descriptions include gritty, grainy, coarse, fibrous and crystalline. Mechanical characteristics relate to the reaction of the food to stress and include qualities such as hardness, cohesiveness, viscosity, elasticity, adhesiveness, brittleness, chewiness and gumminess. Moisture- and fat-related characteristics include dryness/wetness, oiliness and greasiness. To evaluate texture accurately, one should pay careful attention to the time during oral processing when an attribute can be perceived and include this in the quality description. Some researchers now evaluate the 'trajectory' of texture perception qualities during oral processing.

Texture thresholds

The oral cavity is one of the most sensitive regions of the body to touch, with the tip of the tongue and the hard palate having the lowest detection thresholds. Very little research has considered absolute thresholds and differential thresholds for specific food texture stimuli, or differences between individuals in this regard. However, there are large inter-individual differences in the oral physiology parameters (i.e. chewing behaviour, number of chews and rate, tongue movements) that assist oral processing, and there are differences in sensitivity of the somesthetic receptors. It is therefore likely that individual food–subject interactions will lead to differences between individuals in texture perceptions, and this warrants further research. It has been demonstrated that older people are less sensitive to particle size than younger persons, with potential impact on food palatability.

9.7 Role of saliva

Saliva plays an important role in taste function, and moistens and lubricates the food in preparation for swallowing. It contains substances that modulate taste response and acts as a carrier for sapid compounds to the taste buds. Saliva contains a weak solution of NaCl, and ionic constituents of chlorides, phosphates, sulphates and carbonates, as well as other organic components, proteins, enzymes and CO_2. It is capable of buffering acids, and the salivary proteins and muccopolysaccharides give it its slippery and coating properties, which are essential for lubrication of the mouth. The importance of saliva lubrication is most noticeable when it is lost following strong astringent sensation. However, saliva is not necessary for taste response as extensive rinsing of the tongue with deionised water does not inhibit the taste response, but actually sharpens it due to release from adaptation and, for example, the absolute threshold for NaCl is decreased significantly. Saliva is also very important as a solvent that is mixed with food by mastication, aiding food breakdown and bolus preparation. The structural deformation and mixing of food has a significant influence on the release and availability of flavour-active compounds, both sapid and volatile, for sensory stimulation. The structural deformation and mixing of food with saliva, including dilution, will also give rise to differences in texture perception as oral processing progresses. With regard to chemesthesis, there is strong correlation between increased oral chemical irritation and increased salivary flow rate. There are differences between individuals in both saliva flow rate and composition, and this can have a significant impact on the potential of food compounds to stimulate the sensory systems. The initiation of swallowing has been thought to depend on separate thresholds for food particle size and for particle lubrication by saliva. It has also been suggested that swallowing is initiated when a person senses that food particles in the mouth are bound together to form a bolus. However, a person with a relatively high salivary flow rate does not swallow food after fewer chewing cycles than a person with less saliva, although this person will swallow more moistened food.

Astringency is a sensation that does not result from stimulation of the chemical senses per se, although it is caused by chemical stimuli. Astringency sensations are largely tactile and are experienced as a dry and rough mouth, and a drawing, puckering or tightening sensation in the cheeks and muscles of the face. It is believed that tannins or acids binding to salivary proteins and inhibiting their lubricating function cause the dominant astringent sensations. It has also been demonstrated that astringent sensations can result without loss of saliva lubrication for some types of compounds, leading to the conclusion that astringency can result from only the tactile sensation of a precipitate in the mouth. People with a low salivary flow rate have prolonged astringency responses and those with less salivary protein have higher astringency responses.

9.8 Vision

The visual system is our main portal with the outside world and as a result tends to dominate other sensory systems. We use vision to gain information about the colour and appearance (including visual texture) of a food, and also about the immediate environment of the food (from where and from what packaging it comes) before choosing it for consumption. Vision is not directly involved in the evaluation of food palatability, as are taste, olfaction, chemsethesis and somesthesis. Rather visual assessment provides predictive signals for the other senses based on associations that have been learned by experience. For example, anyone familiar with bananas will expect a green banana to have unripe flavours and a firm texture, a blackened banana to be very sweet and soft, whereas a yellow banana will be most suitable for consumption and will probably be chosen as such. This visual dominance, and the expectation that it creates, is easily demonstrated when familiar colour–flavour combinations are confused in a food product, for example when a banana-flavoured food is coloured red or a clear beverage is intensely flavoured.

Anatomy and physiology of the visual system

The visual system consists of the outer eye, or anterior cavity, which includes the cornea, aqueous humour and iris, and the inner eye, which includes the lens, vitreous body and retina, which is connected to the optic nerve. The iris, which is mounted between two ciliary muscles, regulates the amount of light entering the eye (the size of the pupil is determined by the iris) and the lens flexes to focus the image on the retina, accommodating vision of close or far objects. The fundus of the eye includes the retina, macula, fovea, optic disc and retinal vessels. The retina consists of two types of photoreceptor cells (which are the visual receptors): approximately 120 million rods, which are sensitive to low intensity black and white vision (scotopic), and approximately six million cones, which operate at higher light intensities and are sensitive to colour (photopic vision). The optic disc, which is also called the blind spot, is the part of the retina where there are no photoceptors. It is where all of the axons of the ganglion cells exit the retina to form the optic nerve. The macula is

an oval area lateral to the disc used for central vision. The fovea is a small depression in the macula composed almost entirely of cones. The optic nerve leads to the lateral geniculate bodies and then to the cerebral cortex, where visual images are processed.

Visual quality

Colour perception is the brain's response to stimulus of the retina that results from the detection of light after it has interacted with an object. Wavelengths in the visual portion of the electromagnetic spectrum (~380–760 nm) may be refracted, reflected or absorbed by an object that is viewed. It is the reflected light that is seen by the eye. The perceived colour of an object is affected by three entities: the physical and chemical composition of the object, the spectral composition of the light source illuminating the object, and the spectral sensitivity of the viewer's eye. Changing any one of these entities can change the perceived colour of the object. Humans can perceive three primary colours (trichromacy): red, green and blue. This is because cones contain three colour-sensitive pigments, each responding to red (two polymorphic variants at 552 nm and 557 nm), green (at 530 nm) or blue light (at 426 nm) most sensitively. Unlike taste and smell, colour can be relatively easily classified, as all colours consist of a combination of these three primaries.

The colour of an object can also vary in three dimensions. The hue describes the basic 'colour', such as red, green, etc., and is dependent on differences in absorption by the object of various wavelengths. The value describes the relative lightness or darkness, indicating the relationship between reflected and absorbed light without regard for wavelength. The chroma describes the saturation, or the proportion of chromatic content. Chroma determines the purity or vividness of the colour (consider pure green compared with grey green). Verbalisation of colour is subjective for the average person (one who has received no training). However, instrumental measurement of colour is achieved more easily than for flavour and texture because colour is trichromatic. The Commission International de l'Eclairage (CIE) colour system is among the most widely used techniques to define by numbers what a colour 'looks like'. It is based on an additive system, where the principle is to shine the three primaries (red, green and blue) onto a white surface and then vary the amounts of each until an 'unknown' colour is matched. The colour of food is due to compounds (termed pigments) that are contained in the food, such as chlorophylls, carotenoids, anthocyanins or myoglobin, which absorb light of specific wavelengths and reflect other wavelengths. In processed foods, such compounds can be natural (either present naturally in the food or nature-identical but added) or artificial.

The visual sense has a number of characteristics useful for a consistent evaluation of foods in an environment that changes regularly. Object recognition is generally driven by the spatial, temporal and light–dark properties of the object, rather than by its chromatic properties. We can also discount the influences of illumination and recognise a prototypical colour in familiar objects. Objects also have a colour constancy that is served by colour memory and chromatic adaptation.

In addition to colour, we detect appearance attributes that help us to judge food quality. The appearance of an object, its gloss, size, shape and viscosity are determined by the optical properties associated with the object. Light can be distributed over the surface if the object is opaque or within the object if it is translucent. Gloss, transparency, haziness and turbidity are properties attributable to the geometric manner in which light is reflected. Uneven reflection of light from a surface can make an object appear dull or matte. In addition, irregular, patterned or particulate objects reflect light diffusely, whereas smooth objects reflect in a directional manner. Gloss or sheen results where reflection is stronger at a specific angle or in a beam.

As mentioned earlier, humans allow their visual sense to dominate their sensory judgement. This is based on learned experience, as colour is very often related to other sensory attributes, in particular flavour. Red is typical of strawberry, orange is typical of orange citrus, whereas green is typical of lime. Texture contrast, such as lumps, perceived by appearance, will also be perceived in the mouth. The colour of fruit may indicate how ripe it is, and hence its flavour intensity and firmness. The viscosity of a fluid can be assessed visually by pouring the fluid from a container or by tilting the container. However, if the association does not hold in a food due to manufacturing choices, the dominant visual sense can be manifest as a 'halo effect'. Examples of foods where

colour gives an impression that is often not reflected in the sensory properties that are tasted (although most consumers think that it is) include white and yellow margarine or butter, white and red Cheddar cheese, brown and white shelled eggs, or bread made from bleached or unbleached flour. On the other hand, can one imagine eating a meal where foods have been unusually coloured, for example green steak accompanied by brown peas and red French fries. This can be relatively easily achieved using flavourless food colours, but this is certain to reduce the palatability of the familiar meal.

Individual differences

Psycophysical principles apply to vision, as they do to the other senses, and sensitivity to colour and appearance stimuli can be measured, although measurements are relatively complex when all influential factors are taken into account. The best-described differences between individuals are underpinned by physiological differences in the visual system. People lacking one of the three retinal cone pigments fall into various colour-blind categories and comprise 8% of males and 0.44% of females. Colour-blind individuals are classified into different groups. Dichromats lack the ability to see one of the three primary colours (2% of males and 0.03% of females), protanopes have no ability to see red, deuteranopes, comprising about three-quarters of the colour-blind population, have no ability to see green, whereas trianopes have no ability to see blue. The remainder of abnormal persons are protoanomalous and deuteroanomalous trichromats, who have reduced ability to see red and green, respectively. Protanopia and deuteranopia are inherited as recessive, sex-linked characteristics (i.e. they are more common in men than women). Inherited tritanopia is rare and is not sex-linked.

9.9 Adaptation

Adaptation can be defined as the decrement in intensity or sensitivity to a stimulus under constant stimulation by this stimulus. Adaptation results in a higher threshold or a reduced perception of intensity. It is an important operating characteristic of the sensory systems that enables perception of change: the status quo is rarely of interest. We use adaptation constantly to adjust to our changing environment by becoming unresponsive to stimuli that are stable in space and time. An obvious example of adaptation in everyday life is as follows. Consider entering an active kitchen, filled with the odour of food. After a short time there you will no longer notice the odour, which on entering you could perceive strongly. If you leave the kitchen for a time and return again, the odour will be perceived as strongly as before. What is experienced in this example is a feature of all adaptation. Threshold will increase following periods of constant stimulation and ratings of perceived intensity will decrease over time, and may even approach a judgement of 'no sensation'. If the stimulus is removed, then sensitivity returns. The fact that we cannot taste our own saliva, although it contains NaCl and other potentially sapid compounds, is another everyday example of necessary adaptation. Similarly, our odour world is continually filled, so that usually we are at least partially odour-adapted. In terms of visual adaptation, consider walking from a light to a dark room or movie theatre. The adjustment of vision to enable perception is termed dark adaptation. When one returns to the light, leaving the movie theatre, one adapts again; this is termed light adaptation. Chromatic adaptation also occurs where the same object is observed under various sources of illumination. This can be demonstrated by examination of white paper under these conditions, where the paper approximately retains its white colour. Apart from visual texture adaptation, there is little reported regarding adaptation to somesthesis when food is in the mouth. However, it is expected that there will be adaptation, just as we stop feeling our clothes soon after putting them on. Differences have been observed for somesthesis that was direct or indirect; no adaptation was found for roughness perceived by direct touch whereas adaptation was observed for roughness perceived when using a probe.

Adaptation also has a role to play in the perception of mixtures. For example, the sweetness of sucrose and the bitterness of quinine are each partially suppressed when presented in a mixture. However, following adaptation to sucrose, the bitterness of the quinine sucrose mixture will be perceived at a higher intensity, comparable to that of an equimolar unmixed quinine solution. The opposite occurs following adaptation to quinine. Wine has dominant sweet and sour tastes. If wine is consumed with a salad dressed with a vinegar base (which is essentially sour), it will appear sweet to taste. If the same wine is consumed with dessert (which is essentially sweet), it will appear sour to taste. Similar principles hold for odour mixtures. Adaptation to one component of an odour mixture can make another stand out. Returning to wine, differential adaptation may explain why wine character appears to change with time of exposure.

Compounds of the same quality tend to cross-adapt. For example, after adapting to NaCl, the salty taste of other salts is also perceived to be less intense and other taste qualities are unaffected. Adaptation to sucrose reduces sensitivity to other sweet compounds and, similarly, adaptation to one odorant may affect the threshold of another odorant.

9.10 Cross-modal sensory interactions

Cross-modal sensory interactions are often observed when two or more perceptible components of a food system are studied together. The representations from each modality are brought together in multimodal regions of the brain, such as the orbitofrontal cortex, where the signals are integrated to form a complete picture, that is the perception. It is important to identify the nature of these interactions as they may influence consumers' perceptions and preferences in unexpected ways. The factors that cause apparent cross-modal sensory interaction are not always the same. Sensory differences can be caused by interactions between the components of the food prior to introduction to the senses. For example, differences in temperature can change the vapour pressure and partition coefficients of volatile compounds and therefore their release from a solute. Differences in microstructure or viscosity (perceived as texture) can also influence partition and availability of compounds for perception. Changing fat content or salt content also influences the physical chemistry of a food matrix dramatically, changing its flavour significantly. Sensory interactions are also determined by a halo effect, which is due to learning to place greater reliance on one sensory modality over another to make behavioural decisions. This effect is most obvious by the dominance, or bias, of the visual sense over the taste or olfactory sense when familiar colour and flavour combinations are confused, or when the colour intensity is varied beyond expectation (e.g. imagine a dark beverage with no taste). This type of bias can be modified by directing attention to specific characteristics of the product or those of most interest. A true cross-modal sensory interaction is one where the function of one sense (e.g. threshold measures, concentration–response functions) is changed by stimulation of another sense. Some examples of all three interactions that influence sensory perception are given here.

Interactions between the chemical senses of taste and smell have received much attention. Consumers often do not make any distinction between taste and smell, and most often refer to the combined sensation as 'taste'. Incorrect localisation is therefore often misinterpreted as representing interaction. There is in fact very little specific interaction between taste and odour. However, when taste compounds and odour compounds are presented together, the intensity of perception of the combination can be more intense than when either is presented alone. In fact, it has been shown that a below-threshold tastant can be combined with a below-threshold odorant to provide a flavour stimulus above threshold. In addition, sucrose is perceived as sweeter when presented with fruit character odour compounds, but not when presented with savoury character odours. These interactions are learned by experience and the congruency develops from repeatedly experienced pairs, such as for fruity odour and sweet taste.

Interactions between chemesthesis and both odour and taste have been demonstrated. These interactions are truly cross modal, as they are manifest as suppression effects that can be measured using psychophysical functions. When odour molecules and irritant molecules are mixed they produce mutual suppression, much like when odours alone are mixed. As most odorants have irritant effect in addition to their odour quality, suppression may be a common occurrence. If a person has reduced sensitivity to irritation, then the balance of aromatic flavour they perceive may be changed. Capsaicin desensitisation has partial inhibitory effects on sweetness, sourness and bitterness perception, but not on saltiness. However, when capsaicin is presented mixed with these tastants, inhibitory effects are not found. This is most likely because the capsaicin has not had sufficient time to cause desensitisation before the tastants are perceived. There is less evidence to show how tastes can influence the burn of capsaicin, although studies suggest that sweet, sour and salt will reduce the intensity of

burn, with sweet working best. Fat, or fat content, may also reduce burn as capsaicin is highly lipophilic, and fat may remove excess capsaicin that is available for perception. Irritation of various types can also improve preferences significantly. Soft drinks, or sodas, are not particularly pleasant without the fizziness provided by CO_2, and are in fact sweeter to taste.

Interactions between somesthesis, the visual senses and the chemical senses are also common. An intense sweet taste increases the perception of viscosity, although this is observed as a halo effect. The change in perception caused by sweetness intensity may be due to prior association between high levels of sugars and high viscosity. On the other hand, thresholds for the basic tastes, and for most odorants, are higher in solid foods, foams and gels than in water. However, this interaction is most influenced by physico-chemical interactions occurring in the food matrix, rather than effects on the sensory receptors. This influence is particularly so for odour.

Colour has a strong influence on flavour perception. It influences absolute threshold measures, differential threshold measures, discrimination and even the ability of beverages to quench thirst. Darker coloured foods and beverages are rated as having more intense flavour. Uncoloured foods receive lower odour quality ratings, and incorrect identification is common when familiar flavour and colour combinations are confused. These interactions also demonstrate halo effects.

Temperature changes influence intensity of perception for all of the chemical sense modalities. Thresholds for taste compounds are lowest between 22 and 32°C. The effect of temperature can be represented by a U-shaped curve. In practical terms, salted foods taste more salty when they are heated or cooled to the 22–32°C range. Similarly, sweet tasting foods will be most sweet in the 22–32°C range. A good cook knows to adjust seasoning to the temperature at which the food will be served. Temperature also influences chemical irritation perception. The most obvious example is that of the temporary, but significant, relief from chilli burn given by a cold drink.

9.11 Food preferences

Palatability is a term used to describe the hedonic reward provided by the sensory properties of a food or beverage. Evidence shows that a food or beverage that is highly palatable will be consumed in a larger quantity, although palatability also varies depending on the physiological need of the individual that tastes. Palatability is often measured as desire to consume (or eat, or drink).

The palatability of a food is determined by the integrated response to stimulation of all of the senses in combination. It is most logical to refer to palatability when attempting to relate combined chemical sense, somesthetic and visual sense perceptions to preferences, as regular consumers, whose preferences are of most interest, do not normally distinguish between the varied sensory stimuli when they respond to food during consumption.

In developed society, the significance of food has changed from providing basic nutritional needs to providing protocols that define a person, their cultural identity and social standing. In fact, now palatability could be called the social sense because we tend to eat with other people when possible, sharing experiences as we eat. However, when we do share experience, labels are usually prefaced with pleasant or unpleasant remarks. Comments such as 'this soup is too salty' or 'I really like the taste of this sauce' are typical. These labels determine which foods we choose to eat and which we avoid.

With regard to food sensation, there is a strong relationship between sensory perception and hedonic response to food. As the sensory intensity of a given stimulus increases, for example the sweetness of sugar, its hedonic tone becomes increasingly pleasant, reaches a maximum (ideal point) and then decreases in pleasantness to the point of neutral hedonic tone. Further increases in concentration become unpleasant (Figure 9.5). This inverted U-shaped curve is typical of the hedonic response to most chemical stimuli. However, there are many factors that influence an individual person's perception of a food's sensory properties. These include how much has already been eaten, what has already been eaten, and how long ago, past experiences with different foods, individual genomics, nutritional status and, with reference to the preceding paragraph, the culture and personal company that have most influence on a person. Such factors will not negate the relationship between sensory perception and hedonic response described above, but they may alter the shape of psychophysical concentration–response curves, hedonic response curves or both.

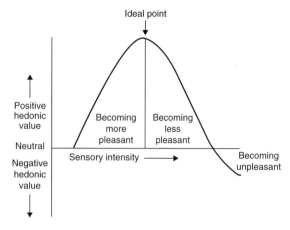

Figure 9.5 The relationship between sensory intensity and hedonic response.

Our reaction to sensory stimulus may be positive when we first try a food, but this positive response may become negative after we have eaten for a while. This change in response can be due to changes in internal state, or satiety, signalling the body to stop eating. However, other factors may also be involved. Consider ordering a dark chocolate pudding, with intense chocolate flavour, at your local café. At first you may feel that the piece you have received is rather small, but you will be doing well to finish it all off, even if you are quite hungry. This latter response is more likely to do with sensory fatigue, or sensory specific satiety, than a signal from inside the body. Sensory specific satiety can be defined as a decrease in the palatability and consumption of a food after it has been consumed, when compared with the palatability and consumption of foods that have not been consumed. This response is common for strongly flavoured foods, but has also been demonstrated for the texture and colour of foods. Beverages, in particular sugar-sweetened beverages, tend to be consumed in excess of nutritional or thirst need. It is likely that the volume of beverage consumed will be negatively correlated with strong flavours, higher viscosity and longer after-taste, and one strategy aimed at achieving satiation in beverages has focused on longer-lasting flavour release. Sensory-specific satiety is also manifest if the same food is presented repeatedly over time to an individual, and can result in reduced intake. This may explain why humans characteristically seek variety in their diet, at least to a point.

People in certain cultures develop preferences for certain foods that are typically associated with that culture: consider the differences between Asian and European cuisines. However, there is little evidence to suggest that peoples of different cultures have different sensitivity to sensory properties. In addition, children, who often avoid unfamiliar foods because of their flavour or texture, come to prefer these foods if repeatedly exposed to them. People also learn to like and to appreciate bitter-tasting foods and beverages such as alcoholic beverages and coffee. People who perform blind preference tests among a range of products within type more often than not choose the product that they are most familiar with or the one that they themselves consume. Evidence suggests that even subtle sensory preferences are learned and are strongly related to past experience with food. However, sensory preferences are not fixed when one reaches a particular point in life. They are continuously changing as experience increases.

Food preferences also demonstrate evolutionary design, instinctive response and adaptive value. At birth, infants prefer sweet taste, which indicates the presence of sugar, an important source of energy. They also tend to dislike bitter taste, which indicates substances that might cause sickness. These responses remain strong throughout life and only change through experience, as referred to above. Salt is liked at low concentrations, but disliked at high concentrations, which makes sense as high intake might disrupt the body's careful osmotic balance. However, rats deprived of salt, a necessary component of their diets, have been shown to compensate and develop a specific hunger for sodium. Food preferences can also be affected by a single pairing of a food with sickness. This response is termed conditioned flavour aversion. There is good evolutionary justification for this extreme response, as sickness was most likely caused by poisoning and conditioned flavour aversion prevents us from making the same mistake again. It has also been demonstrated that acceptance of texture among toddlers is related to experience with texture variety in early infancy and childhood, and that novel colour might be used as a means to overcome established texture and flavour expectations in children.

There are well-documented differences between individuals in ability to taste PROP, and this difference has a genetic cause. Significant individual differences in thresholds to other sapid and odour compounds have also been shown. There are also documented differences in saliva composition and flow rate, mastication behaviour and the quantities of sapid and volatile compounds that individuals can release from their food during eating. With these differences in mind, it may be that some foods taste differently to different people, and that these differences can be genetic. These differences may explain difference in individual food preferences, particularly within cultures.

Memory for taste and smell is particularly durable when compared with that for visual stimuli. Recollection, particularly for smell, is linked to an emotional component that aids the sensory systems in their role as 'gatekeeper'. Long-term memory, often subconscious, enables humans to form associations between tastes and smells and foods that are good and bad to consume, and between tastes and smells and a particular place or occasion. A celebratory meal in a good restaurant will be recalled with more satisfaction than a meal eaten alone or when feeling low. These emotional factors can have a large influence on preferences because of the associative learning. It is important to recognise that these emotions are closely associated with sensory memory, and recent evidence suggests that sensory memory for some tastes and smells is stronger than for others, perhaps referring to physiological need in the past. For example, memory for sweet taste and flavours associated with fats is relatively short term, whereas that for bitterness is longer term. This difference in memory for tastes may have implications for food intake.

9.12 Changing function of the senses across the lifespan

When examining changing function of the senses across the lifespan, it is difficult to distinguish sensitivity from hedonic response. As was discussed in the previous section of this chapter, it is palatability, preferences or hedonic response to stimuli, rather than the stimuli themselves, which determine behaviour towards food and relate best to food intake. To recap: the performance of the senses is responsible for determining initial preferences and may determine how easily new preferences can be learned during life; secondly, the senses constantly maintain their 'gatekeeping' function, screening stimuli to check that they meet preferred criteria, sourcing those that provide positive feelings and rejecting those associated with unhappy experiences or ill-health.

There are several stages of life, from early infancy, through childhood, adolescence, adulthood, middle-age and older people to the oldest old. Food preferences and food intake change across the lifespan. Nutritional requirements also change. Malnutrition, manifest in under-eating, over-eating or insufficient nutrient intake is widespread among almost all age groups or life stages. When one considers the contribution of the human senses to food choice and intake, one should approach the subject from two perspectives. The first is to seek knowledge of how sensitivity and hedonic response change across the lifespan, and ultimately to determine relationships between these factors and eating behaviour that can be exploited in age-appropriate new product development. The other perspective is to understand how society, or the food industry, are currently contributing to incorrect dietary habits and dietary guidance strategy through a lack of understanding of changing sensory function and its significance in helping regulate optimum dietary intake, and to use this knowledge to restrict flavours and textures that cause indulgence and promote flavours (and textures) that signal nutritive value.

Newborn infants can discriminate between basic tastes. They demonstrate this by responding with positive facial expressions to sweet taste and with negative facial expressions to sour and bitter tastes. They are indifferent to salty taste, probably because they are relatively insensitive to it. However, a preference for salt emerges at around 4 months of age due to taste system development. Innate taste preferences remain strong throughout the lifetime, but may be modified by experience, and it is unclear how changes are related to changing sensitivity. For example, salt taste preference can be modified in infants as young as 6 months of age through experience. Children maintain a strong preference for sweet taste, certainly up to 5 years of age, but sweet taste preferences tend to decline between adolescence and adulthood.

The human olfactory system is anatomically complete before birth, and perception of odours via the amniotic fluid and early in infancy may play a role in later responses and preferences to odour stimuli. Studies have shown that newborns can smell and can discriminate between different odours, although they do not demonstrate typical preferences initially.

In fact, infants may like smells that are off-putting for adults, such as those of faecal odours. However, these infants soon learn to develop preferences that are more in keeping with their peers, and by the age of 3 tend to match those of adults. This and other evidence suggests that lifelong preferences and aversions for odours, as well as other strong emotional associations with odours, are formed during infancy and childhood. Preferences for the flavours of fat also appear to be learned, as children may associate specific flavours with high-energy density. Children's preferences for fat are correlated with the BMI of their parents. This suggests a possible genetic link that may also be manifested as 'fat-taste' sensitivity. However, the link may equally be due to the dietary habits these parents give their children. In fact, given the evidence presented, variety of the diet in later life may be compromised by flavour preferences, or food experiences, learned during infancy and in early childhood. This relationship highlights a need to introduce variety in flavours linked to positive nutritional value early in life. Relatively little is known about changes in sensitivity or hedonic response to chemesthesis that accompanies the change from infancy to adolescence and adulthood. Given the impact of chemical irritation on hedonic response, research work is now needed.

In a way that is similar to acquisition of odour preferences through familiarity and associative learning, it is also the case that early experience with texture variety will lead to a greater likelihood of intake of a new food texture. In addition, young children are less dominated by their visual sense, as the associations between appearance and colour and in-mouth perceptions of sensory attributes are not as well formed as those among adults. In many cases children can correctly identify flavour qualities when colours are varied from what is familiar (to an adult). In addition, due to having less-formed associations between appearance and in-mouth perceptions, novel colours may be used to encourage tasting of a (expected) disliked food. This has been demonstrated with new coloured cultivars of vegetables, such as purple cauliflower and yellow beans.

Nutritional disorders may begin during childhood, but are more commonly initiated during the transition from adolescence to adulthood and are established as adulthood progresses. Studies have been conducted to determine whether sensitivity and preferences for sweet taste, the flavour of fat and prevalence of obesity are related. No causal relationship was found, although obese people tend to prefer foods high in sugar and fat, and select fat-rich taste stimuli in sensory tests. Recent evidence suggests a negative correlation between ability to perceive free-fatty acids in the mouth and higher weight status because of greater consumption of energy in fatty foods. Additional factors such as income, socio-economic status, and the availability of sugars and fats were related to intake. On the other hand, women with the eating disorder anorexia nervosa seem to have dissociated taste responsiveness and eating patterns. Their taste preferences for sweet and fat do not differ from other people, but they use them to aid food avoidance rather than selection. Although not conclusive, these studies may demonstrate that it is not sensitivity per se that is important, but how we have learned to use our sensory system as a guide to consumption.

In older people, and in particularly in the oldest old, a new sensory requirement emerges. Older people lose chemical sense function, in parallel with the loss of other biologic functions. This loss is greatest to olfactory function, which is manifest as higher absolute odour thresholds, less ability to perceive differences between suprathreshold odour intensity levels and decreased ability to identify odours. Anatomically, decrement can be seen by morphological change to the olfactory bulb. Taste function, on the other hand, remains relatively intact. Thresholds for salt and bitter taste may increase, whereas sweet and sour thresholds show little change. There are also some intensity decrements to chemesthesis function, although little is known for certain. Chewing efficiency has been demonstrated to decrease among older people, in particular when dental status is also compromised. This loss, and changes in dentition, gives rise to troublesome-to-eat sensory attributes, such as hard and fibrous textures and the presence of peel or seeds. It has also been demonstrated that older people become less sensitive to particle size in-mouth. In general, adaptation proceeds more slowly, recovery from adaptation is lengthier and cross-adaptation is more severe in older people, when compared with the young. In addition, interactions within and between sensory modalities may be effected by a changed contribution of specific compounds or modalities to perception due to differential loss of function. For example, as smell declines at a faster rate, foods that are bitter but have pleasant odour may be experienced as just plain bitter by an older person with poor odour ability. There are also effects of ageing on saliva flow and composition. This change influences ability to break down food, inhibits mixing, retards flavour release and makes swallowing difficult.

Loss of sensory function with ageing may cause older persons to loose interest in food and food-related activities such as cooking or dining out, leading to reduced energy intakes and a reduction in essential nutrient consumption. In addition, the motivation that sensory specific satiety gives to seek variety may be reduced, leading to consumption of a monotonous diet, which can also lead to reduced intake of specific essential nutrients. Losses in ability to sense saltiness can create problems in older hypertensive populations, as they are likely to put more salt in their food. The texture attributes that can become troublesome are often associated with fruits and vegetables, and may lead to avoidance. However, the impact an age-related change in sensory function has on food preferences and food intake is unclear as few studies have demonstrated a causal relationship between sensory impairment, diminished hedonic response and altered food intake in the same group of older people.

In all ages, the perception of food in the mouth signals an innate biological response termed cephalic phase response. This response stimulates saliva flow, and gastric and pancreatic secretions, preparing the gastrointestinal tract for foods that are about to be ingested so that these may be processed efficiently by the digestive system. The extent to which cephalic phase responses change over the lifespan, and the importance of these responses to long-term nutritional status, has yet to be determined. On the other hand, changes in nutritional status, resulting from physiological disturbances that affect nutrient or energy balance, from normal fluctuations in energy status associated with hunger and satiety (sensory-specific satiety was discussed previously) or from modifications in diet (e.g. resulting in specific hunger for salt) can influence sensitivity and hedonic response, although these changes are generally short term. Extreme cases of nutrient deficiency or toxicity can influence the function of the chemical senses. This effect has been observed for vitamins A, B_6 and B_{12}, and for the trace metals zinc and copper. For example, zinc deficiency has been associated with histological changes in taste buds as well as degeneration and loss of taste papillae. Vitamin A deficiency results in gradual, but reversible, loss of taste, although zinc may again be involved as it plays an important role in transporting vitamin A from the liver. Diabetes results in a general reduction in taste sensitivity and losses in ability to sense sweetness may cause diabetics to unwittingly add more sugar to their food. This can create additional nutritional problems, particularly in older people who develop late onset diabetes and find it difficult to manage their diet. Although not directly related to nutrition per se, poor oral and dental health influences sensory function and can also cause dietary restriction if mechanical difficulties or pain are associated with eating of some food types. Medications that are taken for chronic illness also contribute significantly to sensory loss, particularly in older people. The average older person in the USA is taking 3.7 different medications at any one time.

The visual system consists of specialised tissues that are vulnerable to nutritional insults. For example, vitamin A deficiency results in night blindness and xerophthalmia. Thiamin deficiency can result in opthalmoplegia (paralysis of movement of the eye). The eye is also susceptible to damage by toxic material in food and drink. For example, the consumption of methanol results in the formation of formic acid in the body, which damages the retina and can cause blindness; cyanide toxicity can damage the optic nerves and cause amblyopia (dimness of vision without obvious defect or change in the eye). The outer tissues of the eye are susceptible to damage and infection if the production of tears and mucous are affected. The lens of the eye is at risk of developing opacities if the proteins from which it is made become oxidatively damaged. The extremely high oxygen tension within the retina and the high exposure of the eye to ionising radiation also makes it a tissue susceptible to oxidative damage. To protect against free-radical mediated damage, the eye has a number of protective systems to mop up free radicals. With increasing age the effectiveness of this system decreases and two major causes of blindness, cataract and age-related macular degeneration, are consequences.

9.13 Future perspectives

Earlier in this chapter it was stated that the primary function of the human senses (associated with food) are to detect foods that would be bad for the body and should be rejected, and to identify foods that the body needs for survival and that therefore should be consumed. Nevertheless 'what is bad for the body' can be interpreted as flavours and textures that we dislike for whatever personal factors and 'what is good for the body' can be interpreted as those that we like for whatever personal factors. The factors determining personal likes and dislikes for sensory properties (especially flavours) are influenced by genetics, age, nutrition and health status, but most importantly by experience. In addition, individual nutritional status is determined by individual likes and dislikes, and by the quantity of liked foods that is consumed.

The aim of nutritional sciences is to improve dietary quality. Most focus to date has been directed at improving the nutritional quality of foods, by provision of nutritionally enhanced foods and by recommendation of ideal eating habits. Little regard has been given to 'tastes' or 'taste' preferences. To address this, efforts should now be made to develop dietary strategies that take account of the sensory properties of food. Unacceptable flavour, or flavour that does not match individual likes or expectations, is an obstacle to compliance with a recommended change in diet, particularly now that consumers are becoming more affluent and more discerning. The potential nutritional value of functional ingredients may be compromised because they have tastes that do not meet acceptable criteria. For example, phytochemicals, linked with cancer prevention, have a bitter taste for which there is an innate dislike. Sugar, salt and fat replacers do not taste the same as the substances that they seek to replace.

However, the hedonics of palatability, and food preferences, are arguably malleable through experience. As many bitter-tasting compounds are associated with foods that have high nutritive benefit, for example fruits and vegetables, hedonic responses to these bitter tastes need to be adjusted. On the other hand, macronutrients, such as sugar, salt and fat, are generally most liked. As these are linked with chronic disease when consumed in excessive quantities, hedonic response to these flavours needs to be adjusted to reduce consumption. More research attention should be aimed at linking changes in sensory function and food preferences with diet selection and intake under real-life situations. To facilitate this, more work is needed to understand the role of olfaction, chemical irritation and somesthesis in diet selection and food preferences, to compliment that already carried out with taste. More research with real food products is needed, which has greater ecological validity than working with pure tastants or odorants in solution. Nutritional scientists should also recognise the technological challenges facing the food manufacturing industry, as they seek to produce acceptable foods that contain new ingredients and formulations that differ markedly from tradition. In addition, dietary intervention strategies should consider the relationships between sensory likes and dislikes and demographic, economic and sociocultural factors.

It is important to consider sensory requirements and dietary needs in parallel, but at different stages in life. What is the contribution of sensory variety in infancy to lifelong variety seeking behaviour, and do breast-fed and formula-fed infants have different hedonic potential? Although preference studies may show that older-age consumers are satisfied with foods currently available, these foods should be improved to compensate for specific sensory losses, which will, with time, lead to reaquaintance with an increased sensory variety. Given the strong link between sensory properties and digestive response,

this compensation may have unforseen benefits. However, it is important to recognise that the older-age population is very heterogeneous and individual preferences are likely to differ significantly. Responsible nutritional intervention and functional food use may also reduce the need for widespread pharmaceutical use as older age progresses. This will have the added benefit of delaying the adverse effects of medicines on ability to taste and smell, which may contribute to continued good eating habits.

Rather than attempt to play down the importance of the senses to food intake, by demonstrating that, say, price or availability are more significant determinants, it is now time to understand better the development of food palatability and preferences with positive nutrition in mind and to exploit sensory properties to increase intake of foods with high nutritive value. Future research should direct product development for individual nutrition needs, rather than consider sensory quality as part of market positioning after a product has already been produced, which is currently the norm.

Further reading

Engelen L, Van der Bilt A. Oral physiology and texture perception of semisolids. J Text Stud 2008; 39: 83–113.

Finger TE, Silver WL, Restrepo D. The Neurobiology of Taste and Smell, 2nd edn. New York: Wiley–Liss, 2000.

Getchell TV *et al.* Smell and Taste in Health and Disease. New York: Raven Press, 1991.

Lawless HT, Heymann, H. Sensory Evaluation of Foods, Principles and Practices. New York: Chapman & Hall, 1998.

10
The Gastrointestinal Tract

Mariano Mañas, Emilio Martínez de Victoria, Angel Gil, María D Yago and John C Mathers

---

Key messages

- The four basic processes that constitute the functions of the gastrointestinal tract are motility, secretion, digestion and absorption.
- Several nutritional factors can affect gastrointestinal function. Conversely, pathological modifications of this function lead to an altered nutritional state.
- The pancreas is a mixed gland containing both endocrine and exocrine portions. These two parts of the pancreas have a high level of interaction, both in health and in disease conditions.
- The most important digestive function of the liver is the secretion of bile, but it also plays a role in lipid, protein and carbohydrate metabolism as well as the excretion of bile pigments, the storage of several vitamins and minerals, and the processing of hormones, drugs and toxins.

- The intestinal epithelium is a complex system of multiple cell types which maintain precise inter-relationships. The regulatory mechanisms involved with developmental processes are at organism, cellular and molecular levels.
- The primary function of the large bowel is in salvage of energy via bacterial fermentation of food residues, but it also plays a role in the absorption of water and electrolytes, lipid metabolism, the synthesis of certain vitamins and essential amino acids, and the metabolism and absorption of phytochemicals. Bacterial fermentation in this organ may contribute to risk of obesity and influence other aspects of host metabolism and health.

10.1 Introduction

The overall function of the gastrointestinal system is to process ingested foods into molecular forms that can be transferred, along with salts and water, from the external environment to the internal environment of the body. The digestive processes are largely determined by the composition of food ingested. This fact determines the importance of the food and thus the diet, in most aspects of the physiology of the gastrointestinal system, including its regulation.

10.2 Structure and function of the gastrointestinal system

The **structure** of the gastrointestinal system (Figure 10.1) includes the gastrointestinal tract (GIT) and the accessory glands (salivary, exocrine pancreas and liver). The structure of the GIT varies greatly from region to region, but there are common features in the overall organisation of the tissue.

The layered structure of the wall of the GIT (Figure 10.2) includes, from the inside to outside:

- *mucosa*: consists of an epithelium, the lamina propria and the muscularis mucosae.
- *submucosa*: consists largely of loose connective tissue with collagen and elastin fibres. Some submucosal glands are present in some regions. In this layer there is a dense network of highly interconnected nerve cells called the submucosal plexus (Meissner's plexus)
- *muscularis externa*: consists of two substantial layers of smooth muscle cells, an inner circular layer and an outer longitudinal layer. Between both layers there is another prominent network of highly interconnected nerve cells called the myenteric plexus (Auerbach's plexus). Both submucosal and myenteric plexuses (intramural plexuses) constitute, with the other neurons, the enteric nervous

---

Nutrition and Metabolism, Second Edition, edited by S. A. Lanham-New, I. A. Macdonald and H. M. Roche.   © 2011 The Nutrition Society.

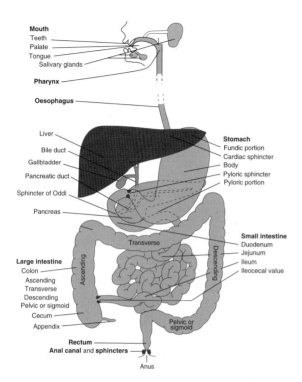

Mouth
Teeth
Palate
Tongue
Salivary glands
Pharynx
Oesophagus
Liver
Bile duct
Gallbladder
Pancreatic duct
Sphincter of Oddi
Pancreas
Stomach
Fundic portion
Cardiac sphincter
Body
Pyloric sphincter
Pyloric portion
Transverse
Ascending
Descending
Small intestine
Duodenum
Jejunum
Ileum
Ileocecal value
Large intestine
Colon
Ascending
Transverse
Descending
Pelvic or sigmoid
Cecum
Appendix
Pelvic or sigmoid
Rectum
Anal canal and **sphincters**
Anus

Figure 10.1 Structure of the gastrointestinal system, including the gastrointestinal tract and accessory glands (salivary, exocrine pancreas and liver).

system. This innervation constitutes the intrinsic innervation (Figure 10.3).

- *serosa*: the outer most layer consists mainly of connective tissue and mesothelial cells.

The gastrointestinal system receives innervations from neurons of the autonomic nervous system, both sympathetic and parasympathetic, which constitutes the extrinsic innervation.

Both types of innervation are important for the regulation of the different functions of the GIT, mainly related to motility and secretion (exocrine and endocrine).

The oral cavity (or mouth) is the first portion of the GIT and is bounded by the lips (anteriorly), the fauces (posteriorly), the cheek (laterally), the palate (superiorly) and a muscular floor (inferiorly). The next structure is the pharynx, which is the common opening of both the digestive and the respiratory systems. The pharynx can be divided into three regions: the nasopharynx, the oropharynx and the laryngopharynx. The first includes the uvula, while the second extends from the uvula to the epiglottis

and communicates with the oral cavity through the fauces. The laryngopharynx extends from the tip of epiglottis to the glottis and oesophagus.

The oesophagus is a segment of the GIT, 25 cm in length, that extends between pharynx and stomach. It lies in the mediastinum, anterior to the vertebrae and posterior to the trachea. It passes through the oesophageal hiatus (opening) of the diaphragm and ends at the cardiac opening of the stomach. The oesophagus has two sphincters, the upper oesophageal sphincter between the pharynx and oesophagus, and the lower oesophageal sphincter between the oesophagus and stomach near the cardiac opening. Both sphincters regulate the movement of the ingested meal into and out of the oesophagus.

The stomach is an enlarged segment of the GIT in the left superior portion of the abdomen. The upper opening from the oesophagus is the gastro-oesophageal or cardiac opening. The region near this opening is called the cardiac region. In the left and upper parts of the cardiac region is the fundus. The body, the largest portion of the stomach, turns to the right, creating a greater curvature and a lesser curvature. The lower opening of the stomach, which communicates with the proximal segment of the small intestine (duodenal bulb), is the pylorus (or pyloric opening). The pylorus is surrounded by a thick ring of smooth muscle, the pyloric sphincter.

The small intestine is a long tube that consists of three portions: the duodenum, the jejunum and the ileum. The large intestine includes the caecum (most proximal), the colon (ascending, transverse, descending and sigmoid), rectum and anal canal. The longitudinal layer of the large intestine is incomplete and forms three bands that are called teniae coli. The contraction of teniae coli causes pouches called haustra along the length of the colon.

The **function** of the GIT includes four general processes: motility, secretion, digestion and absorption (Figure 10.4).

- Motility: includes contractions of the smooth muscle of the GIT wall to mix the luminal contents with the various secretions and move them through the tract from mouth to anus. The components of motility are chewing, swallowing, gastric motility, gastric emptying, small and large intestinal motility, gallbladder contraction and defecation.

Figure 10.2 Layered structure of the gastrointestinal tract. (Modified from Martínez de Victoria E, Mañas M, Yago MD. Capítulo 7, Vol. I. Fisiología digestiva. In: Gil A (ed.) Tratado de Nutrición, 2nd edn. Editorial Medica Panamericana, Madrid, 2010.)

- Secretion: The wall of the GIT and the accessory glands produce several secretions that contribute to the breakdown of ingested food into small molecules. These secretions consist of saliva, pancreatic juice and bile secreted by accessory glands (salivary, pancreas and liver, respectively) and gastric and intestinal juices secreted by the glands lining the wall of the stomach and the small and large intestine.
- Digestion: Most food is ingested as large particles containing macromolecules, such as proteins and polysaccharides, which are unable to cross the wall of the GIT. Before the ingested food can be absorbed, it must be broken down and dissolved. These processes of breakdown and dissolution of the food involve both gastrointestinal motility and

secretion and are termed mechanical and chemical digestion.
- Absorption: The molecules produced by digestion then move from the lumen of the GIT across a layer of epithelial cells and enter the blood or the lymph (internal environment).

These are the four basic processes that, with the mechanisms controlling them, constitute the functions of the gastrointestinal system.

10.3 Motility

Chewing can be carried out voluntarily, but normally is almost entirely under reflex control. Chewing serves to lubricate the food by mixing it with saliva,

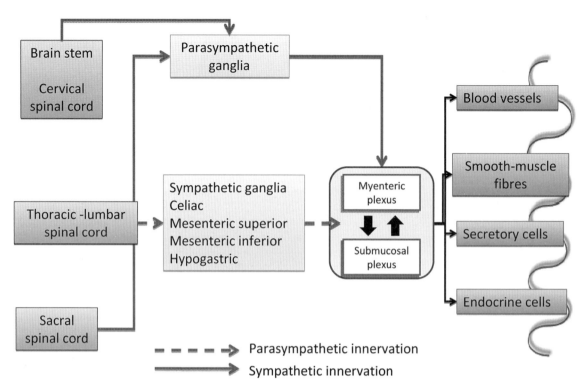

Figure 10.3 Intrinsic and extrinsic innervation of the gastrointestinal tract.

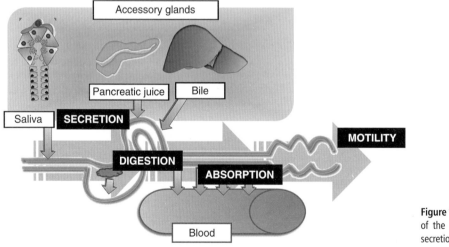

Figure 10.4 The four general functions of the gastrointestinal tract: motility, secretion, digestion and absorption.

to start the starch digestion with ptyalin (α-amylase) and to subdivide the food.

Swallowing is a rigidly ordered reflex that results in the propulsion of food from the mouth to the stomach. The swallowing centre in the medulla and lower pons controls this reflex. There are three phases: oral, pharyngeal and oesophageal. The last phase is carried out by the motor activity of the oesophagus.

Gastric motility serves the following major functions:

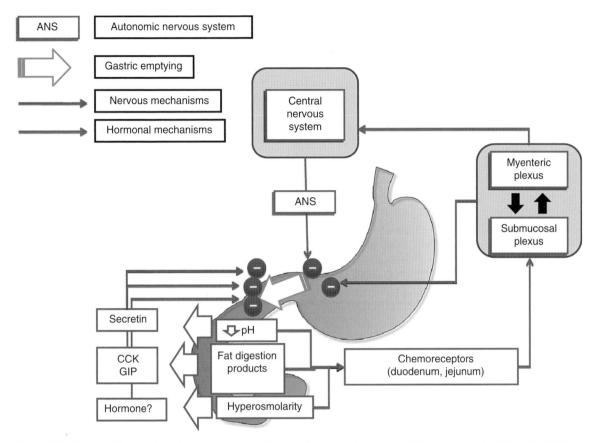

Figure 10.5 Neural and hormonal mechanisms involved in the regulation of gastric emptying. CCK, cholecystokinin; GIP, gastric inhibitory polypeptide. (Modified from Martínez de Victoria E, Mañas M, Yago MD. Capítulo 7, Vol. I. Fisiología digestiva. In: Gil A (ed.) Tratado de Nutrición, 2nd edn. Editorial Medica Panamericana, Madrid, 2010.)

- to allow the stomach to serve as a reservoir for the large volume of food that may be ingested at a single meal
- to fragment food into smaller particles and mix the luminal contents with gastric juice to begin digestion
- to empty gastric contents into the duodenum at a controlled rate.

This last function is closely regulated by several mechanisms so that the chyme is not delivered to the duodenum too rapidly.

The mixing and mechanical fragmentation of the luminal contents and gastric emptying are carried out by peristaltic waves that begin in the pacemaker zone in the middle of the body of the stomach and travel towards the pylorus and through the gastroduodenal

junction. The gastroduodenal junction (pyloric sphincter) allows the carefully regulated emptying of gastric contents to the duodenum for optimal digestion and absorption of nutrients.

Gastric emptying is regulated by both neural and hormonal mechanisms. The signals come from duodenal and jejunal receptors that sense acidity, osmotic pressure and fat content (Figure 10.5).

If the pH of chyme is less than 3.5, the rate of gastric emptying is reduced by neural mechanisms (vagal reflex) and through the release of secretin, an intestinal hormone that inhibits the antral contractions and stimulates the contraction of the pyloric sphincter.

The chyme emptying into the duodenal bulb is usually hypertonic and becomes more hypertonic in the duodenum because of the action of digestive enzymes. The hypertonic duodenal contents slow gastric emptying.

The luminal hypertonic solution releases an unidentified humoral factor (hormone) that diminishes the rate of gastric emptying. A neural component may also be involved. The presence of fat-digestion products (mainly fatty acids and 2-monoglycerides) dramatically decreases the rate of gastric emptying due to an increase in the contractility of the pyloric sphincter. This inhibition of gastric emptying is mediated by both hormonal and neural mechanisms. The effect of unsaturated and long-chain (>14 carbons) fatty acids is greater than that of saturated and medium short-chain fatty acids. Cholecytokinin (CCK) is an intestinal hormone released by the presence of fatty acids and other fat-digestion products. The net effect of CCK is to slow the rate of gastric emptying. Other gastrointestinal hormones, such as gastric inhibitory peptide (GIP) and peptide tyrosine-tyrosine (PYY) are implicated in the slowing of gastric emptying, seen later after food ingestion due to the presence of fatty acids in the ileum ('ileal brake'). The release of glucalgon like peptide-1 (GLP-1) also have a inhibitory role of the gastric emptying.

Finally, the presence of proteins and peptides in the stomach also slows gastric emptying via the release of gastrin. This gastric hormone has a net effect of diminishing gastric emptying. Further inhibition is achieved by the presence of tryptophan, other amino acids and peptides in the duodenum, probably via CCK release.

Motility of the small intestine

The movements of the small intestine can be classified in two major patterns: segmentation, which occurs in the postprandrial period, and the migrating motor complexes (MMCs), which are seen during fasting. The postprandial motility involves alternating contractions of the intestine, which mixes the chyme with digestive secretions, bringing fresh chyme into contact with the mucosal surface for absorption. The interdigestive period consists of bursts of intense electrical and contractile activity separated by longer quiescent periods. This pattern appears to be propagated from the stomach to the terminal ileum. The MMCs sweep the small intestine clean, emptying its contents into the caecum. The mechanisms that regulate the MMCs are both neural (vagal) and hormonal (motilin).

Motility of the colon

There are two major types of movements: segmentation (haustration), with a mixing function, and

Figure 10.6 Neural control of the motility of the gastrointestinal tract.

segmental propulsion, which allows the luminal contents to move to the distal direction.

Control of the contractile activities involves the central nervous system (long reflexes), the intrinsic plexuses of the gut (short reflexes) (Figure 10.6), humoral factors (gastrin, CCK, secretin, etc.) and electrical coupling among the smooth muscle cells.

10.4 Secretion

Salivary secretion

Salivary secretion is produced by the three major salivary glands (parotids, submandibular and sublingual) and other minor glands in the oral mucosa. Saliva lubricates food for swallowing, facilitates speaking and begins the digestion of starch. The functional unit of the salivary gland is the acinus (secretory end-piece). The composition of saliva includes inorganic (salts) and organic (amylase, mucoproteins) components. The primary control of salivary secretion is by the autonomic nervous system, which regulates several gland effectors, including acinar cells, blood vessels, ductular cells and myoepithelial cells.

Gastric secretions

The major secretions of the stomach are hydrochloric acid (HCl), pepsinogens, intrinsic factor and mucus. These components arise from the many secretory glands in the wall of the gastric mucosa. These glands have different cellular types: mucous neck cells (which secrete mucus), parietal or oxyntic cells (which secrete HCl and intrinsic factor), and chief or peptic cells (which secrete pepsinogens). The regulation of gastric secretion is carried out by neural and humoral mechanisms. There are three phases in the regulation process: cephalic, gastric and intestinal. The first is elicited by the sight, smell and taste of food. The second is brought about by the presence of food in the stomach. The last phase is elicited by the presence of chyme in the duodenum.

In the past few years it has been recognised that *Helicobacter pylori*, a Gram-negative microaerophilic flagellated urease-producing rod found in the gastric mucosa, is related to the development of peptic ulcer disease. Studies suggest that *H. pylori* can induce mucosal damage via both direct and indirect mechanisms. The direct mechanisms imply the production by the microorganisms of urease, lipopolysaccharides and cytotoxins that induce mucosal inflammation. The indirect mechanisms include the release of gastrin and somatostatin. The importance of *H. pylori* infection of gastric mucosa has led to the development of treatments of both gastritis and duodenal ulcers with anti-*H. pylori* regimens, such as antacids and antibiotics.

Intestinal secretions

The mucosa of all the segments of the GIT elaborate secretions that contain mucus, electrolytes and water.

Exocrine pancreatic secretion and bile secretion are covered in sections 10.8 and 10.10, respectively.

10.5 Digestion and absorption

Digestion and absorption of carbohydrates

The major source of carbohydrates in the diet is plant starch. The starch is hydrolysed by salivary and pancreatic α-amylase. The further digestion of the oligosaccharides is accomplished by enzymes in the brush-border membrane of the epithelium of the duodenum and jejunum. The major brush-border oligosaccharidases are lactase, sucrase, α-dextrinase and glucoamylase. The end products of the disaccharidases are glucose, galactose and fructose. Several mechanisms transport these products across the intestinal mucosa to the blood, including Na^+-dependent and Na^+-independent active transport.

Digestion and absorption of proteins

The process of digestion of dietary protein begins in the stomach. In the gastric lumen the pepsinogens secreted by the chief cells are activated by hydrogen ions to pepsins, which hydrolyse the proteins to amino acids and small peptides. In the duodenum and small intestine, the proteases secreted by the pancreas play a major role in protein digestion (trypsin, chymotrypsin and carboxypeptidase). The brush border of the small intestine contains a number of peptidases. They reduce the peptides produced by pancreatic enzymes to oligopeptides and amino acids. The principal products of protein digestion are small peptides and amino acids. These products are transported across the intestinal mucosa via specific amino acid and oligopeptide transport systems.

Digestion and absorption of lipids

The digestion of dietary fat is carried out by lipolytic enzymes of the exocrine pancreas (lipase and colipase) and requires the presence of biliary phospholipid and bile salts. The absorption of lipids needs the formation of micelles with bile lecithin, bile salt and products of the fat digestion. Inside the intestinal epithelial cell the lipids are reprocessed and the 2-monoglycerides are reesterified, lysophospholipids are reconverted to phospholipids and most of the cholesterol is reesterified. The reprocessed lipids, along with those that are synthesised *de novo* combine with proteins to form chylomicrons, which enter the bloodstream at the thoracic vena cava, via the lymphatics draining the gut.

Absorption of water and electrolytes

Water movement into or out of the lumen of the GIT is passive. The water moves across the cell plasma membrane or in between cells via paracellular pathways

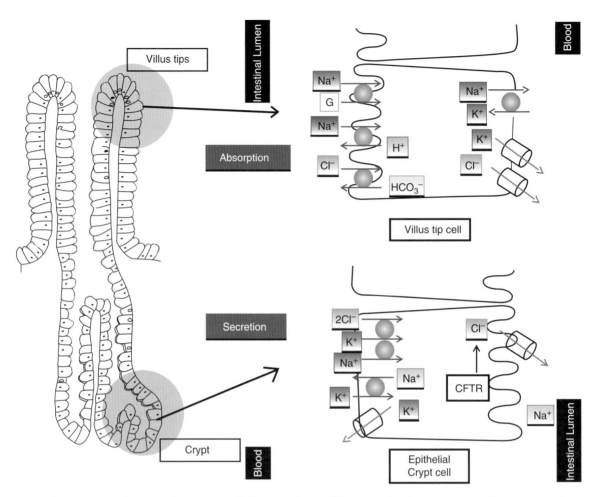

Figure 10.7 Transport mechanisms in the enterocytes of villus tips and crypts of the intestinal epithelium. CFTR, cystic fibrosis transmembrane conductance regulator.

composed of tight junctions and lateral intercellular spaces between epithelial cells. Water molecules follow the osmotic gradients created by electrolyte movement. Electrolytes are transported by both passive and active processes, and these ionic movements control water absorption and secretion.

Net intestinal fluid transport depends on the balance between intestinal water absorption and secretion. The processes are localised to specific regions of the intestinal epithelium. The cells of the villus tip are differentiated so as to promote fluid and solute absorption, whereas those in the crypt region promote fluid and solute secretion. Figure 10.7 shows the transport mechanisms in the enterocytes of both regions (villus tip and crypts).

Na^+ entry into the epithelial cell from the intestinal lumen is passive. This occurs via two mechanisms. One is a Na^+/H^+ antiporter protein that exchanges one sodium ion (in) and one proton (out). The second is the Na^+-glucose co transporter that mediates the coupled entry of Na^+ and glucose into the epithelial cell (1 Na:1 glucose or 2 Na:1 glucose). Na^+ moves down its electrochemical potential gradient and provides energy for moving the sugar into the epithelial cell against a concentration gradient. On the other hand, the presence of glucose in the intestinal lumen enhances Na^+ absorption, which is the basis for the use of glucose in rehydratation solutions during diarrhoea. The absorption of other sugars (galactose) and some neutral and acidic amino acids utilises a similar mechanism.

Figure 10.8 Inputs and outputs of water to and from the gastrointestinal lumen in a healthy adult. (Modified from Martínez de Victoria E, Mañas M, Yago MD. Capítulo 7, Vol. I. Fisiología digestiva. In: Gil A (ed.) Tratado de Nutrición, 2nd edn. Editorial Medica Panamericana, Madrid, 2010.)

Cl^- is absorbed following different pathways. Some Cl^- is absorbed across a paracellular path, some through a cellular pathway composed of an apical $Cl^- - {}^-HCO_3^-$ antiporter and possibly using an unidentified basolateral Cl^- selective channel or a K^+/Cl^- co transporter. There is a linkage between H^+ and ${}^-HCO_3^-$ via carbonic acid and carbonic anhydrase that provides a degree of coupling between the entry of Na^+ and Cl^-.

K^+ is passively absorbed in the small intestine (jejunum and ileum) when its luminal concentration rises because of absorption of water.

10.6 Water balance in the gastrointestinal tract

The water balance in the GIT depends on the input and output of water to and from the gastrointestinal lumen. The water inputs can be exogenous or endogenous. Average oral (i.e. exogenous) intake of water is about 2 l per day. The major components of the endogenous inputs are saliva (1.5 l), gastric juice (2.5 l), bile (0.5 l), pancreatic juice (1.5 l) and intesti-

nal secretions (in normal state 1 l). Thus, the final daily water volume load in the duodenal lumen is 8–10 l. Most of the fluid is absorbed by the small intestine, and about 1 to 1.5 l reaches the colon, which continues to absorb water, reducing faecal water volume to about 100 ml per day (Figure 10.8).

The maximum absorptive capacity of the colon is only about 4 l per day, so if volumes of fluid greater than this enter the small intestine, diarrhoea will ensue despite normal colonic function. The normal intestinal secretion is about 1 l per day but can be as much as 20 l per day. This striking difference between the absorptive and secretory capacity of the small intestine and colon dictates that large volume diarrhoea is most often caused by small intestinal dysfunction.

Diarrhoea

Diarrhoea is a problem of intestinal water and electrolyte balance. It results when excess water and electrolytes are actively transported into the lumen (secretory diarrhoea) or when water is retained in the lumen by osmotically active agents (osmotic diarrhoea).

Another major contributor to diarrhoea is gastrointestinal motility. The rate of transit through the gut determines the time available for intestinal absorption of water and can result in diarrhoea.

Vomiting

Vomiting is a reflex behaviour controlled and co-ordinated by the vomiting centre in the medulla, and involving the somatic and autonomic nervous systems, the oropharynx, the GIT and the skeletal muscles of the thorax and abdomen. It is the expulsion of gastric (or sometimes gastric and duodenal) contents from the GIT via the mouth. This can result from irritation (e.g. overdistension or overexcitation) of both chemoreceptors and mechanoreceptors anywhere along the GIT. It is usually preceded by nausea and retching.

The events of the vomiting reflex are independent of the initiating stimulus and include:

(a) A wave of reverse peristalsis that sweeps from the middle of the small intestine to the duodenum
(b) Xrelaxation of the pylorus and stomach
(c) forced inspiration against a closed glottis
(d) increase in the abdominal pressure owing to diaphragm and abdominal muscle contraction
(e) relaxation of the lower oesophageal sphincter and entry of gastric contents into the oesophagus

(f) forward movement of the hyoid bone and larynx, closure by approximation of the vocal chords and closure of the glottis
(g) projection of gastrointestinal contents into the pharynx and mouth.

Several physiological changes accompany vomiting, including hypersalivation, tachycardia, inhibition of gastric acid secretion and sometimes defecation.

Certain chemicals, called emetics, can elicit vomiting. Their action is mediated by stimulating receptors in the stomach, or more commonly in the duodenum, or by acting in the central nervous system on the chemoreceptor trigger zone near the area postrema in the floor of the fourth ventricle (brainstem).

10.7 The exocrine pancreas

Anatomy and histology of the pancreas

The human pancreas is a pink, soft, elongated organ weighing less than 100 g and lying posterior to the greater curvature of the stomach. It consists of a head, located within the duodenal loop, a body and a tail. The latter extends towards the spleen, onto which it has morphological relations. The pancreas is a mixed gland. It contains both exocrine and endocrine portions (Figure 10.9). The major structural components

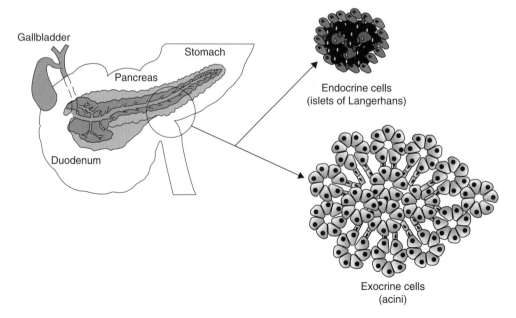

Figure 10.9 Endocrine and exocrine portions of the pancreas.

responsible for the exocrine function of the pancreas are the acinar units (acini) and the duct system, accounting for about 86% of the gland mass. The acini, the enzyme-secreting units of the exocrine pancreas, are round or oval structures composed of epithelial cells (acinar cells) bordering a common luminal space where enzymes are delivered. The acini form lobules that are separated by thin septa. The tiny ducts that drain the acini are called intercalated ducts. Within a lobule, a number of intercalated ducts empty into somewhat larger intralobular ducts. All of the intralobular ducts of a particular lobule then drain into a single extralobular duct; this duct in turn empties into still larger ducts. These larger ducts ultimately converge to form two ducts that drain the secretions into the small intestine. The main duct is called the pancreatic duct (duct of Wirsung), which joins the common bile duct, forming the hepatopancreatic ampulla (ampulla of Vater). The ampulla opens on an elevation of the duodenal mucosa known as the major duodenal papilla. The smaller of the two ducts, the accessory duct (duct of Santorini), leads from the pancreas and empties into the duodenum at the apex of the lesser duodenal papilla.

The endocrine portion of the pancreas is composed of cells organised into clusters called islets of Langerhans. These cells secrete the hormones insulin, glucagon, somatostatin and pancreatic polypeptide. Insulin and glucagon play a major role in the regulation of macronutrient metabolism. The main functions of these hormones are dealt with in other chapters. The functional interactions between the endocrine and exocrine pancreas are discussed in section 10.9.

The pancreas is innervated by the vagus and sympathetic nerves. The vagal fibres innervate both exocrine and endocrine cells, whilst the sympathetic nerves innervate the endocrine cells.

Composition of the pancreatic juice

The exocrine secretion of the pancreas is important in the digestion of foodstuffs. It is made up of an aqueous component and an enzyme component. The enzyme component of pancreatic juice includes enzymes for digesting carbohydrates, proteins, fats and nucleic acids.

The aqueous component of pancreatic juice

This is secreted by the epithelial cells lining the pancreatic ducts and is composed of water, sodium, potassium, bicarbonate and chloride (Figure 10.10). Bicarbonate and chloride are the major anions contained in pancreatic juice. The bicarbonate concentration increases and chloride concentration decreases reciprocally with the rate of secretion.

The primary pancreatic fluid is hypertonic to plasma. Pancreatic duct cells are water permeable and as this primary secretion flows through the ducts water moves into the duct and makes the pancreatic juice isotonic to plasma.

The function of the pancreatic bicarbonate is to neutralise gastric acid entering the duodenum, creating the optimum pH for the action of digestive enzymes in the small intestine.

The hormone secretin is the primary stimulant for bicarbonate secretion. The fluid secreted under secretin stimulation has a higher bicarbonate concentration than that secreted under resting conditions (spontaneous secretion).

Since the function of pancreatic bicarbonate is to neutralise duodenal acidity, it is logical that the acidity of the chyme entering the duodenum stimulates the release of secretin.

The enzyme component of pancreatic juice

The acinar cells secrete the enzyme component of the pancreatic juice. The enzyme component in pancreatic juice includes enzymes for digesting carbohydrates, proteins, fats and nucleic acids (Table 10.1).

The proteases and phospholipases (enzymes that degrade phospholipids) are secreted in the form of zymogen granules; zymogens are inactive precursors of the proteolytic enzymes. In the duodenum inactive pancreatic zymogens are converted to their active form. Enterokinase, an enzyme embedded in the membrane of duodenum epithelial cells, converts the trypsinogen (inactive proteolytic zymogen) to trypsin (Figure 10.11).

The trypsin then activates the other pancreatic zymogens by removing specific peptides from them. A protein present in the pancreatic juice, trypsin inhibitor, prevents the activation of inactive enzymes inside the pancreas. If the pancreatic duct is blocked, the concentration of endogenous trypsin can rise and when the concentration of trypsin inhibitor becomes insufficient the pancreas begins to autodigest (acute pancreatitis).

The major pancreatic proteolytic enzymes are trypsin, chymotrypsin, elastase and carboxypeptidase.

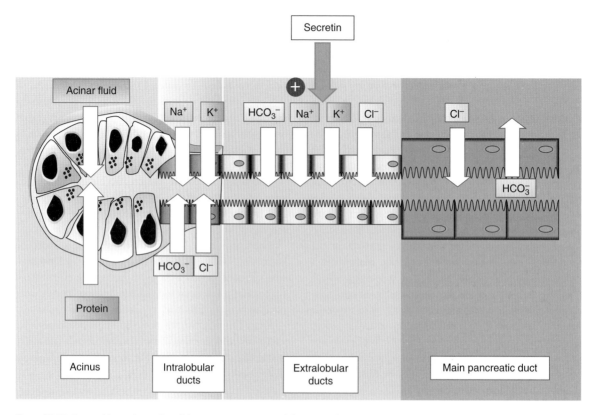

Figure 10.10 Composition and secretion of the aqueous component of the pancreatic juice.

Table 10.1 Enzymes produced in pancreatic juice and the substrate they digest

Enzyme	Substrate
Amylase	Starches (polysaccharides)
Lipase	Tryglicerides
Phospholipase A2	Phospholipids
Carboxypeptidase	Proteins (exopeptidase)
Trypsin	Proteins (endopeptidase)
Chymotripsin	Proteins (endopeptidase)
Elastase	Elastic fibres
Ribonuclease	Ribonucleic acids
Deoxyribonuclease	Deoxyribonucleic acids

The non-proteolytic enzymes are released by the pancreas in their active form. The most important are:

- amylase: carbohydrate-digesting enzyme that degrades starch molecules into oligosaccharides
- ribonuclease and deoxyribonuclease: nucleic acid digesting enzymes

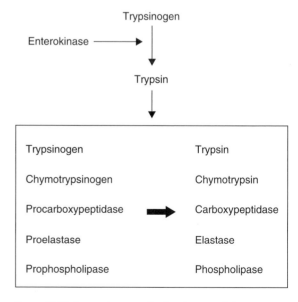

Figure 10.11 Process for converting inactive proteolytic enzymes to their active form.

• lipase: degrades triacylglycerols into fatty acids and glycerol.]

The presence of fat and amino acids in the duodenum is the stimulus for the release of the intestinal hormone cholecystokinin (CCK). This hormone is the most potent stimulus of secretion of the enzymatic component of the pancreatic juice.

The nutrients of the diet initiate, via CCK release, the enzymatic secretion involved in their own digestion.

Regulation of the pancreatic exocrine secretion

Neural and hormonal reflexes regulate pancreatic exocrine secretion (Figure 10.12a–c). The secretion of pancreatic juice occurs in three phases.

• **Cephalic phase**: the taste and the smell of food lead to increased pancreatic secretion via the parasympathetic nerves to the pancreas. The vagal

Figure 10.12 (a) Neural and hormonal reflexes regulating pancreatic exocrine secretion. (b) Neural and hormonal reflexes regulating pancreatic exocrine secretion. (c) Neural and hormonal reflexes regulating pancreatic exocrine secretion. Ach, acetylcholine; CCK, cholecystokinin. (Modified from Martínez de Victoria E, Mañas M, Yago MD. Capítulo 7, Vol. I. Fisiología digestiva. In: Gil A (ed.) Tratado de Nutrición, 2nd edn. Editorial Medica Panamericana, Madrid, 2010.)

impulses stimulate the secretion of the enzyme component of the pancreatic juice.

- **Gastric phase:** the distention of the stomach by food transmits impulses via vagal afferents to the brain, then efferent activity via the vagus nerves to the pancreas increases the enzyme secretion of the pancreas.

During these two phases, vagal impulses, distention of the stomach and the presence of amino acids and peptides in the stomach evoke release of the hormone gastrin, which also stimulates pancreatic secretion. Vagotomy reduces pancreatic exocrine secretion.

- **Intestinal phase:** the acidity of the chyme emptied into the duodenum stimulates the release of secretin. This hormone causes the ductular epithelial cells to secrete a solution high in bicarbonate and in doing so increases the pancreatic flow. Secretin produces a large volume of pancreatic juice with low protein concentration.

CCK is released into the blood by fatty acids and polypeptides in the chyme and stimulates the secretion of digestive enzymes by the acinar cells. CCK potentiates the pancreatic stimulatory effects of secretin and vice versa. Secretin and CCK are released in the mucosa of the duodenum and upper jejunum by enteroendocrine cells and pass into the capillaries and thus into the systemic circulation.

10.8 Diet and exocrine pancreatic function

Adaptation of the exocrine pancreas to diet

The pancreas is very sensitive to a variety of physiological and pathological stimuli, the most important of which are nutritional in origin. Severe alterations in the diet leading to a state of malnutrition are associated with the occurrence of pancreatic injury. This section will focus on the functional changes that may occur when nutritional components in the diet are altered within physiological limits.

Pancreatic adaptation, a phenomenon first noted by Pavlov in the early twentieth century, refers to the ability of the pancreas to modify the volume and composition of its exocrine secretion in response to long-term changes in the levels of nutritional substrates available in the diet. Provided there is an adequate dietary protein supply, the synthesis and content of the major digestive enzymes (proteases, amylase and lipase) change proportionally to the amount of their respective substrates (protein, carbohydrate and fat) in the diet. This adaptation optimises the digestion and utilisation of such substrates.

The pancreatic synthesis and content of trypsinogen and chymotrypsinogen increase in response to high-protein diets. The quality of dietary protein also affects this adaptation. Increasing the intake of high-quality proteins such as casein or fish protein increases chymotrypsinogen, whereas increasing the intake of low-quality proteins such as gelatin or zein does not.

High-carbohydrate diets increase the pancreatic amylase content and synthesis. This effect occurs as the level of dietary carbohydrate increases at the expense of dietary fat or protein, which implies a primary response to the level of carbohydrate.

The intake of high-fat diets enhances the synthesis and content of pancreatic lipase, independently of whether the amount of dietary fat increases at the expense of protein or carbohydrate. Although lipase adapts to increasing dietary fat levels, there may be a threshold of fat content below which there is little adaptation and above which there is significant adaptation. Colipase may adapt to high dietary fat levels, but the response seems to be weaker than that of lipase. Considerable controversy exists over the effects of the type of fat (degree of saturation or major chain length) on the adaptation of pancreatic enzymes.

Most of the information on pancreatic adaptation to diet has been gathered from rats. Only a few studies have evaluated this topic in humans and the results are not conclusive. Investigations in premature infants suggest that adaptive responses occur in humans in a manner similar to that observed in experimental animals. In contrast, altering the quantity of carbohydrate, protein or fat in the diet of adult volunteers for 10 or 15 days failed to induce any changes in the ratios among the enzymes secreted. In humans adapted for 30 days to diets containing either olive oil (rich in oleic acid, a monounsaturated fatty acid) or sunflower oil (rich in linoleic acid, a polyunsaturated fatty acid) as the main source of dietary fat, no differences in the activity of proteases, amylase, lipase and colipase measured in duodenal contents were apparent after the administration of a liquid meal.

Is pancreatic adaptation mediated by specific hormones?

Adaptive changes in pancreatic enzymes are known to be mediated by specific hormones. In most cases the release of these hormones is markedly increased by the nutrients whose digestion they regulate (Table 10.2). The gastrointestinal hormone CCK, which is potently released by ingested protein, dramatically increases the synthesis and tissue level of proteases, so it has been proposed as the mediator of pancreatic adaptation to dietary protein. In many species, CCK release from endocrine I cells in the small intestine is regulated by a luminal negative feedback mechanism. This mechanism, which is important in the normal response of the pancreas to a meal, may also be involved in the pancreatic adaptation to high-protein diets. It is based on the existence of CCK-releasing peptides with the capacity to bind to intestinal endocrine I cells and enhance CCK release. However, because these peptides are sensitive to degradation by pancreatic proteases, only when proteolytic activity is removed (i.e. by administration of protease inhibitors or diversion of pancreatic juice) will they be able to exert this action. In the case of high-protein feeding, abundant protein in the lumen occupies protease active sites, thus preventing the inactivation of CCK-releasing peptides. Several CCK-releasing peptides have been identified in different species: luminal CCK-releasing factor (LCRF) and diazepam-binding inhibitor (DBI), both produced by the intestinal mucosa, and monitor peptide (MP), contained in the pancreatic juice. Figure 10.13 is a schematic diagram of the feedback mechanism.

Table 10.2 Hormonal mediators of pancreatic adaptation to increased nutritional substrates

Substrate	Hormone	(Pro)enzyme synthesis and tissue content
Protein	CCK	↑ Trypsinogen and chymotrypsinogen
Triglyceride	Secretin, GIP	↑ Lipase
Starch	Insulin	↑ Amylase

Figure 10.13 Role of luminal feedback regulation of CCK release in the pancreatic adaptation to high-protein diets. CCK-releasing peptides (either secreted by the exocrine pancreas or by the duodenal mucosa) are protease-sensitive factors that stimulate CCK release from endocrine I-cells in gut epithelium. They are represented by RF (releasing factors) in the diagram. Under conditions of protein fasting, RF are digested and inactivated by pancreatic proteases in the intestinal lumen. In this form, RF are not capable of stimulating CCK release. In contrast, proteases are bound to dietary proteins when these are ingested. RF survive and enhance the release of CCK into the blood circulation. DP, dietary protein. P, proteases.

Secretin and/or gastric inhibitory peptide (GIP), also known as glucose-dependent insulinotropic peptide are believed to mediate pancreatic adaptation to lipid in the diet. Both are produced by cells of the upper intestine and their release is stimulated, among other factors, by the hydrolytic products of fat. Moreover, the administration of either secretin or GIP has proved to augment the synthesis and content of lipase and colipase in pancreatic acinar cells.

A role for insulin in the adaptation of the pancreas to high-carbohydrate diets has been proposed. When animals are rendered diabetic, amylase content, synthesis and mRNA levels fall dramatically, and these parameters are restored following the administration of exogenous insulin. Section 10.9 includes a more detailed discussion about the effects of insulin on the exocrine pancreas.

The type of dietary fat affects the circulating levels of hormones involved in the control of pancreatic secretion, as shown in a study conducted in humans. After a 30-day period on diets containing either olive or sunflower oil as the main source of dietary fat, plasma CCK levels were shown to be higher in the olive oil group than in the sunflower oil group. Also, greater plasma PYY and pancreatic polypeptide (PP) concentrations were found in the subjects who received the olive oil diet. Similar results have been found in dogs adapted for 6 months to diets rich in either of the two same fats. The higher concentrations of inhibiting hormones such as PP and PYY in response to an olive oil diet can explain, at least in part, why long-term adaptation to olive oil leads in this species to an attenuation of the pancreatic response to food compared with the typical one in the animals fed sunflower oil.

Regulation of pancreatic gene expression by long-term dietary changes

Pancreatic adaptation to diet is, at least in the rat, rapid and becomes complete within a week. Changes in pancreatic enzyme content begin within the first 24 h after the dietary change and continue for 5–7 days, when new steady-state levels are reached. Modifications of synthetic rates precede those in content, exhibiting a rapid change in the first few hours after the dietary challenge, and a prolonged, slower one thereafter until days 3–9, when new stable rates are established.

Theoretically, diet can alter the expression of genes encoding specific pancreatic enzymes through mechanisms involving the gene (transcription), its mRNA (processing, extranuclear transport or cytoplasmic stability) and its translation into protein. However, adaptive changes in pancreatic enzymes in animals are clearly associated with changes in specific mRNA levels, suggesting an effect at the transcriptional level. In contrast, shorter-term meal-stimulated protein synthesis in the pancreas (i.e. in the postprandial situation) is regulated primarily at the translational level. Studies using administration of exogenous hormonal mediators support this view, since single periods of hormone stimulation (mimicking the postprandial situation) modify the efficiency of mRNA translation into protein, whereas repeated periods of stimulation (up to 7 days, mimicking the situation after long-term intake of nutrients) lead to changes in mRNA levels. This illustrates the importance of the duration of the adaptation period to a dietary change.

So, how do hormones exert these effects? CCK, secretin and GIP are peptide hormones which interact with specific receptors on the plasma membrane of the pancreatic acinar cell. Their cellular effects are associated with activation of separate intracellular messenger pathways. In rodent acinar cells, the best understood mechanism for the action of CCK (Figure 10.14) involves the hydrolysis of membrane phospholipids known as phosphoinositides and the consequent generation of inositol 1,4,5-trisphosphate (IP_3) and diacylglycerol. IP_3 mobilises cellular calcium (Ca^{2+}) and this ultimately leads to activation of a calmodulin-dependent protein kinase, diacylglycerol activates protein kinase C (PKC). Secretin and GIP evoke increases in the level of cyclic adenosine monophosphate (cAMP), which activates cAMP-dependent protein kinase (Figure 10.15).

Application of Ca^{2+} ionophores, which produces an increase in intracellular Ca^{2+} levels similar to that observed with CCK stimulation, results specifically in increases in the synthesis of pancreatic proteases, the same effect observed after CCK infusion or after adaptation to high-protein diets. Forskolin, a drug that enhances cAMP levels, causes an increase in pancreatic lipase and colipase synthesis similar to that produced by secretin and GIP or by intake of high-fat diets.

Figure 10.14 Signal transduction pathway triggered by cholecystokinin (CCK) in the pancreatic acinar cell. Binding of CCK to its specific receptor (R) activates the Gq class of heterotrimeric G proteins (Gq). The activated Gq then stimulates the activity of phospholipase C (PLC) to hydrolyse the membrane phospholipid phosphatidylinositol 4,5-bisphosphate (PIP_2). This cleavage releases inositol 1,4,5-trisphosphate (IP_3) and diacylglycerol (DAG). IP_3 binds to specific Ca^{2+} channels in the endoplasmic reticulum membrane, causing Ca^{2+} to be released. The rise in cytosolic Ca^{2+} favours the formation of the complex Ca^{2+}-calmodulin, which in turn activates a number of calmodulin-dependent protein kinases (CDPK). In the presence of enhanced Ca^{2+}, protein kinase C (PKC) (which in unstimulated conditions is in the cytosol) also binds Ca^{2+}, and this causes PKC to migrate to the inner surface of the plasma membrane, where it can be activated by the DAG produced by hydrolysis of PIP_2. All PKCs and CDPKs phosphorylate key intracellular enzymes, leading to either activation or inactivation of downstream regulatory proteins and producing the cellular response.

The mechanism by which hormonal mediators regulate the expression of genes for specific enzymes after adaptation to high levels of nutrients has not been completely elucidated. In some cases the genetic elements regulated in the promoter region have been identified, although the full intracellular pathway leading to their regulation is unknown. The process may involve the induction of primary response genes (PRGs, also called immediate–early genes). These genes encode regulatory proteins that control the expression of late response genes (LRGs). Thus, an initial transcription factor (a protein that directly affects gene expression) activated in the signal transduction pathway causes the synthesis of a different transcription factor, which in turn causes the synthesis of additional proteins. In pancreatic acinar cells CCK has been shown to induce the expression of PRGs by increasing their nuclear transcription, and this response occurs at 60 min after the application of the hormone. The role of second

messengers has also been established: increases in intracellular Ca^{2+} or cAMP and direct activation of protein kinase C induces, especially when combined, the expression of PRGs to levels comparable to those observed with CCK stimulation. However, the role of these PRGs in linking second messenger pathways to activation of LRGs has not been determined in this tissue. Figure 10.16 proposes a model to explain the relationships between the transduction pathways and the control of gene expression in the pancreas.

Modification of membrane fatty acid composition as a mechanism for pancreatic adaptation to the type of dietary fat

Investigations of the *in vivo* pancreatic response after medium- or long-term intake of diets differing in the fat source have indicated that pancreatic

Figure 10.15 The cyclic adenosine monophosphate (cAMP) messenger system. After interacting with specific receptors on the plasma membrane, the cellular effects of secretin and glucose-dependent insulinotropic peptide (GIP) are mediated by trimeric G-protein activation (Gs type), which activates the membrane enzyme adenylyl cyclase (AC). The activated AC, the catalytic site for which is located on the cytosolic surface of the plasma membrane, catalyses the conversion of some cytosolic adenosine triphosphate (ATP) molecules to cAMP, which then diffuses throughout the cell to bind and activate the cAMP-dependent protein kinase, also termed protein kinase A (PKA). Similarly to the kinases involved in the CCK pathway, PKA phosphorylates other proteins and the change in the activity of these proteins brings about the response of the cell. Although all of these kinases operate in a similar manner, they are distinct from one another and have their own specific substrates.

adaptation to dietary fat type is mediated, at least in part, by changes in the circulating levels of some gastrointestinal hormones. However, the finding that pancreatic cell membranes are enriched in those fatty acids most abundant in the fat ingested suggests that, in addition to the above mechanism, *in vivo* data may reflect a direct modulatory effect of the type of dietary fat on the secretory activity at the cellular level. Indeed, recent studies with viable pancreatic acinar cells of rats fed over 8 weeks with diets containing either virgin olive oil or sunflower oil as the fat source have shown that dietary-induced changes in the fatty acid profile of pancreatic membranes is associated with modulation of pancreatic cell function as assessed by amylase release and intracellular Ca^{2+} mobilisation in response to CCK-8.

Similar results have been reported in AR42J pancreatoma cells after changing their membrane fatty acid profile by addition of specific fatty acids to the culture medium. Such a direct mechanism for adaptation to dietary fat type seems reasonable when considering the role of membrane fatty acids in cellular signalling. Many steps of the stimulus–secretion coupling process in acinar cells are membrane dependent. Thus, differential enrichment in certain fatty acids may influence the accessibility of secretagogue receptors, the interaction with G proteins, the functionality of enzymes such as phospholipases and protein kinase C (which interact with cell membranes during their activation) or the fatty acyl composition of intracellular messengers like DAG, all of which may imply a different sensitivity of the gland for a given concentration of the hormonal secretagogue in blood.

Effect of pancreatic insufficiency on nutrition

It is clear from the previous sections that a number of nutritional factors can affect exocrine pancreatic function. Conversely, pathological modifications of this function lead to an altered nutritional state.

The pancreas has a reserve capacity that is many times the physiological requirement. Steatorrhea and creatorrhea (excessive amounts of fat and protein, respectively, in the faeces) occur only when the secretion of pancreatic lipase and trypsin is reduced to less than 10% of normal. Patients with severe and chronic pancreatic insufficiency are at high risk for developing different forms of malabsorption, the common end-stage of which is protein–energy malnutrition. Apart from defective absorption of the three major nutrients, there may be other nutritional disorders:

- deficiencies of fat-soluble vitamins (in patients with pancreatic steatorrhea)
- in healthy subjects, a zinc-binding compound of pancreatic origin facilitates intestinal zinc absorption. In chronic pancreatitis, clinically significant malabsorption of zinc may ensue
- vitamin B_{12} deficiency: certain proteins of saliva and gastric juice (R proteins) are able to bind vitamin B_{12}, forming a complex that is not available for absorption. In normal conditions, pancreatic

Figure 10.16 Model for the regulation of pancreatic gene expression by hormones and their intracellular messengers. CCK, cholecystokinin; DAG, diacylglycerol; CDPK, calmodulin-dependent protein kinase; PKC, protein kinase C; GIP, glucose-depend insulinotropic peptide; PKA, protein kinase A; PRGs, primary response genes; LRGs, late response genes.

proteases degrade these proteins, releasing the vitamin. In pancreatic insufficiency due to deficiency of proteases, the amount of vitamin B_{12} absorbed can decrease markedly.

10.9 Interactions between the endocrine and exocrine pancreas

The pancreas is a complex organ that consists of an endocrine part and an exocrine part, which is composed of acini (enzyme secretion) and ducts (fluid and electrolyte secretion). The traditional view of a pancreatic gland with functionally distinct compartments has been proven incorrect and can be now considered obsolete. It has been clearly established that there exists an intensive interaction and integration between the exocrine and endocrine pancreas at morphologic and physiologic levels. These close links play a significant role in pancreatic function not only in normal but also in pathological conditions. Any disease affecting the endocrine pancreas will inevitably affect the exocrine function and *vice versa*.

Anatomical relationships between the exocrine and endocrine pancreas

Associations between acini and endocrine tissue: islet–acinar axis

In the pancreas of humans and other mammals, the islets of Langerhans are scattered among the acinar tissue. The concept of an islet–acinar axis is based morphologically on several facts:

(i) Islets are separated from the acini only by a fine reticular layer, which may allow islet hormones to modulate acinar secretions via a paracrine pathway.

(ii) Most importantly, the existence of a continuous insulo-acinar portal blood system connecting the islets to the surrounding acinar tissue has been demonstrated. This system consists of a rich network of arterioles that reach the islets, form an intra-islet glomerulus and leave the islets as efferent capillaries which subsequently perfuse the exocrine tissue. This means that a large part of the blood arriving to the acini has passed through the islets first. An important consequence is that, under physiological circumstances, the acinar cells are exposed to concentrations of islet hormones that may be much higher (20-fold) than those of peripheral blood.

(iii) The islet–acinar axis is also indicated by other morphological evidences. The acinar cells around the islets (peri-insular) are bigger in size, contain larger nuclei and have more abundant zymogen granules and amylase than those located at a distance from the islet cells (tele-insular). It has been assumed that these differences result from the influence exerted by the islet hormones on the surrounding acinar cells.

Associations between ducts and endocrine tissue

In the rat, at least 75% of islets have multiple connections with the ductal system, mainly centroacinar and/or small intralobular ducts. These connections mainly involve glucagon- and somatostatin-secreting cells because they are located toward the periphery of the islets. However, in some cases ducts penetrate the islets, making extensive contacts with the β-cell core. Evidence seems to confirm that islets and ducts are similarly connected in the adult human pancreas.

Of note, the closest association between ducts and endocrine tissue occurs at the level of endocrine cells not clustered in islets of Langerhans. The existence of single endocrine cells and small 'buds' of endocrine cells has been proved in the pancreas. Single endocrine cells are mainly located scattered within the epithelial lining of the ducts. Most of them face the duct lumen ('open-type' cells). Studies in rats have shown that all four major types of pancreatic endocrine cells [i.e. glucagon-, insulin-, somatostatin- and pancreatic polypeptide-secreting (PP) cells] can be found, with an almost even distribution of insulin- and glucagon-producing cells along the entire duct tree, whereas the incidence of PP and somatostatin-secreting cells gradually increases toward the more distally located portions of the duct system. Information about the human pancreas is less abundant but, interestingly, single insulin-secreting cells associated with the duct system have been shown to account for 15% of all β-cells, whereas they represent only 1% of the total insulin-producing cell population of the rat pancreas.

A third arrangement of endocrine cells associated with the duct system can be found in the adult rat pancreas. This arrangement has been referred to as 'buds'. These consist of small clusters (<20–25 cells) of endocrine cells continuous with the duct lining and predominantly associated with intercalated and intralobular ducts. Buds of endocrine cells are composed mainly of insulin-secreting cells. A similar arrangement also seems to exist in humans.

Bicarbonate secretion is related mainly to centroacinar and terminal duct cells, areas that have been found to make contact with the endocrine tissue. It is therefore likely that a remarkable proportion of bicarbonate-secreting cells are under the paracrine influence of endocrine cell secretion.

Effects of major islet hormones on exocrine function

Trophic effects

In the adult pancreas, cell proliferation is minimal compared with other organs within the gastrointestinal system, except for two circumstances. The first is adaptive growth, which occurs in response to hyperphagia, high-dietary protein, pregnancy and lactation. The second type of growth can be characterised as regeneration and occurs after damage such that as following acute pancreatitis. One of the main mediators of both adaptive and regenerative pancreatic growth is the gastrointestinal hormone CCK. In addition, two islet hormones have been demonstrated to have trophic effects on the exocrine pancreas: insulin and pancreatic polypeptide (PP). Insulin enhances the synthesis and content of pancreatic protein, RNA and DNA. It may intensify the effects of CCK on adaptive pancreatic growth, but a major role for insulin is in regenerative growth. The importance of insulin is shown by the fact that, in diabetic rats, CCK administration fails to induce pancreatic regeneration following pancreatitis unless exogenous insulin is also administered. The role of PP in pancreatic growth is less clear, although it has been suggested that this hormone may exert a local trophic role that protects the pancreas from atrophy in diabetic patients.

Effects on exocrine secretion

Insulin enhances pancreatic enzyme synthesis and content, with emphasis on amylase, and potentiates the stimulatory action of nerves and hormones

(CCK and secretin) on fluid and enzyme secretion. Saturable insulin-binding sites have been demonstrated on both acinar and duct cells in different species, so the effect of the hormone is probably direct. The overall effect of glucagon on pancreatic acinar and duct secretions is, in contrast, inhibitory, although the physiological importance of this action has not been established. Presently, it is not clear whether the effect of glucagon is indirect or due to the direct binding of glucagon to exocrine cells. Somatostatin has an inhibitory effect on the secretion of both acinar and duct cells. Specific somatostatin receptors have been identified on acinar cells and membranes, so it is very likely that pancreatic somatostatin regulates pancreatic enzyme secretion directly as a paracrine messenger or via the insulo-acinar portal system. PP has an inhibitory effect on enzyme secretion, whereas less-convincing evidence supports a similar action on bicarbonate and fluid secretion. The existence of Y4 receptors, highly avid for PP, has been confirmed in the exocrine pancreas, but *in vitro* studies show that PP has no direct action on isolated rat pancreatic acini. Recent studies demonstrate that the primary target of PP appears to be the central nervous system. Hence, the mechanism for PP action on exocrine pancreatic secretion remains elusive.

Exocrine dysfunction in diabetes mellitus

Exocrine pancreatic insufficiency is very frequent in type 1 (about 50%) and type 2 (about 32%) diabetic patients. Impairments of the exocrine pancreatic morphology and function in diabetic patients are frequent and well known. Morphological alterations include a reduction in pancreatic size and alterations of the pancreatic duct system. Histological changes include fibrosis and a moderate degree of acinar atrophy and fatty degeneration. Functional abnormalities include reduced secretagogue-stimulated pancreatic exocrine secretion and reduced enzyme content in the pancreas.

Several mechanisms have been proposed to explain altered exocrine morphology and function in diabetes mellitus:

- Atrophy of the exocrine tissue may be caused by insulin deficiency (lack of trophic effect of high local concentrations of insulin) or related to inadequate blood flow (diabetic microangiopathy).

- Pancreatic fibrosis can result from microangiopathy or from activation of stellate cells by hyperglycaemia.

- Impaired exocrine pancreatic secretion may be due to altered local regulatory function of islet hormones. Low delivery of insulin and elevated glucagon, somatostatin and PP might reduce the response to classical pancreatic secretagogues. Diabetic autonomic neuropathy may lead to impaired enteropancreatic reflexes and thus contribute to exocrine dysfunction.

- As a mechanism, it should also be considered that there may be simultaneous damage of exocrine and endocrine tissue as a net result of a common underlying process affecting the whole pancreas (viral infection, autoimmune-mediated inflammation induced by the presentation of both endocrine and exocrine tissue antigens, or genetic changes affecting the exocrine and endocrine compartments).

- It is also possible that in some patients diabetes has been caused by a previous exocrine disease such as chronic pancreatitis (see below).

Endocrine dysfunction in exocrine pancreatic diseases

Pancreatogenic diabetes mellitus (also named pancreatic, apancreatic or type 3c diabetes mellitus) develops from the impairment of the pancreatic endocrine function due to the progression of a pancreatic disease such as acute and chronic pancreatitis, pancreatic trauma, pancreatic surgery, cystic fibrosis or pancreatic cancer. It is thus regarded as a form of secondary diabetes. Exocrine pancreatic diseases are believed to be responsible for about 0.5–2% of all diabetes mellitus cases. Chronic pancreatitis is one of the most common causes of pancreatogenic diabetes. In fact, about 40–70% of the patients with chronic pancreatitis suffer from diabetes mellitus.

The primary hormonal abnormality in diabetes mellitus associated with chronic pancreatitis is decreased insulin secretion. In chronic pancreatitis, the progressive fibrosis destroys the β-cells and reduces their functional capacity, leading to a deficiency of insulin secretion. In addition, the fibrosis impairs the circulation in the islets, which may result in an impaired delivery of stimulants and attenuated hormonal responses of the islets. Furthermore, pancreatogenic diabetes mellitus is a result not merely of an impaired insulin production, but also of coexisting insulin resistance and alterations

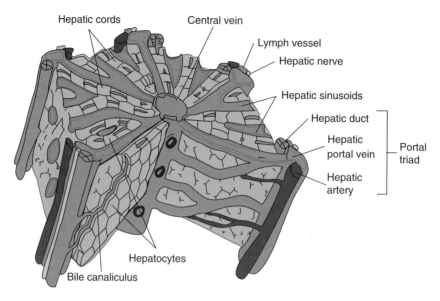

Figure 10.17 Histology and anatomy of the liver.

in insulin action. Loss of hepatic insulin receptor expression caused by PP deficiency and impairment of combined insulin receptor and GLP-2 (glucagon-like peptide 2) endocytosis after insulin binding have been recently demonstrated to contribute to the development of diabetes in chronic pancreatitis.

In conclusion, abundant evidence confirms the influence of the endocrine pancreas on exocrine physiology. Although the possibility that exocrine cells, in turn, influence endocrine function is still at the hypothetical level, the current view of the pancreas is that of an integrated, well-tuned organ in which all the components are functionally related for well-orchestrated functional responses (an endocrine–acinar–ductal axis), a reasonable view if considered that the exocrine portion secretes enzymes and bicarbonate, which affect the digestion and absorption of nutrients, whereas the endocrine part releases hormones that regulate the metabolism and disposal of breakdown products of food within the body.

10.10 Physiology of bile secretion and enterohepatic circulation

The liver of all vertebrates produces and secretes bile. This digestive secretion is elaborated from transport processes in the hepatocyte and is modified along the bile canaliculus and ducts. Finally, in most species bile is stored in the gallbladder and then released into the common hepatic duct and duodenum after a meal.

The liver cells (hepatocytes) are arranged in many functional units called lobules. The lobules are sheets of hepatocytes organised around a central vein (Figure 10.17). Instead of capillaries the liver has large spaces called sinusoids. The sinusoids receive blood containing absorbed nutrients from the hepatic portal vein. The hepatic arterial blood supply to the liver brings oxygen to the liver cells.

Branches of both the hepatic portal vein and the hepatic artery carry blood into the liver sinusoids, where nutrients and oxygen are taken up by the hepatocytes. The liver secretes back into the blood products synthesised by the hepatocytes and nutrients needed by other cells. Blood from both origins leaves the liver in the hepatic vein.

Functions of the liver

The most important digestive function of the liver is the secretion of bile, which is essential for lipid digestion in the intestine. Bile is secreted continuously into specialised ducts, called bile canaliculi, located within each lobule of the liver. These canaliculi empty into bile ducts at the periphery of the lobules. The bile ducts merge and form the right and left hepatic ducts that unite to form a single common hepatic duct. The common hepatic duct is joined by the cystic duct from the gallbladder to form the common bile duct, which empties into the duodenum.

Surrounding the common bile duct at the point where it enters the duodenum is the sphincter of Oddi. When the sphincter is closed the dilute bile secreted by the liver passes into the gallbladder and becomes concentrated until it is needed in the small intestine.

After the beginning of a meal, the sphincter of Oddi relaxes and the gallbladder contracts, discharging concentrated bile into duodenum. The signal for gallbladder contraction is the intestinal hormone CCK. The presence of fat and amino acids in the duodenum is the stimulus for the release of CCK, a hormone that also causes relaxation of the sphincter or Oddi.

Apart from bile secretion the liver has other important functions:

- Lipid metabolism: the hepatocytes synthesise lipoprotein and cholesterol, store some tryglycerides and use cholesterol to synthesise bile acids.
- Carbohydrate metabolism: the liver is one of the major sites of glycogen storage in the body. This occurs after carbohydrate-containing meals and is stimulated by insulin. When blood glucose is low, glycogen is broken down to glucose (glycogenolysis) and the glucose is released into the bloodstream. Under these conditions the liver also synthesises glucose from amino acids and lactic acid (gluconeogenesis).
- Protein metabolism: hepatocytes deaminate amino acids to form ammonia (NH_3), which is converted into a much less toxic product, urea. Urea is excreted in urine.
- The liver synthesises all the major plasma proteins (albumin, globulin, apoproteins, fibrinogen and prothrombin).
- Excretion of bile pigments: bile pigments are derived from the haem portion of haemoglobin in aged erythrocytes. The most important is bilirubin, which is absorbed by the liver from the blood and actively secreted into the bile. After entering the intestinal tract bilirubin is metabolised by bacteria and eliminated in faeces.
- Storage: the liver stores some vitamins (A, D, E, K and B_{12}) and minerals (iron and copper) and participates in the activation of vitamin D.

- Processing of hormones, drugs and toxins: the liver converts these substances to inactive forms in the hepatocytes for subsequent excretion in bile or urine.

Role and composition of the bile

Bile is a mixture of substances synthesised by the liver. It has several components: bile acids, cholesterol, phospholipids (lecithin), bile pigments and small amounts of other metabolic end products, bicarbonate ions and other salts and trace elements. Bile acids are synthesised from cholesterol and before they are secreted are conjugated with the amino acids glycine or taurine. Conjugated bile acids are called bile salts. Bile salts emulsify lipids in the lumen of the small intestine to form micelles, increasing the surface area available to lipolytic enzymes. Micelles transport the products of lipid digestion to the brush-border surface of the epithelial cells, helping the absorption of lipids. Cholesterol is made soluble in bile by bile acids and lecithin.

The epithelial cells lining the ducts secrete a bicarbonate solution, similar to that produced by the pancreas, which contributes to the volume of bile living the liver. This salt solution neutralises acid in the duodenum.

Bile secretion

The hepatocytes produce a primary secretion isotonic to plasma that contains the substances that carry out the main digestive functions (bile acids, cholesterol and lecithin). The bicarbonate-rich fluid secreted by the epithelial cells of the ducts modifies the primary secretion of the liver (Figure 10.18).

Fraction of bile secreted by the hepatocytes

Bile acids, phospholipids, cholesterol, bile pigments and proteins are the most important substances secreted by the hepatocytes into the bile. Bile acids synthesised from cholesterol by the liver are called primary bile acids (cholic acid and chenodeoxycholic acid). The bacteria of the small intestine dehydroxylate primary bile acids to form secondary bile acids (deoxycholic acid and lithocholic acid).

Before they are secreted, bile acids are conjugated with the amino acids glycine or taurine to make them more water soluble. Bacteria in the intestine

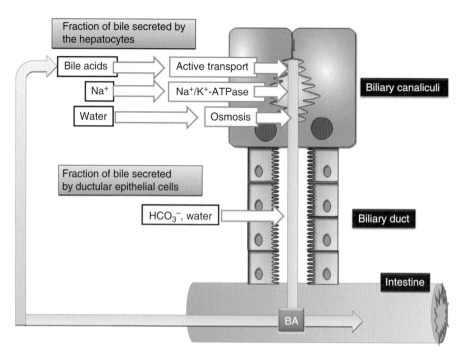

Figure 10.18 Process of bile secretion in the hepatocytes of the liver. (Modified from Martínez de Victoria E, Mañas M, Yago MD. Capítulo 7, Vol. I. Fisiología digestiva. In: Gil A (ed.) Tratado de Nutrición, 2nd edn. Editorial Medica Panamericana, Madrid, 2010.)

deconjugate bile salts into bile acids, which are absorbed in the ileum and go back to the liver, where they are converted into bile salts again and secreted along with newly synthesised bile acids. The uptake of bile acids by the liver stimulates bile salts release. This process is known as the enterohepatic recirculation of bile salts (Figure 10.19).

Hepatocytes secrete phospholipids, especially lecithin, which help to solubilise fat, cholesterol and bile pigments in the small intestine. The synthesis of bile acids from cholesterol and the excretion of cholesterol and bile acids in faeces is one of the mechanisms to maintain cholesterol homeostasis. Hepatocytes remove bilirubin from the bloodstream attached to glucuronic acid molecules. The resultant conjugated bilirubin is secreted into the bile.

Fraction of bile secreted by ductular epithelial cells

These cells secrete a bicarbonate-rich salt solution that accounts for about half of the total bile volume. The concentration of HCO_3 is greater than in the plasma and helps to neutralise the intestinal acid.

This secretion is stimulated by secretin in response to the presence of acid in the duodenum.

Bile concentration and storage in the gallbladder

Between meals the sphincter of Oddi is closed and the dilute bile secreted by the liver passes through the cystic duct into the gallbladder and becomes concentrated. The gallbladder mucosa absorbs water and ions (Na^+, Cl^-, HCO_3^-) and can concentrate bile salts 10-fold. The active transport of Na^+ into the interstitial space produces an elevated osmolarity in this region and the osmotic flow of water across the epithelium; HCO_3^- and Cl^- are transported to the interstitial space to preserve electroneutrality.

Regulation of bile secretion

Several factors increase the production or release of bile (Figure 10.20):

- The rate of return of the bile acids to the liver via portal blood affects the rate of secretion of bile

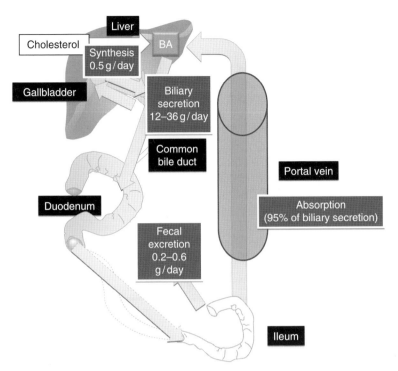

Figure 10.19 Enterohepatic circulation of bile acids (BA). (Modified from Martínez de Victoria E, Mañas M, Yago, MD. Capítulo 7, Vol. I. Fisiología digestiva. In: Gil A (ed.) Tratado de Nutrición, 2nd edn. Editorial Medica Panamericana, Madrid, 2010.)

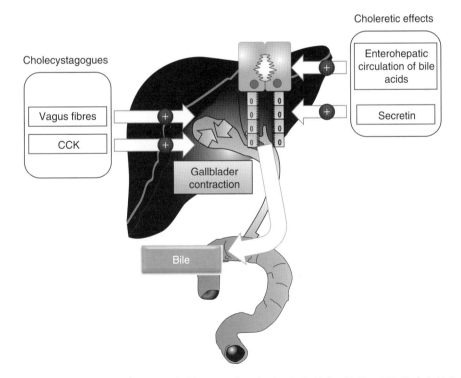

Figure 10.20 Factors controlling bile secretion. (Modified from Martínez de Victoria E, Mañas M, Yago MD. Capítulo 7, Vol. I. Fisiología digestiva. In: Gil A (ed.) Tratado de Nutrición, 2nd edn. Editorial Panamericana, Madrid, 2010.)

acids. Bile acids stimulate bile production and secretion, in fact there is a linear relationship between bile acids secretion rate and bile flow. Bile acids increase bile flow because they provide an osmotic driving force for filtration of water and electrolytes (choleretic effect).

- During a meal CCK is released into the blood by fatty acids and polypeptides in the chyme. This causes contraction of the gallbladder and release of concentrated bile. CCK also relaxes the sphincter of Oddi, allowing the flow of bile, rich in bile salts, into the duodenum. These bile salts return via the enterohepatic circulation to the liver, further stimulating bile acid secretion and bile flow. CCK also directly stimulates the primary secretion by the liver.
- Parasympathetic impulses along the vagus nerve (cephalic influences) also cause contraction of the gallbladder.
- The acidity of the chyme emptying to the duodenum stimulates the release of secretin. This hormone causes the ductular epithelial cells to secrete a solution high in bicarbonate and doing so increases the bile flow.

10.11 Adaptation of the biliary response to the diet

There is abundant information on adaptation of the pancreatic exocrine secretion in response to the composition of the diet. The physiological significance of this adaptation is to optimise the digestion and utilisation of macronutrients. Reports about the role of major dietary components in bile secretion, on the other hand, are relatively scarce, in spite of the fact that this secretion is essential for lipid digestion.

Bile salts are synthesised and secreted by the liver, stored and concentrated in the gallbladder, and delivered into the duodenum in response to a meal. Postprandial gallbladder contraction and sphincter of Oddi relaxation is mainly regulated by CCK. This hormone is released into blood by the products of digestion of macronutrients. Changing the composition of macronutrients in the diet may evoke different plasma levels of CCK and thus modify the bile flow, the supply of bile salts into the duodenum, the enterohepatic circulation, the hepatic synthesis of bile acids and the amount excreted into the bile.

In healthy subjects, higher CCK release in response to food has been associated with stronger gallbladder emptying. There is a positive linear relationship between CCK release and gallbladder contraction. Meals differing in either the type or the amount of fat, protein or carbohydrates may be effective in stimulating CCK release and biliary secretion to varying degrees.

In addition, decreased postprandial gallbladder emptying has been suggested to play a major role in the development of gallstones in humans, therefore dietary factors may be important in the pathogenesis of gallbladder stasis.

Major dietary components, CCK release and gallbladder contraction

Carbohydrates

Carbohydrates seem to have no influence on bile secretion when they constitute the standard proportion of the diet. Institution of a 95% carbohydrate diet reduces gallbladder emptying and diminishes bile salt pool size and bile acid secretion. Fat is the stronger stimulant for the release of CCK. Diets very rich in carbohydrates and with an adequate protein supply are very low in fat and these diets have been shown to be especially ineffective in the stimulation of CCK secretion and gallbladder contraction.

Protein

Several studies have shown that the amount and type of dietary protein influences biliary secretion. High-protein diets have been shown to increase bile acid secretion and the presence of bile salts in the lumen of the small intestine and have been shown to stimulate plasma CCK secretion. The effect of low-protein diets on the postprandial emptying of the gallbladder has also been examined. A 3-day low-protein/low-fat diet increased fasting gallbladder volume and significantly decreased fasting plasma CCK levels in humans. This suggests that CCK secretion regulates fasting gallbladder volume and that basal CCK release depends on diet composition. This diminished gallbladder stimulation affects bile flow and bile acid secretion in resting conditions and in response to food. The quality of the dietary protein also affects CCK release. Animal studies have demonstrated this, although more human studies in this area are necessary before the relationship between biliary response to a meal and protein quality is fully understood.

Intravenous infusion of amino acid solutions appears to have different effects on gallbladder contraction and CCK secretion depending on the amino acid composition. Tryptophan and phenylalanine appear to be the most potent stimulants to CCK secretion and gallbladder contraction in humans.

Fat

The amount and type of dietary fat ingested also affects biliary secretion. In general, when the amount of fat ingested increases, the biliary response shows a marked rise in bile acid concentration and output. It has been suggested that this response is an adaptation process ensuring adequate fat digestion. In humans, CCK release and gallbladder contraction after a meal depend mainly on fat intake. Low-fat and fat-free diets decrease gallbladder emptying and CCK levels when compared to a normal mixed diet. High-fat diets produce opposite results. Some studies suggest that meals high in long-chain triacylglycerols (LCT) produce a postprandial increase in plasma CCK concentration while meals containing medium-chain triacylglycerols (MCT) inhibit CCK release.

The type of dietary fat also affects gallbladder emptying. Oleic acid, the major fatty acid in olive oil, is one of the most potent stimulators of CCK release known. In human subjects fed for 30 days diets containing either olive oil or sunflower oil as the main source of dietary fat, it was confirmed that the type of dietary fat affects the plasma levels of CCK. Postprandial CCK plasma levels were higher in the olive oil group, so a first option to explain the mechanisms of the biliary adaptation to dietary fat involves the existence of hormonal mediators. However, whether or not the secretory activity of liver cells is influenced directly by dietary fat alteration is unknown.

The biological effects of dietary fatty acids are partly due to their incorporation into the cellular structures of organs and tissues. In different tissues there is evidence that the lipid profile of the diet can influence the fatty acid composition of cell membranes, this being associated with a modification of cell function. This is not an unexpected finding since there is growing evidence that fatty acids, in addition to their role in determining membrane structure and fluidity, can participate in intracellular processes as diverse as signal transduction or the regulation of gene expression.

The plasma membranes of tissues and organs differ, however, in their adaptation to dietary fat type. The liver, for instance, is very sensitive to dietary changes. In contrast, other tissues, such as the brain, skeletal muscle and heart, seem to show relatively minor adaptive alterations in the lipid composition of their membranes. A second possibility to explain the mechanisms of biliary adaptation is that dietary fat composition may change the responsiveness of the liver to circulating secretagogues and/or to alter calcium signalling as a consequence of the modification of the fatty acid composition of the liver membranes, as explained in the pancreas section.

10.12 Growth, development and differentiation of the gastrointestinal tract

The intestinal epithelium is a complex equilibrium system of multiple cell types undergoing continual renewal while maintaining precise interrelationships. The crypt-villous axis is composed of a dynamic cell population in perpetual change from a crypt proliferative and undifferentiated stage to a mature villous stage. The migration of crypt cells is accompanied by cellular differentiation, which leads to morphological and functional changes.

The regulatory mechanisms involved with developmental processes are at organism, cellular and molecular levels. At the organism level there is an expanded array of hormones and dietary effects that modulate the ontogeny of the intestine. The adult phenotype of the small intestine is established via a series of developmental transitions resulting from the interaction of visceral endoderm and mesoderm.

During development and in adult epithelium, cellular phenotypes are defined by the expression of specific sets of genes in individual cells. The regulation of those genes is mainly done at the transcriptional level, although some genes may be regulated after initiation of the transcription during translation or even by late modifications of synthesised proteins in the endoplasmic reticulum and Golgi system. The particular set of genes expressed in a single cell type has recently been referred to as the 'transcriptome'. Intestinal epithelial cell transcriptomes shift in well-orchestrated patterns during the development, differentiation and adaptive processes of the intestinal mucosa. In addition to this intrinsic gene programme, intestinal epithelial cells respond to extrinsic signals, including nutrients and other dietary components, by producing various molecules. Using different experimental approaches, recent studies have further characterised intestinal epithelial-cell biology and provided evidence of its polyvalent nature and important role in gut homeostasis.

Ontogeny of digestive and absorptive functions in humans

By the time of birth, all mammals must be able to digest all the nutritional components of their mother's milk. Lactose is the primary carbohydrate in the diet of the infant until the time of weaning. Lactase, sucrase and maltase activities appear between 8 and 9 weeks of gestational age in the jejunum. The greatest increase in lactase activity occurs during the third trimester, while at 20 weeks sucrase and maltase activities are already 50–75% of those found in term infants and adults. The appearance of lactase coincides with the appearance of microvilli. Unlike other species in which lactase activity declines at weaning, in the human it is maintained well beyond the weaning period. However, a decline occurs between 3 and 5 years of life. Sucrase and maltase activities are maintained throughout life.

Glucoamylase is the most important enzyme for digestion of complex carbohydrates. This enzyme is detectable by 20 weeks of gestational age and the greatest increase occurs between the period of foetal development and early postnatal development. Its activity in infants less than 1 year is comparable to that of adolescents.

Alkaline phosphatase is detectable by 7 weeks of gestation but levels in newborns are substantially less than in adults.

As for sucrase and maltase, most brush-border peptidases appear to mature more rapidly in humans than in rats. γ-Glutamyl transpeptidase (γ-GT) activity increases more than twofold between 13 and 20 weeks of gestational age and its activity is higher in foetuses than in infants and adults. Aminopeptidase activity appears at 8 weeks of gestation, and adult values are attained by 14 weeks. Oligoaminopeptidase, dipeptidylamino peptidase IV and carboxypeptidase increase in activity from 8 to 22 weeks of gestational

age and are present in infants. Lysosomal enzymes undergo little ontogenic change in the human.

Longitudinal distribution of the various enzymes along the small intestine often varies with the stage of development. Lactase and sucrase show a proximo-distal gradient through adulthood, and glucoamylase and γ-GT activities are fairly uniform throughout the small intestine.

Active transport of glucose is demonstrable by 10 weeks of life in the jejunum and by 12 weeks in the ileum. *In vivo* data suggest that little change occurs between 30 weeks and term. A high-affinity, low-capacity Na–glucose cotransport system along the length of the small intestine and a low-affinity, high-capacity system in the proximal intestine, have been found in human foetuses. Glucose absorptive capacity seems to increase as a function of age from foetal life to adulthood.

Amino acid transport can also be demonstrated by 12 weeks of gestational age. Amino acid uptake is accomplished by sodium-dependent and -independent transport mechanisms. The Na-dependent pathways include the NBB and Phe systems for neutral amino acids, the Xag system for acidic amino acids, and the amino system for proline and hydroxyproline. The Na-independent pathways include the L system for neutral amino acids and y+ system for basic amino acids. The NBB system, which transports leucine, is demonstrable in the entire small intestine of both infants and adults.

Macromolecules are also capable of crossing the small intestinal mucosa. The pathway of macromolecular uptake in the human is unclear, although endocytic and pinocytic processes can occur. The ability of the human intestinal mucosa to take up macromolecules is increased in infancy and during episodes of intestinal injury, such as diarrhoea and malnutrition. The intestinal closure is enhanced in breast-fed infants compared to those fed formula milk.

Calcium absorptive capacity in preterm infants is greater than 50% of adult levels. In agreement with the needs of the growing infant, iron absorption is more efficient in infants than in adults, although iron bioavailability is fairly dependent on dietary components, that is the presence of lactoferrin in human milk.

By 8–11 weeks of gestational age, gastrin, secretin, motilin, gastric inhibitory peptide (GIP), enteroglucagon, somatostatin, vasoactive intestinal peptide (VIP), gastrin and cholecystokinin are demonstrable. The concentrations of these peptides increase throughout gestation and are at adult levels between 31 and 40 weeks gestational age. Gastrin, secretin, motilin and GIP are localised to the duodenum and jejunum, whereas enteroglucagon, neurotensin, somatostatin and VIP are distributed throughout the small intestine.

Hormonal and dietary regulation of ontogenic changes in the small intestine

Administration of exogenous glucocorticoids during the first or second postnatal week causes precocious maturation of intestinal structure and function. In the absence of glucocorticoids, there is a dramatic reduction in the rate of maturation. Glucocorticoids cause intestinal maturation by transcriptional changes but hormones may also have post-translational effects on proteins of the microvillous membrane as a result of their capacity to alter membrane fluidity and glycosylation patterns. Glucocorticoids are capable of eliciting terminal maturation of the human intestine in a manner analogous to their effects in the rat. These hormones increase the lactase activity *in vitro*. In addition, retrospective and prospective studies have shown that prenatal corticosteroid treatment is associated with a significantly reduced incidence of necrotising enterocolitis in preterm infants.

Thyroxine (T_4) is a reasonable candidate for mediating the ontogeny of enzyme changes in the human small intestine, and total and free serum T_4 increase during the latter half of gestation. Insulin levels increase just prior to ontogenic changes in disaccharidase activities. For example, in the human amniotic fluid insulin directly reflects foetal insulin output, and the concentration increases during the last trimester. The rise in insulin precedes the prenatal increase in lactase activity that occurs in the third trimester.

Other hormones and substances have been proposed to play a role in the regulation of intestinal mucosal ontogeny. Many of them are known growth factors, but their direct effects on intestinal maturation are largely unknown.

In preterm infants the provision of small amounts of milk enterally within the first week of life shortens the time it takes for infants to be able to tolerate all nutrients. Early introduction of feeding also appears to enhance the development of a more mature small intestinal motility pattern and improve enteral feeding tolerance. In addition, water feeding is not as effective as formula feeding in stimulating the release of gastrointestinal peptides in the premature infant.

Epithelial growth and differentiation

The small intestinal epithelium originates from stem cells that give rise to four different cell lineages:

- absorptive enterocytes
- mucus-producing goblet cells
- enteroendocrine cells
- Paneth's cells.

The first three cell types migrate towards the villi, whereas Paneth's cells migrate downwards to the crypt base. The intestinal epithelial cells form intimate contacts with T lymphocytes, which in turn may regulate epithelial cell growth and barrier function. The intestinal epithelium provides unique opportunities for the study of cell differentiation and apoptosis. The gut epithelium along the crypt–villus axis is dynamic, with equilibrium between crypt cell production and the senescence and exfoliation of differentiated cells. Regulation of normal intestinal epithelial growth is thought to be dependent on mesenchymal–epithelial interactions as well as interactions with extracellular matrix proteins. Mesenchymal fibroblasts secrete growth factors that influence intestinal epithelial cell migration, proliferation and differentiation. As mature epithelial cells are produced, they express a variety of intestine-specific gene products involved in digestive, absorptive, cell migratory and cell protection functions.

Proteinase-activated receptors (PARs) are a family of G-coupled receptors for serine protease. PAR-2 has been recently found to be expressed in the villi and crypt region of the rat small intestine and in the basolateral and apical membrane of the rat enterocytes. Trypsin at physiological concentrations activates PAR-2, which triggers the release of inositol triphosphate, arachidonic acid and prostaglandin E_2 and F_{1a}, therefore luminal trypsin may serve as a signalling protein for enterocyte activation via PAR-2.

Protein kinase C (PKC) is involved in cell growth and differentiation in various cell types. PKCα expression is increased in Caco-2 spontaneous cell differentiation, although levels of other kinases remain unchanged in postconfluent cells. Concurrently, expression of PKCα regulated cyclin-dependent kinase inhibitor p21^{wafl} increases in differentiated cells, therefore the PKCα and p21^{wafl} cascade could direct a signal that influences the differentiation status of intestinal epithelial cells. Paneth's cells are likely to play a role in secretion and protection against microflora. Paneth's cell allocation occurs early during epithelial cytodifferentiation and crypt formation and leads to the production of marker proteins such as phospholipase A2 (Pla2s), cryptidins and lysozyme.

Transforming growth factor-α (TGF-α) and TGF-β, as well as epidermal growth factor (EGF) and hepatocyte growth factor (HGF), are potent multifunctional growth factors that appear to play critical roles in the intestine under normal development and during injury. Using immunohistochemistry, TGF-β$_1$ has been localised to the smooth muscle cells of the muscularis propria in the human foetal intestine. In untreated adult rats TGF-α expression has been also demonstrated in the epithelial cells at the villous tip and TGF-β expression in epithelial cells in the upper crypt. TGF-α and TGF-β may accelerate wound healing in the intestine. Polyamines and ornithine decarboxylase-dependent cations have been demonstrated to be crucial for the migration of epithelial cells into regions of damaged tissue to promote early mucosal repair. Insulin-like growth factor (IGF) peptides are known to stimulate gastrointestinal growth in normal adult rats and IGF-I has been shown to selectively stimulate intestinal growth in developing rats.

Brush-border hydrolases

Lactase and sucrase isomaltase
The developmental expression of lactase and sucrase-isomaltase (SI) enzyme activity correlates with the change in diet at the time of weaning from predominantly lactose-containing milk to non-lactose-containing foods. The expression of the two enzymes appears to be largely genetically determined and transcriptionally regulated. However, the profiles are markedly different, with lactase mRNA appearing before SI mRNA, peaking earlier and then rapidly declining. SI mRNA peaks later and is then maintained at 70% of its peak value. A second major determinant of enzyme activity is the stability of the proteins, with lactase having a longer half-life than SI.

There is strong support for additional independent transcription factors to allow for the differential regulation of these two genes. Further support for differential regulation is provided by the observation that increased cyclic AMP levels increase lactase biosynthesis and mRNA levels but inhibit SI synthesis. Transgenic mouse experiments show that the patterns of SI gene expression are regulated by multiple functional cis-acting DNA elements. There are at least three groups of transcriptional factors involved in SI promoter activation, including hepatocyte nuclear factor 1 (HNF-1), Cdx proteins and nuclear proteins that interact with a GATA binding site. There is little correlation of SI transcription with the expression of these transcription factors, which is apparently due to the differential expression of coactivator proteins that thereby modulate the activation of the SI promoter.

Each of the intestinal epithelial cell lineages contains the necessary components for SI expression, and normal enterocyte-specific expression probably involves a repression mechanism in the goblet, enteroendocrine and Paneth's cell lineages.

Peptidases
γ-GT catalyses the transfer of glutamic acid from a donor molecule such as glutathione to an acceptor molecule such as a peptide. The mouse γ-GT gene is unique since it has seven different promoters and contains six 5′-exons. The combination of different promoter usage along with alternative splicing generates tissue specific mRNAs from this single gene.

Enterokinase is a hydrolase that activates latent hydrolytic enzymes in the intestinal lumen by proteolytic cleavage of the proenzymes. The cloning of the bovine enterokinase has revealed a complex protease with multiple domains. Its amino acid sequence suggests that the enterokinase is activated by an unidentified protease and therefore is not the first enzyme of the intestinal digestive hydrolase cascade. The regulation of the expression of the enterokinase gene is largely unknown.

Dipeptidyl peptidase IV (DPP-IV), a brush-border hydrolase, is identical to the T-cell activation molecule CD26. It is a member of the prolyl oligopeptidase family of serine proteases that plays an important role in the hydrolysis of proline-rich peptides. Differential expression of DPP-IV has been reported along the vertical villous axis, with high levels of expression in the villous cells and lower levels in the crypt cells and horizontal axis.

Alkaline phosphatase

Intestinal alkaline phosphatase (IAP) is a brush-border enzyme that is secreted into the serum and lumen, and undergoes extensive postnatal developmental regulation of expression. The adult rat intestine expresses two IAP mRNAs, IAP-I and IAP-II, which have about 70% nucleotide sequence identity with complete divergence at the carboxy terminus.

Transporters

The Na-dependent glucose co transporter (SGLT1) and seven facilitative glucose transporters (GLUT-1 to GLUT-7) have been cloned. SGLT1, GLUT-2 and GLUT-5 are expressed in the small intestine. SGLT1 is located in the apical membrane of the enterocytes, GLUT-2 is anchored to the basolateral membrane and GLUT-5 appears to function as an intestinal fructose transporter.

The Na-dependent uptake of bile is also developmentally regulated, with a marked increase at weaning. This co-transporter is regulated at the transcriptional level at the time of weaning with subsequent changes in the apparent molecular weight of the protein after weaning.

Regulatory peptides

Pituitary adenylate cyclase-activating peptide (PACAP) is a neuropeptide that exists in two functional forms and is a member of a group of regulatory peptides that includes secretin, glucagons, gastric inhibitory peptide, growth hormone-releasing factor and vasoactive intestinal peptide (VIP). PACAP receptors have tissue-specific affinity for both PACAP and VIP. PACAP nerves exist within the myenteric plexus, deep muscular plexus and submucosal plexus in the canine terminal ileum. In addition, PACAP receptors are present in deep muscular plexus and circular muscular fibres.

Uroguanylin and guanylin are endogenous proteins that regulate intestinal chloride secretion by binding to the guanylate cyclase C, and guanylin also has been shown to be involved in duodenal bicarbonate secretion. Uroguanylin is expressed throughout the intestinal tract and in the kidney. This gene is predominantly expressed in the villous. Guanilyn, however, is localised

to the distal small intestine and proximal colon and is expressed in both the crypt and villous.

Intestinal cytoprotection

Cyclooxygenases

Two cyclooxygenase (Cox) isoforms, Cox-1 and Cox-2, catalyse the synthesis of prostaglandins. Cox-1 is expressed constitutively in most mammalian tissues and prostaglandins produced by Cox-1 are thought to play a major role in the maintenance of gastrointestinal homeostasis, including gastric cytoprotection and blood flow. Cox-2 is induced in monocytes and macrophages by proinflammatory cytokines, mitogens, serum and endotoxin. Prostaglandins synthesised by Cox-2 mediate the inflammatory response. Cox-2 is expressed at very low levels in the intestinal epithelium but is expressed at high levels in human colon cancers and adenomas and in spontaneous adenomas in mice that carry a mutant APC gene. In the normal colonic epithelium there is not significant Cox-2 expression, but in ulcerative colitis and Crohn's disease Cox-2 is expressed in epithelial cells in upper crypts and on the surface but not in the lower crypts.

The area of Cox-1 expression in the small and large intestine corresponds to the area of epithelial proliferation in the crypt. As the epithelial cell migrates up out of the crypt and onto the villous it differentiates and stops expressing Cox-1.

Trefoil peptides

Trefoil peptides contain a unique motif with six cysteine residues and three intrachain disulphide bonds, resulting in a three-loop structure. They are expressed highly in gastrointestinal mucosa and are resistant to protease digestion in the lumen, probably due to their unusual trefoil domain. Known members of the trefoil peptide family include pS2, spasmolitic peptide (SP) and intestinal trefoil factor (ITF), all cloned from several species. The stomach secretes pS2, the stomach and duodenum secrete SP and the small and large intestine secrete ITF. Although the exact function of these proteins has not yet been determined, they are found in high levels at the edges of healing ulcers and are believed to be involved in the protective function of the mucosal barrier.

Mucins

Mucins are a key component of the protective gel layer that coats the mucosal surface. Whether secretory or membrane bound, mucins contain diverse, highly *O*-glycosylated repeat amino acid residues. Mucin expression is known to be both cell-type and tissue specific as different mucins have been localised to specific regions of the gastrointestinal tract. Mucin precursors for mucins, MUC2–MUC6, have been identified from the stomach to the small and large intestine, MUC3 from the small intestine, MUC4 from the large intestine, and both MUC5AC and MUC6 from the stomach. Little is known about the specific function of individual MUCs, but the site-specific expression of these molecules suggests that the composition of MUC5AC and MUC6 is beneficial in protecting the stomach from acid-induced damage.

Human MUC2 is expressed almost exclusively in goblet cells and may be abnormally expressed in colon cancer. The gene for human MUC2 maps to chromosome 11p15 and analysis of the locus reveals two regulatory elements, an enhancer and an inhibitor, upstream from the MUC2 translation start site. MUC-1 protein expression has been located to microvilli on the luminal surface of the epithelial cell in the intestine.

Regulation of intestinal tract gene expression mediated by nutrients

Traditionally it has been assumed that gene expression in higher eukaryotes was not directly influenced by food components but by the action of hormones, growth factors and cytokines. However, it is now known that diet is a powerful means to modify the cellular environment of the gastrointestinal tract. Dietary regulation of the genes expressed by the epithelium confers three fundamental advantages for mammals. It enables the epithelium to adapt to the luminal environment to better digest and absorb nutrients; it provides the means whereby breast milk can influence the development of the gastrointestinal tract, and when the proteins expressed by the epithelium act on the immune system, it constitutes a signalling mechanism from the intestinal lumen to the body's defences. Each of these mechanisms is amenable to manipulation for therapeutic purposes. Major nutrients, that is glucose and fatty acids, as well as minor nutrients, that is liposoluble vitamins A and D, hydrosoluble vitamins B_1, B_6, C and biotin, and minerals (iron, zinc, copper and selenium), influence the expression of a number of genes directly or in a concerted action with hormones.

The regulation of genes by nutrients requires that some enzymes, transporters and membrane receptors interact with the particular nutrient, resulting in a series of cellular events that lead to modulation of the transcriptional or translational gene processes. Production and secretion of insulin from the β-cells of the pancreas is crucial in maintaining normoglycaemia. This is achieved by tight regulation of insulin synthesis and exocytosis from the β-cells in response to changes in blood glucose levels. The synthesis of insulin is regulated by blood glucose levels at the transcriptional and post-transcriptional levels. Although many transcription factors have been implicated in the regulation of insulin gene transcription, three β-cell-specific transcriptional regulators, Pdx-1 (pancreatic and duodenal homeobox-1), NeuroD1 (neurogenic differentiation 1) and MafA (V-maf musculoaponeurotic fibrosarcoma oncogene homologue A), have been shown to play a crucial role in glucose induction of insulin gene transcription and pancreatic β-cell function. These three transcription factors activate insulin gene expression in a co-ordinated and synergistic manner in response to increasing glucose levels. It has been shown that changes in glucose concentrations modulate the function of these β-cells.

The transcriptional role of glucose has largely been investigated in liver, where involvement of the lipogenic pathway is prominent. In the presence of insulin, which is required to activate glucose metabolism in hepatocytes, high glucose concentrations induce expression of genes that encode glucose transporters and glycolytic and lipogenic enzymes [e.g. L-type pyruvate kinase (L-PK), acetyl-coenzyme A carboxylase (ACC) fatty acid synthase (FAS) and malic enzyme] and down-regulate genes of gluconeogenesis, such as the phosphoenolpyruvate carboxykinase gene (PEPCK). Recently, using microarrays, 283 glucose-responsive genes in rat hepatocytes that are essentially involved in carbohydrate metabolism and *de-novo* lipogenesis have been identified. Promoter analysis of glucose-regulated genes (e.g. those encoding acetyl-coenzyme A carboxylase, FAS, L-PK and Spot 14) allowed investigators to identify a carbohydrate response element (ChORE) that is constituted by two E-boxes separated by five nucleotides. A member of the basic helix–loop–helix leucine zipper family of transcription factors that can bind this DNA motif was purified and named ChORE binding protein (ChREBP). ChREBP is abundant in tissues where lipogenesis is highly active, such as liver, small intestine, and white and brown adipose tissue, whereas its expression is low in skeletal muscle.

A growing number of reports clearly demonstrate that amino acids are able to control physiological functions at different levels, including the initiation of protein translation, mRNA stabilisation and gene transcription. Extensive studies on the asparagine synthetase (*ASNS*) and C/EBP homology binding protein (*CHOP*) genes allowed characterisation of specific responsive sequences in their promoter, which were named either nutrient-sensing response elements (NSRE) or amino acid responsive elements (AARE). Specific transcription factors involved in the amino acid response pathway (AAR) have also been identified, and are members of the basic region/ leucine zipper superfamily of transcription factors. In parallel, some amino acids involved in many cellular functions, particularly glutamine and leucine, have been shown to exert a wide range of effects via the activation of different signalling pathways and transcription factors. Although the molecular details of these effects are not completely known, the heterogeneity of the involved factors might suggest multiple amino acid response pathways depending on the amino acid studied, the cell type used and the gene promoter configuration.

The glutamine-responsive genes and the transcription factors involved correspond tightly to the specific effects of this amino acid in the inflammatory response, cell proliferation, differentiation and survival, and metabolic functions. Indeed, in addition to the major role played by nuclear factor-κB (NF-κB) in the anti-inflammatory action of glutamine, the stimulatory role of activating protein-1 and the inhibitory role of CHOP in growth-promotion, and the role of c-myc in cell survival, many other transcription factors are also involved in the action of glutamine to regulate apoptosis and intermediary metabolism in different cell types and tissues. The signalling pathways leading to the activation of transcription factors suggest that several kinases are involved, particularly mitogen-activated protein kinases (MAPK).

The stimulatory effect of leucine on protein synthesis is mediated through up-regulation of the initiation of mRNA translation. A number of mechanisms, including phosphorylation of ribosomal protein S6 kinase, eukaryotic initiation factor (eIF)4E binding protein-1 (4E-BP) and eIF4G, contribute to the effect of leucine on translation initiation. These mechanisms not only promote global translation of mRNA but also contribute to processes that mediate discrimination in the selection of mRNA for translation. A key component in a signalling pathway controlling these phosphorylation-induced mechanisms is the protein kinase, termed the mammalian target of rapamycin (mTOR). The activity of mTOR toward downstream targets is controlled in part through its interaction with the regulatory-associated protein of mTOR (known as raptor) and the G protein b-subunit-like protein. Signalling through mTOR is also controlled by upstream members of the pathway such as the Ras homologue enriched in brain (Rheb), a GTPase that activates mTOR and tuberin (also known as TSC2), a GTPase-activating protein, which, with its binding partner hamartin (also known as TSC1), acts to repress mTOR. The Rag proteins, a family of four related small GTPases, interact with mTOR in an amino acid sensitive manner and seem to be both necessary and sufficient for mediating amino acid signalling to mTOR.

In addition to EGF, insulin and other growth factors and nutrients, human milk contains some nutrients that influence gene expression. Lactoferrin, a protein involved in Fe bioavailability, is a proliferative factor for lymphocytes, embryonic fibroblasts and human intestinal HT-29 cells. It also increases sucrase and alkaline phosphatase activities in intestinal cells. These data suggest that lactoferrin may affect intestinal growth and differentiation, probably by internalisation of the lactoferrin–receptor complex.

Soluble nucleotides are present in milk from various mammals, contributing up to 20% of the non-protein nitrogen. Although nucleotide deficiency has not been related to any particular disease, dietary nucleotides are reportedly beneficial for infants since they positively influence lipid metabolism, immunity and tissue growth, development and repair. Nucleotides are naturally present in all foods of animal and vegetable origin as free nucleotides and nucleic acids. Concentrations of RNA and DNA in foods depend mainly on their cell density, whereas

```
┌─────────────────────────────────────┐
│ Increased rate of protein synthesis │
│ Ribosomal aggregation               │
│ Increased rRNA                      │
│ Modification of nucleotide          │
│ intracellular pool                  │
└─────────────────────────────────────┘
                  ↑
        ┌────────────────────┐
        │  Dietary Nucleotides │
        └────────────────────┘
                  ↓
      Modulation of gene expression
```

Hepatic genes	Intestinal and Immune Systems
Acyl CoA desaturases	HPRT, APRT
Collagens	Disacharidases
Laminin	Alkaline phosphatase
Fibronectin	Differentiation genes (RHO E)
Metaloproteases	Cytokines
TIMPs	Surface antigens
	Immunoglobulins
	CNT1 and CNT2 nucleoside transporters

Figure 10.21 Modulation of gene expression by dietary nucleotides. TIMPs: HPRT, hypoxanthine phosphoribosyl transferase; APRT, aderine phosphoribosyl transferase; CNT, concentrative nucleoside transporters.

the content of free nucleotides is species specific. Thus, meat, fish and seeds have a high content of nucleic acids, and milk, eggs, and fruits have relatively lower levels. Milk has a specific free-nucleotide profile for each species. The nucleotide content of colostrum is qualitatively similar but quantitatively distinct in human and ruminants. In general, total colostrum nucleotide content increases immediately after parturition, reaches maximum levels from 24 to 48 h after birth and decreases thereafter with advancing lactation. Dietary nucleotides appear to modulate lipoprotein and fatty acid metabolism in human early life, and affect the growth, development and repair of the small intestine and liver in experimental animals. Moreover, dietary nucleotides modify the intestinal ecology of newborn infants, enhancing the growth of bifidobacteria and limiting that of enterobacteria, and have a role in the maintenance of the immune response in both animals and human neonates.

Erythrocytes and lymphocytes, enterocytes and glial cells have a common characteristic: their ability to synthesise nucleotides by the *de novo* pathway is very low. Thus, an external supply of nucleosides seems to be needed for optimal functioning. Several investigations support the hypothesis that the enterocyte is not fully capable of developing the *de novo*

purine synthesis and that this metabolic pathway may be inactive unless it is induced by a purine deficient diet. The purine salvage pathway, as measured by the activity of its rate-limiting enzyme hypoxanthine phosphoribosyl transferase (HGPRT), is highest in the small intestine relative to liver and colon; moreover, a purine free diet lowers HGPRT activity.

A number of studies have demonstrated that dietary nucleotides in part regulate gene expression in the intestine (Figure 10.21). Intestinal mRNA levels of the enzymes HGPRT and APRT declined in response to nucleotide restriction in the diet. Nuclear 'run-on' assays both in nuclei isolated from the small intestine and from an intestinal epithelial cell line (IEC-18) demonstrated that dietary-nucleotide restriction significantly altered the transcription rate. A 35-bp region (HCRE) in the promoter of the HPGRT gene has been identified as the element necessary to this response, and the protein that interacts with this region has been identified and purified. Recently, it has been shown that the addition of nucleosides to Caco-2 cells increased the expression and activity of the general transcription factors activating enhancer binding protein 2 alpha (TFAP2A) and CCAAT displacement protein (CUX1) and v-ets avian erythroblastosis virus E26 oncogene homologue 1 (ETS1), and SMAD family member 2. In

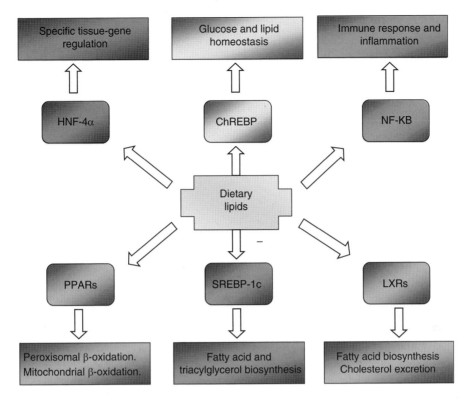

Figure 10.22 Transcription factors and metabolic pathways affected by dietary lipids. ChREBP, carbohydrate response element binding protein; HNF-4, hepatic nuclear factor-4; LXR, liver X receptors; NF-κB, nuclear factor κB; PPAR, peroxisome proliferator receptor; SREBP, sterol response element binding protein.

contrast, these nucleosides decreased the expression and activity of the general upstream stimulatory factor 1 (USF1) and the cAMP response element-binding protein 1 (CREB), glucocorticoid receptor (NR3C1), nuclear factor erythroid (NFE2), NFKB and tumour protein p53. These data suggest that exogenous nucleosides affect the expression and activity of several transcription factors involved in cell growth, differentiation and apoptosis, and in immune response and inflammation.

Glucose, fructose, sucrose, galactose and glycerol increase the expression of lactase in rat jejunum homogenates. Long-chain fatty acids decrease the lactase expression, whereas high-starch diets increase its expression. In mice, the expression of the glucose–sodium cotransporter SGLT1 is increased by dietary carbohydrates and the effect is apparent only in the crypts. In addition high-fructose diets increase the expression of GLUT-5.

Dietary fat plays a key role in the regulation of gene expression in many tissues controlling the activity or abundance of key transcription factors (Figure 10.22). A number of transcription factors, including peroxisome proliferator receptors (PPAR), hepatocyte nuclear factor 4 (HNF4), liver X receptors (LXR), steroid response binding proteins (SREBP) 1a, 1c and 2, and NFκB have been shown to be modulated by dietary fat components, particularly fatty acids and cholesterol, and some of their derivatives, namely eicosanoids and oxidised sterols.

In vivo studies established that PPAR-α- and SREBP-1c-regulated genes are key targets for polyunsaturated fatty acid (PUFA) control of hepatic gene expression. PUFAs activate PPAR-α by direct binding, leading to the induction of hepatic fatty acid oxidation. PUFAs inhibit hepatic fatty acid synthesis by suppressing SREBP-1c nuclear abundance through several mechanisms, including suppression of SREBP-1c gene transcription and enhancement of proteasomal degradation and mRNA SREBP1c decay. Changes in intracellular non-esterified fatty acids (NEFA) correlate well with changes in PPAR-α

Figure 10.23 Regulation of gene expression mediated by vitamin D. AP, alkaline phosphatase; Gla, Galactooxidase; 24-OHase, 24-calciferol hydroxylase.

activity and mRNASREBP-1c abundance. Several mechanisms regulate intracellular NEFA composition, including fatty acid transport, acyl CoA synthetases and thioesterases, fatty acid elongases and desaturases, neutral and polar lipid lipases, and fatty acid oxidation. Many of these mechanisms are regulated by PPARα or SREBP-1c. Together, these mechanisms control hepatic lipid composition and affect whole-body lipid composition.

Changes in diet greatly affect the mucosal immune system and alterations in the luminal environment of the intestine regulate the expression of genes in the enterocyte responsible for signalling to immune cells. Genes expressed by the epithelium orchestrate leukocytes in the lamina propria. For example, chemokine expression in the mouse intestinal epithelium, through transgenic means, induced the recruitment of neutrophils and lymphocytes into intestinal tissues. Diet alters the expression of the genes responsible for signalling by a variety of pathways. The introduction of a normal diet to a weanling mouse up-regulates major histocompatibility complex (MHC) class II expression through a particular iso-

form of the class II transactivator, a protein that acts in the nucleus. Short-chain fatty acid (SCFA) concentrations in the intestinal lumen vary markedly with diet. SCFAs increase IL-8 and insulin-like growth factor binding protein-2 (ILGFBP2) expression by inhibiting histone deacetylase activity in the enterocyte. Down-regulation of gene expression by butyrate can act through acetylation of the inhibitory transcription factor Sp3. Myofibroblasts enhance enterocyte chemotactic activity by cleaving inactive precursors; and myofibroblast genes also are regulated by SCFA.

Vitamins D and A acts as true hormones and their action on the expression of many genes occurs via binding to nuclear receptors in many organs, including the intestine (Figure 10.23). In addition, other vitamins, such as biotin and vitamin B$_6$, are also involved in the regulation of gene expression, and it is well known that metals can influence the regulation of some genes. For example, the post-transcriptional regulation of ferritin and transferrin receptor by dietary iron levels is well recognised.

10.13 The large bowel

Until the 1980s, the large bowel was a relatively neglected organ, once described as a 'sophisticated way of producing manure' which, unfortunately, was inclined to go wrong, resulting in common diseases and disorders such as constipation, ulcerative colitis and colorectal cancer. Fortunately, recent investigations on the aetiology, prevention and treatment of these diseases and disorders have illuminated the structure and function of the large bowel and it is now clear that the colorectum is much more than just the last part of the gastrointestinal tract where stool is formed. From a nutritional perspective, recognition that the primary function of this organ is salvage of energy via bacterial fermentation of food residues has revolutionised understanding of this area of the body. The human body contains about 10^{15} cells, of which only one-tenth are human. The remainder are bacterial cells, most of which are found in the colon, where they dominate metabolic processes. As discussed later, there is emerging evidence that these bacterial cells and their metabolic processes make important contributions to the physiology and health of the human host and may have implications for the development of obesity and of obesity-related diseases.

Structure

The large bowel forms the last 1.5 m of the intestine and is divided into the appendix, cecum, transverse colon, descending colon, sigmoid colon and rectum. It is about 6 cm in diameter, becoming narrower towards the rectum. With the exception of the rectum (the final 12 cm of the intestine), the large bowel has a complex mesentery supplying blood from the superior and inferior mesenteric arteries. Blood drained from the colon reaches the liver via the portal vein. As with the more proximal regions of the intestine, the large bowel has two layers of muscle, an outer longitudinal layer and an inner circular layer, which work together to sequester and move digesta along the tract. Although food residues travel through the small bowel in just a few hours, digesta may be retained in the large bowel for 2–4 days or longer. The colon has a sacculated appearance composed of pouches known as haustra. These are formed by the organisation of the outer longitudinal smooth-muscle layer into three bands called the taeniae coli (which are shorter than the other longitudinal muscles) and by segmental thickening of the inner circular smooth muscles.

The parasympathetic vagus nerve innervates the ascending colon and most of the transverse colon, with the pelvic nerves innervating the more distal regions. There are also connections to the colon from the lower thoracic and upper lumbar segments of the spinal cord via noradrenergic sympathetic nerves.

The mucosa of the colon consists of a single layer of columnar epithelial cells which are derived from stem cells located at or near the base of the crypts. Unlike the small bowel, there are no villi, so that the inner surface of the colon is relatively flat, which may have contributed to the misapprehension that this organ is unimportant in digestion and absorption. There is a higher density of goblet cells than in the small intestine, producing mucus that both protects the colonic surface and coats the increasingly more solid faeces as it is propelled through the large bowel. The water content of the gut decreases from about 85% in the cecum to 77% in the sigmoid colon. Immune protection extends into the large intestine with the presence of gut-associated lymphoid tissue (GALT) in nodules within the mucosa and extending into the submucosa.

Functions of the large bowel

Energy salvage

Many animal species have evolved a symbiotic relationship with microorganisms which allows them to extract energy from food materials that otherwise would be indigestible by the animal's enzymes. This is best exemplified by mammalian herbivores, which may obtain up to three-quarters of their energy as the by-products of anaerobic fermentation in specialised sacs before the gastric stomach (e.g. in ruminants) or in a massively enlarged large bowel (e.g. in equids, members of the horse family). In each case, commensal bacteria (and sometimes other microorganisms, such as protozoa and fungi) proliferate by fermenting plant matter in specialised regions of the intestine that do not secrete digestive enzymes. The energy-containing end-products of this fermentation, principally SCFAs, are absorbed readily and metabolised. For those animals in which fermentation precedes the gastric stomach or where there is ingestion of faeces (best described for lagomorphs such as the rabbit) the bacterial biomass is also an important source of nutrients.

In humans consuming westernised diets, the equivalent of 50–60 g dry weight of food residues and endogenous material dissolved and suspended in approximately 1–1.5 l of fluid flow into the cecum from the ileum every day. For those eating low-fat diets with lots of plant foods rich in carbohydrates, which are poorly, or not at all, digested in the small bowel (e.g. non-starch polysaccharides and resistant starch), considerably more carbohydrate and other energy-containing food components escape into the colon. In a world with an increasing proportion of obese people, loss of this potential energy would not be a problem, but throughout human history shortage of food has been much more common, therefore the ability to salvage as much energy as possible from food will have been an evolutionary advantage and may have made the difference between survival and death. This energy salvage is achieved by bacterial fermentation of carbohydrates and, to a lesser extent, proteins. Bacterial cells make up at least 50% by weight of colonic contents, where they are present at concentrations of about 10^{10}–10^{11} cells/g wet matter. Relatively few bacterial phyla have been found in the human gut with about 90% of the organisms being Firmicutes or Gram-negative Bacteriodetes. However, there are a huge number of individual bacterial species (approximately 2000) in the human gut and this complex microbiota has the ability to hydrolyse much of the polymeric food residues and to ferment the resulting sugars and other small molecules that flow into the large bowel (see Table 10.3 for examples). Until recently, this great diversity of bacterial species, together with the inability to grow some of the organisms in pure culture, has proved a big challenge for conventional bacteriology. However, the application of modern molecular biological techniques, including the use of 16S-rRNA probes and associated bioinformatics tools and databases, has proved very effective in beginning to characterise the colonic microflora.

The virtual absence of oxygen in the anaerobic conditions in the lumen of the large bowel means that the bacterial inhabitants cannot oxidise organic matter using the Krebs cycle and oxidative phosphorylation. Instead, reduced dinucleotides, generated via the glycolytic pathway, are converted to

Table 10.3 Examples of major bacterial species found in the human colon and their characteristic substrates

Bacterial species	Characteristic polymeric substrate
Bacteriodetes	
Bacteroides thetaiotaomicron	Starch
Bacteroides celluloslyticus	Cellulose
Bacteroides ovatus	Xylan
Firmicutes	
Roseburia intestinalis	Xylan, starch
Roseburia inulinivorans	Inulin, starch
Eubacterium rectale	Starch
Actinobacteria	
Bifidobacterium adolescentis	Starch

their oxidised counterparts via metabolism of pyruvate to SCFAs. In this way, most of the energy present in the intractable carbohydrates escaping small bowel digestion is absorbed across the colonic epithelial cells as the SCFAs acetate, propionate and butyrate. SCFA absorption is largely by transcellular mechanisms, including carrier-mediated transport and non-ionic diffusion. Only a very small proportion, usually much less than 5%, of SCFA production is lost in the faeces. The principal gaseous end-products of large bowel fermentation are carbon dioxide, hydrogen and methane, with everyone generating carbon dioxide and hydrogen, but only 30–40% of people producing significant quantities of methane. These gases are released in the flatus (about 500 ml/day) or absorbed and excreted via the lungs.

It appears that the colonic microflora preferentially ferment carbohydrates, switching to proteins and other nitrogenous substrates only in the more distal large bowel when accessible carbohydrates become exhausted. Degradation of the 10–12 g of nitrogenous compounds entering the colon from the small bowel daily yields a range of quantitatively minor end-products, including branched-chain and longer-chain SCFAs, ammonia, hydrogen sulphide, indole, skatole and volatile amines. However, several of these compounds are implicated in colonic diseases; for example hydrogen sulphide is believed to contribute to the aetiology or recurrence of ulcerative colitis, while ammonia and sulphide may play a part in damaging colonocytes, leading to increased risk of colorectal cancer.

Absorption of water and electrolytes

Daily faecal output is highly variable, but is in the order of 100–150 g stool containing about 25 g dry matter. This means that the large bowel absorbs approximately 1 l of water every day. Water is absorbed down an osmotic gradient, mainly from the proximal colon, following the absorption of sodium and chloride ions and of SCFAs. Sodium uptake is driven by an active process powered by a Na^+/K^+-ATPase pump situated on the basolateral membrane of the colonocyte. Chloride ions are absorbed passively in exchange for bicarbonate ions. Water absorption is under both neural (via the enteric nerve plexus) and hormonal control. Aldosterone, angiotensin and the glucocorticoids stimulate water absorption, while the antidiuretic hormone, vasopressin, decreases water absorption. An unpleasant side-effect of treatment with some antibiotics can be the development of diarrhoea as a result of suppression of colonic bacteria and subsequent reduction in SCFA production. However, such observations have led to improved therapies for diarrhoeal diseases. Addition of resistant starch to oral rehydration preparations has been shown to reduce the duration of diarrhoeal episodes. Whilst the mechanism responsible for this improved therapy remains to be confirmed, it seems likely that the absorption of the enhanced SCFA production from starch fermentation results in greater water absorption and so a shorter duration of loose stools.

Lipid metabolism

The most extensively studied aspect of lipid metabolism in the colon is the bacterial transformation of the up to 5% of bile salts that are not absorbed in the ileum. Bile salts are deconjugated (removal of glycine and taurine residues) and, depending on the pH of the digesta (which ranges from about 5.5 in the cecum to 6.5 in the distal colon), the primary bile acids may be converted to secondary bile acids by dehydroxylation. The latter are more lipid soluble and are absorbed by passive diffusion (probably about 50 mg/day) then returned to the liver, where they have an important role in regulating bile acid synthesis. Most of the cholesterol entering the colon is excreted as such in faeces, but some is metabolised to the relatively insoluble derivatives coprostanol and coprostanone, which are not absorbed. The anaerobic nature of the colonic lumen does not allow the oxidation of long-chain fatty acids, which explains why diseases causing fat malabsorption in the small intestine result in greatly increased excretion of fat in the faeces (steatorrhea). A similar effect is seen with anti-obesity drugs such as Orlistat (available on prescription as Xenical or, in some countries, as the over-the-counter preparation sold as Alli), which act by inhibiting gastric and pancreatic lipases. As a result, dietary triacylglycerols flow into the colon and give rise to the well-described side effects of steatorrhea and, in some cases, faecal incontinence. In the anaerobic conditions of the colon, unsaturated fatty acids may be biohydrogenated using the reducing power (H_2) generated as a by-product of carbohydrate fermentation.

Synthesis of vitamins and essential amino acids

Although it has been known for more than 50 years that the bacteria in the large bowel synthesise a wide range of vitamins, in particular several of the B vitamins and vitamin K, there is rather poor understanding of the nutritional significance of this synthesis. In part this is due to the considerable technical difficulty in making quantitative measurements of vitamin absorption from the human colon. The presence of menaquinones (bacterially derived forms of vitamin K) in human blood and tissues attests to uptake of these substances from the human gut, but there is only modest experimental evidence for the frequently cited assertion that about half of vitamin K needs can be obtained by colonic synthesis. The observation that low intakes of folate are associated with an increased risk of colorectal cancer and the accumulating evidence that low folate status can compromise the integrity of the genome are stimulating interest in factors (dietary or otherwise) that may modulate folate synthesis in the large intestine. It is possible that bacterially synthesised folate could be absorbed and utilised by colonocytes (affording protection against colorectal cancer) with or without an impact on folate status elsewhere in the body.

In the same way that colonic bacteria synthesise vitamins for their own use, they synthesise amino acids, including the essential amino acids. Some of the nitrogen required for this synthesis is derived from urea circulating in the bloodstream, which diffuses readily into the bowel where it is hydrolysed by the gut microflora to ammonia. It has been proposed that intestinally synthesised amino acids may make a significant contribution to the amino acid needs of children and adults on very low protein intakes. However, quantifying this contribution remains a tough challenge. The factors that lead to effective salvage by the colon of nitrogen as amino acids are unknown, but may include adequate supplies of ammonia and carbohydrate to stimulate colonic bacterial proliferation. Even if the colonic bacteria can be encouraged to produce extra essential amino acids it is not clear how those amino acids are transferred from the bacteria to, and taken up by, colonocytes. This is an important research area with potentially profound implications for the understanding of colonic physiology and for the derivation of human protein and amino acid needs.

Metabolism and absorption of phytochemicals

The strong epidemiological evidence that those consuming diets rich in vegetables and fruits have a lower risk of developing several common non-communicable diseases, including cardiovascular disease and cancer, has stimulated research on the components of these plant foods that may be protective. There is particular interest in the non-nutrient secondary metabolites of plants described collectively as phytochemicals or phytoprotectants, which have bioactivity when consumed by humans. To be effective in protecting human cells against oxidative damage, for example, these compounds must be released from the plant tissue, absorbed across the intestinal mucosa and transported in sufficient concentrations to their site of action. Disruption of plant cells by cooking may help to release phytochemicals, but for uncooked foods degradation of plant cell walls and release of their phytochemical contents is aided greatly by bacterial fermentation in the colon. Phytochemicals are chemically diverse, but a large proportion are found naturally as glycosides. In many cases, these must be converted to the aglycone derivatives (a process that is accomplished readily by colonic bacteria) before they can be absorbed. Bacterial metabolism is also believed to be responsible for the production of the active derivatives of some phytochemicals. Among the best known are enterolactone and enterodiol, which are oestrogen-like compounds derived by bacterial degradation of the plant lignans matairesinol and secoisolariciresinol, respectively. There is some epidemiological evidence that these lignans may contribute to protection against hormone-related cancers and cardiovascular disease.

Manipulation of the large bowel to enhance or protect health

An unpleasant side-effect of treatment with some antibiotics can be the development of diarrhoea as a result of suppression of colonic bacteria and subsequent reduction in SCFA production. This is one of the most frequent, albeit unwanted, illustrations of the ease with which the colonic flora can be manipulated. The recognition that the balance of microflora within the large bowel may influence health has stimulated attempts to manipulate the flora in health-promoting ways using two main approaches.

Probiotics

A probiotic is a live microbial food ingredient that is beneficial to health. The concept is quite straightforward. All one needs is a 'gut-friendly' bacterium that is both demonstrably safe and beneficial to health and that can be consumed in an attractive food product. Several probiotic products (mostly fermented milk-based products) are on the market in Japan, Europe and elsewhere. Some potential probiotic species may help to overcome pathogenic bacteria such as *Clostridium difficile*, which can become dominant if the endogenous flora is disturbed, such as by the use of broad-spectrum antibiotics. Other potential probiotics are intended to improve immune defences, for example by direct interaction with the GALT or the production of 'protective' end-products such as butyrate. In addition to finding microbes that produce demonstrable benefits to human health *in vivo*, there have been challenges in the development of delivery systems (foods) that have both a good shelf-life and ensure that an appropriate and effective dose of bacteria reaches the large bowel (or other site of activity). Despite these challenges, there is now good evidence that probiotics are effective in the prevention of traveller's diarrhoea and probiotics show promise in the prevention of antibiotic-associated diarrhoea in children. In addition, there is accumulating evidence that probiotics may have a role in alleviating some of the symptoms of irritable bowel syndrome (IBS) but more research is needed to determine the optimal dose of probiotics and the subgroups of IBS patients likely to benefit most.

It is possible using genetic engineering to tailor the potential benefit of probiotic organisms. For example, a food-grade *Lactococcus lactis* was engineered to secrete the anti-inflammatory cytokine interleukin-10 and was as effective as conventional steroid drugs in the treatment of inflammatory bowel disease in mice. Whether such approaches are developed as far as food products will depend on the public's acceptance or otherwise of genetically modified food ingredients and the demonstration that such products are safe and effective for human use.

Prebiotics

Prebiotics are food ingredients that stimulate selectively the growth and activity of bifidobacteria and lactobacteria in the gut and thereby have the potential to benefit health. Given the difficulty of delivering enough 'gut-friendly' bacteria in foods in the form of probiotics, an alternative approach is to augment the numbers of the desired bacteria in the large bowel by supplying them with substrates that give them a competitive advantage. All prebiotics developed to date are relatively small carbohydrates (degree of polymerisation 2–60), which are essentially indigestible by mammalian enzymes and so are delivered in digesta to the colon. There is good evidence that some of these oligosaccharides can produce significant shifts in the balance of bacterial species in the human colon, but how they do so is not yet certain. For example, consumption of 15 g/day of the probiotic oligofructose for 15 days increased bifidobacteria and decreased bacteroides, clostridia and fusobacteria in the faeces (Gibson *et al.*, 1995). Because many of them are present in commonly used foods such as onions and some cereal products, it is probable that such carbohydrates are safe in the amounts likely to be eaten. However, research to obtain sound evidence for the effectiveness of prebiotics in protecting or enhancing health is in its early stages.

Colonic bacteria and obesity

There is growing evidence that the mixture of bacterial species (the microbiome) in the colon of obese people differs from the microbiome of those who are leaner. Obesity is associated with a reduction in bacterial diversity with a lower proportion of bacteriodetes and higher proportion of actinobacteria. At first sight one might imagine that these differences in the microbiome of obese individuals were a conse-quence of different dietary choices or of being obese *per se* but, most intriguingly, it now appears that the large bowel micobiota may play a causal role in the development of obesity. In studies of the large intestinal microflora of genetically obese *ob/ob* mice, lean *ob/+* and wild-type siblings all fed the same diet, the *ob/ob* mice had only half the proportion of bacteriodetes but a greater abundance of firmicutes than their lean siblings. When germ-free mice were colonised with the gut flora from obese mice, they became fatter than equivalent mice colonised by flora from lean animals, which suggests that the microbiota may play a causal role in the development of obesity. The mechanism(s) through which the microbiota may modulate adiposity are poorly understood but the dominant current hypothesis is that the flora associated with obesity are more efficient at harvesting energy from the food residues that flow into the large bowel.

Given the continuing rise in the proportion of the population which is overweight or obese, the discovery that the intestinal flora may contribute to obesity risk opens the way for research on innovative approaches for the prevention or treatment of obesity based on manipulation of the bacteria resident in our colon. It seems likely that this apparent link with obesity risk will be a considerable incentive for the development of better tools for studying the gut microbiota and for systematic study of the consequences of altered flora for human health and well-being. It is well established that differences in food intake are associated with alterations in the balance of species within the microbiota and in the patterns of end-products of large bowel fermentation but there is little understanding of the underlying mechanisms which limit the ability to use food (or food components) to change the flora to improve health. In contrast with the old idea that the colon is simply a 'sophisticated way of producing manure', the current revolution in knowledge about this organ places the colon centre stage in understanding diet and health and further discoveries of its importance are anticipated.

10.14 Future directions

Over the past years, the hypothesis has emerged that digestive end products and/or their metabolic derivatives may regulate pancreatic gene expression directly and independently of hormone stimulation. The quantity, type (mainly degree of unsaturation) and duration of the fat ingested affects the final response. The role of fatty acids in the control of gene expression is now at an early stage of understanding and whether or not this mechanism is related to pancreatic adaptation to dietary fat is unknown and will have to be defined by additional research.

The pancreas appears at present to be an integrated organ in which all the three components (islets, acini and ducts) are anatomically and functionally related. Abundant evidence confirms the influence of the endocrine pancreas on exocrine physiology. The interesting additional possibility is that exocrine cells, in turn, can influence endocrine function. Duct cells can secrete regulatory factors such as cytokines and eicosanoids, which might affect islet cell function, so the hypothesis is worth further investigation.

Current information on developmental gene expression in the intestine as well as the dietary regulation of genes expressed in the developing intestinal epithelium is limited to only a handful of genes, which are primarily highly expressed genes involved in differentiated cellular functions. However, in the future expression patterns of transcriptional regulatory

factors and signalling proteins involved in the regulation of intestinal transcriptomes will enable the assessment of the entire transcriptome of each cell type of the intestinal mucosa.

Further reading

Beger HG *et al*. The Pancreas, 2nd Edn. London: Blackwell, 2008.

Bertelli E, Bendayan M. Association between endocrine pancreas and ductal system. More than an epiphenomenon of endocrine differentiation and development? J Histochem Cytochem 2005; 53: 1071–1086.

Gibson GR *et al*. Selective stimulation of bifidobacteria in the human colon by oligofructose and inulin. Gastroenterology 1995; 108: 975–982.

Jackson AA. Salvage of urea-nitrogen and protein requirements. Proc Nutr Soc 1995; 54: 535–547.

Macfarlane GT, Gibson GR Microbiological aspects of the production of short-chain fatty acids in the large bowel. In Physiological and Clinical Aspects of Short-chain Fatty Acids. (Cummings JH, Rombeau JL, Sakata T, eds). Cambridge: Cambridge University Press, 1995: pp. 87–105.

Sandford PA. Digestive System Physiology, 2nd edn. London: Edward Arnold, 1992.

Smith ME, Morton DG. The Digestive System. Edinburgh: Churchill Livingstone, 2001.

Steidler L et al. Treatment of murine colitis by Lactococcus lactis secreting interleukin-10. Science 2000; 289; 1352–1355.

Tilg H, Moschen AR, Kaser A. Obesity and the microbiota. Gastroenterology 2009; 136: 1476–1483.

11
The Cardiovascular System

Gabriele Riccardi, Angela A Rivellese and Christine M Williams

Key messages

- Raised plasma low-density lipoprotein (LDL) cholesterol, raised triacylglycerol (TAG), raised blood pressure and reduced levels of high-density lipoprotein (HDL) cholesterol are established independent risk factors for cardiovascular disease (CVD).
- Raised levels of the clotting factors (factor VII, fibrinogen and von Willebrand factor) and reduced activation of the fibrinolytic system (tissue plasminogen activator and plasminogen activator inhibitor-1) have been shown to be independent risk factors for CVD.
- Diabetes and visceral obesity are associated with an increased risk of CVD due in part to elevated glucose levels and the blood lipoprotein abnormalities that occur in insulin resistance.
- There is general agreement that a reduced intake of saturated fat is essential to decrease LDL cholesterol levels and related cardiovascular risk. Replacing saturated fat with monounsaturated or

n-6 polyunsaturated fatty acids (PUFA) induces a similar decrease in LDL cholesterol.
- Among the different types of fatty acids, long-chain n-3 fatty acids, at a dosage of 2–3 g/day, have the most relevant hypotriacylglycerolaemic effect. Modest intakes of long-chain n-3 PUFA significantly reduce the risk of CVD without affecting plasma lipid levels.
- Carbohydrate increases plasma TAG, but dietary fibre counteracts this negative effect.
- *Trans*-fatty acids have a clear negative effect on HDL cholesterol; replacing dietary fat with dietary carbohydrates reduces HDL levels; moderate alcohol intake raises them.
- A combination diet that includes increased fruit and vegetables, reduced salt and reduced total and saturated fat intakes has a more powerful effect on blood pressure than a single-nutrient intervention.

11.1 Introduction

Epidemiological research in the 1950s began to show quite clearly that diseases of the vascular system, particularly coronary heart disease and stroke, have a strong root in lifestyle factors. As our knowledge of epidemiological predictors of heart disease, now referred to as risk factors, grew, so too did our understanding of how specific nutrients can influence their manifestation. This chapter aims to provide the reader with an overview of this large and complex topic. The first part of the chapter examines pathophysiological aspects of the cardiovascular system, while the second part examines the roles of specific nutrients in modifying the risk factors for cardiovascular disease (CVD).

Section 11.2 discusses the physiological factors involved in maintaining a healthy vascular system and which, by definition, lead to morbidity and mortality

when they operate outside the norms of physiology. Section 11.3 examines the pathology of CVD and the concept of risk factors, and Section 11.4 describes the manner in which each of the factors involved in vascular function contributes to risk of disease. Subsequent sections examine the role of individual dietary components in CVD. The key areas of metabolism that need to be considered when studying nutrition and the cardiovascular system are plasma lipids, blood pressure, endothelial function, the haemostatic and fibrinolytic pathways, and insulin sensitivity.

11.2 Factors involved in a healthy vascular system

Lipids [cholesterol, triacylglycerol (TAG) and phospholipids] are transported in blood plasma as lipoprotein particles, consisting of a neutral lipid core

Nutrition and Metabolism, Second Edition, edited by S. A. Lanham-New, I. A. Macdonald and H. M. Roche. © 2011 The Nutrition Society.

(TAG and esterified cholesterol) surrounded by a coating of the more hydrophilic phospholipids and free cholesterol (Figure 11.1). The lipoproteins present in plasma are of varying density and size according to the relative amounts of lipid and protein present in the particle (Table 11.1). Cholesterol is carried in the smaller, denser particles, low-density lipoprotein (LDL) and high-density lipoprotein (HDL) cholesterol. TAG is carried in the larger, less-dense particles, very low-density lipoprotein (VLDL) and chylomicrons. Because raised levels of LDL cholesterol and TAG, and reduced levels of HDL cholesterol, have been identified as risk factors for

cardiovascular disease, an understanding of their normal metabolism is important to appreciate the way in which diet and other lifestyle factors can influence the circulating concentrations of these lipoprotein particles.

Low-density lipoprotein metabolism

LDL particles are largely formed within the circulation from VLDL particles secreted by the liver (Figure 11.2). Through the action of lipoprotein lipase (LPL, an enzyme present in muscle and adipose tissue), TAG is progressively removed from the VLDL particle. The fatty acids that are released by the action of the lipase are taken up and used as an energy substrate by tissues (especially skeletal and cardiac muscles) or are stored within adipose tissue. This progressive removal of TAG from the core of the VLDL particle leads to the formation of a smaller, more cholesterol-rich particle, sometimes referred to as intermediate-density lipoprotein (IDL). IDL may be removed from the circulation by the liver or, by the further action of LPL, may be converted to LDL cholesterol. The essential function of LDL is the transport of cholesterol to peripheral tissues for the formation of cell membranes and synthesis of steroid hormones. LDL formed from VLDL and IDL is taken up by specific receptors (LDL or apoB/E receptors) present on all cell membranes. When the levels of cholesterol within cells are high, the LDL receptors are reduced in number (down-regulated) to prevent excessive uptake of cholesterol. Under such

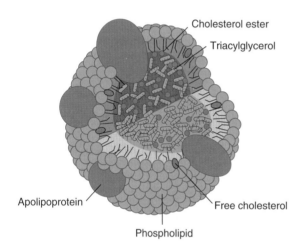

Figure 11.1 Diagrammatic representation of a typical lipoprotein particle showing the major lipid and protein components.

Table 11.1 Characteristics of the major lipoprotein classes

Fraction	Diameter (nm)	Site of synthesis	Function of major lipids	Major apolipoproteins	Composition (% by weight)			
					Protein	TAG	TC	PL
Chylomicron	80–1000	Gut	Transport of dietary fat	B48, A1, A2, C	1	90	5	4
VLDL	30–80	Gut, liver	Transport of endogenous fat from liver	B100, C	10	65	13	13
LDL	20–22	Capillaries of peripheral tissue, liver	Transport of cholesterol to peripheral tissues	B100	20	10	45	23
HDL	9–15	Gut, liver	Removal of cholesterol from peripheral tissues to liver	A1, A2, C	50	2	18	30

TAG, triacylglycerol; TC, total cholesterol; PL, phospholipid; VLDL, very low-density lipoprotein; LDL, low-density lipoprotein; HDL, high-density lipoprotein. The proportions shown are approximate only and vary within each major class.

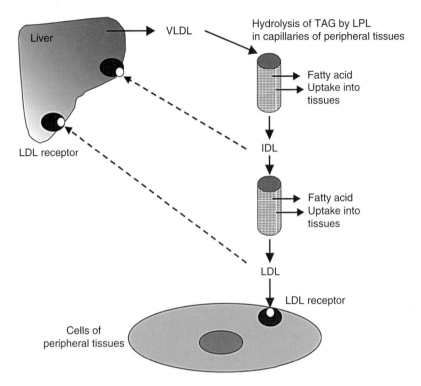

Figure 11.2 Pathway of low-density lipoprotein (LDL) metabolism from production of very low-density lipoprotein (VLDL) particles in liver, their hydrolysis by lipoprotein lipase (LPL) in capillaries of peripheral tissues with progressive removal of triacylglycerol (TAG) to form intermediate-density lipoprotein (IDL) and then LDL. LDL is removed from circulation via LDL receptors on all cell membranes, with the highest density of receptors found in the liver.

circumstances, LDL particles remain within the circulation. It is clear from this that the major factors that will determine the concentration of LDL in the circulation are:

- the rate of formation of VLDL and its conversion to LDL in the circulation
- the density of the LDL receptor on cell membranes.

Since half of the body's LDL receptors are present in the liver, it follows that hepatic LDL receptor density is a major determinant of circulating LDL concentrations. The majority of cholesterol carried by LDL is endogenously synthesised in the liver. The rate-limiting enzyme in cholesterol biosynthesis, 3-hydroxy-3-methylglutamyl-coenzyme A (HMG-CoA) reductase, can be regulated to a very significant extent by a family of drugs known as statins, as well as by dietary fats. Another route to the lowering of blood cholesterol is the plant sterols, which are not capable of being incorporated into micellar lipid and thus create a pool of unabsorbed lipid in the distal gut in which some ingested cholesterol becomes trapped. Equally, gut sequestration of bile acids by dietary fibre disrupts the enterohepatic recirculation of bile acids back to the liver and thus requires a greater diversion of hepatic cholesterol to bile acids. This reduces the flow of hepatic free cholesterol to LDL cholesterol for export to plasma.

High-density lipoprotein metabolism

Precursor HDL particles are formed in the small intestine and the liver, and consist of small amounts of cholesterol and phospholipid complexed with a transport protein, apolipoprotein A1 (apo A1). HDL particles play a central role in reverse cholesterol transport (Figure 11.3), whereby cholesterol is transported back from peripheral tissues to liver for oxidation and removal. Although peripheral cells can synthesise cholesterol, they are unable to oxidise the

Figure 11.3 Major steps in reverse cholesterol transport. Small high-density lipoprotein (HDL) receives free cholesterol secreted by peripheral cells. By the action of lecithin cholesterol acyl transferase (LCAT), free cholesterol is esterified on HDL to form the large HDL particle. HDL returns cholesterol to the liver, either directly via uptake on HDL receptors or indirectly via transfer of cholesterol onto very low-density lipoprotein (VLDL) and chylomicron (CM) remnant particles in exchange for triacylglycerol (TAG). The latter step is catalysed by cholesterol ester transfer protein (CETP), a circulating enzyme associated with lipoprotein particles. Cholesterol-enriched VLDL and CM remnants are taken up by remnant receptors or by the low-density lipoprotein (LDL) receptor on the liver.

cholesterol molecule. Excess cholesterol is therefore removed from cells and transported to the liver for oxidation and excretion via reverse cholesterol transport. This is one of the prime functions of the HDL particle. Cells secrete excess cholesterol in the free unesterified form. This is initially taken up by the precursor HDL particle. By the action of lecithin cholesterol acyl transferase (LCAT), a fatty acid (usually linoleic acid) is removed from lecithin and transferred to cholesterol on HDL, forming the more stable and hydrophobic cholesterol ester, which migrates to the hydrophobic HDL core. HDL, now enriched with cholesterol ester, can be removed directly by the liver through the action of a putative receptor that has not yet been isolated. However, an alternative and more active pathway appears to be the transfer of cholesterol ester from HDL onto the TAG-rich particles, VLDL and CMs. In return, TAG is transferred onto the HDL particles. The reciprocal transfer of cholesterol ester and TAG between HDL

and TAG-rich particles is catalysed by the action of cholesterol ester transfer protein (CETP). The cholesterol ester that is transferred onto VLDL and chylomicron particles is rapidly removed by the liver when these particles are taken up by hepatic receptors. Because the remnants of VLDL and chylomicron particles are removed by the liver via high-throughput remnant receptors as well as by the LDL receptor, this mechanism provides a very efficient means of returning excess cholesterol to the liver for excretion. In simple terms the HDL particle uses the TAG-rich particles as vehicles for transferring the excess cholesterol removed from cells back to the liver for conversion to bile acids.

Very low-density lipoprotein and chylomicron metabolism

For convenience it is useful to consider the metabolism of chylomicron particles as the exogenous pathway and of VLDL particles as the endogenous

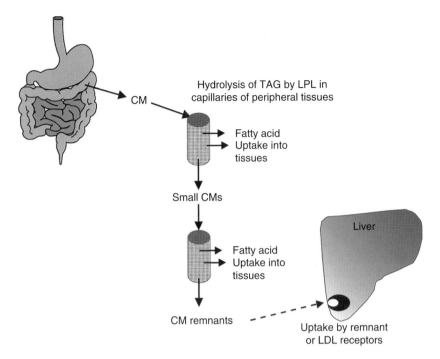

Figure 11.4 Outline of the exogenous pathway of triacylglycerol (TAG) metabolism. Chylomicron (CM) particles are formed in the enterocyte following the digestion and absorption of dietary fat and are secreted for 4–8 h after a fat-containing meal. The particles are hydrolysed by lipoprotein lipase (LPL, present on the capillary lining of blood vessels supplying adipose tissue, skeletal muscle and heart), with removal of TAG and eventual removal of smaller delipidated particles (remnants) via specific remnant receptors or by the low-density lipoprotein (LDL) receptor.

pathway, although in essence they form part of a continuous common transport system for TAG-rich lipoproteins.

Exogenous pathway

Dietary TAG is hydrolysed in the small intestine to form free fatty acids and monoacyl glycerol. Once absorbed across the brush-border membrane of the enterocyte, monoacylglycerol and free fatty acids are re-esterified to form TAG. The mature chylomicron particle is formed when TAG combines with cholesterol and the transport protein apo B-48 in the endoplasmic reticulum. A surface coating of phospholipid and free cholesterol increases the water solubility of the particles, which are then secreted into the lacteals and, via the lymphatic system, enter the blood circulation via the thoracic duct. It is clear from this account that dietary fat, unlike other digested nutrients, does not enter the circulation via the portal vein and liver, but bypasses the liver and enters directly from the gut. This means that dietary TAG can be directly taken up from the circulating chylomicron particles into adipose tissue, skeletal and cardiac muscle (Figure 11.4). These tissues possess LPL. Following a fat-containing meal the amount of LPL on adipose tissue capillary endothelial cell membranes is increased (by the action of insulin). This activates the enzyme and allows hydrolysis of TAG on chylomicron particles. The particles become progressively smaller as TAG is gradually removed. Eventually the action of lipoprotein lipase on chylomicrons is terminated and the smaller particles, known as chylomicron remnants, are removed by the liver via the remnant or the LDL receptors. Whereas this is the pathway followed by most dietary fatty acids, the medium-chain and short-chain fatty acids ($\leq$ C12: 0) pass directly to the liver in the portal vein rather than being absorbed via the lymphatic system. This is a consequence of their higher water solubility and, thus, the complex pathway for water-insoluble fatty acids is not needed. It follows that these fatty acids do not contribute to the increase in blood TAG (postprandial lipaemia) that occurs following ingestion of a fat-containing meal.

Endogenous pathway

The endogenous pathway of TAG metabolism involves the hepatic synthesis, secretion and subsequent metabolism of the VLDL particles. VLDL synthesis is stimulated in the liver by increased availability of free fatty acids (FFA). Increased FFA delivery to the liver occurs either in the fed state, when large amounts of FFA are being released from circulating chylomicrons, or in the fasted state, when there is breakdown of stored TAG from adipose tissue. The FFA are delivered to the liver and through the action of insulin are re-esterified to TAG. As in the enterocyte, the TAG combines with cholesterol and a specific apolipoprotein (in this case apo B-100), together with a surface coating of phospholipid and cholesterol ester, to form the mature VLDL particles. The secretion of VLDL is regulated by insulin, being inhibited by high levels of insulin and stimulated when insulin levels begin to fall. Following a meal, therefore, increased secretion of VLDL tends to occur 2–3 h after meal consumption when insulin levels are beginning to fall.

In the fasted state most of the circulating TAG-rich particles are VLDL. In the fed state after a fat-containing meal, chylomicrons begin to enter the circulation within 30 min and reach their highest concentration 2–4 h after the meal. During this time, VLDL secretion tends to be low owing to the high circulating insulin concentrations. However, as insulin falls the secretion of VLDL particles from the liver increases and these particles become the dominant TAG-rich particle in the late postprandial stage after a meal. VLDL metabolism is very similar to that outlined for chylomicrons above. VLDL particles are hydrolysed by LPL. Hydrolysis of TAG and uptake of FFA into tissues proceeds in the same way as for chylomicrons, but VLDL appear to be a better substrate for skeletal muscle lipase than for adipose tissue. Partial removal of TAG results in the formation of the VLDL remnant (also known as IDL); complete removal leads to the formation of circulating LDL as outlined in the section above (Figure 11.2).

Blood pressure

Blood pressure is the force that causes blood to flow through the arteries and capillaries, and finally via the veins back to the heart. Blood pressure is maintained by regulation of cardiac output and peripheral resistance at the arterioles, postcapillary venules and heart. Blood pressure is regulated by central as well as peripheral neuronal mechanisms, by capillary fluid shifts and by central and local hormone secretions. The kidney also contributes to maintenance of blood pressure by regulating blood volume. The autonomic nervous system is the most rapidly responding regulator of blood pressure and receives continuous information from the baroreceptors (pressure-sensitive nerve endings) situated in the carotid sinus and the aortic arch. This information is relayed to the vasomotor centre in the brainstem. A decrease in blood pressure causes activation of the sympathetic nervous system, resulting in increased contractility of the heart (via β-adrenoceptors) and vasoconstriction of both the arterial and venous side of the circulation (via α-adrenoceptors). The capillary fluid shift mechanism refers to the exchange of fluid that occurs across the capillary membrane between the blood and the interstitial fluid. This fluid movement is controlled by the capillary blood pressure, the interstitial fluid pressure and the colloid osmotic pressure of the plasma. Hormonal mechanisms operate in various ways to maintain blood pressure, including vasoconstriction, vasodilatation and alteration of blood volume. The principal hormones involved in raising blood pressure are epinephrine and norepinephrine, secreted from the adrenal medulla in response to sympathetic nervous system stimulation. They increase cardiac output and cause vasoconstriction and act very rapidly. Renin release from the kidney increases in states such as hypotension because of both sympathetic nerve stimulation of the kidneys and a reduction in glomerular filtration. Renin stimulates the conversion of angiotensinogen to angiotensin, both in the circulation and in vascular tissue. Plasma angiotensin is converted in the lung to angiotensin II, which is a potent vasoconstrictor. In addition, angiotensin II stimulates the production of aldosterone from the adrenal cortex, which decreases urinary fluid and electrolyte (sodium) loss from the body. The kidneys help to regulate the blood pressure by increasing or decreasing the blood volume via alterations in water and sodium reabsorption in the kidney tubules, and also by the renin–angiotensin system, and are consequently the most important organs for long-term blood pressure regulation.

The vascular endothelium

Damage to the vascular endothelium appears to be the unifying pathophysiological event through which the adverse effects of raised circulating blood lipids, glucose, homocysteine and thrombotic factors result in atherosclerosis and thrombosis. The vascular endothelium should be considered not only as a barrier against large circulating molecules, but also as an organ regulating vascular tone through its response to, and production of, vasodilator and vasoconstrictor substances. Moreover, it regulates the balance between thrombosis and fibrinolysis, and platelet aggregation, through the production of prostacyclin and other bioactive substances. The adhesion of monocytes to the endothelium is mediated in part through the presence of adhesion molecules [intercellular adhesion molecule-1 (ICAM-1), vascular cell adhesion molecule (VCAM)] on the surface of the endothelial cell. The key regulatory component of the endothelial cell is nitric oxide (NO), the production of which is central to all of the above functions. NO is formed from L-arginine by nitric oxide synthase. NO is a vasodilator, it inhibits platelet aggregation and smooth muscle cell proliferation and reduces adhesion of monocytes to the endothelium. When there is impaired endothelial function, the vasodilatory response to standard drugs is impaired; this is now used as a dynamic *in vivo* measure of endothelial dysfunction. Other measures of endothelial dysfunction include measurement of circulating proteins that are derived from the endothelium [e.g. endothelin, von Willebrand factor (vWf), ICAM-1, VCAM and plasminogen activator inhibitor-1 (PAI-1)].

The haemostatic system

The haemostatic system coordinates a finely regulated series of reactions that occur at the surface of damaged blood vessels to reduce or terminate bleeding following tissue injury. Cessation of bleeding occurs via three overlapping pathways. First, there is adhesion and aggregation of blood platelets at the site of injury. Secondly, there is conversion of soluble protein fibrinogen to its insoluble product, the fibrin fibril, by activation of the clotting pathway and generation of the clotting enzyme, thrombin, which in turn triggers platelet activation and aggregation. Finally, the fibrin fibrils cross-link with the aid of factor XIII (FXIII), thereby 'wringing' the clot of plasma and increasing its firmness by retraction. The cessation of clot formation is achieved via activation of another pathway, the fibrinolytic pathway, which prevents excessive clot formation in response to activation of the clotting cascade.

The following sections outline the major steps involved in coagulation, platelet aggregation and fibrinolysis.

Coagulation (clotting) pathway

As shown in outline in Figure 11.5, this pathway comprises two separate activation pathways (the intrinsic and extrinsic pathways), which feed into the final common pathway leading to thrombin generation and fibrin production. Although the pathways are activated separately there are many cross-reactions between them that provide autoregulation.

The extrinsic and final common pathways

The main trigger of coagulation is a protein called tissue factor, which is exposed on the blood vessel wall when there is injury. Cellular tissue factor then initiates coagulation through interactions with a circulating clotting protein called factor VII (FVII). Once FVII binds to accessible tissue factor it undergoes a single cleavage that converts it to its active enzyme, FVIIa (the 'a' suffix indicates the activated state). Cleavage is performed either by autoactivation (by FVIIa already present and bound to tissue factor) or by activated factor IX (FIXa) or activated factor X (FXa). Coagulation occurs when the initial stimulus is sufficient to cause conversion of activity in the pathway from a basal or steady state to a 'cascade' of activation. As amplification occurs at each step of the pathway, one molecule of FVIIa–tissue factor complex is responsible for many thousands of molecules of thrombin generated from prothrombin. Thus, in secondary haemostasis, FVIIa–tissue factor activates FIX and FX. Plasma FIXa, with its cofactor vWf (VIIIa), also activates FX. Plasma FXa, with its cofactor factor Va, then cleaves prothrombin to thrombin.

The intrinsic pathway and the contact system

The four proteins of the contact system are factor XII (FXII), factor XI (FXI), prekallikrein (PK) and high molecular weight kininogen (HMK). The proteins play major roles in coagulation, with their activation

Figure 11.5 Outline of the intrinsic and extrinsic pathways of coagulation. Exposure of blood to negatively charged non-membranous surfaces activates the intrinsic pathway. The extrinsic pathway is activated when blood comes into contact with cell membranes, exposing tissue factor (TF). The sequence of protein activations are dependent on phospholipids and take place on cell membrane surfaces. HMK, high molecular weight kininogen; TM, thrombomodulin. 'a' denotes the enzyme product of the inactive precursor protein.

at negatively charged surfaces leading to formation of FXIIa and FXIa. Likely activators of the intrinsic pathway include collagen (like tissue factor, collagen is exposed on blood-vessel walls on tissue damage), heparans and FFA. Surface-bound FXIa then activates FIX, and FIXa will activate FVII and FX. *In vitro* studies show long-chain saturated fatty acids such as stearate (C18) to be potent activators of the intrinsic system, while unsaturated fatty acids such as oleate are ineffective.

Platelets

Platelets are formed from the megakaryocytes of the bone marrow, each of which releases about 4000 platelets on maturation. On stimulation, platelets form aggregates as a result of exposure, on their surface membranes, of binding sites that allow adjacent platelets to adhere to one another. The exposure of

'sticky' binding sites on the platelet comes about as the result of activation of platelet receptors by aggregating factors (thrombin, collagen), clotting factors (vWf, fibrinogen) and inhibitors. Running through the platelet is an open canalicular system of invaginated plasma membrane, thus increasing the effective platelet surface area many-fold. In the platelet interior are dense granules packed with adenosine diphosphate (ADP) and serotonin. Other granules (α-granules) contain many compounds, including platelet-derived growth factor (PDGF), fibrinogen, vWf and factor V. Adhesion of platelets to the endothelium triggers intracellular signals, which result in release of active compounds (e.g. ADP) that release the contents of the granules, promote striking shape change and favouring aggregation. For example, collagen binding and binding of thrombin to its platelet receptors trigger platelet synthesis of

Figure 11.6 Outline of the role of homocysteine in the remethylation pathway. The vitamin B_{12}-dependent enzyme methionine synthase catalyses the methylation of homocysteine to methionine. Conversion of methionine to S-adenosylmethionine and its subsequent demethylation to S-adenosylhomocysteine generate methyl groups essential to the synthesis of phospholipids, DNA, etc. Further methylation of homocysteine required to sustain the remethylation pathway is through the action of methylene tetrahydrofolate reductase (MTHFR), which generates the methyl donor 5-methyltetrahydrofolate from 5,10-methylene tetrahydrofolate. The latter is in turn dependent on the dietary supply of folic acid.

prostaglandins from membrane arachidonic acid. The product, thromboxane A_2, initiates the release reaction, thereby encouraging aggregation of activated platelets. With sustained activation, a plug of aggregated platelets incorporating fibrin and entrapped red and white blood cells results in the formation of a clot or thrombus.

Fibrinolytic pathway
The fibrinolytic pathway operates as a feedback system to prevent excessive activation of fibrinogen and regulate the extent of clot formation. The main regulatory steps lead to the conversion of inactive plasminogen to the active enzyme, plasmin, which activates the breakdown of fibrin. Plasminogen activation is achieved by a number of different plasminogen activators, the most important of which is tissue plasminogen activator (tPA), the release of which from vascular endothelial cells is stimulated by a variety of agents. When a fibrin clot is evolving, tPA and plasminogen bind sequentially to fibrin, thereby providing the conditions for rapid generation of plasmin. By the lytic action of plasmin, a complex

array of fibrin and fibrinogen degradation products is generated and clot formation terminated. An important regulatory component of this complex system is PAI-1, activation of which prevents conversion of plasminogen to plasmin, thereby reducing fibrinolysis.

Homocysteine

Homocysteine is a sulphur-containing amino acid found in all cells, where it plays a role in the generation of methyl groups, which are required for a range of essential functions, particularly in DNA synthesis. Its relevance with respect to the functioning of the cardiovascular system is that elevated levels of homocysteine appear to cause damage to the vascular endothelium and may play a primary role in initiating the damage that leads to atherosclerosis. Homocysteine is an intermediate in one-carbon metabolism, lying between two connected metabolic cycles (remethylation and trans-sulphuration). In the remethylation reaction (Figure 11.6), homocysteine accepts a methyl group from methyl tetrahydrofolate to form methionine. Methionine, in turn, is converted to *S*-adenosylmethionine (SAM), which is the main donor of methyl groups in the synthesis of DNA, proteins and phospholipids. The micronutrients folic acid and vitamin B_{12} play an important part in this cycle, folate as a component part of methyl tetrahydrofolate, and vitamin B_{12} as a cofactor for the enzyme methionine synthase, the enzyme that catalyses the remethylation step. Another enzyme, methylene tetrahydrofolate reductase (MTHFR), plays an important role by supplying methyl tetrahydrofolate for the remethylation step.

Insulin sensitivity

Insulin is a metabolic hormone secreted by the β-cells of the pancreas in response to food ingestion. The main stimulus for insulin release is the increase in blood glucose that occurs within a few minutes of ingesting a carbohydrate-containing meal. Insulin has a wide variety of actions on cellular glucose metabolism (see Chapter 5), but its main effects are to decrease blood glucose following a meal, thereby maintaining circulating glucose concentrations within narrow normal limits (4–10 mmol/l). However, insulin also has important effects on protein metabolism – stimulating its synthesis and inhibiting its catabolism – and on lipid metabolism. Through its actions in stimulating hydrolysis of circulating TAGs, and uptake of the released FFAs into adipose tissue, skeletal and cardiac muscle, this hormone plays a central role in maintaining plasma TAG concentrations within normal limits during the fasted and postprandial states (0.5–4 mmol/l).

11.3 Pathogenesis of cardiovascular disease

Atherogenesis is a very complex and slowly progressive process involving several pathophysiological systems, on which both genetic and environmental factors act. This process occurs in the intima and media of large and medium-sized arteries and leads to the formation of focal lesions (plaques), which might be complicated by intraplaque haemorrhage, rupture and overimposed thrombosis that causes ischaemia in the region supplied by the artery.

In the twentieth century, two major hypotheses – the thrombogenic and the lipidic – were postulated for the origin of CVD. The two theories can be unified into a single multifactorial theory involving one common step represented by endothelial dysfunction. This widely accepted theory is generally called the response to injury hypothesis and its main steps are summarised in Figure 11.7. Different risk factors (hyperlipidaemia, LDL oxidation, hypertension, etc.) induce endothelial injury, leading to compensatory responses that alter the normal homeostatic functions of the endothelium. This occurs particularly at certain areas of the coronary tree such as the branching points, where blood turbulence is high. In particular, a variety of forms of injury increase the permeability of the endothelium to lipids and proteins, and increase the adhesion to monocytes and platelets. This in turn induces the endothelium to have procoagulant instead of anticoagulant properties and to form vasoactive molecules, such as cytokines and growth factors, which promote the migration and internalisation of monocytes and proliferation of vascular smooth-muscle cells. These, together with increased lipid accumulation and increased connective tissue synthesis, lead to the formation of atheromas. If the atherogenic process continues, there will be cycles of accumulation and activation of mononuclear cells, migration and proliferation of smooth-muscle cells with cell necrosis and formation of fibrous tissue, which eventually lead to the formation of advanced lesions, the fibrous atheromas. Fibroatheromas grow slowly and can induce arterial stenosis, but often represent an unstable lesion that can be complicated by intraplaque haemorrhage and rupture. Plaque rupture is followed by blood entry into the plaque core from the lumen, with activation of platelets and the coagulation cascade. This leads to the formation of a thrombus, which can cause acute ischaemia. The primary cause of arterial thrombosis involves tissue factors, which are present in normal adventitia and atherosclerotic plaques and which, as mentioned in the previous sections, are able to initiate the extrinsic clotting cascade. The general hypercoagulable or prothrombotic state of subjects with atherosclerosis is of great importance in the final stages leading to myocardial infarction or stroke. As a consequence, these individuals have increased plasma levels of clotting factors (fibrinogen, factor VII, vWf), enhanced platelet reactivity and reduced fibrinolysis.

When the arterial lumen is significantly narrowed or closed following the progressive increase in arterial

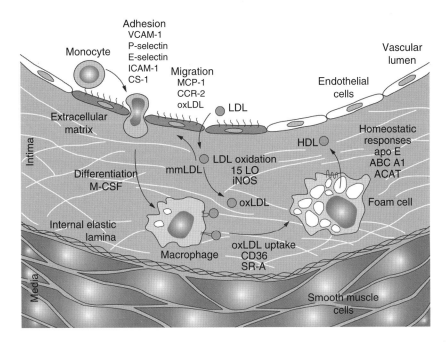

Figure 11.7 The response to injury hypothesis. LDL, low-density lipoprotein; HDL, high-density lipoprotein; VCAM-1, vascular cell adhesion molecule-1; ICAM-1, intercellular adhesion molecule-1; CS-1, connecting segment-1; MCP-1, monocyte chemoattractant protein-1; CCR-2, chemokine receptor-2; M-CSF, macrophage-chemokine stimulating factor; 15 LO, 15 lipoxygenase; iNO,: inducible nitric oxide synthatase; apoE, apolipoprotein E; MMLDL, minimally modified LDL: ABC A1, ATP binding cassette A1; ACAT, acylcholesterol acyltransferase; SR-A, scavenger receptor A. (Reprinted from Cell, 104(4) Glass CK, Witztum JI, Atherosclerosis: the road ahead, 503–516 Copyright © (2001), with permission from Elsevier.)

stenosis or, more frequently, the formation of thrombus, atherosclerosis becomes clinically manifest: depending on the arteries involved in this process, the individual will suffer from myocardial or cerebral infarction, peripheral vascular disease or mesenteric ischaemia. The progression of the atherosclerotic lesions throughout life is highly variable, partly because of the presence and severity of different cardiovascular risk factors.

Cardiovascular risk factors

The term cardiovascular risk factor is used to identify factors predicting an increased likelihood of developing CVD. Many of these factors have been identified (Table 11.2); some of these factors are modifiable (lifestyle, e.g. diet, exercise and smoking), while others are not (gender, age and genetic traits). The following section will focus on the main cardiovascular risk factors and their normal physiology and metabolism. Section 11.5 will consider the extent to which specific nutrients influence the functioning of these risk factors.

Table 11.2 Risk factors for cardiovascular diseases

Untreatable	Potentially treatable
Men	Cigarette smoking
Age >45 years for men, after menopause for women	Dyslipidaemia: increased cholesterol, fasting and postprandial triacylglycerol, low-density and very low-density lipoproteins levels, decreased high-density lipoprotein levels
Genetic traits	Oxidisability of low-density lipoproteins
	Obesity, especially visceral obesity
Psychosocial	Hypertension
Low socio-economic class	Hyperglycaemia, diabetes and the metabolic syndrome
Stressful situations	Prothrombotic factors
Coronary-prone behaviour patterns, type A behaviour	High homocysteine levels
	Lp(a)
	Subclinical inflammation

11.4 Risk factors for cardiovascular disease

Plasma cholesterol and cardiovascular disease risk

Increased plasma cholesterol levels, particularly LDL cholesterol, are undoubtedly one of the most important risk factors for CVD. This is true not only for very high cholesterol levels, such as those occurring in genetically determined lipid disorders (familial hypercholesterolaemia, familial combined hyperlipidaemia, type III hyperlipidaemia), but also in a large majority of people (about half the adult population in high-risk countries) with only moderately high plasma cholesterol levels. Familial hypercholesterolaemia is a rare genetic condition caused by a defect in the gene that codes for the LDL receptor. Homozygous individuals have no LDL receptors, while heterozygotes have half the normal number of LDL receptors. Because the hepatic LDL receptors are reduced in number or absent, these individuals cannot regulate their circulating LDL levels and develop extremely high plasma LDL cholesterol concentrations at a very young age. However, in most individuals raised levels of LDL cholesterol are determined by an interaction between genetically transmitted, but relatively minor, metabolic abnormalities (often multiple genes are involved) and lifestyle-related factors (polygenic or common hypercholesterolaemia). All the cross-sectional and prospective studies on this topic have clearly shown that the association between plasma total cholesterol levels and coronary heart disease (CHD) mortality is very strong, is independent of other risk factors and is characterised by increased risk with increasing plasma cholesterol concentrations, starting even at 'low' cholesterol levels. The causal relationship with atherosclerosis has also been proven by the fact that interventions that reduce total and LDL cholesterol significantly reduce total and CHD mortality.

Although the concentration of LDL in the circulation is important in determining its uptake into the endothelium, other factors, including the oxidative modification of LDL in the arterial wall, appear to be just as important. LDL particles are taken up by macrophages, especially after being oxidised or otherwise modified, and may then be deposited in the arterial intima, thus leading to the formation of atheroma.

Thus, oxidation and other modifications of LDL seem to play an important role within the pathogenic mechanisms of atherosclerosis. The dietary relevance of oxidised LDL is clear, since the capacity of LDL to resist oxidation is dependent on the type of fatty acids present and the antioxidant content of the particle.

High-density lipoprotein cholesterol and cardiovascular disease risk

The inverse association between HDL cholesterol levels and incidence of CVD has so far been confirmed by many cross-sectional and prospective studies. Low HDL levels are now considered a strong risk factor for CVD and the LDL:HDL cholesterol ratio a much stronger predictor of risk than an elevated LDL cholesterol level alone. However, it should be stated that low HDL levels often occur along with moderately raised plasma TAG and, indeed, a low HDL level may be a marker for the presence of the metabolic syndrome. This is a syndrome that is characterised by a collection of abnormalities, including raised blood glucose, raised TAG, low HDL, visceral obesity and raised blood pressure. The underlying cause of the abnormalities appears to be insulin resistance, whereby increased secretion of insulin fails to return circulating glucose and TAG to normal concentrations owing to resistance to the actions of insulin in peripheral cells and the liver (see Chapter 16).

A complete identification of the mechanisms through which HDL protects against CVD is lacking, although it is clear from the account of the role of HDL in maintaining normal reverse cholesterol transport (Section 11.2) that reduced circulating levels of HDL will have severely compromised the ability to maintain cellular and circulating cholesterol homeostasis. In particular, there will be reduced ability to remove excess cholesterol from cells leading to accumulation of cholesterol in peripheral cells. There is also evidence that HDL acts as an antioxidant and protects LDL from oxidation.

Plasma triacylglycerol and cardiovascular disease risk

Many studies have shown an association between high levels of plasma TAG and CVD. However, what has been disputed over the years is whether hypertriacylglycerolaemia represents a risk factor independent of other factors that are often associated with it (e.g. obesity, hyperglycaemia, low HDL cholesterol levels, hypertension, abnormalities in coagulation factors). The role of TAGs as an independent risk factor seems more consistent in people with diabetes. Moreover, in cross-sectional and prospective studies, higher levels of TAGs and chylomicron remnants in the postprandial period have been found to be associated with higher risk of CHD. In particular, two recent very large prospective studies have clearly shown that postprandial TAG levels (2–4 h after a meal) are associated with a higher risk of cardiovascular events, more than fasting TAG and independently of other cardiovascular risk factors.

Intervention trials have shown that hypertriacylglycerolaemia is indeed an important modifiable risk factor. There are a number of mechanisms by which elevated plasma TAG may lead to an increased risk of CVD. Some studies have shown that chylomicron and VLDL remnants that are enriched with cholesterol can be taken up by monocytes in a similar manner to LDL and form the characteristic foam cell of the atherosclerotic lesion. However, elevated TAG levels have also been shown to lead to adverse changes in LDL and HDL cholesterol via excessive transfer of TAG onto the HDL and LDL particles via the CETP-catalysed reaction (Figure 11.3). When LDL and HDL acquire large amounts of TAG from the TAG-rich lipoproteins, the TAG undergoes hydrolysis by the hepatic lipase. Removal of TAG from LDL and HDL leads to the formation of small dense LDL and HDL particles. Small dense HDL particles are rapidly catabolised by the liver, leading to reductions in circulating HDL concentrations. Conversely, small dense LDL is poorly recognised by the normal LDL receptor and remains in the circulation longer than normal. Because of its smaller size and longer half-life, small dense LDL is more able to penetrate the endothelium and contribute to atherogenesis.

Many studies have shown raised levels of fasting and postprandial TAG, small dense LDL and lowered levels of HDL in type 2 diabetes and in subjects with insulin resistance. These abnormalities in lipoprotein concentration and composition are likely to be the one of the main causes of the greater risk of CVD that is associated with these conditions. The atherogenic consequences of raised plasma TAG therefore include direct atherogenic effects of chylomicron and VLDL remnant particles, reduced levels of HDL and raised levels of the atherogenic small dense LDL. In addition to these atherogenic actions, raised TAG, particularly in the postprandial state, may be prothrombotic since it has been shown to lead to the activation of factor VII, part of the extrinsic pathway of blood clotting.

Blood pressure and cardiovascular disease risk

High blood pressure is a reversible risk factor for CVD for which a strong causal relationship has been found. The positive relationship between both systolic and diastolic blood pressure and CVD is found not only among hypertensive individuals but also among those considered to be normotensive. Studies have suggested that even small reductions in blood pressure can have large beneficial effects on the risk of CVD. The relationship of blood pressure to CVD risk is important with respect to potential preventive nutritional strategies, since high blood pressure is one of the 'deadly quartet' of visceral obesity, hyperlipidaemia, hypertension and hyperinsulinaemia that make up the metabolic syndrome. This syndrome has repeatedly been linked with modern lifestyles characterised by high levels of stress, inappropriate diets and lack of exercise. The well-known roles of ions such as sodium, potassium, calcium, magnesium and chloride in regulating blood volume, vascular tone and membrane ion-channel activity also indicate the potential role of micronutrients as well as macronutrients in blood-pressure regulation.

Diabetes, the metabolic syndrome and cardiovascular disease risk

Diabetic patients are characterised by very high cardiovascular risk. Hyperglycaemia and, in particular, other cardiovascular risk factors – in primis dyslipidaemia and hypertension – are very often present in these patients, and contribute to their very high cardiovascular risk. Individuals with the metabolic syndrome also have a high cardiovascular risk. It is still debated whether this high risk is only due to the clustering of the cardiovascular risk factors characterising this syndrome or also to insulin resistance *per se*, which is considered one of the main pathogenetic mechanisms leading to the metabolic syndrome. As a matter of fact, visceral obesity, insulin resistance and hyperglycaemia are all associated with a pro-inflammatory state activated by adipocyte hypertrophy in visceral adipose tissue (release of macrophage chemoattractant proteins) and by the proinflammatory activity of raised FFA plasma levels. In the presence of a pro-inflammatory state, atherogenesis is accelerated as a consequence of the endothelial dysfunction induced by c-reactive protein and other inflammatory cytokines. Moreover, atherosclerotic plaques become enriched with macrophages, thus becoming more instable and, therefore, leading to higher risk of cardiovascular events.

Endothelial dysfunction and cardiovascular disease risk

Because endothelial dysfunction is an important early step in atherogenesis, measurement of endothelial function *in vivo* is being studied as a means of risk assessment. Some of the early studies indicate that these new measurements may prove useful in identifying subjects at risk of CVD, but it is not yet known whether they will prove to be more valuable than the conventional risk factors such as serum cholesterol and blood pressure that are currently used.

Homocysteine and cardiovascular disease risk

Very high homocysteine levels, due to inborn errors of the metabolism of this amino acid, cause severe atherosclerosis with clinical manifestations at a very early age. However, the importance of more moderately raised levels of homocysteine as a risk factor for CVD remains uncertain. Although retrospective epidemiological studies have suggested a strong association between raised homocysteine and CVD risk, recent prospective studies suggest that the risk may be smaller. The issue is important for the dietary prevention of CVD since moderate hyperhomocysteinaemia is due in part to inadequate dietary intake of folic acid and vitamins B_6 and B_{12}. The adverse effects of low folate intakes appear to be particularly important for those individuals (30% of most populations) who carry a variant form of the MTHFR enzyme and who demonstrate elevated homocysteine levels. The exact mechanism by which elevated homocysteine levels may cause vascular disease are uncertain but may involve disruption of normal endothelial physiology. The endothelial dysfunction leads to multiple biological effects as described above, including abnormal vasoconstriction, platelet aggregation, monocyte adhesion and procoagulation.

Coagulation, platelets and fibrinolytic factors and cardiovascular disease risk

Prospective epidemiological studies have shown that raised concentrations of specific clotting and antifibrinolytic factors are predictive of CHD. Plasma FVIIc has been found to be a marker of risk of fatal, but not non-fatal, CVD. Many studies have found plasma fibrinogen concentration to be a strongly positive predictor of CHD, and vWf has also been shown to be an independent risk factor in a number of studies. Elevated levels of these clotting factors in people at risk of CVD are believed to reflect a prothrombotic state that could contribute to their increased risk. In the fibrinolytic system, both low tPA and high PAI-1 are risk factors for CHD. Both are believed to be markers of hypofibrinolysis.

Although the platelet plays a central role in thrombosis, and platelet hyperactivation is believed to be one of the mechanisms involved in inducing a prothrombotic state, platelet hyperreactivity is not established as a strong risk factor, largely because of difficulties in carrying out measurements of platelet aggregability *in vitro*.

11.5 Dietary components and their effect on plasma lipids

Cholesterol levels

The effects of different dietary components on plasma cholesterol levels have been studied for many years, so a large body of data exists in the literature on the effect of different types of nutrients on plasma cholesterol (Table 11.3). However, many of these studies, especially the older ones, have only taken into account the effects of diet on total plasma

Table 11.3 Effects of different dietary components on low-density lipoprotein (LDL) cholesterol

Nutrients	Effect on LDL cholesterol
Saturated fatty acids	↑↑
Trans-fatty acids	↑↑
Dietary cholesterol	↑
Plant sterols	↓
MUFA	—
n-6 PUFA	↓ (high amounts)
n-3 PUFA	↑ (high amounts)
Soy protein	↓ —
Carbohydrate	—
Fibre	↓↓
Alcohol	—

↑, increase; ↓, decrease; —, no effect. MUFA, monounsaturated fatty acid; PUFA, polyunsaturated fatty acid.

cholesterol, without differentiating between the cholesterol present in LDL and that present in HDL. This is of fundamental importance, as indicated in the previous section, since the two lipoproteins have opposite effects on CVD.

Saturated fatty acids

Epidemiological studies have consistently shown that the intake of saturated fatty acids is directly correlated with plasma cholesterol levels and with mortality from coronary artery disease. All the intervention studies performed on humans since the early 1950s have shown that saturated fatty acids are the key dietary factor responsible for increased plasma cholesterol, and that this effect is largely due to increased LDL cholesterol. Although the increase in LDL cholesterol during high saturated fat diets is greater in subjects with higher baseline cholesterol levels, it is still of significance even in normocholesterolaemic individuals.

Recently there has been increased emphasis on the possible difference between the individual saturated fatty acids and plasma cholesterol fractions. Among the saturated fatty acids, the most hypercholesterolaemic are C14:0 (myristic acid) and C16:0 (palmitic acid), while stearic acid (C18:0) appears to be neutral or even hypocholesterolaemic. However, this evidence is based on a limited number of studies and requires further research before conclusions can be drawn and recommendations made. The ability of saturated fatty acids to raise LDL cholesterol levels appears to be due to the effect of these fatty acids in

regulating the expression of the LDL receptor on hepatic cell membranes. When levels of these fatty acids in hepatic cell membranes are high there is down-regulation of the LDL receptor protein and thus a reduced rate of removal of LDL from the circulation. The neutral or even hypocholesterolaemic effect of stearic acid seems to be due to its high rate of conversion to 20:1 monounsaturated fatty acid.

Unsaturated fatty acids

In the past 30 years, many intervention studies have been performed to investigate the possible hypocholesterolaemic effect of the unsaturated fatty acids [monounsaturated fatty acids (MUFA) and n-6 polyunsaturated fatty acids (PUFA)]. From the results of these studies some definite conclusions can be drawn. Both MUFA and PUFA are able to reduce total and, in particular, LDL cholesterol. It is now possible to derive equations that predict the hypocholesterolaemic effect of MUFA or n-6 PUFA. According to these equations, if 10% of the dietary energy derived from SFA were replaced by MUFA or n-6 PUFA, LDL cholesterol would decrease by 0.39 mmol/l (15 mg/dl) and by 0.42 mmol/l (18 mg/dl), respectively. Therefore, the effects of MUFA and PUFA on LDL cholesterol are quite similar.

In relation to the effects of long-chain n-3 PUFA on LDL cholesterol, a review of all the controlled studies performed clearly showed that doses of approximately 3 g/day of n-3 PUFA given as supplements increase LDL cholesterol by 5–10%, especially in hypertriacylglycerolaemic patients. These responses have also been reported in healthy people and may be more common in certain susceptible genotypes. These reported LDL-raising effects of n-3 PUFA have been observed with fish oil supplements but not with fish. Nevertheless, whether intakes of the long-chain n-3 PUFA are increased via fish or fish oils, pronounced cardiovascular benefits of modest increases in intakes of long-chain n-3 PUFA have been observed in secondary prevention trials. Two recent studies have shown that intakes of approximately 1 g/day of long-chain n-3 PUFA reduce the rate of cardiovascular mortality by 30–45%. In both studies there were very limited effects on plasma lipid levels and the decreased risk of cardiovascular mortality was probably due to the beneficial influence of n-3 PUFA on thrombosis or on cardiac arrhythmias.

Unlike saturated fatty acids, which cause down-regulation of the LDL receptor and reduced rates of LDL removal from the circulation, unsaturated fatty acids increase the expression of the LDL receptor protein, causing a greater rate of removal of LDL from the circulation. In this respect, unsaturated fatty acids act like the statin drugs, which lower LDL cholesterol through their actions on genes that regulate hepatic lipid metabolism. These drugs reduce rates of hepatic cholesterol synthesis and increase rates of LDL removal from the circulation by up-regulation of the LDL receptor.

Trans-fatty acids

Trans-unsaturated fatty acids are produced in the rumen during ruminant fermentation and are therefore found in meat and dairy products. They are also produced commercially in large quantities by partial hydrogenation of vegetable oil in the preparation of shortening and margarine.

All the metabolic studies on *trans*-fatty acids have clearly shown that they significantly increase LDL cholesterol levels and decrease HDL cholesterol levels. A meta-analysis of all these studies indicates that replacing 1% of dietary energy derived from oleic acid or polyunsaturated fats with *trans*-fatty acids induces an average LDL cholesterol increase of about 0.05 mmol/l (2 mg/dl) and, contrary to what happens with saturated fatty acids, a significant decrease also of HDL cholesterol levels. These two opposite effects imply an increase in the LDL:HDL cholesterol ratio (Table 11.3), with possible effects in increasing the risk of CHD, as reported by both cross-sectional and prospective studies.

Dietary cholesterol

Prospective studies have shown a positive significant correlation between cholesterol intake and CHD mortality, which is partly independent of plasma cholesterol levels. Several intervention studies on humans have evaluated the effects of dietary cholesterol on lipid metabolism, and the most consistent results on LDL levels can be summarised as follows.

There is great variability among individuals. Some people are able to reduce their endogenous cholesterol synthesis in response to an increase in cholesterol intake, without changing their levels of LDL cholesterol (the 'compensators'). Others do not have this ability and their plasma cholesterol levels increase after a cholesterol-rich diet (the 'non-compensators'). Unfortunately, there are no simple markers, clinical or otherwise, that allow these two types of individuals to be differentiated. Moreover, for very high levels of dietary cholesterol (>850–1000 mg/day), the ability of compensators to maintain normal plasma cholesterol levels may be overcome.

In practice, high levels of dietary cholesterol are generally associated with high levels of saturated fat and often the more powerful effect of the latter is dominant. The increase in LDL cholesterol in response to a diet high in cholesterol is usually more consistent in high-risk individuals, such as hyperlipidaemic and diabetic patients.

Besides dietary cholesterol, plant sterols and their saturated derivatives – stanols – may reduce LDL cholesterol levels (a 5–10% reduction with an intake of 2 g/day) since they are poorly absorbed and are able to inhibit cholesterol absorption.

Carbohydrates and dietary fibre

Carbohydrates do not have a direct and independent effect on LDL cholesterol and therefore it can be said that they are 'neutral' in this respect. However, foods rich in carbohydrates represent one of the easiest ways to replace saturated fats and are thus very important for practical reasons. On the other hand, dietary fibre, which is naturally present in carbohydrate-rich foods, has a direct hypocholesterolaemic effect. In fact, the studies performed either with diets naturally rich in fibre, especially soluble fibre, or with different types of fibre added to foods (guar, psillium, oats, etc.) have consistently shown that dietary fibre *per se*, independently of other dietary changes, is able to reduce LDL cholesterol. This happens mainly because dietary fibre is able to reduce cholesterol absorption and bile acids reabsorption in the intestinal lumen. The hypocholesterolaemic effect of dietary fibre is present in healthy people, patients with hyperlipidaemia and those with diabetes, and is still more evident in patients with both hyperlipidaemia and diabetes.

Proteins

In the context of dietary proteins and lipid metabolism, a brief mention of soy protein is merited. A meta-analysis on this topic has indicated that soy protein has a mild lowering effect on LDL cholesterol in hypercholesterolaemic subjects, while in those with normal lipid values there is an irrelevant effect.

Dietary composition and plasma triacylglycerol levels

Fatty acids

Among the fatty acids, the most relevant hypotri-acylglycerolaemic effect is observed with the long-chain n-3 fatty acids. In fact, supplementation with long-chain n-3 fatty acids (even by as little as 2–3 g/day) can reduce TAG levels by 25–30% in both normoli-pidaemic and hyperlipidaemic individuals. The precursor n-3 fatty acid (α-linolenic acid, present in some plants and oils) is also able to reduce TAG levels, although the magnitude of the effect seems smaller. Long-chain n-3 fatty acids have also been reported to reduce the postprandial lipaemic response, with a reduction particularly in chylomi-cron and chylomicron remnants. The effects of the other fatty acids on postprandial lipaemia are less well defined; however, the available evidence indicates that the amount of fat, rather than its composition, is the most important determinant of postprandial chylomicron response. Chronic and acute ingestion of food enriched with saturated fat produces enhanced postprandial lipaemia in comparison with MUFA and n-6 PUFA. Only a few studies have compared these two types of fatty acid (MUFA versus n-6 PUFA) on postprandial lipaemia, and their results are variable.

Carbohydrates and dietary fibre

The majority of intervention studies that have examined the effect of high-carbohydrate, low-fat diets on plasma TAG levels have shown that such diets lead to an elevation of plasma TAG. This is accompanied by a fall in plasma HDL levels and an increase in the percentage of LDL as small dense particles. It is important to note that whereas the majority of studies have recorded these effects, not all have done so. It is also important to note that these effects occur with diets varying in the ratio of simple to complex carbohydrates. These potentially adverse effects of high-carbohydrate, low-fat diets have led many eminent nutritionists to advocate a more vigorous pursuit of changing the composition of the dietary fat, while paying less attention to changing total fat level. However, the potential adverse effects of low-fat, high-carbohydrate diets should be seen in the wider context of public health nutrition strategies to reduce CVD. An increase in physical activity, a reduction in body-fat content and increased intake of long-chain

Table 11.4 Effects of different dietary components on plasma triacylglycerol (TAG)

	Fasting TAG	Postprandial TAG
Saturated fatty acids	—	↑
MUFA	—	?
n-6 PUFA	↓	?
n-3 PUFA	↓↓	↓
Carbohydrate	↑	↑
Fibre	—	or ↓↓
Alcohol	↑	↑

↑, increase; ↓, decrease; —, no effect; ?, no sound data. MUFA, monounsaturated fatty acid; PUFA, polyunsaturated fatty acid.

n-3 PUFA will all lead to reduced TAG levels and increased HDL levels, thus overcoming the effect observed in narrow, single-factor intervention studies. No doubt this area will be one to watch for the future.

Dietary fibre does not seem to have direct effects on TAG levels. However, it counteracts the possible negative effect of carbohydrates on trygliceride metabolism. Moreover, a diet rich in carbohydrates and rich in fibre is able to reduce postprandial TAG response. The data on dietary effects on TAG are summarised in Table 11.4.

Diet and high-density lipoprotein cholesterol levels

In comparison with the effects of diet on LDL cholesterol, less is known of the influence of dietary components on HDL cholesterol, since little attention has been paid to this powerful cardiovascular risk factor until recently (Table 11.5).

Fatty acids

Saturated fatty acids, considered as a group or as individual fatty acids, do not reduce HDL cholesterol and most studies show that saturated fats increase this cholesterol fraction. However, these data have to be seen in the context of the very deleterious effects of saturated fatty acids on LDL cholesterol. In contrast, *trans*-fatty acids have a combined negative effect on both LDL and HDL cholesterol, since they increase the former and reduce the latter.

MUFA and n-6 PUFA have almost comparable effects on HDL cholesterol, based on studies in which moderate amounts of PUFA have been used (<10% of total energy intake). In fact, with higher levels of PUFA in the diet (>10%, an amount no longer recommended because of a putative effect on

Table 11.5 Effects of different dietary components on high-density lipoprotein (HDL) cholesterol

Nutrients	Effect on HDL cholesterol
Saturated fatty acids	↑
Dietary cholesterol	— or ↑
MUFA	—
Trans-fatty acids	↓
n-6 PUFA	↓ (high amount)
n-3 PUFA	—
Carbohydrate	— or ↓
Fibre	—
Alcohol	↑

↑, increase; ↓, decrease; —, no effect. MUFA, monounsaturated fatty acid; PUFA, polyunsaturated fatty acid.

Table 11.6 Nutritional recommendations for the treatment of hyperlipidaemia

Saturated fat	<7% of total calories
Monounsaturated fat	15–20% of total calories
Polyunsaturated fat	≤10% of total calories
Total fat	30–35% of total calories
Cholesterol	<200 mg/day
Carbohydrate	50–60% of total calories
Fibre	30 g/day
Protein	≈15% of total calories
Total calories[a]	Balanced between energy intake and expenditure to maintain body weight/prevent weight gain

National Cholesterol Education Programme (NCEP), Adult Panel Treatment III. The National Heart, Lung and Blood Institute.
[a] Daily energy expenditure should include at least moderate physical activity, contributing approximately 200 kcal/day.

carcinogenesis and gallstones), reductions in HDL cholesterol have been observed. Finally, n-3 fatty acids, both long and short chain, do not seem to have significant and relevant effects on HDL cholesterol levels.

Carbohydrate and dietary fibre

In contrast to what happens with plasma TAG levels, the effects of dietary carbohydrate on HDL cholesterol levels are quite variable. However, in general, the isocaloric replacement of dietary fat with carbohydrate leads to a reduction in HDL. The magnitude of the reduction probably depends on the type of carbohydrate (carbohydrate with high glycaemic index versus carbohydrate with low glycaemic index). In support of this observation, a prospective study in a middle-aged population has shown that a higher glycaemic index of foods consumed is the only independent determinant of lower HDL cholesterol levels. In this context, dietary fibre influences HDL cholesterol indirectly through its effect on the glycaemic index of the foods.

Alcohol and plasma lipids

The effects of alcohol on plasma lipids are quite contradictory. On the one hand, alcohol increases plasma TAG levels (a negative effect). On the other, it increases HDL cholesterol levels (a positive effect). The latter effect seems to be one of the possible mechanisms accounting, at least in part, for the protective effect of moderate alcohol consumption on the risk of CHD that has been shown in many epidemiological studies.

Taking into account the energy intake deriving from alcohol and its possible influence on plasma TAG levels and body weight, a moderate consumption of alcohol (two or three drinks/day) may have beneficial cardiovascular effects by means of the increased HDL levels that it causes.

On the basis of the effects of the different dietary components on plasma lipids so far reviewed, nutritional recommendations for the treatment of hyperlipidaemia have been given, and these are summarised in Table 11.6.

11.6 Diet and blood pressure

Hypertension is one of the major cardiovascular risk factors, and many intervention studies have clearly shown that reducing blood pressure leads to a significant reduction in the incidence of CHD, congestive heart failure, stroke and renal disease, and mortality rates.

The prevalence of hypertension in Western countries is very high, with about 50–60% of individuals above 55 years being classified as hypertensive (systolic/diastolic blood pressure >[ησ]140/90). Although genetic, hormonal and metabolic factors play a significant role in determining who will become hypertensive, lifestyle factors contribute strongly to the high prevalence of hypertension. This section will focus on the possible role of micronutrients and macronutrients on blood pressure regulation.

Dietary macronutrient composition and blood pressure

Fat, particularly the type of fat rather than the total amount consumed, seems to be the most important macronutrient in relation to blood pressure regulation. All of the available evidence (cross-sectional studies and controlled clinical trials) fails to support any relationship between average total fat intake and average blood pressure. However, there is evidence that n-3 PUFA and MUFA have some influence on blood pressure. Supplementation with n-3 fatty acids reduces blood pressure in hypertensive subjects but not in normotensive ones. For significant effects to occur, doses above 3.3 g/day are needed, and this intake can only be achieved through n-3 fatty acid supplementation.

Data on MUFA are somewhat contradictory, as some show a blood pressure reduction in both hypertensive and normotensive individuals, and others no effect. However, a recent multicentre intervention trial has shown a significant reduction of systolic and diastolic blood pressure (an average of 3 mmHg) in healthy normotensive people when moderate amounts of saturated fat were replaced with monounsaturated fat.

There are various possible explanations for the blood pressure-modulating effects induced by the different types of fat: the incorporation of unsaturated fat into lipid cell membranes increases the membrane permeability, thereby stimulating sodium and cation transport. Increased synthesis of related prostaglandins, with a possible influence on factors such as arterial vasodilatation, electrolyte balance and renal renin secretion, may also play a role.

Besides the type of fat, dietary fibre may have some effects on blood pressure. Two metaanalyses show a significant reduction of blood pressure, particularly systolic blood pressure, with increased intake of dietary fibre. This effect is more evident in hypertensive individuals.

Moreover, some epidemiological and intervention studies have provided evidence that dietary proteins also have a beneficial effect on blood pressure. This effect could be due to the degradation of some proteins into peptides with antihypertensive properties such as those deriving from milk and dairy products, which may act through angiotensin-converting enzymes inhibition.

Alcohol and blood pressure

All of the available evidence shows that there is a significant direct relationship between alcohol intake and blood pressure, with an increase especially for intakes above three or four drinks per day. As a reduction in alcohol intake improves blood pressure, the recommendation for the management of hypertension is to limit daily alcohol intake to no more than 30 ml for men and 15 ml for women.

Minerals and blood pressure

Sodium intake

Epidemiological studies have shown a positive association between dietary salt intake, blood-pressure levels and the prevalence of hypertension. Most intervention trials indicate that a reduction in salt intake significantly reduces both systolic and diastolic blood pressure. This effect is more evident in hypertensive, diabetic, obese and elderly subjects, and in certain populations such as African–Americans, while it is less evident in normotensive people. Some studies in normotensive people failed to find a significant reduction in diastolic blood pressure, but it is important to remember that the response to salt intake reduction is highly variable among individuals and this different response may be modulated by genetic factors. Considering all the available evidence, the recommendations are to reduce sodium intake to no more than 100 mmol/day (approximately 6 g of sodium chloride or 2.4 g/day of sodium).

Potassium intake

Epidemiological studies show an inverse correlation between blood-pressure levels and potassium intake. Almost all of the intervention trials performed have shown a significant reduction in systolic and diastolic blood pressure with potassium supplementation. Again, as for salt, this effect is more evident in hypertensive than in normotensive people and in studies where participants were accustomed to high salt intake. Potassium may act on blood-pressure regulation through its natriuretic effect or its possible effect on vascular smooth-muscle cells.

The daily dietary recommended intake for potassium is generally 120 mmol/day (4.7 g/day).

Calcium intake

Calcium supplementation has not been shown to have a significant effect on blood-pressure reduction in subjects with adequate calcium intake. However, epidemiological studies have shown an inverse association between calcium intake and blood pressure, and some of the beneficial effects of dairy products on blood pressure levels may be mediated through their high calcium content.

Multiple dietary changes and recommendations

Since a variety of macronutrients and micronutrients is involved in the regulation of blood pressure, it is likely that a 'combination diet' that includes changes in overall dietary habits could have a more powerful effect on blood pressure than the modulation of individual dietary constituents. This hypothesis has been validated by the Dietary Approaches to Stop Hypertension (DASH) study, where a diet rich in fruit and vegetables (to increase potassium and fibre intake), low in saturated and total fat, and rich in low-fat dairy products (to increase calcium intake and dairy peptides) was able to decrease significantly systolic and diastolic blood pressure, compared with a 'Western' diet, in both normotensive and mildly hypertensive individuals. It has been shown that if these combined diets also include a reduction in salt intake, systolic and diastolic blood pressure can be reduced even further.

11.7 Effects of dietary factors on coagulation and fibrinolysis

While it is probable that diet interacts with both coagulation and fibrinolysis, the exact nature of this is not yet completely understood. Much of the information in relation to the effect of dietary factors on coagulation and fibrinolysis derives from animal studies and epidemiological observations. To date, few properly controlled human dietary intervention studies have examined the effect of dietary components on haemostasis. Many of the human studies provide conflicting results. These divergent results probably reflect the fact that many studies have used different biochemical indices to measure coagulation and fibrinolysis. In addition, the assays used to measure coagulation and fibrinolysis are rather crude and it is unlikely that they reflect the true state *in vivo*. For example, platelet aggregation is often measured in platelet-rich plasma, but *in vivo* platelet aggregation is a very complex process that represents the interaction of the platelet with several other components of

the blood and the vascular endothelium. The effect of dietary fat on coagulation and fibrinolysis has been widely studied, but there is little consistent information in relation to the effects of other nutrients and non-nutritive food components. Dietary intervention studies show that dietary fatty acids have a minimal effect on plasma fibrinogen levels. It has been shown that very high intake of saturated fat, particularly stearic acid, induces a modest increase in plasma fibrinogen concentrations, but the biological significance of this effect is questionable. Epidemiological studies have shown a negative relationship between plasma fibrinogen and n-3 PUFA intake. Several intervention studies investigated the potential effects of increasing dietary n-3 PUFA in lowering fibrinogen levels, but the results have been inconsistent.

In contrast, several epidemiological and human intervention studies have shown a consistent effect of dietary fat on coagulation factor VII. The level and activity of factor VII are affected by the amount of dietary fat consumed. It is reduced by low-fat diets and increased when high-fat diets are consumed. Factor VII activity is also related to postprandial lipid metabolism, whereby it is activated during the postprandial state following the ingestion of a meal containing fat. This effect is probably related to the presence of greater levels of TAG-rich lipoproteins (chylomicrons and VLDL), which provide a surface capable of activating the protein. Dietary fatty acid composition may also affect factor VII activity. Although short-term experiments show little effect, there is evidence from longer human dietary intervention studies that habitual high intake of saturated fat increase factor VII, compared with monounsaturated fat. There is considerable variability in terms of how studies have measured factor VII, and not all assays reflect the true state *in vivo*. Factor VII assays can measure the amount of the protein or the activation status; the latter is probably more relevant since it is only the active proportion of factor VII that contributes to coagulation.

Fibrinolysis is influenced by dietary factors, particularly by dietary fat. tPA is a major initiator of fibrinolysis in the normal circulation. It binds to the fibrin in a clot and promotes the generation of plasmin, which promotes clot dissolution. tPA activity is increased by a low-fat, high-fibre diet. In general, dietary fat composition does not have a major influence on tPA activity. Conversely, dietary fat composition has important effects on PAI-1. PAI-1 is increased by a high intake of n-3 PUFA and decreased when the diet is rich in oleic acid. PAI-1 activity is also increased by dietary carbohydrate intake, more if the carbohydrate-rich foods have a high glycaemic index.

Platelets are important contributors to both coagulation and fibrinolysis. Platelet procoagulant activity, also called platelet factor 3, is closely related to platelet aggregation. Dietary fatty acid composition can have significant effects on platelet membrane fatty acid composition. For example, n-3 PUFA supplementation will lead to a significant increase in platelet phospholipid eicosapenatenoic and docosahexaenoic acids levels. There is no doubt that altered platelet membrane fatty acid composition affects the activation of coagulation and fibrinolysis, nevertheless the exact nature of this is not fully understood. However, there is some evidence that saturated fatty acids promote a prothrombotic state. Again, the true nature of this effect is unknown because it is very difficult to measure platelet activity *ex vivo* in a manner that accurately reflects the *in vivo* situation.

11.8 Homocysteine

Homocysteine is a central metabolic intermediate in the metabolism of sulphur-containing amino acids. Homocysteine, which is formed as a result of the breakdown of dietary methionine, can be converted to either methionine (by the remethylation pathway) or cysteine (by the *trans*-sulphuration pathway) (Figure 11.6). These pathways are dependent on up to four B-vitamins: folate, vitamin B_{12}, vitamin B_6 and riboflavin. In recent years, evidence has been accumulating implicating elevated plasma homocysteine (hyperhomocysteinaemia) as an independent risk factor for occlusive CVD.

The causes of hyperhomocysteinaemia are both nutritional and genetic. In the extreme, patients with rare inborn errors of metabolism that impair *trans*-sulphuration (cystathionine β-synthetase deficiency) have profoundly elevated homocysteine in plasma and urine (homocysteinuria), and develop occlusive vascular disease in early adulthood or even childhood. Although such inborn errors are extremely rare, genetically inherited functional variants of the enzymes involved in homocysteine metabolism are commonly found in the general population, and are associated with mild to moderate elevations in homocysteine. However, the most common cause of elevated homocysteine is low status of one or more of the B vitamins associated with its metabolism.

Vitamin therapy with folic acid, alone or in combination with vitamins B_6 and B_{12}, and dietary supplementation with cereal products fortified with these vitamins can significantly lower plasma homocysteine levels. As a consequence of the introduction of a mandatory folic acid fortification policy in the USA, plasma homocysteine levels in the population have declined considerably in recent years.

However, the intervention studies so far carried out with supplements of folic acids in combination with vitamins B_6 and B_{12} do not show any benefits in terms of cardiac event reduction.

11.9 Diet and antioxidant function

As a by-product of oxygen metabolism and transport, the cells of the human body produce oxidants – reactive oxygen species (ROS) – that damage biological macromolecules such as DNA, proteins, lipids and carbohydrates. However, cells also contain complex defence systems against the actions of ROS, comprising different antioxidants, some of endogenous origin (superoxide dismutases to remove the superoxide anion, enzymes for removing hydrogen peroxide and organic peroxides, such as glutathione peroxidase) and some derive from the diet (e.g. vitamins C and E, β-carotene). In general, there is a balance between oxidant production and antioxidant defence: the imbalance between the two induces 'oxidative stress', which is now considered to be a very important process in the development of atherosclerosis. Oxidised LDL, more than native LDL, is involved in several steps of atherosclerosis, such as endothelial injury, monocyte chemotaxis, perturbation of vascular tone, growth factor synthesis and antibody formation. Moreover, aside from LDL oxidation, oxidative stress could be important in the development of atherosclerosis through other mechanisms, such as activation or repression of gene expression, apoptosis and cell death. Lipoprotein oxidation, in particular the susceptibility of LDL to oxidation, may be influenced also by the type of the diet, in particular by the type of fats. The few studies performed on this topic have shown that a diet rich in n-6 polyunsaturated fat increases *ex vivo* LDL oxidation in comparison to monounsaturated fat, which is more stable and, therefore, less liable to be oxidised. The few data on the effect of n-3 polyunsaturated fat on LDL oxidation are very discordant, as some of them show no effect and others increased or even decreased *ex vivo* susceptibility of LDL to oxidation. It should be stated that, although the role of LDL oxidation in the pathogenesis of atherosclerosis is well accepted, there is much debate as to the physiological relevance of *ex vivo* measurements of LDL oxidation and its use as a risk for CVD.

If oxidative stress is so important, the supply of antioxidants through the diet, as well as the choice of nutrients capable of reducing oxidation, could be crucial in the prevention of CVD. The antioxidant hypothesis proposes that antioxidant vitamins may slow the progression of atherosclerosis by blocking the oxidative modification of LDL cholesterol and thus decreasing its uptake into the arterial lumen. The most important dietary antioxidants are vitamins C and E and β-carotene (provitamin A). All of these vitamins are able to reduce oxidation of LDL *in vitro*, but their effectiveness in preventing CVD is yet unresolved. Most observational epidemiological studies support a cardioprotective effect of carotenoids and vitamin E, whereas the relationship between vitamin C intake and the risk of heart disease is weak and inconsistent. However, intervention studies with vitamin E and β-carotene, both in primary and secondary prevention, have failed to show a significant benefit of these vitamins taken as a dietary supplement for the prevention of CHD.

11.10 Insulin sensitivity

Diet composition and insulin sensitivity

The effects of insulin on lipid, carbohydrate and protein metabolism depend not only on insulin concentrations at the level of the target organ, but also on the cells' ability to transmit insulin signalling (insulin sensitivity). Impaired insulin sensitivity not only is associated with type 2 diabetes but also facilitates the occurrence of metabolic abnormalities and CVD risk factors that, in turn, predispose to ischaemic cardiovascular disease (the metabolic syndrome). Weight reduction represents the most effective means to improve insulin sensitivity in overweight individuals.

Even a modest weight reduction (4.5 kg) is able to improve significantly insulin's action in relation to glucose, lipid and protein metabolism, and, moreover, to reduce the risk of diabetes. Weight reduction has a strong beneficial effect on all the cardiovascular risk factors associated with insulin resistance, namely hyperglycaemia, hypertension, dyslipidaemia (high TAG and low HDL) and inflammation endothelial dysfunction.

Insulin sensitivity can be influenced not only by total energy intake, but also by dietary composition. In this respect, of great interest are the specific effects of the quality of dietary fat, as there is considerable evidence in experimental animals that the increased amounts of saturated fat in the diet may lead to insulin resistance. In humans, there is indirect evidence for the same effect: a higher saturated fat intake is associated with impaired insulin action. Human studies have also attempted to evaluate the relationship between total fat intake and insulin sensitivity. Many epidemiological studies, both cross-sectional and prospective, are now available showing that fat intake is correlated with both plasma insulin values (positively) and insulin sensitivity (negatively). These correlations are largely mediated by body weight, which may explain why in these studies saturated and unsaturated fats (which have identical energy content) show similar relationships with insulin sensitivity. If the effect of total fat intake on body weight is properly accounted for, the relationship between dietary fat and insulin sensitivity becomes less consistent.

A more appropriate study design to evaluate the effect of fat intake, both in terms of total amount and quality, on insulin sensitivity independently of all possible confounders is the intervention trial. Few such studies are available in the literature, but these studies are consistent in showing that when total fat intake is increased from 20 to 40% no major effect is observed on insulin sensitivity. Only more extreme experimental conditions, such as when fat intake varies from almost 0% to as much as 55%, may be able to modify insulin sensitivity. Concerning the effect of quality of fat, a large multicentre intervention study undertaken in healthy individuals given either a high saturated fat or a high monounsaturated fat diet for 3 months showed that a high monounsaturated fat diet significantly improved insulin sensitivity compared with a high saturated fat diet. However, this beneficial effect of monounsaturated fat disappears in individuals whose total fat intake is high (35–40% of total energy). Similar beneficial effects on insulin sensitivity have been shown in overweight and type 2 diabetic patients, when saturated fat was replaced with n-6 polyunsaturated fat. At odds with data in animals, n-3 fatty acids supplementation does not have any influence on insulin sensitivity in humans.

By and large, there are insufficient data available to draw any firm conclusions as to whether and how insulin sensitivity may be influenced by the glycaemic index of diets, alcohol and micronutrient intakes.

Nutritional influence on fasting and postprandial blood glucose levels

Although closely related, fasting and postprandial blood glucose levels are regulated by mechanisms that are, to some extent, different. While postprandial blood glucose concentrations depend largely on meal composition, fasting values are only minimally influenced by the amount and/or rate of glucose absorption during the previous meal, and reflect the rate of glucose production in the liver by means of two key processes, glycogenolysis and gluconeogenesis, which are regulated by insulin secretion and insulin sensitivity.

Diabetes is a disease that results from either a failure in insulin secretion (type 1 diabetes or a failure in the sensitivity to insulin (type 2 diabetes). Although both types of diabetes increase the risk of CVD, less severe forms of insulin resistance, which manifest as disturbed lipid metabolism in the absence of overt hyperglycaemia, are present in a significant proportion of middle-aged adults in developed countries and also confer increased cardiovascular risk.

Of course, all the nutritional factors acting on insulin sensitivity may also influence blood glucose levels both at fasting and postprandially; the latter is also affected by the amount of carbohydrates in a meal, their quality and the quantity of dietary fibre.

11.11 Perspectives on the future

Lipids, genetics and cardiovascular disease

A great many of the advances in our understanding of the role of lipids in the pathophysiology of cardiovascular disease have arisen from the study of rare mutations such as those of genes coding for proteins involved in the LDL receptor pathway. However, as pointed out in Chapter 2, more commonly genetic variation plays a significant role in determining individual responsiveness to diet. Numerous apolipoproteins (e.g. apoE, apoA1,2, apoC1,2,3, apoB-48, apoB-100), enzymes (e.g. LPL, CETP, HMG-CoA reductase), receptors (e.g. LDL receptor, remnant receptor) and transcription factors (e.g. PPAR-α, PPAR-γ, SREBP) are involved in lipid and lipoprotein metabolism. It is likely that polymorphisms in these and other regulatory proteins will prove to be responsible for modifying both the risk of CVD and interindividual responsiveness to dietary components that can modify CVD risk.

One of the most widely studied polymorphisms is that of the apoE gene, which produces three main isoforms: E_2, E_3 and E_4. The prevalence of these alleles varies between populations, but is generally in the region of 14% (E_2), 60% (E_3) and 26% (E_4). The apoE isoforms represent examples of single nucleotide polymorphisms (SNPs) which, in the case of E_4, involves an arginine for cysteine substitution at residue 112, whereas E_2 involves a cysteine for arginine substitution at residue 158. Some 2% of the population are homozygous for E_2 and display markedly delayed chylomicron clearance, while 14% are heterozygous and show much less effect on chylomicron clearance. In contrast, the E_4 allele is associated with an increased risk of CVD, higher LDL cholesterol and greater than average responsiveness in terms of LDL cholesterol to dietary saturated fat but not statin therapy. Given the number of potential SNPs in the large number of proteins involved in lipid and lipoprotein metabolism that could confer variability in dietary responsiveness, it is clear that the big challenge for the future will be in exploiting the forthcoming explosion of data in this area, arising from the application of technology for high-throughput genomic analysis and the advances in the understanding of the huge array of data that will arrive through bioinformatics. It is probable that this will lead to the ability to predict an individual's responsiveness to a particular dietary change and thereby provide customised dietary advice based on their particular gene profile. There are enormous social and economic benefits to accurately titrating the proper effective diet to an individual's needs.

Table 11.7 Dietary components with known or putative cardioprotective effects

Component	Effect
Known effects	
Long-chain n-3 PUFA	Prevention of secondary cardiovascular disease
PUFA, MUFA (in place of SAFA)	LDL cholesterol reduction
Plant sterols	LDL cholesterol reduction
Dietary fibre	LDL cholesterol reduction
Putative effects	
Soy protein	LDL reduction cholesterol
Milk peptides	Reduction of blood pressure
Isoflavones, long-chain n-3	Reduction of endothelial dysfunction
PUFA, MUFA (in place of SAFA)	Reduction of platelet aggregation
Carotenoids, vitamin E,	Reduction of susceptibility of
flavonoids, e.g. reservatrol	LDL to oxidation
Quercetin	Reduction of platelet aggregation

PUFA, polyunsaturated fatty acid; MUFA, monounsaturated fatty acid; CLA, conjugated linoleic acid; LDL, low-density lipoprotein; HDL, high-density lipoprotein.

While this might be true of all diseases, the high social and economic cost of diseases of the cardiovascular system will put CVD in the front line of this technology, which, however, has not yet shown any relevant clinical usefulness besides the diagnosis of the genetic forms of hyperlipidaemia.

Bioactive microcomponents in foods and their effects on cardiovascular disease risk factors: role of gene expression screening

Recognition of the potential cardioprotective effects of many nutrient and non-nutrient components of foods in recent years (Table 11.7) has led to the introduction of the concept of 'functional foods' (or nutraceuticals): foods in which normal levels of these bioactive compounds are increased, either through their enrichment at source [e.g. increased levels of conjugated linoleic acid (CLA) in milk] or through their addition during the manufacturing process (e.g. plant sterols in spreads and margarines). The dietary compounds for which cardioprotective effects have been suggested are exceedingly diverse and include possible blood pressure-lowering peptides in milk, cholesterol-lowering effects of soy proteins and plant isoflavones, antioxidant effects of

flavonoids found in wine and tea, and platelet antiaggregating effects of quercetin found in onions (see Chapter 14). Not all of the studies conducted in human volunteers have provided conclusive or convincing findings, but considerable research effort is currently being applied and is likely to reveal that at least some of the compounds have potential application for the prevention of CVD. Already it is clear from secondary prevention trials that modest amounts of eicosapentaenoic and docosahexaenoic acid have powerful cardioprotective effects that could be harnessed via their enrichment in the diet. There has been considerable research into the effects of CLA on risk factors for atherosclerosis. CLA is a mix of conjugated isomers of all-*cis* C18:2n–6 and the different isomers have different and sometimes divergent effects. Whereas CLA is the focus of present attention, there are almost certainly likely to be other conjugated isomers of very biologically active fatty acids such as arachidonic, eicosapentaenoic or docosahexaenoic acids that may prove to be even more potent than the parent compounds.

Two of the factors that have limited the development of this exciting area are the cost and complexity of conducting intervention trials in human volunteers. Compromise of cost over study design means that many trials are too small to demonstrate statistically significant findings. However, the availability of high-throughput microarray technology (genomics) and proteomics, applied to cell-culture models, will enable putative bioactive compounds to be screened for their ability to influence the expression of target genes. This will allow nutritional trials to be limited to compounds already shown to influence key pathways in relevant cell systems.

Further reading

Arshag D *et al.* The effect of select nutrients on serum high-density lipoprotein cholesterol and apolipoprotein A-I levels. Endocrine Rev 2006; 27: 2–16.

Glass CK, Witztum JL. Atherosclerosis: the road ahead. Cell 2001; 104(4): 503–516.

Hermansen K. Diet, blood pressure and hypertension. Br J Nutr 2000; 83 (Suppl 1): s113–s119.

Hornstra G, Barth CA, Galli C. Functional food science and the cardiovascular system. Br J Nutr 1998 (Suppl 1): s113–s146.

Houston MC, Harper KJ. Potassium, magnesium, and calcium: their role in both the cause and treatment of hypertension. J. Clin. Hypert. 2008 (Suppl.10): 2–11.

Kris-Etherton PM, Shaomey Y. Individual fatty acid effects on plasma lipids and lipoproteins: human studies. Am J Clin Nutr 1997; 65 (Suppl): 1628s–1644s.

NHLBI. Third Report of the Expert Panel on Detection Evaluation and Treatment of High Blood Cholesterol in Adults. National Cholesterol Education, 2001.

Riccardi G, Rivellese AA. Dietary treatment of the metabolic syndrome: the optimal diet. Br J Nutr 2000; 83 (Suppl 1): s143–s148.

Riccardi G, Rivellese AA, Giacco R. Role of glycemic index and glycemic load in the healthy state, in prediabetes, and in diabetes. Am J Clin Nutr. 2008 Jan; 87(1): 269S–274S.

Risérus U, Willett WC, Hu FB. Dietary fats and prevention of type 2 diabetes. Prog Lipid Res 2009; 48: 44–51.

Zaman AG et al. The role of plaque rupture and thrombosis in coronary artery diseases. Atherosclerosis 2000; 149: 251–266.

12
The Skeletal System

John M Pettifor, Ann Prentice, Kate Ward and Peter Cleaton-Jones

Key messages

- Bone provides important supportive and protective functions for the body, and its constituent cells are in close relationship with those of the bone marrow, from which they are derived.
- Bone is a dynamic tissue, which is continually being resorbed and replaced (the process of remodelling). The rate of remodelling is influenced by a number of different factors, including circulating hormones such as sex steroids and parathyroid hormone. Bone formation and resorption can be measured by various different biochemical assays, which may be of use in assessing bone and mineral metabolism.
- Bone mass can be accurately measured by several techniques, including dual-energy X-ray absorptiometry (DXA) and computed tomography. Each method has its advantages and disadvantages, which may complicate the interpretation of the results.
- Peak bone mass, which is reached in early adulthood, is influenced by different factors, including heredity, gender, nutrition,

hormonal status and lifestyle patterns. Peak bone mass may influence the prevalence of fragility fractures occurring in later life.
- Important metabolic bone diseases include osteomalacia/rickets and osteoporosis. The former is common in infants, young children and the elderly in a number of developing and developed countries owing to vitamin D deficiency, while the latter is becoming an increasingly severe problem in the ageing population of developed countries.
- Several nutritional factors play permissive roles in ensuring optimal bone health. Among the most important of these are vitamin D and calcium, but many other nutrients, singly or in combination, may influence bone and mineral homeostasis.
- The nutritional factors influencing tooth development and dental caries are less well understood, but it appears that genetic factors combine with nutritional patterns to influence caries prevalence.

12.1 Introduction

Rickets and osteoporosis are two diseases of bone which have major impacts on the state of health and quality of life of young and old, respectively, in both developing and industrialised countries. Nutritional factors play important roles in determining the prevalence of these two diseases. This chapter sets the scene for the reader by providing an overview of the structure and physiology of bone, and of the factors that determine bone and tooth growth and development. The physiological changes that occur during pregnancy and lactation and with ageing are discussed and the factors that may influence these changes are described. This chapter should be read in conjunction with other chapters in other books in this series.

12.2 Bone architecture and physiology

The skeletal system plays a number of important physiological roles, thus its integrity must be maintained for the normal function of the human body. These physiological functions include:

- *support* for the body: in this role the skeleton is responsible for posture, for allowing normal joint movement and muscle activity through providing the levers on which muscles act, and for withstanding functional load bearing
- *protection* of organs, such as the brain and lungs
- *providing a reservoir* of calcium
- *acting as a buffer* to maintain normal acid–base balance

Nutrition and Metabolism, Second Edition, edited by S. A. Lanham-New, I. A. Macdonald and H. M. Roche. © 2011 The Nutrition Society.

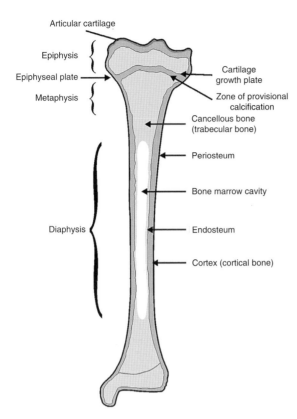

Figure 12.1 Schematic representation of a long bone with the important anatomical areas labelled.

Bone composition

Unlike most other tissues, which are composed mainly of cells, bone is mainly composed of an extracellular matrix. The cells that maintain this matrix are relatively sparse, being present only on the various surfaces of the calcified matrix and scattered within the matrix that makes up cortical bone. Bone thus consists of a non-cellular calcified matrix and the cells that maintain this matrix. As shown in Box 12.1, mineral is the major constituent of bone.

Bone matrix

The matrix is made up of both *collagenous* and *non-collagenous* proteins, with type I collagen making up 90% of total bone protein (Box 12.2). The fibrous nature of collagen provides elasticity and flexibility to bone as well as the scaffolding on which mineralisation can occur. The collagen fibres are oriented in directions influenced by the stresses and strains experienced by the developing bone through weight bearing, and the attachments of muscles, tendons and ligaments. Type I collagen is a triple-helical molecule containing two identical α_1 (I) chains and an α_2 (I) chain. These chains are rich in lysine and proline, which undergo post-translational modifications, including hydroxylation of lysyl and prolyl residues (which requires vitamin C), glycosylation of lysyl and hydroxylysyl residues, and the formation of intramolecular and intermolecular covalent cross-links (Figure 12.2). These post-translational modifications are important in ensuring the linkage of the collagen molecules into fibrils, thus increasing the strength of the collagen network. The collagen molecules are linked end to end and side to side in a staggered pattern, resulting in gaps between the molecules, where mineral deposition occurs. Measurement of these various collagen cross-links has been used successfully to assess the rate of bone resorption in the clinical situation.

- through its close relationship with bone marrow, *maintaining a normal haemopoietic and immune system.*

Bone may be divided into compact (cortical) bone, which provides mainly the supporting and protective functions of bone and makes up approximately 85% of bone tissue, and trabecular, cancellous or spongy bone, which is composed of thin calcified trabeculae enclosing the haemopoietic bone marrow and adipose tissue and comprises only 15% of the skeleton. Trabecular bone is considered to be physiologically more active than cortical bone because of its larger surface area. The internal trabecular structure of bones such as that found in the vertebral bodies and femoral neck plays an important supportive role, preventing collapse or fracture. Figure 12.1 schematically depicts a long bone such as the femur or tibia and highlights the various anatomical regions of the bone.

Box 12.2 Bone matrix

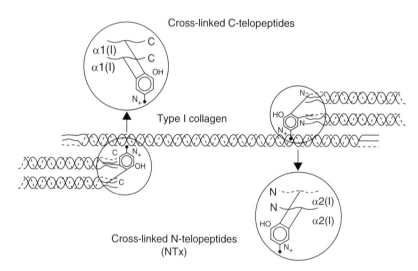

Figure 12.2 Schematic diagram of type I collagen, highlighting its linkages with other fibres. (Reproduced with permission from Calvo S *et al.*, Molecular basis and clinical application of biological markers of bone turnover. Endocrine Review 1996: 17: 333–68 © The Endocrine Society.)

The non-collagenous proteins make up only approximately 10% of total bone protein and can be divided into three major groups:

- proteoglycans
- glycosylated proteins
- γ-carboxylated proteins.

The proteoglycans molecules may be important regulators of bone formation, but their physiological functions in bone have not been clearly elucidated. The *glycosylated proteins*, such as alkaline phosphatase, osteonectin, osteopontin, fibronectin and bone sialoprotein, probably play a number of different roles, which for many of the proteins have not been well established, but they may be important in

regulating matrix mineralisation, bone cell growth and proliferation, and in osteoblast differentiation and maturation. Alkaline phosphatase, which is a zinc-containing metalloenzyme, is an essential enzyme for the normal mineralisation of bone. Inherited defects in the molecule result in the condition of hereditary hypophosphatasia, which in its most severe form is lethal in infancy. Zinc deficiency is associated with low circulating levels of alkaline phosphatase.

The *γ-carboxylated proteins* osteocalcin, matrix-Gla-protein and protein S are post-translationally modified by the action of vitamin K-dependent γ-carboxylases to form dicarboxylic glutamyl (Gla) residues, which enhance calcium binding. The actual role of these proteins in bone is unclear, but they may inhibit mineral deposition. The measurement of serum levels of osteocalcin is increasingly used as a measure of osteoblastic activity. Clinical vitamin K deficiency reduces the number of carboxylated glutamic acid residues per molecule of osteocalcin.

The *mineral component* of bone is mainly in the form of hydroxyapatite $[Ca_{10}(PO_4)_6(OH)_2]$, which provides stiffness and load-bearing strength to bone. The crystals of hydroxyapatite are approximately 200 Å in length, and form in and around the collagen fibrils, where they grow both by increasing in size and by aggregation. The mechanism by which mineralisation occurs is not well understood, although it is believed that extracellular matrix vesicles (produced by osteoblasts) initiate mineralisation either by removing inhibitors of mineralisation, such as pyrophosphate and adenosine triphosphate (ATP), present in the matrix, or by increasing calcium and phosphate concentrations locally to allow crystallisation to occur. Although the exact role of alkaline phosphatase produced by osteoblasts in the mineralisation process is unclear, it is essential for normal mineralisation, as evidenced by the severe mineralisation defect seen in children with hypophosphatasia, a disease caused by genetic mutations in the alkaline phosphatase gene.

The hydroxyapatite crystal may take up dietary cations and anions into its lattice. Magnesium or strontium may replace calcium in the crystal lattice, resulting in smaller, less perfect crystals, while fluoride incorporation increases crystal size and decreases solubility. Bisphosphonates, a family of antiresorptive agents, bind to the surface of apatite crystals, preventing resorption. Tetracycline, an antibiotic, also binds avidly to newly formed apatite crystals, resulting in fluorescence of newly deposited bone and tooth mineral. This characteristic of tetracycline is used clinically to measure bone mineralisation rates and the extent of bone surface undergoing mineralisation in histological sections. If taken during the formation of teeth, tetracyclines result in staining of teeth through their incorporation in the mineralising enamel.

Bone cells

The important bone cells are *stromal osteoprogenitor cells*, *osteoblasts*, *osteocytes*, *lining cells* and *osteoclasts* and their precursors. However, it is becoming increasingly apparent that there is a close inter-relationship between the various haemopoietic cells in the bone marrow and bone cells, not only because precursors of bone cells may reside within the marrow but also because of the cross-talk between the various cell types.

Osteoprogenitor cells are found in the periosteum and bone marrow. These mesenchymal stem cells may develop through appropriate stimuli into two very different cell types: adipocytes (fat cells) or osteoblast precursors. Various growth factors, cytokines and hormones [including transforming growth factor-β_1 (TGF-β_1), fibroblast growth factor (FGF), a number of bone morphogenetic proteins and parathyroid hormone (PTH)] are responsible for controlling the proliferation and differentiation of these mesenchymal cells into preosteoblasts, osteoblasts and osteocytes. Both PTH and the active form of vitamin D, 1,25-dihydroxyvitamin D [1,25(OH)$_2$D], are important in controlling the proliferation and differentiation of these bone-forming cells. The control of the development of these cells is complex and beyond the scope of this chapter; the reader is referred to a number of reviews for further information.

Osteoblasts are responsible for the secretion of bone matrix and for the production of matrix vesicles, which probably initiate mineralisation of the preformed osteoid. During the maturation of the osteoblast, the cell initially secretes collagen and is rich in alkaline phosphatase, but later produces osteocalcin and other matrix proteins, such as osteopontin. As the osteoblast becomes encircled by matrix, it transforms into an osteocyte.

Osteocytes are known as the mechanosensing cells and constitute 90–95% of all bone cells within the adult. They have cytoplasmic extensions which lie in canaliculi though the bone matrix. These extensions connect with adjacent cells (osteocytes, osteoblasts and lining cells) and extend into the bone marrow. Osteocytes sense changes in strain within the matrix and signal to both osteoclasts and osteoblasts to stimulate bone resorption or formation. These mechanosensing cells are thus vital to the process of bone remodelling. The exact mechanism by which the osteocyte senses strain changes *in vivo* is not fully understood, but is thought to be related to changes in fluid flow shear stress at the cell membrane. Recent evidence suggests that factors secreted by the osteocytes, such as FGF23 and sclerostin, have endocrine, paracrine and autocrine actions.

Osteoclasts (bone-resorbing cells) are derived from haemopoietic stem cells, which have the potential to become macrophages or multinucleated osteoclasts depending on the stimuli received during development. Osteoclasts lie in contact with the mineralised trabecular surface or in Howship's lacunae. These cells are rich in endoplasmic reticulum and Golgi complexes. The cell membrane adjacent to the bone matrix is characterised by a peripheral sealing zone that is rich in integrins, and a central ruffled border that forms a space between the osteoclast and the bone matrix into which lysosomal enzymes (such as tartrate-resistant acid phosphatase and cathepsin K), proteinases (such as collagenase) and hydrogen ions are secreted. The hydrogen ions and enzymes dissolve the mineral and digest the demineralised matrix, the products of which are internalised into the osteoclast, transported across the cell into the extracellular fluid or released through the sealing zone. Hormones that stimulate osteoclast number and activity include parathyroid hormone, $1,25(OH)_2D$ and a number of inflammatory cytokines, while calcitonin reduces osteoclastic activity.

Bone remodelling

Bone is not a dead organ; rather it is continually being resorbed and replaced. This process is known as bone remodelling (Figure 12.3) and it not only helps to maintain bone in optimal condition through repairing microfractures but is also important in serum calcium homeostasis. Bone turnover occurs in discrete packages throughout the skeleton, and the process of resorption followed by replacement is tightly coupled so that in the healthy young adult there is no net loss or gain in bone. As one grows older, and particularly in the postmenopausal period, progressive bone loss occurs as a result of incomplete replacement of the bone that has been resorbed. The control of the rate of bone remodelling, the mechanisms by which the osteoclasts are activated and how the whole process is coupled are areas of intensive investigation, which still have many unanswered questions. The balance between bone formation and resorption is essential in maintaining bone mass (Figure 12.4). Recent studies have provided a better understanding of how the various bone cells interact. For example, osteoblasts control osteoclast precursor development through the production of RANK-ligand, which binds to RANK on osteoclast precursors and stimulates osteoclast

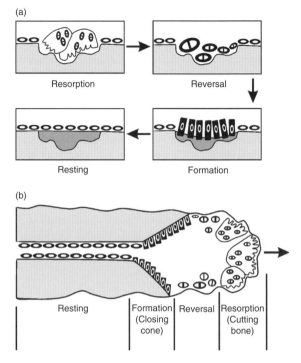

Figure 12.3 The bone remodelling cycle. (a) Remodelling at the trabecular bone surface. (b) Remodelling occurring in cortical bone. (Reproduced from the Primer on the metabolic Bone Diseases and Disorders with the permission from the American Society of Bone and Mineral Research.)

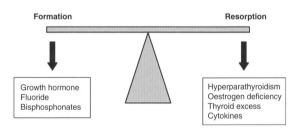

Figure 12.4 Balance between bone formation and resorption, which is essential to maintain bone mass.

proliferation. Osteoprotogerin, a circulating binder of RANK-ligand, reduces the amount of RANK-ligand available to bind to osteoclast precursors, thus reducing osteoclast production.

The whole process of remodelling of a particular package of bone takes about 3–4 months, with the resorption process lasting about 10 days and the filling in of the cavity taking about 3 months. Systemic hormones, such as PTH, $1,25-(OH)_2D$ and calcitonin, alter bone remodelling mainly through inducing more or fewer remodelling sites in the skeleton. Oestrogen deficiency, as occurs at the time of the menopause, causes bone loss mainly through its effect on the osteoblast, preventing complete filling in of the resorption cavity that develops during the remodelling cycle. Excessive bone resorption, either through the formation of excessively deep resorption cavities or through the progressive thinning of trabecular bone with each remodelling cycle, will result in weakening of the trabecular bone structure owing to the loss of connectivity between the various rods and plates that make up the trabecular scaffolding, resulting in progressive risk of minimal trauma fractures. States of very high bone turnover, which may occur in diseases such as Paget's disease or severe primary or secondary hyperparathyroidism, result in the formation of woven rather than lamellar bone. In woven bone the collagen fibres are laid down in a disorganised fashion, resulting in the loss of the normal lamellar structure with a resultant loss in bone strength.

Biochemical assessment of bone remodelling

Since the early 1990s great strides have been made in the development of assays for the measurement of both serum and urine markers of bone formation and resorption, and these have helped in noninvasively assessing bone turnover.

Markers of bone formation

Table 12.1 lists the bone biochemical markers currently available for the assessment of bone turnover.

Total alkaline phosphatase has until recently been the only marker of osteoblastic activity available, but as serum total alkaline phosphatase also reflects that produced at other sites, in particular the liver, elevated total levels do not necessarily reflect an increase in osteoblastic activity. Alkaline phosphatase concentrations are characteristically elevated in all forms of osteomalacia and rickets, in hyperparathyroidism and in Paget's disease. The measurement of *bone-specific alkaline phosphatase* (BSAP) utilises specific monoclonal antibodies to detect the bone component of the tissue non-specific alkaline phosphatase isoenzyme and more accurately reflects an increase in osteoblastic activity. Depressed levels of alkaline phosphatase may occur in zinc deficiency and protein–energy malnutrition, and in inherited disorders of the alkaline

Table 12.1 Biochemical markers of bone turnover

Formation
- Serum
  - Total alkaline phosphatase (AP)
  - Bone-specific alkaline phosphatase (BSAP)
  - Osteocalcin (OC)
  - Carboxy-terminal propeptide of type I collagen (PICP)
  - Amino-terminal propeptide of type I collagen (PINP)

Resorption
- Serum
  - Cross-linked C-telopeptide of type I collagen (ICTP)
  - Tartrate-resistant acid phosphatase (TRAP)
- Urine
  - Hydroxyproline
  - Free and total pyridinolines (Pyd)
  - Free and total deoxypyridinolines (Dpd)
  - N-telopeptide of collagen cross-links (NTx)
  - C-telopeptide of collagen cross-links (CTx)

phosphatase gene (hereditary hypophosphatasia). *Osteocalcin* is a non-collagenous protein secreted by the mature osteoblast. Thus, serum levels should reflect osteoblastic activity and bone formation. In general, BSAP and osteocalcin values correlate; however, some studies suggest that osteocalcin levels may be normal in patients with rickets despite markedly elevated alkaline phosphatase values. The reasons for this dissociation are unclear.

The *amino- and carboxy-terminal propeptides of type I collagen* (PINP and PICP, respectively) are cleaved and excreted during collagen biosynthesis. Assays for the determination of the propeptides at both the N- and C-terminals have been developed, but they do not appear to be as useful as either BSAP or osteocalcin in assessing bone formation and osteoblastic activity.

Markers of bone resorption

Unlike the assessment of bone formation, which generally uses serum, the assessment of bone resorption usually requires the measurement of products excreted in urine. The most useful markers are those derived from the breakdown of type I collagen, which occurs during the resorption of bone matrix. The measurement of hydroxyproline excretion in urine has until recently been the gold standard; however, hydroxyproline is found not only in collagen derived from bone, but also in collagen from tendons, cartilage and soft tissues. Thus, the amount excreted in urine may reflect the breakdown of other tissues besides bone and that ingested in the diet.

The measurement of hydroxyproline has over the past few years been replaced by the measurement of the *pyridinoline and deoxypyridinoline cross-links of collagen* (Pyd and Dpd, respectively). Dpd is more specific for bone than Pyd, but is less abundant. Currently, the generally used immunoassays measure free Pyd and Dpd, rather than the protein-bound molecules, which may make the interpretation of results difficult if storage or biological variations alter the ratio of free to protein-bound molecules. Assays have also been developed to measure the *N- and C-terminal telopeptides of collagen* in urine.

In serum, an assay is available to measure cross-linked *C-terminal telopeptide of type I collagen*, but the assay does not appear to be as useful as the measurement of the urinary markers of bone resorption. A reasonably specific marker of osteoclast activity is *tartrate-resistant acid phosphatase* (TRAP), which is secreted into serum. Its measurement is limited by its instability in serum and by the fact that it is not entirely specific for osteoclasts.

Clinical usefulness of biochemical markers of bone turnover

Bone markers are useful in assisting in the diagnosis of metabolic bone disease, such as osteomalacia and rickets, and hyperparathyroidism but they have little or no use in the diagnosis of osteoporosis, although they may help in understanding the pathogenesis of osteoporosis and monitoring the response to therapy.

One of the major problems with the use of most of the bone resorption markers is their great variability from day to day as a result of the need to measure their excretion in urine. Twenty-four-hour urine samples are notoriously difficult to collect accurately, and are thus generally avoided. If one uses a fasting urine specimen, then one needs to relate the excretion of the urine marker to the excretion of creatinine in the same sample. However, creatinine measurements have a built-in variability and vary depending on muscle mass and nutritional status. Compounding the problem is the fact that a number of bone turnover markers have a circadian rhythm, thus specimens collected at different times of the day or night may vary markedly. Samples should therefore be collected at a constant time during the day,

and if they are being collected with specimens to assess calcium homeostasis, they should be collected in a fasting state.

Bone turnover markers are probably most useful as a research tool to assess rates of bone turnover in groups of subjects, and in clinical medicine to determine the bone response to an intervention such as drug therapy. They are also most useful when groups of subjects are compared, rather than when using them to determine the bone turnover status of an individual.

Assessment of bone mass

One of the techniques used to assess bone health is the measurement of the amount of mineral present in the bone. Before the advent of more advanced techniques, the usual method to assess the amount of mineral in bone was to use radiographs of the lumbar spine or hips and judge whether the radiographic density appeared to be normal, increased or decreased. The problem with this technique is that one needs to have lost some 30% of bone mineral before it becomes obvious on the routine radiograph and the interpretation is open to considerable subjectivity. The loss of radio-density on radiographs is termed *osteopenia*, which could be due to a loss of bone (matrix and mineral; osteoporosis) or a failure of mineralisation of normal amounts of matrix (osteomalacia).

Advances in technology since the early 1980s have resulted in the availability of rapid and accurate methods of assessing bone mass. A number of different techniques have been used to determine bone mass (Table 12.2), but dual-energy X-ray absorptiometry (DXA) is the most widely accepted (Figure 12.5). Measurement of bone mass is relevant to assess the degree of osteoporosis/osteopenia, to determine possible fracture risk and to assess response to therapy or the effect of disease on bone mass.

DXA is generally accepted as the gold standard against which other techniques are measured and has replaced the other techniques in most cases. It measures bone mineral content (BMC) in grams and bone area in cm^2. From these two measurements the so-called bone mineral density (BMD) in g/cm^2 is calculated (Box 12.3). It should be noted that the BMD is an areal bone density and does not measure true volumetric density of bone. Thus, unlike true density, BMD is influenced not only by

Table 12.2 Techniques used to measure bone mass

Technique	Sites measured	Precision (% CV)	Radiation dose (μSv)
Single X-ray absorptiometry (SXA)[a]	Forearm	~1	<1
Dual-energy X-ray densitometry (DXA)[a]	Spine, hip, forearm, whole body	1–2.5 depending on site	~1–3
Peripheral DXA	Forearm, calcaneus, phalanges	1–1.7	<1
Quantitative computed tomography (QCT)	Spine	2–4	~50
Peripheral QCT (pQCT) single slice	Radius, tibia, femur	~1–2	~1
High resolution pQCT	Distal radius and tibia	<4%	<3
Quantitative ultrasound (QUS)	Calcaneus, tibia, phalanx	0.3–5	0

[a] Earlier versions were single and dual photon absorptiometry, which were superseded due to poorer precision and technical limitations such as decay of isotope sources.

Figure 12.6 The concept of areal bone mineral density (BMD). The three blocks (a), (b) and (c) represent three blocks of bone of the same volumetric density of x g/cm^3. The projected area of block (a) is 1 cm^2, block (b) 2 cm^2 and block (c) 1 cm^2. Thus the BMD measured by DXA would be x g/cm^2 for blocks (a) and (b), but 2x g/cm^2 for block (c) as it is twice as thick as blocks (a) and (b). Note that BMD measured by DXA is dependent not only on the true bone density (volumetric) but also on the thickness of the bone, which is not measured by DXA. The dashed arrow represents the path of the X-ray beam through the three blocks.

Figure 12.5 Schematic diagram of a dual-energy X-ray densitometer. Note the collimated X-ray beam moves through body from inferior to superior. Using this method, whole body, lumbar spine, femoral and radial bone mineral content and area may be measured and bone mineral density calculated.

Box 12.3 Definitions used in densitometry (DXA)

Bone mineral content: The total bone mineral present in a defined area. It is measured in grams (g).
Bone area: The projected area of bone detected by the attenuation of the X-ray beam. It is measured in cm^2.
Bone mineral density: This represents bone mineral content per unit bone area. Thus, it represents an areal bone density and not a volumetric density as the thickness of bone is not determined by DXA. The units are g/cm^2.

---

the true density of bone but also by the volume of bone (Figure 12.6).

An understanding of this is important, as bones with the same volumetric bone density but different volumes will have different BMDs. BMD will increase with increasing bone size without a change in the true bone density. Furthermore, BMD reflects the average areal bone density of all the constituents of the particular bone being measured, thus the value will depend on amount of cortical as well as trabecular bone. Quantitative computed tomography (QCT) has an advantage in that it measures the volumetric density of bone. Furthermore, regions of bone, such as the cortical or trabecular regions, can be selected, thus allowing an assessment of the differential effects of a disease or treatment on the different types of bone.

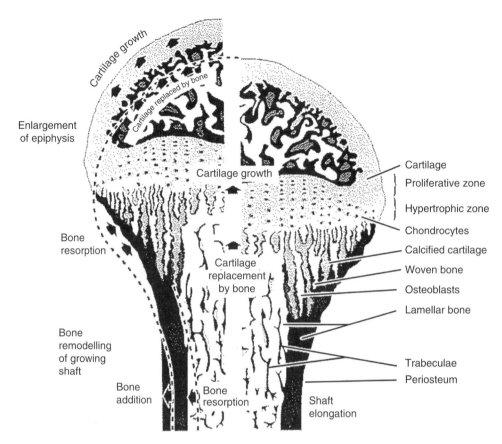

Figure 12.7 Changes associated with longitudinal growth of a long bone. Note the modelling that needs to take place in order for the bone the same shape but larger. (This figure was published in Vitamin D, 1st edn. Fieldman D, Glorieux FH and Pike JW. Copyright © Elsevier 2007.)

QCT is not more widely used because of the expense of the equipment, its lack of portability and the relatively high radiation dose. Portable peripheral devices (pQCT) are available, which measure bone geometry and strength, and the volumetric bone density of cortical and trabecular bone in the appendicular skeleton (forearm and tibia). More recently high-resolution pQCT has allowed *in vivo* assessment of bone microarchitecture at the distal radius and tibia.

12.3 Bone growth

Bone growth during foetal, childhood and adolescent periods involves not only elongation of long bones by proliferation of the growth plate cartilage, but also growth at the periosteal surfaces of both the long bones and membranous bones. Thus, as bones enlarge they undergo modelling, which involves the resorption of

bone in one area and the deposition of bone in another. From the time of birth to closure of the epiphyses and cessation of growth during adolescence, the skeleton increases in length by about three-fold, with quite marked changes in skeletal proportions, with limb length increasing more than trunk length (Figure 12.7).

Skeletal growth rates are not constant throughout childhood. After birth there is a marked deceleration in growth until 3 years of age, when the growth rate plateaus until the onset of puberty. Girls have their growth spurt approximately 2 years before boys and fuse their epiphyses earlier than boys.

Hormonal control of skeletal growth

Postnatally, the most important hormones regulating skeletal growth are growth hormone, insulin-like growth factor-1 (IGF-1), thyroid hormone and the sex steroids (Box 12.4).

Box 12.4 Important hormonal regulators of bone growth

- Growth hormone
- Insulin-like growth factor-1
- Thyroid hormone
- Sex hormones, especially oestrogen

The control of foetal growth is less clearly under-stood, but considerable interest in this area has been generated by the important role foetal growth has not only in adult size, but also in the future risk for car-diovascular disease, hypertension and non-insulin-dependent diabetes mellitus. Although genetic factors play a role in determining foetal growth, the predomi-nant factor is the nutritional, oxygen and hormonal milieu in which the foetus develops. Both IGF-1 and IGF-2 are necessary to achieve normal foetal growth, but the effect of IGF-1 deficiency during foetal life is more severe than that of IGF-2 deficiency.

Growth hormone probably induces most of its effect on growth through the stimulation of IGF-1 secretion both from the liver and in the growth plate, where it stimulates the proliferation of cartilage cells, resulting in an elongation of long bones. It is possible that the paracrine actions of IGF-1 in the growth plate are more important than the hormonal effects of IGF-1 pro-duced in the liver, as studies using a targeted knockout of the IGF-1 gene in the liver did not show a reduction in the growth-promoting actions of growth hormone. Unlike congenital deficiency of IGF-1, which manifests during foetal development, congenital growth hor-mone deficiency manifests postnatally with a falling off of growth velocity around 12 months of age. Nutritional deprivation probably causes a reduction in growth velocity through reducing IGF-1 production.

It also appears that IGF-1 may be an important mediator of the effect of sex steroids on bone growth during puberty, as both growth hormone and IGF-1 levels rise during puberty. The rise in growth hor-mone during puberty is a result of an increase in cir-culating oestrogen concentrations in both boys and girls. In boys it is likely that the increase in oestrogens is through the aromatisation of testosterone.

Sex steroids play an essential role not only in the growth spurt that occurs during puberty but also in the cessation of growth through the closure of the epiphyses. It appears that at physiological levels cir-culating oestrogen stimulates growth, while at phar-

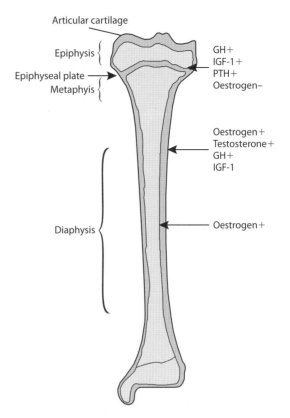

Figure 12.8 Sites of hormone actions on the growing long bone. Stimulation of bone growth is indicated by +, while inhibition of growth is indicated by −. GH, growth hormone; IGF-1, insulin-like growth factor-1; PTH, parathyroid hormone.

macological levels it suppresses longitudinal growth, possibly through reducing IGF-1 levels. Oestrogen is responsible for epiphyseal closure in both boys and girls. Sex steroids have effects not only on the growth plate, but also on the endosteal and periosteal bone surfaces, resulting in an increase in cross-sectional diameter of the long bones. It appears that androgens and oestrogen may have different effects on these bone surfaces. Both androgens and oestrogen cause an increase in periosteal new bone formation, with resultant widening of the bone, but only oestrogen has an effect on the endosteal bone surface, with a consequent increase in cortical bone thickness. Thus after puberty, boys have wider bones than girls, and girls have a narrower endosteal diameter due to bone deposition on the endosteal surface (Figure 12.8).

Thyroid hormone is essential for the normal pro-liferation and maturation of the growth plate.

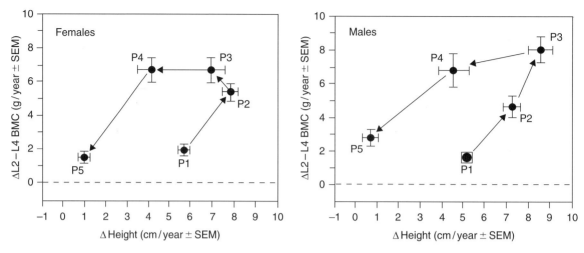

Figure 12.9 Relationship between changes in the bone mineral content (BMC) and height in adolescents grouped according to pubertal stages. Note that in the early stage of puberty (P1) height gain is good but changes in BMC lag behind, while the reverse holds true in the later stages of puberty. (Reproduced with permission from Thientz G *et al.*, Longitudinal monitoring of bone mass accumulation in healthy adolescents: evidence for a marked reduction after 16 years of age at the level of the lumbar spine and femoral neck in female subjects. J Clin Endocrinol Metab 1992; 75: 1060–5 Copyright © The Endocrine Society.)

Cretinism or congenital thyroid deficiency is associated with abnormalities of the epiphyses and marked short stature. From a nutritional standpoint, severe iodide deficiency in the mother and infant will manifest with growth failure.

Bone mass accumulation during childhood and adolescence

The skeleton increases its calcium content from birth to the end of adolescence by about 40 times (from 25 to 1000 g). A large proportion of this deposition occurs during puberty, but the proportions gained by boys and girls during this period differ as girls enter puberty earlier than boys. It is estimated that 50% of the total bone mass of the adult female is laid down during puberty, whereas the figure for men is 20%. In Caucasian children, maximal gain in bone mass occurs between 11 and 14 years of age in girls and between 13 and 17 years of age in boys.

The pattern of bone mass accumulation during childhood is similar to that of growth in height, as bone growth accounts for the majority of bone mass accumulation. However, the relationship between BMC and height gain during puberty is not linear, but rather follows a loop pattern (Figure 12.9).

The dissociation between the rates of statural growth and mineral mass accumulation during puberty could be viewed as a period of relatively low bone mass (Figure 12.10) and may account for the increase in fracture incidence that occurs round this time. As linear growth slows, bone mass accumulation continues to occur and the deficit is made up.

Peak bone mass

Although longitudinal growth of bone ceases with the fusion of the epiphyses, bone mass continues to accumulate as bone consolidates and periosteal new bone formation continues. The concept of peak bone mass, which is defined as the amount of bone tissue present at the end of skeletal maturation, has assumed considerable significance as there is good evidence that the risk of osteoporotic fractures in later life is inversely related to the amount of bone accumulated during maturation (Box 12.5). Skeletal maturation is considered to occur early in the third decade of life, although the timing of the achievement of peak bone mass may vary slightly between different skeletal sites.

Factors known to influence peak bone mass include heredity, gender, race, nutrition, hormonal status (in particular the sex steroids and IGF-1), exercise and physical weight. By far the most important is the genetic influence, with 50–85% of the variance in peak bone mass at different sites

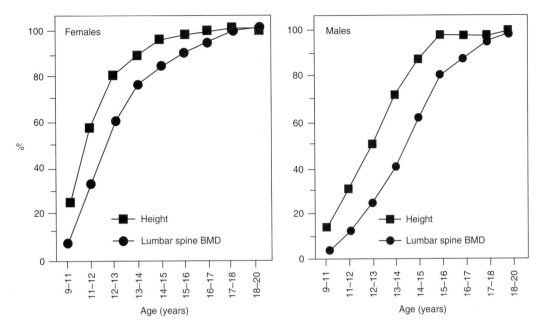

Figure 12.10 Comparison in cumulative gain between lumbar spine bone mineral density (BMD) and standing height during adolescence. The values are expressed as the percentage difference between 18–20-year-old and 9–11-year-old groups. (With kind permission from Springer Science + Business Media: Osteoporosis International, Asynchrony between the rates of standing height gain and bone mass accumulation during puberty vol 7 (1997) 525–32 Fournier PE *et al.* Copyright © Springer Ltd.)

Box 12.5 Factors influencing peak bone mass

- Genetic
- Race (African–Americans > Caucasians)
- Gender
- Nutritional, for example calcium intake
- Physical exercise
- Hormonal status
- Body weight

---

being accounted for by heritability. The role of nutrition and in particular dietary calcium intake during childhood in influencing peak bone mass has been an area of intense investigation and will be discussed later in this chapter. However, a definitive answer on the role of dietary calcium is not yet available. Exercise has been shown to have a modulating influence on peak bone mass, with weight-bearing exercises being the most effective, but the effect of exercise is relatively small (3–5%). Although small, on a population basis an increase in peak bone mass of this magnitude might have a considerable influence on fracture rates in later life.

There is an increasing gradient of fracture risk with decrease in bone mass, such, for example, that a reduction at the femoral neck of one standard deviation below the young adult mean increases the relative risk of hip fracture by 2.6. Consequently, both peak bone mass and the rate of subsequent bone loss are major determinants of osteoporotic fracture risk in later life. The maximisation of peak bone mass by optimising environmental factors that influence skeletal development during childhood and adolescence is regarded as an important preventive strategy against future fractures.

Conceptually, peak bone mass, as defined by BMC or BMD, contains elements related to the size of the skeleton, to the amount of bony tissue contained within it, to the mineral content of that tissue, and to the degree to which the bony tissue is actively undergoing remodelling. It is, as yet, unclear which of these aspects is most influential in determining future fracture risk.

Gender and ethnic differences in bone mass

Peak bone mass is significantly greater in adult males than females (Figure 12.11). This difference is due to

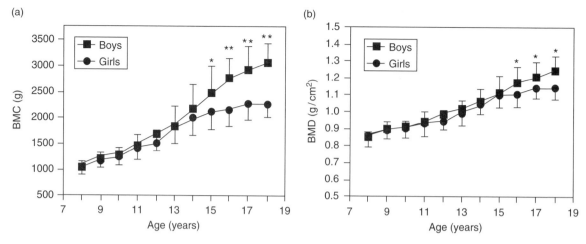

Figure 12.11 (a) Total body bone mineral content (BMC) and (b) areal bone mineral density (BMD) in Caucasian boys and girls from 8 to 18 years of age. Note the divergence of values between boys and girls developing after the onset of puberty. The effect is more marked for BMC than BMD as true volumetric bone density is similar in boys and girls, the difference in BMD being mainly due to a difference in bone size. (Reproduced with permission from Maynard LM *et al*. Total body and regional bone mineral content and areal bone mineral density in children aged 8–18y: the Fels longitudinal study. American Journal of Clinical Nutrition 1998; 68: 1111–7. Copyright © American Society for Nutrition.)

a greater bone size in males than females, rather than due to a difference in true bone density. At birth, boys and girls have similar bone masses and it is only at the onset of puberty that these gender differences develop, owing to the delayed and more prolonged growth spurt in boys.

Ethnic differences in bone mass have been consistently found in studies conducted in the USA, with African–Americans having approximately 5–15% greater bone mass at all measured sites than white Americans, after adjusting for body size. These differences are present before the onset of puberty. Thus, it is often assumed that black Africans have similarly elevated bone mass values. Studies in both The Gambia and South Africa have been unable to confirm this generalised increase in bone mass. Studies of other ethnic groups have been less detailed, but it appears that Asian women from the Indian subcontinent have similar or lower bone mass than American or European Caucasian women.

Skeletal changes during pregnancy and lactation

Pregnancy and lactation are associated with alterations in calcium and bone metabolism that temporarily affect the mineral content of the skeleton (Box 12.6). Both the foetus and the nursing infant increase calcium demands on the pregnant and lac-

> **Box 12.6 Skeletal and mineral changes during pregnancy**
>
> - Increased bone turnover
> - Increased intestinal calcium absorption
> - Increased urinary calcium loss
> - Increase in serum 1,25-$(OH)_2$D
> - Variable changes in bone mineral content

tating woman. These changes are evident from early to mid-gestation and continue through and beyond lactation. In pregnancy, bone resorption and formation rates are increased by 50–200%, and maternal calcium intestinal absorption efficiency and urinary calcium excretion are elevated. In lactation, calcium absorption efficiency returns to normal, but there is evidence of renal conservation of calcium in some women. Bone turnover continues to be elevated and differences in the timing of the skeletal response in terms of resorption and formation favour the release of calcium from the skeleton during early lactation, with restitution during and after weaning.

Direct studies of changes in BMC using densitometry have been largely restricted to lactating women because of the small radiation dose involved. Such studies have demonstrated striking reductions in BMC after 3–6 months of lactation, particularly in

Figure 12.12 Changes in bone mineral content of the lumbar spine during lactation and after weaning. Data are adjusted for scanned bone area. □, Mothers who breast-fed for >9 months (n = 20); △, Mothers who breast-fed for 3–6 months (n = 13); ○: Mothers who formula-fed (n = 11). (Reproduced with permission from Laskey MA, Prentice A. Bone mineral changes during and after lactation. Obstet Gynecol 1999; 94: 606–15.)

axial regions of the skeleton, such as the lumbar spine and femoral neck, where decreases average 3–5% (Figure 12.12).

Lactation-associated reductions in BMC are remarkable given that the rate of postmenopausal bone loss is typically 1–3% per year. BMC is recovered later in lactation or after weaning, and at some sites exceeds that measured after parturition. Lactational amenorrhea, the length of lactation and other aspects of infant-feeding behaviour influence the magnitude and temporal pattern of the skeletal response experienced by breast-feeding women. However, the final outcome appears to be similar irrespective of duration of lactation, or indeed whether the woman breast-fed or not.

Studies in women in which measurements were made before conception and after delivery also demonstrate reductions in whole body and regional BMC sufficient to make a sizeable contribution to maternal and foetal calcium economy. In contrast, substantial increases have been reported in women entering pregnancy while still breast-feeding, suggesting that skeletal changes during pregnancy may depend on the status of the maternal skeleton before conception.

The mechanisms underlying the effects of pregnancy and lactation on calcium and bone metabolism are not fully understood. Originally, it was considered that the observed metabolic changes were due to physiological hyperparathyroidism, driven by the inability of the dietary calcium supply to meet the high calcium requirement for foetal growth and breast-milk production. For this reason, women in the past were advised to increase their calcium intake during pregnancy and lactation. It is, however, now generally accepted that this is not the case, first, because PTH concentrations are not elevated during pregnancy and lactation; secondly, because the metabolic changes precede the increased requirement for calcium; and thirdly, because the effects appear to be independent of calcium intake. The fact that the metabolic and skeletal responses to lactation are not related to dietary calcium intake has been confirmed by calcium supplementation studies in populations accustomed to low and medium-to-high calcium intakes. As a consequence of these latest findings, it is no longer considered necessary for a woman to increase her calcium intake during pregnancy and lactation, and this is reflected in recent dietary recommendations, for example by the Department of Health (UK) and the Institute of Medicine Food and Nutrition Board (US/Canada).

Osteoporosis with fractures is a rare complication of pregnancy and lactation. When it does occur, the condition frequently involves the hip or spine, is more common in the first pregnancy and usually resolves spontaneously. The cause is unknown, and most cases are either idiopathic or secondary to warfarin or corticosteroid therapy. There is no evidence that osteoporosis of pregnancy and lactation is a consequence of nutrient deficiencies or that it can be prevented by changes in diet and lifestyle.

12.4 Teeth

Anatomy and development

Humans have two dentitions. The primary dentition, also known as the deciduous dentition, has 20 teeth in four quadrants each with two incisors, one canine and two molars. The permanent dentition contains 32 teeth: each quadrant has two incisors, one canine, two premolars and three molars. The incisors, canines and premolars succeed the overlying primary teeth, but the permanent molar teeth have no predecessors,

Table 12.3 Timings of tooth formation and eruption based on Ash's figures

Dentition	Jaw	Order of eruption	Calcification first seen	Crown completed	Eruption	Root completed
Primary	Mandible and maxilla	Central incisor	14 weeks[a]	1½–2½ months	8–10 months	1½ months
		Lateral incisor	16 weeks[a]	2½–3 months	11–13 months	1½–2 months
		First molar	15.5 weeks[a]	5½–6 months	16 months	2¼–2½ months
		Canine	17 weeks[a]	9 months	19–20 months	3¼ months
		Second molar	19 weeks[a]	10–11 months	27–29 months	3 months
Permanent	Mandible		At birth			
		First molar	3–4 months	2½–3 years	6–7 years	9–10 years
		Central incisor	3–4 months	4–5 years	6–7 years	9 years
		Lateral incisor	4–5 months	4–5 years	7–8 years	10 years
		Canine	1¼–2 years	6–7 years	9–10 years	12–14 years
		First premolar	2¼–2½ years	5–6 years	10–12 years	12–13 years
		Second premolar	2½–3 years	6–7 years	11–12 years	13–14 years
		Second molar	8–10 years	7–8 years	11–13 years	14–15 years
		Third molar		12–16 years	17–21 years	18–25 years
	Maxilla		At birth			
		First molar	3–4 months	2½–3 years	6–7 years	9–10 years
		Central incisor	10–12 months	4–5 years	7–8 years	10 years
		Lateral incisor	1½–1¾ years	4–5 years	8–9 years	11 years
		First premolar	2–2¼ years	5–6 years	10–11 years	12–13 years
		Second premolar	4–5 months	6–7 years	10–12 years	12–14 years
		Canine	2½–3 years	6–7 years	11–12 years	13–15 years
		Second molar	7–9 years	7–8 years	12–13 years	14–16 years
		Third molar		12–16 years	17–21 years	18–25 years

[a] *In utero.*

they develop as the jaws grow beyond the size that accommodates the primary teeth.

Teeth erupt over a wide period, earlier in some individuals than in others. They also erupt in a different sequence in the primary and permanent dentitions, and in the latter between the jaws. In general, mandibular teeth erupt before maxillary teeth. In this chapter mean timings of tooth formation have been rounded off to make them easier to remember (Table 12.3). There is a considerable range of values depending on the researcher. As a rule of thumb, the normal range of values in months is about 1 month either side of the mean; year values range about 1 year either side of the mean. Notice in Table 12.3 that calcification of the crowns of primary teeth begins *in utero*.

The anatomy of a typical tooth cross-section is shown in Figure 12.13. A tooth is divided into an anatomical crown and an anatomical root that meet at the neck (cervix). The anatomical crown is that part covered by enamel and the anatomical root is that part covered by cementum. The clinical crown is the portion of the anatomical crown visible in the

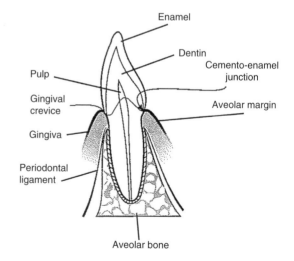

Figure 12.13 Diagram of a longitudinal section of an incisor.

mouth. The bulk of the tooth consists of calcified enamel and dentin, with a central uncalcified pulp that contains loose connective tissue, nerves and blood vessels.

Composition of enamel, dentin and cementum

Enamel is formed by ectodermal cells (ameloblasts) that disappear once enamel formation is complete. It is highly calcified, approximately 96% inorganic material, 0.8% organic and 3.2% water, arranged as crystals of calcium hydroxyapatite (see section on bone matrix). Because the ameloblasts disappear at the completion of enamel formation, if enamel is damaged it cannot re-form. During enamel formation anything that interferes with the ameloblasts or with calcification will produce poorer quality enamel shown by two visible defects. Hypoplasia is present when the enamel matrix has been poorly formed; it presents as a pit or fissure on the enamel surface. If calcification has been altered hypocalcification will be seen as opaque, white areas ranging in size from a spot to an entire surface. Highly calcified enamel is transparent, allowing the yellow colour of the underlying dentin to be seen; less calcified areas lack this transparency.

The position of enamel hypoplasia or hypocalcification on individual teeth, or on combinations of teeth, in both primary and permanent dentitions, can give a reasonable indication of when development was abnormal. What caused the defect is not so easily decided. Current thought is that excess fluoride is the only nutritional cause that can be diagnosed with reasonable certainty; the majority of other enamel defects are said to be due to transient infections, chronic illness or metabolic conditions such as rickets, but a clear link to the cause is rarely possible. Whatever the cause, there is interference with ameloblast and odontoblast function.

Dentin and cementum are similar in composition to bone, and are less calcified than enamel, being approximately 68% inorganic material, 22% organic and 10% water. Dentin is formed by mesodermal cells (odontoblasts) that retreat towards the pulp as dentin is laid down. They remain after tooth formation is complete and so can form more dentin, called secondary dentin, in response to an irritant such as dental caries or a filling. Secondary dentin and calcifications called pulp stones may also be formed by multipotential cells in the pulp tissue. Dentin itself contains no cells but has fine tubules that contain a portion of the odontoblasts (odontoblast process) left there as the cells retreated towards the pulp while laying down dentin. Secondary dentin may contain trapped cells and does not have tubules. Cementum

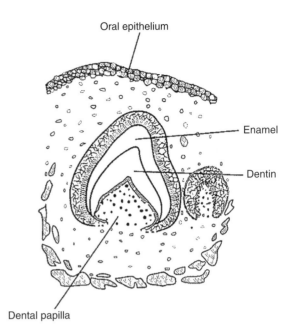

Figure 12.14 Diagram of the developmental stages of a tooth.

looks similar to bone and contains entrapped cells (cementoblasts). Cementum attaches the periodontal ligament to the root surface. There is remodelling of the alveolar bone supporting the teeth, as happens elsewhere in the skeleton, but no similar remodelling of tooth tissues takes place.

Development of teeth

The teeth develop from two of the three primary germ layers, ectoderm and mesoderm. Ectoderm gives rise to the enamel of teeth; mesoderm provides the dentin, pulp, cementum and periodontal ligament. By the 37th day of development there is a horseshoe-shaped epithelial thickening in each jaw (the dental lamina). At intervals along this, thickenings develop (the tooth germs). The bottom part of these invaginates to form a bell-shaped structure around the inner tissue, called the dental papilla. A double layer of cells lining the inner aspect of the bell develops into the outer ameloblasts that lay down enamel from the inside out, and the inner odontoblasts that form dentin as they retreat towards the dental papilla, which is the future pulp area. As these two tissues are deposited the cell layers move apart, the gap being filled with the developing crown. Once the crown is formed the root develops (Figure 12.14).

Table 12.4 Recommended dietary fluoride supplement dosage according to drinking water fluoride concentration

Age	Water fluoride (ppm)		
	<0.3	0.3–0.6	>0.6
Birth–6 months	0.25	0	0
6 months–3 years	0.25	0	0
3–6 years	0.50	0.25	0
6–16 years	1.00	0.50	0

The amounts are in milligrams of fluoride per day (2.2 mg sodium fluoride = 1 mg fluoride ion).

Eruption

The mechanisms of tooth eruption are complex and still not completely solved. Teeth eventually appear in the mouth through a combination of growth of supporting bone, elongation of the tooth root and growth of the pulp.

Nutrition and teeth

Prenatal nutrition and developing teeth

Surprisingly, prenatal nutrition has very little effect on the developing teeth. Since all of the primary teeth begin to calcify *in utero* they are relatively protected from a lack of calcium; the mother supplies all of the calcium needed whether or not she gains or looses bone during pregnancy.

The movement of tetracyclines and fluoride across the placental barrier has been studied in depth. Current opinion is that tetracyclines easily cross the placenta for deposition in the dentin and cementum to produce visible discoloration. In contrast, fluoride does not cross the placenta easily. Fluoride ingestion by the mother must be very high, >3 ppm/day, to produce even mild fluorosis of the primary dentition, and if the mother ingests the usual upper therapeutic supplemental dose of 0.5 mg to 1.0 mg per day (Table 12.4) this does not raise fluoride levels in the primary teeth developing *in utero*.

Postnatal nutrition and developing teeth

Postnatal nutrition has been shown to affect developing teeth in animal experiments, but effects on humans are less clear. Ingested tetracycline is deposited in developing dentin and cementum to produce a greengray discoloration that can be seen through the overlying enamel and fluoresces in ultraviolet light.

Adequate calcium in a balanced diet has been stressed to be essential for tooth development after birth, but evidence to support this is lacking. In the 1920s vitamin D deficiency was postulated to produce a 'poorer quality' enamel, but modern research does not support this. Osteoporosis has no effect on the teeth.

Nutrition and dental caries

A direct cause-and-effect relationship between nutritional status and dental caries has not been demonstrated. Both wasting and stunting are associated with retarded exfoliation of the primary teeth and with increased caries rates. What is not clear is whether the increased caries rate is because teeth are present for longer in the mouth and therefore have a longer chance of developing caries, or because the teeth are more susceptible to the disease. Regarding the permanent teeth in the same children, surprisingly, accelerated tooth eruption is seen but still with an increased caries rate. It is believed that a single moderate malnutrition episode under the age of 1 year may alter enamel formation sufficiently to be associated with increased caries later in life, but firm evidence to support this is lacking.

Fluoride and dental fluorosis

Fluoride is regarded by dental associations, dental research organisations and the World Health Organisation (WHO) as an essential nutrient that reduces susceptibility to dental caries. The mechanism is complex, but includes formation of calcium fluroapatite through displacement of hydroxyl ions and interference with the metabolism of cariogenic organisms present in dental plaque. Some 70% of ingested fluoride is excreted in the urine over 24 h. Current opinion is that the preventive effect in dental enamel is topical, through adsorption onto enamel crystals in the outer few micrometres of enamel, rather than a systemic deposition into enamel and dentin during tooth development. A modern development is to provide a continuous low concentration of fluoride in the mouth through slow release fluoride devices attached to teeth.

Sources of fluoride intake are drinking water and food, as well as fluoridated salt, milk and fluoride-containing dental products such toothpastes or gels applied topically to teeth. The optimal oral intake of fluoride ion, that is, the level that gives good protection against dental caries with a low level of dental fluorosis, is approximately 0.5 mg/day. The most cost-effective source, in public health terms, is from fluoridated drinking water. For many years the recommended

Figure 12.15 (a) Limb deformities in children living in an area associated with endemic fluorosis. (b) Teeth staining due to endemic fluorosis.

concentration for fluoridated water in temperate climates has been a concentration of 1 ppm of fluoride ion, but because of increased intake from other sources such as fluoridated toothpastes it is now felt that this should be lower to reduce the rate of dental fluorosis. There is not yet general agreement on the level for water fluoridation, other than it will be lower in hot climates in which more water is drunk than the 1 ppm concentration recommended for temperate climates. Regarding fluoride supplementation from tablets, the recommendation of the American Dental Association's Council on Dental Therapeutics is shown in Table 12.4.

Excess fluoride over a period of time can result in endemic fluorosis which may present with generalised bone abnormalities (osteosclerosis and osteoporosis) and deformities suggestive of rickets (see section 12.5) (Figure 12.15a). Especially during the first 3 years of life, excess of fluoride produces dental fluorosis, comprising mottling and staining of teeth as well as surface pitting (Figure 12.15b); the severity of the mottling increases with rising fluoride intake. At a water fluoride ion concentration of 1 ppm about 10% of individuals will show mild mottling

(occasional white patches on enamel); the rate is about 20% at a concentration of 2 ppm, thereafter it rises exponentially to 100% at 3 ppm. When very severe mottling is present, enamel is particularly brittle and flakes off the underlying dentin. Caries in such teeth is more frequent than at lower levels of dental fluorosis.

Dental caries

Dental caries is a multifactorial disease. Figure 12.16 summarises the interaction of teeth, fermentable foods and bacteria that must occur in dental plaque for sufficient time, influenced by an individual's resistance to the disease, for caries to develop.

Bacteria in dental plaque metabolise fermentable carbohydrates into organic acids which demineralise enamel, as well as dentin if in contact with that. The critical pH below which demineralisation occurs is pH 5.7. Subsequently, proteolytic enzymes break down the organic component. Remineralisation, aided by saliva and fluoride, may happen in the early stages before proteolysis. The more rapidly a food is fermented and the longer a tooth is exposed to a pH

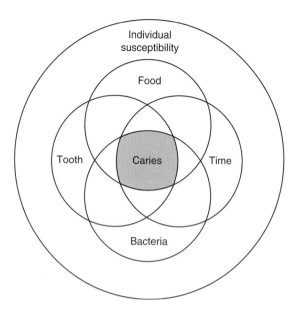

Figure 12.16 Interactions necessary for the development of dental caries.

Figure 12.17 Stephan curve after 10% sucrose rinse and 24 h-old dental plaque.

24-h-old plaque. After a 1-min rinse there is a rapid drop in pH within 3 min, followed by a gradual rise back to resting levels over the next 30 min. The return to resting levels is produced by flow of saliva, the buffering action of the salts in saliva and the removal of the food from the mouth. Non-fermentable foods that stimulate saliva flow do not drop the pH below 5.7 and may actually increase it, as in the case of peanuts (Figure 12.17). Since all meals are mixtures of many foods the pH response is complex. Traditional research has reported on eating of single foods and on sequences of food, but not on food mixtures.

The more often the plaque pH is below 5.7, and the longer it remains there, the greater the potential for demineralisation and dental caries. Lessening of this risk is the basis for the preventive advice to restrict intake of sticky, fermentable foods to three meals and two snacks per day, together with a reduction in cariogenic organisms in contact with teeth through removal of dental plaque at least once per day.

That sugars, as fermentable carbohydrates, play an aetiological role in dental caries is universally accepted, but beyond that statement there is uncertainty on their precise relationship with the disease. In the 1940s results from prospective dietary studies in a Swedish mental institution and an orphanage in Australia, together with national patterns of reduced caries associated with reduced sucrose consumption in Europe during World War II, suggested a direct causal relationship between sugars, particularly sucrose, and dental caries. This belief has persisted among some scientists to the present day, to the extent that the Committee on Medical Aspects of Food Policy in Great Britain (COMA) recommended that consumption of extrinsic non-milk sugars should not exceed 60 g per person per day. Contrary views are that the Swedish study was far removed from normal eating, and the Australian and World War II results were due to replacement of a highly refined diet with a less refined diet, possibly including protective factors. More recent prospective epidemiological studies have not shown that reductions in fermentable carbohydrates in the general population are accompanied by reductions in dental caries. Indeed, general reductions in dental caries that have occurred over the past 20 years in industrialised countries have happened as fermentable carbohydrate intake has either remained the same or increased. This reduction is held to be the effect of fluoride in toothpastes. The national policies

below 5.7, the worse is the potential damage. The length of exposure is influenced by a food's inherent retention in the mouth. For example, liquids are cleared from the mouth more rapidly than solids, and foods that stimulate salivary flow though their consistency or chemical properties are cleared more rapidly than bland foods.

The change in pH that is typical is the pattern after a rinse with sucrose. Figure 12.17 shows this Stephan curve after a 10% sucrose rinse in the presence of

Table 12.5 Differences between osteoporosis and rickets

	Osteoporosis	Nutritional rickets
Age of presentation	Older and postmenopausal women	Infants and young children
Pathology	Loss of bone (mineral: matrix normal)	Failure to mineralise bone matrix (mineral: matrix decreased)
Speed of onset/development	Slow	Rapid
Presentation	Pathological fractures	Limb deformities
Diagnosis	Densitometry assessment or biopsy	Radiographs
Biochemistry	Typically normal	Hypocalcaemia, hypophosphataemia and elevated alkaline phosphatase and parathyroid hormone[a]

[a]Hyperparathyroidism is variable in dietary calcium deficiency. In stages 2 and 3 of vitamin D deficiency elevated PTH concentrations are invariable.

to limit sugar intake that some scientists favour are likely to be unattainable, expensive, ineffective and even harmful through an increased intake of fats.

Since the introduction of Cochrane-type systematic reviews of published evidence, a more objective evaluation of the association between dental caries and sucrose intake is possible. The most recent such review did not demonstrate a relationship between quantity of sucrose ingested and dental caries but did find a moderately significant association of frequency of sucrose intake with dental caries.

A fair summary of the relationship between fermentable carbohydrates and dental caries is that intake of these in a person at high risk of dental caries plays a more powerful role than in someone at low risk of dental caries. The problem is that risk of dental caries (or resistance to the disease) is a much talked about but ill-understood concept. What is clear from many studies around the world is that about 60% of dental caries occurs in about 20% of people. The reason for this is not known. Targeting of such high-risk persons should be the most cost-effective way of preventing the disease, but as yet identification of high-risk people before dental caries develops remains elusive.

12.5 Nutritional rickets

Nutritional rickets occurs in the paediatric age range, especially in the infant and young child. Although rickets may have a number of different aetiologies, nutritional causes are by far the most important globally and constitute a major public health problem in a number

of countries. Despite the ease of its prevention, and the rapidity of its response to treatment, the disease does not receive the attention it should from international agencies and national governments, so children are being left physically handicapped and stunted unnecessarily. In this section the causes, presentation and biochemical and radiological changes associated with nutritional rickets are presented. A brief overview of its treatment and prevention is also provided.

Rickets is a clinical syndrome characterised by a delay in or failure of mineralisation of the cartilaginous growth plates in the growing child. These abnormalities result in deformities at the growth plates of rapidly growing bones. Accompanying these changes, there is also a delay in mineralisation of newly formed osteoid at the endosteal and periosteal bone surfaces, resulting in an increase in osteoid seam width. These latter abnormalities are features of osteomalacia, which is also characterised by an increase in osteoid surface and volume, an increase in the mineralisation lag time and a decrease in tetracycline uptake at the mineralisation front. Thus, the disease of rickets is associated with clinical features related to both the growth plate abnormalities of rickets and those of osteomalacia at the various bone surfaces.

The differences between osteoporosis and rickets are listed in Table 12.5.

Causes of rickets

As mentioned above, rickets is primarily a disease characterised by a failure of mineralisation of preformed matrix. For bone or cartilage matrix to

Table 12.6 Classification of the causes of rickets

Calciopenic rickets	Phosphopenic rickets	Inhibition of mineralisation
Vitamin D deficiency	Dietary deficiency, e.g. breast-fed very low-birthweight infant	Aluminium toxicity
Increased vitamin D metabolite catabolism	Inhibition of intestinal phosphate absorption	Fluoride excess
1α-Hydroxylase deficiency	Increased renal loss of phosphate:	Hereditary hypophosphatasia
Renal failure	X-linked hypophosphataemia	First generation bisphosphonates
Abnormalities of the vitamin D receptor	Fanconi's syndrome distal renal tubular acidosis tumour associated	
Dietary calcium deficiency		

The table is not a comprehensive list, but it does highlight the numerous causes of rickets.

mineralise, the concentrations of both calcium and phosphorus at the mineralisation site must be sufficient for the growth and aggregation of the hydroxyapatite crystals, the formation of which are facilitated by the matrix vesicles (from osteoblasts), which actively accumulate calcium and phosphorus ions and remove inhibitors of crystal formation.

Thus, the causes of rickets may be broadly classified into three large groups: those related to an inability to maintain adequate calcium concentrations at the mineralising bone surface or growth plate (calciopenic rickets), those related to an inability to maintain appropriate phosphorus concentrations (phosphopenic rickets) and those that directly inhibit the process of mineralisation (Table 12.6).

From Table 12.6 it is clear that there are numerous causes of rickets, the majority of which are not nutritional in origin and thus will not be considered in this chapter. Nevertheless, nutritional rickets remains the most common form of rickets globally. Until recently, nutritional rickets has been considered to be synonymous with vitamin D-deficiency rickets, but recent studies suggest that not only is vitamin D deficiency an important cause but so too is a low dietary calcium intake, and the two may act synergistically to exacerbate the risk of developing rickets.

Nutritional rickets: a global perspective

Despite advances in our understanding of calcium homeostasis (see *Introduction to Human Nutrition*, Chapter 9) and vitamin D metabolism (see *Introduction to Human Nutrition*, Chapter 8), nutritional rickets remains a major cause of morbidity and mortality in children in many parts of the world.

Although rickets has been thought of as a disease that originated with the Industrial Revolution in Europe, descriptions of rickets have been attributed to both Homer (900 BC) and Soranus Ephesius (AD 130). Before the Industrial Revolution, rickets was a disease of the children of the aristocracy, as they were frequently kept indoors and excessively clothed if venturing outside. With the rapid growth of cities associated with urban migration, which accompanied the Industrial Revolution, urban slums rapidly developed. The excessive pollution, narrow streets and overcrowding resulted in most young children living in these appalling conditions receiving little or no sunshine. Their mothers likewise were often vitamin D deficient and suffering from osteomalacia, resulting in obstructed labour and neonates being born with no vitamin D stores. In the late nineteenth and early twentieth century several studies described the almost universal prevalence of rickets in young children in Europe. The importance of ultraviolet light in the prevention and treatment of rickets was appreciated in the first quarter of the twentieth century, and with the discovery of vitamin D and its role in the aetiology of rickets, the stage was set for the almost complete elimination of vitamin D-deficiency rickets from a number of developed countries through programmes of food fortification, vitamin D supplementation and education.

During World War II, the UK introduced vitamin D fortification of a number of foods including milk, cereals and bread. The incidence of rickets fell dramatically, but the programme fell into disrepute because of uncontrolled fortification, which was thought to have resulted in an increase in idiopathic hypocalcaemia in young infants, although this association has not been conclusively proven. Since then the incidence of nutritional rickets has risen and is particularly a problem among Asian immigrants living in the northern cities of the UK.

In North America, the prevention of rickets through fortification has been more successful. The universal fortification of milk with vitamin D at 400 IU/quart (32 fl oz, approximately 900 ml) since the 1930s has almost eradicated the disease in young children, except in those who are exclusively breast-fed or who are on milk-free diets. However, since the 1980s there have been reports of a resurgence of rickets in at-risk families, in particular in infants who are breast-fed for prolonged periods, in vegan and vegetarian families, and in infants of African–American mothers.

In central Europe and Algeria, rickets has been successfully prevented in infants and young children by the administration of high doses of vitamin D every 3–5 months for the first 2 years of life (*stosstherapie*). Despite the advances that have been made in the prevention of rickets in young children in many developed countries, the disease remains a major problem in a number of these countries. Not surprisingly, nutritional rickets is more common in those countries at the extremes of latitude, as ultraviolet light exposure is limited for large parts of the year and the cold weather necessitates wearing clothes that cover the majority of the skin surface. Thus, the prevalence of clinical rickets in Tibet has been estimated to be over 60% in children, and similar figures have been obtained from surveys in Mongolia and northern China. Nutritional rickets remains a problem in many countries, even those closer to the equator with larger amounts of sunshine than the countries mentioned above. These countries include Sudan, Ethiopia, Nigeria, Algeria, Saudi Arabia, Kuwait and other countries in the Middle East, India and Bangladesh. Furthermore, a high prevalence of rickets has been described in young children in areas of Greece and Turkey. Thus, there must be other factors beside high latitude that contribute to predisposing a child to rickets. A number of studies have highlighted poverty, malnutrition, maternal vitamin D deficiency, prolonged breast-feeding and overcrowding as important risk factors (Box 12.7).

Box 12.7   Factors predisposing a child to vitamin D-deficiency rickets

- Living in a country at high latitude
- Lack of sunlight exposure through overcrowding, social customs, clothing or pollution
- Infants whose mothers lacked vitamin D in pregnancy
- Prolonged breast-feeding without vitamin D supplementation or appropriate UVB exposure
- Low dietary calcium intake
- Increased melanin pigmentation

Cultural and social customs may also aggravate the problem. Several countries have large Muslim communities, which practise 'purdah', thus increasing the risk of vitamin D deficiency in mothers and their young children.

Although the typical age of presentation of vitamin D-deficiency rickets is during the second 6 months of life, reports from a number of developing countries describe clinical signs of rickets in children over the age of 2 years. It is possible that many of these children are suffering from the residual effects of earlier active, but now healed, rickets. However, recent studies from Nigeria, South Africa and Bangladesh have suggested that children outside the infant age group with clinical signs of rickets may be suffering not from vitamin D deficiency, but rather from the effects of low dietary calcium intakes. The calcium intakes of affected children are remarkably similar in the different countries, with intakes estimated to be approximately 200 mg/day. The characteristic features of the diets are the high cereal content and the lack of variety and of dairy product intake. It is unclear how widespread this form of nutritional rickets is, but low dietary calcium intakes may also exacerbate the severity of vitamin D-deficiency rickets by increasing the catabolism of vitamin D and thus increasing the requirements of vitamin D.

The burden that nutritional rickets places on children globally is unclear, but in those countries in which there is a high prevalence of rickets, a significant proportion of the infant mortality may be directly or indirectly due to the disease. This has clearly been shown in Ethiopia, where it has been estimated that children with rickets have a 13 times higher incidence of pneumonia, which is associated with a 40% mortality. The long-term sequelae of severe rickets are difficult to quantitate, but short stature, residual limb deformities resulting in early osteoarthritis and pelvic deformities in women leading to a high incidence of obstructed labour are some of the problems.

In addition to rickets, recent evidence suggests that vitamin D deficiency may also have wider complications, such as impairing immunity and increasing tuberculosis infection, increasing the risk of type I diabetes and possibly increasing allergic diseases in children.

Pathogenesis of vitamin D-deficiency rickets

As mentioned in the section above, the most common cause of nutritional rickets is vitamin D deficiency. To maintain vitamin D sufficiency, people are largely dependent on the conversion in the skin of 7-dehydrocholesterol to vitamin D_3 through the photochemical action of ultraviolet light, as the normal unfortified diet is generally deficient in vitamin D (see *Introduction to Human Nutrition*, Chapter 8). Thus, vitamin D deficiency is most common at the two extremes of life: in young infants who are unable to walk and in older people who are infirm and are unable to go out of doors.

Vitamin D-deficiency rickets is most prevalent in infants and toddlers between the ages of 3 and 18 months, although it may occur at any age if social customs, skin pigmentation and living in countries at extremes of latitude combine to prevent adequate ultraviolet B (UV-B) exposure of the skin. It is uncommon under 3 months of age because the newborn infant is provided with some vitamin D stores as 25-hydroxyvitamin D (25-OHD) crosses the placenta, umbilical cord values being approximately two-thirds of maternal concentrations. However, the half-life of 25-OHD is only 3–4 weeks, so values fall rapid after birth unless the infant is exposed to ultraviolet light or receives a dietary source of vitamin D. Furthermore, these stores may be inadequate if the mother is vitamin D deficient, resulting in an earlier presentation of rickets or, in rare cases, of the neonate being born with rickets.

Human breast milk typically contains very little of the parent vitamin D or its metabolites. It has been estimated that normal human milk contains the equivalent of approximately 40–60 IU/l. Assuming that an infant consumes about 650 ml of breast milk daily, the vitamin D intake from that source would only amount to 26–39 IU/day, thus contributing little to the maintenance of the vitamin D status of the exclusively breast-fed infant. Supporting the above conclusions is the finding that serum levels of 25-OHD in exclusively breast-fed infants correlate with their sunshine exposure, highlighting the importance of UV-B exposure, rather than diet, in preventing rickets in breast-fed infants. The amount of sunlight needed to maintain normal serum concentrations of 25-OHD in the infant appears to be very little, although it will vary according to latitude and season. In Cincinnati, USA, during summer, it has been estimated to vary between 20 min a week for an infant in a nappy only to 2 h a week for an infant fully clothed but without a cap. The reliance on sunlight exposure and the intradermal formation of vitamin D for the maintenance of vitamin D sufficiency in exclusively breast-fed infants has resulted in the presentation of clinical rickets having a strong seasonality in most studies. Rickets is most prevalent in late winter and the early spring months (Figure 12.18).

Before the introduction of formula milks for the feeding of non-breast-fed infants, breast-feeding was noted to reduce the risk of rickets in young infants compared to those fed diluted cow's milk. More recent studies, however, consider breast-feeding to be a risk factor in infants whose mothers lacked vitamin D in pregnancy. An explanation for this apparent paradox is that breast-milk substitutes are now all required to be vitamin D fortified, thus protecting against vitamin D deficiency. Before the introduction of modified cow's milk formulae, non-breast-fed infants were fed unmodified or diluted cow's milk which, like breast milk, contains very little vitamin D. Furthermore, the calcium:phosphorus ratio of 1:1 and the high phosphate content of cow's milk both adversely affect calcium homeostasis in the relatively vitamin D-deficient infant, resulting in a higher prevalence of clinical rickets.

Although vitamin D deficiency is the ultimate cause of rickets in the Asian community in the UK, it is likely that several of the factors mentioned earlier combine to exacerbate the low vitamin D concentrations and the development of rickets. These factors include decreased vitamin D formation in the skin owing to increased skin coverage by clothing and a greater degree of melanin pigmentation than the Caucasian population, a low vitamin D intake, a low

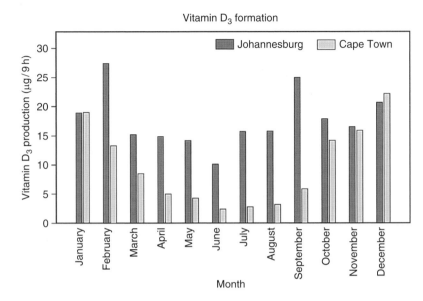

Figure 12.18 Seasonal variation in the production by sunlight of vitamin D$_3$ from 7-dehydrocholesterol *in vitro* in two cities at different latitudes in the southern hemisphere (Johannesburg 26°S and Cape Town 32°S). Note the production of vitamin D in the two cities during the summer months is similar, but during the autumn and winter months (March–September) vitamin D production is minimal in the more southerly city of Cape Town. (Reproduced with permission from Pettifor JM *et al.* The effect of season and latitude on in vitro vitamin D formation by sunlight in South Africa. S Afr Med J 1996; 86: 1270–2.)

dietary calcium content of the mainly vegetarian diet, and poor intestinal absorption of calcium because of the high phytate content of the diet. Low calcium intakes and impaired calcium absorption have been shown to increase vitamin D requirements through an increase in its catabolism as a result of the elevated 1,25-(OH)$_2$D concentrations (Figure 12.19). Thus, these mechanisms push mild vitamin D insufficiency into frank vitamin D deficiency and rickets unless vitamin D intake or skin exposure to sunlight is increased (Box 12.7). Recommended vitamin D intakes are summarised in Table 12.7. Possible strategies to prevent vitamin D deficiency are summarised in Box 12.8.

Biochemical changes associated with vitamin D-deficiency rickets

As discussed in Chapter 8 of *Introduction to Human Nutrition*, in this series, vitamin D plays an important role in maintaining normal calcium homeostasis, mainly through optimising intestinal calcium absorption. The biochemical hallmark of vitamin D deficiency is a low circulating concentration of 25-OHD, which is the major circulating form of the vitamin. In the majority of studies of vitamin D levels in vitamin D-deficiency rickets, 25-OHD concentrations are reported to be less than 4 ng/ml (<10 nmol/l). The lower threshold of vitamin D adequacy used to set dietary recommendations has to date been based on a plasma concentration of 25-(OH)D, which ensures the absence of rickets, in

Figure 12.19 Possible pathogenesis of rickets in the Asian immigrant community in northern Europe. The disease is thought to be the result of a combination of relative vitamin D insufficiency and inadequate intestinal calcium absorption. PTH, parathyroid hormone.

the UK this level is >10 ng/ml (>25 nmol/l) and the USA it is 11 ng/ml (>27.5 nmol/l). However, there is considerable debate around whether this should be revised upwards to take account of other potential health requirements of vitamin D. Higher thresholds, for example 40, 50 and 80 nmol/l, have been proposed but at present there is no consensus. As 1,25-(OH)$_2$D is considered to be the physiologically active metabolite of vitamin D, low levels would be expected to be reported in active vitamin D-deficiency rickets. However, serum 1,25-(OH)$_2$D concentrations are not consistent and low, normal or raised levels have been found in patients. It is sug-

gested that the elevated levels are due to a slight increase in substrate, perhaps through sunlight exposure or dietary intake, causing a transient elevation in 1,25-(OH)$_2$D concentrations. Rapid rises in 1,25-(OH)$_2$D to supraphysiological levels have been documented in vitamin D-deficient subjects after the administration of very small doses of vitamin D or exposure to sunlight.

The biochemical progression of vitamin D deficiency has been divided into three biochemical stages, although there are no sharp boundaries between the stages (Table 12.8). Stage I is the earliest stage and is characterised by hypocalcaemia with normal serum phosphorus, alkaline phosphatase and PTH values. During this phase, the infant may present with features of hypocalcaemia without clinical or radiological signs of rickets being found. Frequently, this stage is not detected clinically as the infant may pass through this stage to stage II without clinical symptoms. In stage II, secondary hyperparathyroidism develops and partially corrects the hypocalcaemia, thus serum calcium concentrations may be within the low normal range, but serum phosphorus values are low and alkaline phosphatase concentrations are elevated. In this stage, the typical radiographic features of rickets are found. Stage III is associated with severe clinical and radiological rickets, with hypocalcaemia once again occurring and alkaline phosphatase values reaching even higher levels. Recently attention has been drawn to vitamin D deficiency with hypocalcaemia presenting rarely in young infants as a cardiomyopathy.

Other biochemical features found in vitamin D-deficiency rickets include decreased urinary calcium excretion, decreased renal tubular reabsorption of phosphorus, increased urinary adenosine monophosphate (cAMP) excretion, generalised aminoaciduria and impaired acid excretion, which are all features of

Table 12.7 Dietary intakes of vitamin D recommended by British and American expert committees (the North American recommendations are currently being reviewed)

Age group	UK reference nutrient intake (μg (IU)/day)	American adequate intake (μg (IU)/day)
0–6 months	8.5 (340)	5.0 (200)
7 months and older toddlers	7 (280)	5.0 (200)
Children and adults	0[a]	5.0 (200)[b]
>65 years (UK) or >70 years (USA)	10 (400)	15 (600)
Pregnancy and lactation	10 (400)	5.0 (200)

[a] 10 μg/day for general population (<50 years) with limited skin sunshine exposure.
[b] For those (<50 years) in the population with limited or uncertain skin sunshine exposure, 10 μg/day aged 50 to 70 years.

Box 12.8 Possible strategies to prevent vitamin D deficiency

- Ensure regular skin exposure to sunlight
- Regular vitamin D supplementation
- Intermittent high-dose supplementation (*stosstherapie*)
- Food fortification

Table 12.8 Progression of the biochemical and radiological changes in untreated vitamin D deficiency

	Stage I	Stage II	Stage III
X-ray changes	Nil to slight osteopenia	Mild to moderate changes of rickets	Severe changes of rickets
Serum calcium	Low	Low to normal	Very low
Serum phosphorus	May be normal	Low	Low
Alkaline phosphatase	Normal to mildly elevated	Raised	Very raised
Parathyroid hormone	Normal to mildly elevated	Raised	Very raised

Figure 12.20 Radiographic changes of rickets. Note the progressive improvement in the radiographic picture from left to right in response to vitamin D treatment over a period of 3 months. (Reproduced with permission from Pettifor JM Calcium, phosphorus and vitamin D. In: Clinical Nutrition of the Young Child, vol 2. (A Ballibriga, O Brusner, J Dobbings *et al*. eds.), 1994 Copyright © New York/Vevey: Raven Press/Nestec Ltd.)

hyperparathyroidism. Bone turnover markers are typically increased, with increased excretion of urinary hydroxyproline and pyridinoline cross-links. Characteristically, alkaline phosphatase values are elevated, but serum osteocalcin has been reported to be within the normal range in untreated rickets.

Histological changes of bone

Histological changes in vitamin D-deficiency rickets occur both at the growth plate and at the endosteal and periosteal bone surfaces. At the growth plate there is a failure of calcification of the longitudinal septa surrounding cartilage cells in the lower hypertrophic zone and the cells fail to undergo apoptosis, while cells in the proliferative zone continue to divide. Blood vessels invading the zone of provisional calcification also cease to proliferate. Thus, the growth plate widens and with the effect of weight bearing and continued proliferation the longitudinal rows of cartilage cells and thus the growth plate become distorted and splayed.

At the endosteal bone surface, newly formed osteoid fails to mineralise; thus, the trabecular surface covered by unmineralised osteoid increases and the osteoid seams widen. Although these features are typical of osteomalacia, they are not pathognomonic unless they are accompanied by the finding of an increase in the mineralisation lag time (the time taken for newly laid osteoid to mineralise).

Radiological changes of bone

The radiological changes of rickets are typically seen best at the growth plates of rapidly growing bones, thus the distal radius and ulna, and the femoral and tibial growth plates at the knee are the usual sites examined (Figure 12.20). The characteristic changes include a loss of the provisional zone of calcification and thus blurring of the demarcation between the metaphysis and the cartilaginous growth plate, widening of the growth plate, and cupping and splaying of the distal metaphysis. The epiphyses typically are poorly mineralised and underdeveloped, resulting in a delay in the bone age compared with chronological age. In older children and adolescents features of osteomalacia, such as Looser zones or pseudofractures, may predominate.

The type and position of deformities of the long bones vary depending on the age of the child, the degree of weight bearing and the severity of the rickets. If hypotonia is severe, deformities might not develop until weight bearing occurs with the commencement of treatment. Genu varum (bow legs) tends to occur in young children who develop rickets, as this age group tends to have a normal physiological bowing. In the older child, genu valgum (knock knees) is more common.

Once treatment has commenced, the initiation of radiological healing may be seen within 3 weeks, with the appearance of a broad band of increased density occurring at the position of the provisional zone of calcification at the distal end of the metaphysis (Figure 12.20). Over the following weeks, the epiphyseal plates narrow, the epiphyses mineralise and cortices thicken. Modelling of deformities occurs so that in many situations apparently severe deformities disappear over a period of months.

Clinical presentation

The clinical picture of rickets depends to a certain extent on the age of the child at presentation. Clinical features of hypocalcaemia may occur at any age, but are more common in the young infant, when they may present with apneic attacks, tetany, convulsions or stridor. Delay in motor milestones and hypotonia are common presentations. Typically, the infant is floppy and sweating and has a protuberant abdomen (Figure 12.21). In severe rickets, hepatosplenomegaly may be present, partially pushed down by the flattened diaphragm, but also enlarged by extramedullary erythropoiesis.

The clinical picture of hypocalcaemia and rickets is covered in greater detail in the *Clinical Nutrition* textbook of this series.

Dietary calcium deficiency

Studies conducted since the 1970s in a number of countries, including South Africa, Nigeria, The Gambia, Bangladesh and India, have highlighted the importance of low dietary calcium intakes in the pathogenesis of nutritional rickets in vitamin D-replete children outside the infant age group. Prior to these studies, it was believed that low dietary calcium intakes were not responsible for rickets in children, except in a few very unusual situations, when young children with gastrointestinal problems were placed on very restricted diets that were very low in calcium (Figure 12.22).

The hallmark of rickets due to dietary calcium deficiency rather than vitamin D deficiency is the finding of 25-OHD values within the normal range and elevated 1,25-$(OH)_2$D concentrations in children who are older than those normally at risk of developing vitamin D deficiency (Table 12.9). Further dietary calcium intakes are characteristically low, at about 200 mg/day, and diets are devoid of dairy products, and high in phytates and oxalates. In South Africa, the children are usually aged between 6 and 16 years and

Figure 12.21 Clinical features of vitamin D deficiency rickets in an 8-month-old child. Note the marked chest deformities and the rather protuberant abdomen. (This figure was published in Vitamin D, vol. 1, Vitamin D deficiency and nutritional rickets in children 294–294. Copyright Elsevier.)

live in rural parts of the country. Unlike those with vitamin D deficiency, the children with dietary calcium deficiency do not have muscle weakness. In Nigeria, the children are younger than those described from South Africa. They tend to present around 4 years of age, having had symptoms for approximately 2 years. In both countries, medical assistance is generally sought because of progressive lower limb deformities.

Support for the hypothesis that dietary calcium deficiency plays an important role in the pathogenesis of rickets in these children comes from the therapeutic response to calcium supplements (Figure 12.23).

It is not known how widespread the problem of dietary calcium deficiency is. It is likely that children with dietary calcium deficiency have been and

Figure 12.22 Lower limb deformities in children in South Africa with dietary calcium-deficiency rickets. (Reproduced with permission from Pettifor JM. Dietary calcium deficiency. In: Rickets (FH Glorieux ed.), Copyright New York/Vevey: Raven Press/Nestec Ltd, 1994.)

Table 12.9 Differentiating features between vitamin D deficiency and dietary calcium deficiency rickets

	Vitamin D deficiency	Dietary calcium deficiency
Onset	Usually between 6 and 18 months	Usually after weaning (>2 years)
Hypotonia	Present	Usually not present
Biochemistry:		
25-OHD	Usually <10 nmol/l	Usually >25 nmol/l
1,25-(OH)$_2$D	Variable (may be low, normal or elevated)	Elevated
Dietary calcium intake	Variable (usual close to RDA)	Low (usually ~200 mg/day)

continue to be diagnosed as vitamin D deficient and treated with vitamin D and calcium supplements. On this regimen the bone disease will respond, and thus the incidence of dietary calcium deficiency will be severely underestimated. Nevertheless, the apparent scarcity of the clinical disease needs to be confirmed by more detailed studies in developing countries where maize (corn) forms a major part of the cereal staple. Although in both Nigeria and South Africa maize is the staple, in Bangladesh rice is the cereal staple, and it has been suggested that the low dietary calcium intakes associated with its almost exclusive

consumption may be responsible for an apparent increase in the incidence of rickets in children since the 1980s (Figure 12.24).

Rickets of prematurity

Over the past few decades, rapid advances have been made in the management of very low-birthweight infants, resulting in a marked improvement in survival rates, particularly for infants weighing less than 1000 g at birth. Associated with the increased survival has been an increase in clinical and biochemical evidence of metabolic bone disease in these infants

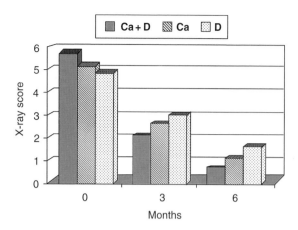

Figure 12.23 Response of randomly assigned Nigerian children with active rickets to treatment with calcium supplements (1000 mg/day), vitamin D (600,000 IU 3 monthly, or a combination of both over 6 months. The X-ray score reflects the severity of radiographic changes at the wrist and knee (Maximum score = 10). The children who received the calcium supplements with or without vitamin D responded significantly better than those receiving vitamin D alone.

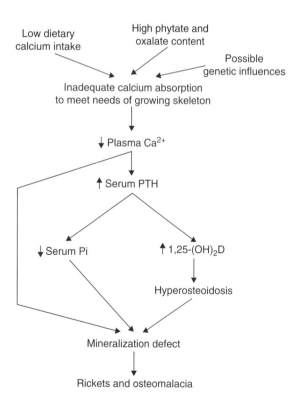

Figure 12.24 Proposed pathogenesis of dietary calcium deficiency rickets. Note that a combination of factors may play a role in the pathogenesis. PTH, parathyroid hormone; Pi, inorganic phosphate; 1,25-(OH)$_2$D, 1,25-dihydroxyvitamin D.

Box 12.9 Biochemical features of metabolic bone disease in preterm infants

- Hypophosphataemia
- Normal or increased serum calcium levels
- Elevated 1,25-(OH)$_2$D concentrations
- Raised alkaline phosphatase concentrations
- Normal parathyroid hormone concentrations
- Hypercalciuria
- Reduced urinary phosphate excretion

(Box 12.9). The bone disease encompasses a range of abnormalities from radiographic osteopenia to frank rickets and pathological fractures. The major risk factor associated with the development of the disorder is severe immaturity (<1000 g) accompanied by breast-milk or soy formula feeding and prolonged illness. Although the pathogenesis is multifactorial, phosphorus depletion due to an inadequate intake plays a major role.

Supplementation of the breast-milk-fed infant with phosphorus rapidly improves the retention of both calcium and phosphorus, and corrects the biochemical picture of the phosphorus depletion syndrome. Once an adequate phosphorus intake is assured, the calcium content of breast milk may become a limiting factor, so simultaneous calcium supplementation is often recommended. Care, however, should be exercised as supplemental calcium may precipitate out before being administered to the baby. As vitamin D stores in the newborn infant are limited and many of these very premature low-birthweight infants spend prolonged periods in intensive care units and neonatal nurseries, an adequate vitamin D intake needs to be ensured. It is recommended that vitamin D 800–1000 IU/daily should be provided as a supplement.

12.6 Bone loss with ageing

Osteoporosis: a global perspective

The WHO has defined osteoporosis as a condition characterised by low bone mass and microarchitectural deterioration of bone tissue that leads to enhanced bone fragility and a consequent increase in fracture risk. These fractures occur most commonly in the wrist, spinal vertebrae and hip, but they can occur elsewhere in the skeleton. Osteoporosis is further defined by the WHO as a BMC or BMD, measured

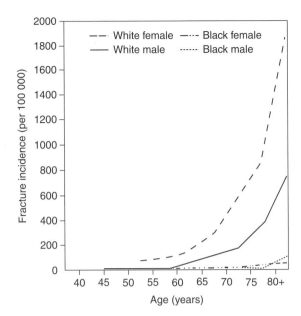

Figure 12.25 Annual incidence of femoral neck fractures in the Johannesburg population over 40 years of age. The marked ethnic differences in incidence are apparent. (Reprinted from The Lancet vol ii Bone Density in aging Caucasian and African Populations 1326–8 Copyright (1979), with permission from Elsevier.)

by absorptiometry, of more than 2.5 standard deviations below the young adult mean. Fractures are the clinically important manifestation of osteoporosis, whereas low bone mass classifies those at risk.

Osteoporosis is a major health problem among older adults. In the UK, over 3 million people are currently affected and approximately 60 000 hip fractures, 50 000 wrist fractures and at least 40 000 vertebral fractures occur each year. One in two British women and one in 5 men over the age of 50 years can expect to experience an osteoporotic fracture during their remaining years. Similarly high fracture rates occur in white populations of northern Europe, the USA and Australasia. However, in other populations, such as those of Africa and China, the incidence is much lower, at least in terms of hip fracture, which is the most reliable statistic available (Figure 12.25). In countries where hip fracture rates are high, women are at greater risk than men, while in countries where the incidence of hip fracture is low, men and women are at approximately equal risk. Within countries there are differences between ethnic groups in hip fracture risk. For example, African–Americans and New Zealand Maoris are at lower risk than their

Box 12.10 Important facts about osteoporosis

- Major public health problem in many countries
- Prevalence varies with ethnicity
- Incidence rising in most countries
- Lifestyle factors probably play an important role in the pathogenesis

Caucasian counterparts, while the incidence of hip fractures in Singapore is highest in the Indian community. However, within all regions and ethnic groups, hip fracture incidence is increasing because of the rise in the number of people surviving to an age when hip fractures are more common. It has been estimated that the global incidence will increase from 1.66 million in 1990 to 6.26 million in 2050 because of the change in demographic profile (Box 12.10).

The pathogenesis of osteoporosis is still a matter of intensive research. Factors that have been implicated include low sex hormone concentrations, especially oestrogen withdrawal at the menopause, compromised supply or metabolic handling of calcium and other nutrients, poor vitamin D status and physical inactivity. Low bone mass and propensity to fracture are heritable traits, which makes it likely that there is a strong genetic component in the pathogenesis of the disease. The involvement of a number of candidate genes has been proposed and polymorphisms in these genes are associated with differences in phenotype or gene expression. Examples include the genes encoding for the vitamin D receptor, the oestrogen receptor, collagen-1-α_1 and IGF-1. At present, however, there is no convincing evidence of an association between any of these polymorphisms and fracture risk.

There are no accepted explanations for the geographical and ethnic differences in fracture incidence. Effects of differences in diet, sunlight exposure and activity levels have been suggested, as well as genetic influences. The variation in fracture incidence is unlikely to be related to low bone mass per se, since Asian and African people generally have lower BMC than their Western counterparts. This is partly, but not entirely, related to their smaller body, and therefore bone, size. Global variations in osteoporosis cannot be explained by differences in calcium intake because hip fracture incidence is greatest in countries with the highest calcium intakes, such as those of northern Europe. Differences in skeletal anatomy, metabolism and microarchitecture may be important, such as the shorter hip axis length of Asian and African people relative to their height, and the higher bone turnover and greater trabecular width in the spines of black South Africans.

Postmenopausal osteoporosis

After the attainment of peak bone mass during the second to third decade of life, bone tissue is gradually lost from the skeleton in both men and women. Periosteal bone growth continues, and the tissue that is lost is from endosteal surfaces. In women, this bone loss is accentuated in the 10–15 years that follow oestrogen withdrawal at the menopause, when approximately one-third of cortical bone tissue and one-half of cancellous bone tissue is lost.

Bone loss is the net consequence of imbalances between bone resorption and formation resulting from changes in the recruitment, activity and lifespan of osteoclasts and osteoblasts. Two types of bone loss are often distinguished, postmenopausal (type I) and age-related (type II) osteoporosis, the first being characterised by a relative increase in osteoclast numbers, the latter by a relative decrease in osteoblast numbers. However, the classification of osteoporosis is not clear-cut; both types may coexist or may represent parts of the same continuum. The features of postmenopausal osteoporosis are summarised in Box 12.11.

Postmenopausal, or type I, osteoporosis affects individuals aged 50–75 years and is more common in women than in men. Accelerated bone loss is associated with reductions in calcium absorption and in circulating concentrations of PTH and $1,25\text{-}(OH)_2D$. Fractures occur most commonly at the distal radius (Colles' fracture of the wrist) and in the spinal vertebrae (crush fracture), regions rich in cancellous bone. Oestrogen deficiency is regarded as the main pathogenetic factor; of type I osteoporosis at the cellular level, oestrogen withdrawal produces a greater number of active osteoclasts, more bone remodelling sites and deeper excavation of resorption cavities. Trabeculae become perforated and may disappear altogether, which reduces the strength of cancellous bone to withstand compressive forces. A number of antiresorptive agents are available for the treatment of postmenopausal osteoporosis, primarily bisphosphonates.

Age-related osteoporosis

Age-related, or type II, osteoporosis affects women and men over about the age of 70 (ratio 2: 1). In general, bone loss is not accelerated and bone turnover may be reduced. Calcium absorption is reduced, $1,25\text{-}(OH)_2D$ concentrations may be low but PTH levels may be increased. Fractures occur commonly in the proximal femur (hip) and spinal vertebrae (wedge fracture). They are associated with trabecular thinning in cancellous bone and the presence of giant resorption cavities in cortical bone.

Ageing is associated with several factors that may result in bone loss and increased bone fragility. These include decreases in physical activity and muscle strength that have direct effects on the skeleton, and also indirect factors via impaired neuromuscular protective mechanisms, which increase the likelihood of falling and of a fall resulting in fracture. Age-related low oestrogen and growth hormone concentrations may impair the function and senescence of osteoblasts, resulting in declining bone turnover and osteocyte numbers, which may reduce the ability to repair fatigue microdamage. Secondary hyperparathyroidism caused by declining renal function and compromised vitamin D status may also be important, via direct effects on the skeleton and indirect effects on calcium handling. Calcium and vitamin D supplementation has been shown to reduce the incidence of non-vertebral fractures in older men and women. The features of age-related osteoporosis are summarised in Box 12.12.

Box 12.11 Features of postmenopausal osteoporosis

- Occurs between 50 and 75 years of age
- Female:male ratio 6:1
- Associated with fractures of the distal forearm and vertebrae
- Associated with oestrogen withdrawal
- Associated with excessive osteoclast activity
- Prevented by oestrogen replacement

Box 12.12 Features of age-related osteoporosis

- Occurs generally in people over 70 years of age
- Male:female ratio 2:1
- Involves fractures of the hip and vertebrae
- Associated with impaired osteoblast function
- Associated with decreased intestinal calcium absorption, hyperparathyroidism and poor vitamin D status

Low circulating levels of endogenous oestrogens are produced in women even though they are many years postmenopause and these may continue to play an important role in the bone health of older women. Current oestrogen use in women aged 65 and older, for example, has been associated with a decreased risk of non-vertebral fractures, especially at the wrist. Similarly in men, some of the skeletal effects of testosterone appear to be mediated through its conversion by aromatase to oestrodiol, and this may be one factor involved in male osteoporosis associated with low testosterone concentrations. Recently, it has been proposed that oestrogen deficiency is the underlying cause of the late, slow phase of bone loss in postmenopausal women and the continuous phase of bone loss in ageing men in addition to the early, accelerated bone loss post menopause.

Role of vitamin D deficiency

Poor vitamin D status may have a role in the pathogenesis of age-related bone loss and fracture, although frank osteomalacia is rarely implicated. It is thought that the mechanism for the increase in bone loss and fractures is via the resulting secondary hyperparathyroidism, although the muscle weakness and depression associated with vitamin D deficiency may also be important.

Vitamin D is obtained either from the diet or by endogenous production in the skin by the action of sunlight (see Chapter 8 in *Introduction to Human Nutrition*). The intermediate metabolite 25-OHD, produced from vitamin D in the liver, is a useful status marker, being responsive to changes in dietary vitamin D and to sunlight exposure. Plasma 25-OHD concentrations decline with age, as a result of decreased endogenous production of the vitamin caused by reduction in the exposure to sunlight, in the tissue content of the precursor, 7-dehydrocholesterol, and in the efficiency of the synthetic process.

Associations have been reported between 25-OHD concentration and BMD in middle-aged and older women. However, vitamin D intervention trials of older people with either bone loss or fracture as outcome have met with mixed success, possibly reflecting differing degrees of vitamin D insufficiency in the various study populations. Trials of calcium and vitamin D together have resulted in a decreased incidence of non-vertebral

---

> **Box 12.13 Vitamin D and older people**
>
> - High prevalence of poor vitamin D status in older people
> - Poor vitamin D status associated with decreased sunlight exposure, low 7-dehydrocholesterol levels in the skin, poor vitamin D intakes, decreased kidney and liver function for conversion of vitamin D to active metabolites and obesity
> - Vitamin D and calcium supplements reduce fracture risk
> - Reduced kidney/liver function affecting vitamin D status in older people

---

fractures, but not consistently in the attenuation of bone loss (Box 12.13).

Traditionally, a serum 25-OHD concentration of 25 nmol/l has been used to define the lower end of the normal range, a value higher than that at which clinical osteomalacia is usually seen. Using this cut-off, a significant prevalence of vitamin D insufficiency has been recognised in the older populations of UK and elsewhere in Europe, particularly those in residential accommodation. Several recent studies have reported inverse relationships between plasma concentrations of 25-OHD and PTH, suggesting that the rise in PTH that accompanies declining vitamin D status may occur at plasma 25-OHD concentrations higher than the traditional cut-off, especially in older age groups. There are calls to increase the lower cut-off of normality for 25-OHD to match a putative threshold below which the concentration of PTH would be expected to rise. Such a change would substantially increase the numbers of people classified as vitamin D deficient and would, perhaps, prompt greater action to improve vitamin D status. However, on a population basis, there is a wide variation in PTH concentration at any given 25-OHD level and such a threshold has yet to be defined with any certainty. In addition, in the context of age-related bone loss and fragility fractures, it is, as yet, unclear what concentrations of PTH, and hence of 25-OHD, are optimal for long-term bone health.

12.7 Specific nutrients and their effects on bone health

In this section the effects of specific nutrients on bone health will be discussed. It should be borne in mind that isolated nutrient deficiencies are unusual; rather, they reflect an unbalanced diet and therefore

Table 12.10 Dietary intakes of calcium reference by the British and American expert committees

	UK reference nutrient intake mg (mmol)/day	American adequate intake mg (mmol)/day
Infants	525 (13.1)	210–270 (5.3–6.8)
Children	350–550 (8.8–13.8)	500–800 (12.5–20.0)
Adolescents		1300 (32.5)
Males	1000 (25.0)	
Females	800 (20.0)	
Adults	700 (17.5)	1000 (25)
Postmenopausal	700 (17.5)	1200 (30)
Pregnancy	700 (17.5)	1000 (25)
Lactation	1250 (31.25)[a]	1000 (25)

[a] May not be necessary.

may be associated with other less obvious nutrient or energy deficiencies, which could mask or aggravate the apparent effects on bone.

Calcium

Calcium is one of the main bone-forming minerals (99% of the body's approximately 1000 g of calcium is in bone), so an appropriate supply to bone is essential at all stages of life. Only approximately one-third of dietary calcium from a Western-style diet is absorbed, and calcium is lost from the body by urinary excretion and in dermal and gastrointestinal secretions. In estimating calcium requirements, most committees have used either a factorial approach, where calculations of skeletal accretion and turnover rates are combined with typical values for calcium absorption and excretion, or a variety of methods based on experimentally derived balance data. Reference calcium intakes are shown in Table 12.10. There has been considerable debate about whether current reference intakes are adequate to maximise peak bone mass and to minimise bone loss and fracture risk in later life, and the controversies continue.

Calcium intake and foetal and infant growth
Direct evidence from supplementation studies in pregnancy on the maternal and foetal skeleton is lacking but in a population with low calcium intake, calcium supplementation through pregnancy has been shown to have no effect on foetal and infant bone mineral accretion or on breast milk calcium concentration.

Calcium intake and peak bone mass
Correlations between calcium intake and adult BMC/BMD have been reported from a large number of cross-sectional and retrospective studies, although there are many other studies where no such association has been observed. Meta-analyses have concluded that calcium intake is a significant determinant of BMD, but the magnitude of the effect is small, about 1% of the population variance. Interpretation of this association is difficult, however, because few studies have adjusted adequately for the confounding effects of body size.

Supplementation of children with calcium salts results in an increase in bone mineral accompanied by a decrease in bone turnover, possibly indicating fewer remodelling sites at the tissue level, while supplementation with milk appears to increase bone mineral by promoting skeletal growth. Whether either of these interventions ultimately alters peak bone mass and, if so, whether later fracture risk is reduced, has yet to be determined. Some studies suggest that an adequate calcium intake is required to optimise the effect of physical activity on bone mass in the child and adolescent.

Calcium and the postmenopausal period
Calcium supplementation given to women around the time of the menopause has little or no effect on the BMD of cancellous regions of the skeleton, where the greatest loss of bone is occurring at that time, but may cause a modest increase in regions rich in cortical bone.

Calcium intake and bone loss during ageing
In older women, calcium supplementation is associated with a higher BMD, by around 1–3%, and with reductions in bone loss in the first 1–2 years after supplementation is started, although it does not prevent some loss from occurring. Longitudinal studies, which follow people prospectively over time, have shown a relationship between customary calcium intake and bone loss in some studies but not others. Case-control studies in Britain, Australia and Canada, populations with medium to high average calcium intakes, have reported no relationship between customary calcium intake and the risk of hip fracture, whereas studies in Hong Kong and southern Europe, where average calcium intakes are lower, have observed an increase in hip fracture risk with declining calcium

intake. Cohort studies give similar results. While meta-analyses have suggested an increase in hip fracture incidence with declining calcium intake, this effect appears to be strongest in populations with a comparatively low average calcium intake and suggests that there is a threshold of increasing risk below around 400–500 mg/day.

Long-term studies suggest that the effects of calcium supplementation occur largely in the first 1–2 years. Calcium has antiresorptive properties, and the increase in BMD that accompanies calcium supplementation is thought to reflect a reduction in the activation of new bone remodelling sites, the infilling of current resorption cavities and an increase in the reversible calcium space. Once this process is complete and a new steady state has been achieved, no further increase in BMD occurs and bone loss continues at a similar rate to before. A similar mechanism is thought to underlie the increase in BMD observed during supplementation of children and adolescents with calcium salts. There have been only a few calcium supplementation trials with fracture as an end-point. Results have been modest and inconsistent, but sample sizes have been small. Larger trials of calcium and vitamin D supplementation in older people have demonstrated reductions in the incidence of non-vertebral fractures.

In general, the effect of customary calcium intake on the outcome of calcium supplementation has not been investigated. In those studies where it has, no relationship has been noted, except in a study of American women 6 or more years postmenopause, where the effect on BMD and on bone loss was limited to those with a daily calcium intake below 400 mg/day. Taken together with the observational data, this suggests, for women living in Western-style environments, that customary calcium intakes below the UK lower reference nutrient intake (LRNI) of 400 mg/day may not be compatible with long-term bone health. There is, however, no evidence of beneficial skeletal effects of a customary calcium intake above the current UK reference nutrient intake (RNI) for any age group, although calcium supplementation is a recognised adjunct in the treatment of bone loss and the prevention of fracture in vulnerable individuals. Recent committees reviewing the evidence have felt unable to use bone health and fracture outcomes as criteria for calculating RNI values.

Phosphorus

Phosphorus is an essential bone-forming element and, as with calcium, an adequate supply of phosphorus to bone is necessary throughout life. Both calcium and phosphorus are required for the appropriate mineralisation of the skeleton, and a depletion of serum phosphate leads to impaired bone mineralisation and compromised osteoblast function. However, there is little evidence that, in healthy individuals, the dietary intake of phosphorus limits good bone health, except in the special case of very low-birthweight infants. Although there is a set proportion of calcium and phosphorus in bone (Ca:P = 10:6), the ratio of calcium to phosphorus in the diet can vary over a wide range with no detectable effects on the absorption and retention of either mineral. Reports of correlations between phosphorus intake and BMD are inconsistent and likely to be affected by size-confounding. Concerns have been expressed about the possible adverse effects of the increasingly high intake of phosphorus in Western-style diets, especially in relation to the consumption of phosphate-based carbonated drinks. At present, it seems unlikely that high phosphorus intakes have consequences for long-term bone health.

Magnesium

Magnesium is involved in bone and mineral homeostasis and is important in bone crystal growth and stabilisation. In a limited number of studies, magnesium intake has been reported to be positively associated with both BMD and excretion of bone resorption markers in middle-aged women, and short-term increases in BMD have been observed with magnesium supplementation. However, the influence of magnesium nutrition, within the range of normal customary intakes, on long-term bone health is unknown. Magnesium is one of a number of nutrients found in fruit and vegetables which contribute to an alkaline environment and which may promote bone health by a variety of mechanisms (see later in this section), making it difficult to examine the effects of magnesium alone.

Protein intake

High protein intake

On a worldwide basis, high protein intakes have been linked with hip fracture because the consumption of protein, particularly as meat and dairy products, is greatest in countries where hip fractures are common. Protein intake is a determinant of urinary calcium excretion, and animal protein, which is rich in sulphur-containing amino acids, and contributes to an acidic environment (see later in this section). There are concerns, but no evidence, that high protein intakes are inadvisable for long-term bone health. For example, when meat is the protein source, the hyper-calciuric effect of protein is offset by the hypocalciuric effect of meat phosphorus and calcium balance is not affected by high-meat diets. Conversely, there are data which suggest a positive interaction between physical activity and protein intake during growth.

Protein deficiency

Protein deficiency very seldom occurs as an isolated nutrient deficiency; thus it is difficult to separate out the effects of protein deficiency from those of other nutrient deficiencies that occur in protein energy malnutrition. In children, protein–energy malnutrition is associated with osteopenia and decreased bone growth, which manifests clinically as stunting, a decrease in cortical thickness and a loss of trabecular bone. There is also a delay in bone age due to a delay in the mineralisation of the ossification centres, but the epiphyseal plates are narrowed owing to a reduction in cartilage cell proliferation. In older people, protein supplements may reduce bone loss, possibly through increasing IGF-1 levels. Several studies have suggested that low protein intakes (but not at levels seen in protein energy malnutrition) might influence bone mass both in children and older people.

In protein–energy malnutrition, the biochemical markers of bone turnover are reduced, as evidenced by a reduction in serum alkaline phosphatase levels and urinary hydroxyproline excretion. A similar reduction in bone turnover is seen at the histological level, with a reduction in osteoblastic and osteoclastic surfaces. Total serum calcium concentrations are often low, in keeping with the reduction in serum albumin values, and serum phosphorus levels may also be markedly reduced. The pathogenesis of the latter changes is ill-understood, although there is evidence of poor renal conservation of phosphate in the child with kwashiorkor.

The long-term consequences of protein deprivation in infancy and childhood on bone health have not been studied, but it appears as though there are few detrimental consequences, as in most countries that have high malnutrition rates, osteoporosis and fractures in adulthood are uncommon.

Vitamin C

Ascorbic acid acts as a cofactor in the hydroxylation of lysine and proline, which are major constituents of collagen. Hydroxylation is important in the formation of cross-links between the collagen fibres and the formation of mature collagen. A severe nutritional deficiency of ascorbic acid leads to the clinical picture of scurvy (Figure 12.26), but the florid syndrome is rarely seen today.

Vitamin K

Vitamin K plays a major role in the γ-carboxylation of glutamic acid residues on a number of proteins (the vitamin K-dependent proteins). The best known of these proteins are the vitamin K-dependent coagulation proteins, but there are also three such proteins in bone: osteocalcin, matrix Gla protein and protein S. The best studied of these is osteocalcin, which, unlike the other two bone vitamin K-dependent proteins, is found only in mineralised tissue and synthesised only by osteoblasts and odontoblasts. The characteristic of the γ-carboxylated proteins is their calcium-binding activity, thus osteocalcin is found bound to mineralised matrix. The physiological role of these bone Gla proteins is unclear, but it has been suggested that osteocalcin may inhibit hydroxyapatite formation or control bone resorption.

From a clinical perspective, there are data to suggest that there is an inverse relationship between vitamin K intake and the prevalence of fractures in older people. Furthermore, several studies have shown an increase in under-carboxylated osteocalcin (a measure of vitamin K deficiency) in older people, and a relationship between the concentration of undercarboxylated osteocalcin and hip fracture rates and BMD. As yet, the data are limited and inconsistent, and no firm conclusions can be drawn.

Similarly, conflicting results have been reported from studies investigating whether or not warfarin, a vitamin K antagonist, is associated with a decrease in bone density and an increased risk of fractures. A supplementation study using vitamin K_2 (menatetranone) in older osteoporotic patients demonstrated a decrease in clinical fractures and a reduction in the loss of BMD at the lumbar spine over a 2-year period.

(a)

(b)

(c)

Figure 12.26 Radiographic changes associated with scurvy in children. Advanced scurvy with fractures of thickened, brittle provisional zones of calcification. (a) Multiple infractions in the provisional zone, with peripheral spurring and early subperiosteal calcification. (b) Longitudinal fractures of the provisional zones of calcification. (c) Crumpling fractures of the provisional zones of calcification. (Reproduced with permission from Silverman FH ed. Caffey's Pediatric X-ray Diagnosis, 8th edn. Copyright (1985) Year Book Publishers, Chicago, USA.)

Fluoride

The role of fluoride in bone health remains controversial, but its role in preventing dental caries is not disputed. Over the past 20 years, considerable interest has been generated in the therapeutic role of fluoride in the management of osteoporosis. Although high doses of fluoride increase bone mass and density through stimulating osteoblastic activity and preventing crystal dissolution, there is little evidence at present that it reduces fracture rates.

Some 50% of ingested fluoride is deposited in bone or teeth, where it displaces bicarbonate or hydroxyl ions in hydroxyapatite to form fluoroapatite. Its incorporation in the apatite crystal reduces the ability of the crystal to dissolve, thus in teeth reducing the risk of caries and in bone causing an increase in bone mass. In bone, however, there is little evidence that at physiological concentrations fluoride has any effect on bone mass.

At pharmacological doses, fluoride (approximately 50 mg of sodium fluoride) increases BMD by stimulating bone formation. At higher doses bone formation is abnormal, with features of woven bone appearing. Despite the increase in BMD, particularly at the lumbar vertebrae, there is no conclusive evidence that fracture rates are reduced.

In a number of areas in the world, such as India, South Africa and Tanzania, endemic fluorosis has been reported due to the chronic ingestion of borehole water with high fluoride concentrations (8–20 mg/l). Typically, the features of endemic fluorosis include joint stiffness, limb deformities and staining of the teeth (Figure 12.15a and b). In children, features of rickets may be seen. Radiologically, there may be osteopenia of the distal ends of the long bones, but the axial skeleton shows osteosclerosis with ligamentous calcification around the joints. The biochemical changes are usually minimal, although hypocalcaemia and elevated alkaline phosphatase and parathyroid concentrations have been reported.

Other dietary factors

Many other nutrients and dietary factors may be important for long-term bone health. Among the essential nutrients, plausible hypotheses for involvement with skeletal health, based on biochemical and metabolic evidence, can be made for zinc, copper, manganese, boron, vitamin A, B vitamins, potassium and sodium. Evidence from physiological and clinical studies is largely lacking. Zinc nutrition is important in infant growth, and associations with BMD have been noted in middle-aged premenopausal women. Copper supplementation ameliorated bone loss in one study of perimenopausal women. A high intake of vitamin A as retinol was associated with hip fracture in Sweden. A higher BMD has been associated with a higher dietary potassium intake, along with other nutrients associated with fruit and vegetable intake. It is suggested that the skeleton may act as a reservoir of alkaline salts for the maintenance of adequate acid–base homeostasis, and foods that promote an alkaline environment, such as fruit and vegetables, may diminish the demand for skeletal salts to balance acid generated from foods such as meat. Sodium is intimately involved in the excretion of calcium through the renal tubules, and a direct relationship is found between urinary sodium and calcium excretion in free-living populations. A high sodium intake may reduce BMD and exacerbate age-related bone loss, but the evidence is not conclusive.

Other components of the diet could also influence bone health. Of these, phytoestrogens are generating interest in that they are naturally occurring plant chemicals with weak oestrogenic properties. Phytoestrogens include soy-derived isoflavones, such as genistein and daidzein, and lignans derived from cereals, fruit and vegetables. These compounds are able to bind to both the α- and β-oestrogen receptors, and may act as receptor agonists or antagonists depending on the tissue. Studies in animal models suggest that phytoestrogens may prevent bone loss after ovarectomy but, as yet, data from human studies are inconclusive.

Although the evidence of a link between intakes of these dietary components and bone health is not sufficiently secure for firm dietary recommendations, the accumulating picture suggests that current healthy-eating advice to increase potassium intake, to decrease sodium intake and to consume more fresh fruit and vegetables is unlikely to be detrimental to bone health and may be beneficial.

12.8   Lifestyle factors and bone health

Alcohol

Ethanol use increases the risk of fracture through several direct and indirect mechanisms, for example through an increased risk of falls, reduced nutrient intakes with associated malnutrition, increased prevalence of heavy smoking, hypogonadism and a direct inhibition of bone formation. Thus, studies of patients suffering from alcoholism have shown reduced bone density and histological evidence of osteoporosis. Biochemically, the characteristic feature is a reduction in serum osteocalcin, but reduced serum calcium and vitamin D levels have also been reported.

Whether social drinking (1–2 units/day) is associated with an effect on bone is unclear and inconsistent, with some studies suggesting a positive effect and others suggesting negative effects.

Smoking

Smoking is associated with a small but significant reduction in BMD, particularly in older men and women when compared with age-matched controls in the majority of studies. The mechanisms by which smoking reduces bone density are unclear, although a number of possibilities exist, including depression of the vitamin D–PTH system, increased alcohol consumption, decreased exercise, reduced free oestradiol and decreased body mass.

Physical activity and exercise

Physical activity is an important modulator of bone mass, not only during childhood but also during adulthood and in older people. Complete immobilisation may result in a loss of some 40% of bone mass. However, exercise added to the normal routine of daily activity may only add a few per cent onto the average bone mass of children and adults. In a meta-analysis of randomised and non-randomised controlled trials conducted over a 30-year period, exercise training programmes were found to prevent or reverse bone loss of almost 1% per year in both the lumbar spine and femoral neck in pre- and postmenopausal women. The osteogenic effects of exercise are specific to the anatomical sites at which the mechanical strain occurs. Thus, tennis players have greater bone density in the dominant than in the non-dominant arm. The type of exercise may also make a difference, as swimmers have lower bone density at axial sites than other athletes.

Eating disorders and malabsorption syndromes

Eating disorders (anorexia nervosa and bulimia) are becoming major problems among the adolescent and young adult population of the most developed

Box 12.14 Possible factors responsible for bone loss in anorexia nervosa

- Oestrogen deficiency
- Dehydroepiandrosterone deficiency
- Undernutrition with associated protein, mineral and vitamin deficiencies
- Insulin-like growth factor-1 deficiency
- Increased cortisol levels
- Excessive exercise

nations of the world. Besides the obvious adverse effects on nutritional status, these disorders have varying adverse effects on bone. Studies suggest that anorexia nervosa carries with it more severe consequences for bone health than bulimia. Bone loss occurs in the majority of anorexic subjects, with over 50% having bone densities more than two standard deviations below age-matched controls. Non-spinal fractures are reported to have a seven-fold increase. It appears that trabecular bone is more severely affected than cortical bone. The pathogenesis of bone loss in anorexia nervosa is multifactorial (Box 12.14), but oestrogen deficiency associated with amenorrhea probably plays a central role. Other contributing factors include malnutrition, IGF-1 deficiency, dehydroepiandrosterone deficiency, increased cortisol levels and possibly associated excessive exercise.

As mentioned earlier, bulimia appears to affect bone mass less severely than anorexia nervosa. In general, women with bulimia are not as wasted or undernourished as anorectic subjects, nor do they have the same prevalence of amenorrhea. They also appear to be less obsessive about the need for exercise, as in one study only 30% of bulimics exercised regularly, compared with 100% of anorectics. Bulimic subjects who exercise maintain their BMD at weight-bearing sites better than sedentary peers, and have higher BMD than anorectic subjects.

Malabsorption syndromes such as cystic fibrosis (see *Clinical Nutrition* textbook) and celiac disease are associated with an increased risk of osteoporosis through associated malnutrition, and calcium and vitamin D malabsorption. As life expectancy in subjects with cystic fibrosis increases with the advances that have been made in the control of respiratory complications, minimal trauma fractures are becoming more common.

Inflammatory bowel disease is also associated with an increase in osteoporosis, with approximately 50% of patients estimated to suffer from osteopenia. Factors aggravating the condition include undernutrition, high levels of circulating inflammatory cytokines, lack of exercise and the use of corticosteroids.

Vegetarianism

There is no evidence that a lactovegetarian diet is associated with differences, either detrimental or beneficial, in BMD or fracture risk. There have been few investigations of individuals consuming vegan or macrobiotic diets, but there is some evidence that these may be associated with low BMD. However, interpretation of studies is difficult because of other differences that may be associated with a vegetarian lifestyle that may affect bone health, such as body weight, smoking habits, physical activity patterns and socioeconomic status. Infants weaned onto macrobiotic diets are at risk of growth retardation and rickets.

Lactose intolerance

Lactose has long been thought to enhance the absorption of calcium, based on animal studies. However, data from human investigations have been inconsistent and recent work suggests that lactose does not have an effect on either calcium absorption or excretion in healthy humans. Lactose intolerance is associated with a low calcium intake because of avoidance of milk and milk products, and is regarded as a likely risk factor for osteoporosis. Studies with fracture or bone loss as an outcome have produced an inconsistent picture, with some suggesting a modest risk for those with lactose intolerance, but not others.

Body weight, body composition and obesity

Body weight and height are major determinants of BMC and BMD. Small build is a risk factor for vertebral fracture, while tall individuals are more prone to hip fracture (see section 12.3). Anatomical variations between adults may reflect the impact of environmental effects at different stages of skeletal development and these may influence later predisposition to fractures. Size in infancy predicts adult BMC, suggesting that the environment *in utero* and early life may be an important modulating factor. Low body weight, especially in connection with anorexia nervosa and the frailty of old age, is associated with an increased risk of fractures, and being overweight with reduced risk. In contrast obesity is a recognised risk factor for fracture in children, with obese individuals having inappropriately low BMC/BMD for their weight. Recent evidence also suggests obesity to be a risk factor for fracture in older people. It should be remembered that obesity is associated with a higher prevalence of poor vitamin D status, and this may also contribute to the negative effect of fat mass on bone mass. In young people and men, studies of body composition suggest that for the same body weight, leanness (a higher lean-to-fat ratio) is associated with higher bone mineral mass, whereas in postmenopausal women, it is fatness (a lower lean-to-fat ratio) that is positively related to bone mineral mass. Various interpretations have been put forward to explain this dichotomy, including the osteogenic effects of muscle in younger people, the shock-absorbing effects of adipose tissue in older people and the possible endogenous production of oestrogens by adipose tissue, which may be particularly important in women after the menopause. Recent animal studies have suggested a role for leptin in the control of bone mass. Situations associated with poor leptin signalling are associated with high bone mass.

12.9 Perspectives on the future

Bone research has progressed in leaps and bounds since the 1980s and in the next decade it is likely that a much greater understanding of the genetic and biochemical factors that are important in controlling bone mass and thus the incidence of fragility fractures will develop. These developments will probably offer the pharmaceutical industry an enormous spectrum of therapeutic possibilities for the optimisation of bone mass and the treatment of osteoporosis.

From a more nutritional point of view, a lot more needs to be learnt about the factors responsible for bone mass accretion during childhood and adolescence, the development of peak bone mass and bone health in older people. Furthermore, the interaction of nutrients, nutritional status, lifestyle, and paracrine and endocrine factors on bone homeostasis need to be explored in greater depth at all stages of the human life cycle. Of increasing interest is the role of micronutrients and non-nutritional compounds in fruit and vegetables, such as vitamin K, phytoestrogens and acid–base balance, on bone homeostasis.

Further reading

Amid I *et al*. Fluoride supplements, dental caries and fluorosis: a systematic review. J Am Dent Assoc 2008; 139: 1457–1468.

Anderson CA *et al*. Sucrose and dental caries: a review of the evidence. Obesity Rev 2009; 10 (Suppl 1) 41–54.

Ash MM Jr. Wheeler's Dental Anatomy, Physiology and Occlusion, 7th edn. Philadelphia, PA: WB Saunders, 1993.

Bonewald LF. Osteocytes as dynamic multifunctional cells. Ann NY Acad Sci 2007; 1116: 281–290.

Burt BA, Szpunar SM. The Michigan study: the relationship between sugar intake and dental caries over three years. Int Dent J 1994; 44: 230–240.

Chevalley T *et al*. High-protein intake enhances the positive impact of physical activity on BMC in prepubertal boys. J Bone Miner Res 2008; 23: 131–142.

Cummings SR, Melton LJ. Epidemiology and outcomes of osteoporotic fractures. Lancet 2002; 359: 1761–1767.

Department of Health. Nutritional Aspects of Bone Health: with Particular Reference to Calcium and Vitamin D. Report of the Subgroup on Bone Health, Working Group on the Nutritional Status of the Population of the Committee on Medical Aspects of Food and Nutrition Policy. London: The Stationery Office, 1998.

Dietary sugars and human disease. Report on Health and Social Subjects No. 37. London: Committee on Medical Aspects of Food Policy, 1989.

Goulding A. Risk factors for fractures in normally active children and adolescents. Med Sport Sci 2007; 51: 102–120.

Heaney R *et al*. Peak bone mass. Osteoporosis Int 2000; 11: 985–1009.

Kanis JA *et al*. European guidance for the diagnosis and management of osteoporosis in postmenopausal women. Osteoporos Int 2008; 19: 399–428.

Pessan JP *et al*. Slow release fluoride devices: a literature review. J Appl Oral Sci 2008; 16: 238–240.

Pettifor JM. Vitamin D deficiency and nutritional rickets in children. In: Vitamin D, 2nd edn. (Feldman D, Glorieux FH, Pike JW, eds). Elsevier, San Diego. 2005; pp. 1065–1083.

Preface. Dosage schedule for dietary fluoride supplements. J Pub Health Dent 1999; 59: 203–204.

Prentice A. Diet, nutrition and the prevention of osteoporosis. Public Health Nutr 2004; 7: 227–243.

Prentice A. Vitamin D deficiency: a global perspective. Nutr Rev 2008; 66: S153–S164.

Prentice A. Pregnancy and Lactation. In: Pediatric Bone – Biology and Diseases (Glorieux FH, Juppner H, Pettifor J, eds). Elsevier, San Diego. 2003; pp. 249–269.

Prentice A *et al*. Nutrition and bone growth and development. Proc Nutr Soc 2006; 65: 348–360.

Rauch F, Schonau E. Changes in bone density during childhood and adolescence: An approach based on bone's biological organization. J Bone Miner Res 2001; 16: 597–604.

Rosen CJ, ed. Primer on the Metabolic Bone Diseases and Disorders of Mineral Metabolism. 7th edn. Washington: American Society for Bone and Mineral Research, 2008.

Scientific Advisory Committee on Nutrition. Update on Vitamin D. London: The Stationery Office, 2007.

Seeman E. An Exercise in geometry. J Bone Miner Res 2002; 17: 373–380.

Seeman E. Pathogenesis of bone fragility in women and men. Lancet 2002; 359: 1841–1850.

Seeman E. Periosteal bone formation–a neglected determinant of bone strength. N Engl J Med 2003; 349: 320–323.

Sperber GH. Craniofacial Embryology. Dental Practitioner Handbook No. 15, 4th edn. London: Wright, 1989.

Standing Committee on the Scientific Evaluation of Dietary Reference Intakes, Food and Nutrition Board, Institute of Medicine. Dietary Reference Intakes for Calcium, Phosphorus, Vitamin D and Fluoride. Washington, DC: National Academy Press, 1997.

Symposia of developmental defects of enamel. Adv Dent Res 1989; 3: 87–271.

Thandrayen K, Norris SA, Pettifor JM. Childhood fracture rates in South Africans of different ethnic origins: The Birth to Twenty Cohort. Osteoporos Int 2009; 20: 47–52.

Van Staa TP *et al*. Epidemiology of fractures in England and Wales. Bone 2001; 29: 517–522.

13
The Immune and Inflammatory Systems

Parveen Yaqoob and Philip C Calder

Key messages

- There is a bidirectional interaction between nutrition, infection and immunity, whereby undernutrition decreases immune defences against invading pathogens, making an individual more susceptible to infection, but the immune response to an infection can itself impair nutritional status and alter body composition.
- Practically all forms of immunity are affected by protein–energy malnutrition, but non-specific defences and cell-mediated immunity are more severely affected than humoral (antibody) responses.
- Micronutrients are required for an efficient immune response and deficiencies in one or more of these nutrients diminish immune function, providing a window of opportunity for infectious agents. However, excessive intakes of some micronutrients may also impair immune function.
- Essential fatty acids have an important role to play in the regulation of immune responses, since they provide precursors for the synthesis of eicosanoids. The balance between n-6 and n-3 polyunsaturated fatty acids may influence the development of immunologically based diseases (particularly inflammatory diseases), although research in this area is not conclusive.

- Deficiencies in essential amino acids are likely to impair immune function, but some non-essential amino acids (e.g. arginine and glutamine) may become conditionally essential in stressful situations.
- Probiotic bacteria have been shown to enhance immune function in laboratory animals and may do so in humans. Prebiotics may also have these effects, but research in this area is not conclusive.
- Breast milk has a composition that promotes the development of the neonatal immune response and may protect against infectious diseases.
- There appears to be a range of nutrient intakes over which the immune system functions optimally, but the exact nature of this range is not clear. It is often assumed when defining the relationship between nutrient intake and immune function that all components of the immune system will respond in the same dose-dependent fashion to a given nutrient. This is not correct, at least as far as some nutrients are concerned, and it appears likely that different components of the immune system show an individual dose–response relationship to the availability of a given nutrient.

13.1 Introduction

Associations between famine and epidemics of infectious disease have been noted throughout history: Hippocrates recognised that poorly nourished people are more susceptible to infectious disease as early as 370 BC. In general, undernutrition impairs the immune system, suppressing immune functions that are fundamental to host protection against pathogenic organisms. Undernutrition leading to impairment of immune function can be due to insufficient intake of energy and macronutrients and/or deficiencies in specific micronutrients (vitamins and minerals). Often these occur in combination: this is particularly notable for protein–energy malnutrition

and deficiencies in micronutrients such as vitamin A, iron, zinc and iodine. Clearly, the impact of undernutrition is greatest in developing countries, but it is also important in developed countries, especially among the elderly, individuals with eating disorders, alcoholics, patients with certain diseases, premature babies and those born small for gestational age. The precise effects of individual nutrients on different aspects of immune function have been notoriously difficult to study. However, it is becoming clear that many nutrients have defined roles in the immune response and that each nutrient has a distinct range of concentrations over which it supports optimal immune function. Lowering the level of the nutrient below this range or increasing it in excess of the range

---

Nutrition and Metabolism, Second Edition, edited by S. A. Lanham-New, I. A. Macdonald and H. M. Roche.   © 2011 The Nutrition Society.

can impair immune function. Thus, the functioning of the immune system is influenced by nutrients consumed as normal components of the diet and appropriate nutrition is required for the host to maintain adequate immune defences towards bacteria, viruses, fungi and parasites.

Unfortunately, the immune system can become dysfunctional or dysregulated, resulting in inappropriate activation of some components. In some individuals the immune system recognises a host (self) antigen and then proceeds to direct its destructive activities against host tissues. These diseases are termed chronic inflammatory diseases, and examples are rheumatoid arthritis, psoriasis, systemic lupus erythmatosus, multiple sclerosis, ulcerative colitis and Crohn's disease. In some other individuals the immune system becomes inappropriately sensitised to a normally benign antigen, termed an allergen, and so reacts vigorously when that antigen is encountered. These are the atopic diseases, which include allergies, asthma and atopic eczema. It is now recognised that atherosclerosis has an immunological component and some cancers arise and develop as a result of diminished immuno-surveillance. Thus, modulation of immune function by dietary components might be an effective means for altering the course of these diseases. Furthermore, diet may underlie the development of some of these diseases.

This chapter begins with an overview of the key components of the immune system, concentrating on the cells that participate in immune responses, the mechanisms by which they communicate and how the system operates in health and disease. The role of nutrients in the immune system is examined using specific examples, and the cyclic relationship between infection and nutritional status discussed. The main body of the chapter is devoted to an evaluation of the influence of individual macronutrients and micronutrients on immune function.

13.2 The immune system

Innate immunity

The immune system acts to protect the host from infectious agents that exist in the environment (bacteria, viruses, fungi, parasites) and from other noxious insults. The immune system has two functional divisions: the innate (or natural) immune system and the acquired (also termed specific or adaptive) immune system (see Figure 13.1). Innate immunity consists of physical barriers, soluble factors and phagocytic cells, which include granulocytes (neutrophils, basophils, eosinophils), monocytes and macrophages (Table 13.1). Innate immunity has no memory and is therefore not influenced by prior exposure to an organism. Phagocytic cells, the main effectors of innate immunity, express surface receptors that recognise certain structures on bacteria. Binding of bacteria to the receptors triggers phagocytosis and subsequent destruction of the pathogenic microorganism by toxic chemicals, such as superoxide radicals and hydrogen peroxide. Natural killer cells also possess surface receptors and destroy their target cells by the release of cytotoxic proteins. In this way, innate immunity provides a first line of defence against invading pathogens. However, an immune response often requires the coordinated actions of both innate immunity and the more powerful and flexible acquired immunity.

Acquired immunity

Acquired immunity involves the specific recognition of molecules (antigens) on an invading pathogen which distinguish it as being foreign to the host. Lymphocytes, which are classified into T- and B-lymphocytes, affect this form of immunity (Figure 13.1). All lymphocytes (indeed all cells of the immune system) originate in the bone marrow. B-lymphocytes undergo further development and maturation in the bone marrow before being released into the circulation, while T-lymphocytes mature in the thymus. From the bloodstream, lymphocytes can enter peripheral lymphoid organs, which include lymph nodes, the spleen, mucosal lymphoid tissue, tonsils and gut-associated lymphoid tissue. Immune responses occur largely in these lymphoid organs, which are highly organised to promote the interaction of cells and invading pathogens.

The acquired immune system is highly specific, since each lymphocyte carries surface receptors for a single antigen. However, acquired immunity is extremely diverse; the lymphocyte repertoire in humans has been estimated at recognition of approximately 10^{11} antigens. The high degree of specificity, combined with the huge lymphocyte repertoire, means that only a relatively small number of lymphocytes will be able to recognise any given antigen. The acquired immune system has developed the ability for

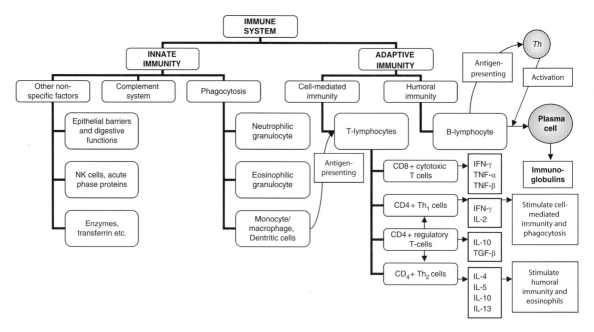

Figure 13.1 Overview of the immune system. (With permission from CAB Reviews.)

Table 13.1 Components of innate and acquired immunity

	Innate	Acquired
Physicochemical barriers	Skin	Cutaneous and
	Mucous membranes	mucosal immune
	Lysozyme	systems
		Antibodies in mucosal
		secretions
	Stomach acid	
	Commensal bacteria	
Circulating molecules	Complement	Antibodies
	Granulocytes	Lymphocytes (T and B)
Cells	Monocytes/	
	macrophages	
	Natural killer cells	
Soluble mediators	Macrophage-derived	Lymphocyte-derived
	cytokines	cytokines

Box 13.1 Features of the acquired immune response

- Specificity
- Diversity
- Memory
- Self-regulation

clonal expansion to deal with this. Clonal expansion involves the proliferation of a lymphocyte once an interaction with its specific antigen has occurred, so that a single lymphocyte gives rise to a clone of lymphocytes, all of which have the ability to recognise the antigen causing the initial response. This feature of acquired immunity has often been likened to building up an army to fight a foreign invasion. The acquired immune response becomes effective over several days after the initial activation, but it also persists for some

time after the removal of the initiating antigen. This persistence gives rise to immunological memory, which is also a characteristic feature of acquired immunity. It is the basis for the stronger, more effective immune response to re-exposure to an antigen (i.e. reinfection with the same pathogen) and is the basis for vaccination. Eventually, the immune system will re-establish homeostasis using self-regulatory mechanisms involving communication between cells. The major features of the acquired immune response are summarised in Box 13.1.

B- and T-lymphocytes

B-lymphocytes are characterised by their ability to produce antibodies (soluble antigen-specific immunoglobulins) which confer antigen specificity to the acquired immune system (i.e. the antibodies produced by B-lymphocytes are specific for individual antigens). This form of protection is termed humoral immunity. B-lymphocytes carry immunoglobulins, which are capable of binding an antigen, on their cell surfaces (Figure 13.1). Binding of immunoglobulin with antigen causes proliferation of the B-lymphocyte and subsequent transformation into plasma cells, which secrete large amounts of antibody with the same specificity as the parent cell.

Immunoglobulins (antibodies) are proteins consisting of two identical heavy chains and two identical light chains. Five different types of heavy chain give rise to five major classes of immunoglobulin, IgA, IgD, IgG, IgM and IgE, each of which elicits different components of the humoral immune response. Antibodies work in several ways to combat invading pathogens. They can 'neutralise' toxins or microorganisms by binding to them and preventing their attachment to host cells, and they can activate complement proteins in plasma, which in turn promote the destruction of bacteria by phagocytes. Since they have binding sites for both an antigen and for receptors on phagocytic cells, antibodies can also promote the interaction of the two components by forming physical 'bridges', a process known as opsonisation. The type of phagocytic cell bound by the antibody will be determined by the antibody class: macrophages and neutrophils are specific for IgM and IgG, while eosinophils are specific for IgE. In this way, antibodies are a form of communication between the acquired and the innate immune response; they are elicited through highly specific mechanisms, but are ultimately translated to a form that can be interpreted by the innate immune system, enabling it to destroy the pathogen.

Humoral immunity deals with extracellular pathogens. However, some pathogens, particularly viruses, but also some bacteria, infect individuals by entering cells. These pathogens will escape humoral immunity and are instead dealt with by cell-mediated immunity, which is conferred by T-lymphocytes. T-lymphocytes express antigen-specific T-cell receptors (TCR) on their surface, which have an enormous antigen repertoire. However, unlike B-lymphocytes, they are only able to recognise antigens that are presented to them on a cell surface (the cell presenting the antigen to the T-lymphocyte is termed an antigen presenting cell); this is the distinguishing feature between humoral and cell-mediated immunity. Activation of the TCR results in entry of T-lymphocytes into the cell cycle and, ultimately, proliferation. Activated T-lymphocytes

also begin to synthesise and secrete the cytokine interleukin-2 (IL-2), which further promotes proliferation and differentiation by autocrine mechanisms. Thus, the expansion of T-lymphocytes builds up an army of T-lymphocytes in much the same way as that of B-lymphocytes. Effector T-lymphocytes have the ability to migrate to sites of infection, injury or tissue damage. There are three principal types of T lymphocytes: cytotoxic T-cells, T helper cells and regulatory T-cells. Cytotoxic T-lymphocytes carry the surface protein marker $CD8^+$ and kill infected cells and tumour cells by secretion of cytotoxic enzymes, which cause lysis of the target cell, or secretion of the antiviral cytokine interferon-γ (IFN-γ) or inducing apoptosis (suicide) of target cells. Helper ($CD4^+$) T-lymphocytes eliminate pathogens by stimulating the phagocytic activity of macrophages and the proliferation of, and antibody secretion by, B-lymphocytes. Regulatory T-cells ($CD4^+CD25^+FoxP3^+$) suppress the activities of B-cells and other T-cells and prevent inappropriate activation.

In delayed-type hypersensitivity (DTH), antigen-activated $CD4^+$ T-lymphocytes secrete cytokines, which have several effects, including recruitment of neutrophils and monocytes from the blood to the site of antigen challenge and activation of monocytes to effect elimination of the antigen. This type of cell-mediated immunity forms the primary defence mechanism against intracellular bacteria, such as *Listeria monocytogenes*. The DTH reaction can be induced in humans by contact sensitisation with chemicals and environmental antigens or by intradermal injection of microbial antigens, and as such has been widely used as a rapid *in vivo* marker of cell-mediated immunity. Approximately 4 h after initiation, neutrophils infiltrate the site, but this rapidly subsides and by 12 h T-lymphocytes migrate from blood vessels and accumulate in the epidermis. By 48 h macrophages are present in all areas and spongiosis (swelling and thickening of the skin) occurs. The degree of the DTH reaction can be assessed by measuring the thickening of the skin, normally 48 h after exposure to the antigen.

While effective immune responses are highly desirable, some aspects of immunity have undesirable consequences. For example, bactericidal and inflammatory mediators secreted by macrophages are toxic not only to pathogens, but also to host tissues, resulting in unavoidable tissue damage. For this reason, immune responses, and macrophage responses in particular, need to be tightly controlled and the self-regulatory properties of the immune system highly effective; regulatory T-cells are thought to be an important part of this self-regulatory activity.

Gut-associated immune system

The immune system of the gut (sometimes termed gut-associated lymphoid tissue) is extensive and includes the physical barrier of the intestine, as well as components of innate and adaptive immune responses. The physical barrier includes acid in the stomach, peristalsis, mucus secretion and tightly connected epithelial cells, which collectively prevent the entry of pathogens. The cells of the immune system are organised into specialised lymphoid tissue, termed Peyer's patches, which are located directly beneath the epithelium in the lamina propria. This also contains M-cells, which sample small particles from the gut lumen. Other lymphocytes are also present in the lamina propria, as well as being associated with the epithelium itself.

Because the gut-associated immune system is inaccessible and requires invasive techniques for study, it is relatively poorly understood and much of our understanding of the influence of nutrition on this aspect of immunity comes from animal studies. Endoscopy and biopsy of gut-associated immune tissues is possible, but data from this type of study are very limited. The most useful practical marker of the gut-associated immune system is salivary IgA (see section B-and T-lymphocytes), although this relies on the assumption that secretion of Ig in saliva reflects that of the rest of the gut-associated system. There are also some markers available for measuring inflammation in the intestine; these include components of neutrophils in stools and markers of protein loss. New technologies are likely to employ capsules, which travel through the gut transmitting images and sampling tissue from selected sites. Such techniques could revolutionise our understanding of gut immunity, but may not be available for some time yet.

Communication within the immune system: cytokines

Communication within the acquired immune system and between the innate and acquired systems is brought about by direct cell-to-cell contact involving adhesion molecules and by the production of chemical messengers, which send signals from one cell to another. Chief among these chemical messengers are proteins called cytokines, which can act to regulate the activity of the cell that produced the cytokine or of other cells. Each cytokine can have multiple activities on different cell types. Cytokines act by binding to specific receptors on the cell surface and thereby induce changes in the growth, development or activity of the target cell.

Tumour necrosis factor-α (TNF-α), IL-1 and IL-6 are among the most important cytokines produced by monocytes and macrophages. These cytokines activate neutrophils, monocytes and macrophages to initiate bacterial and tumour cell killing, increase adhesion molecule expression on the surface of neutrophils and endothelial cells, stimulate T- and B-lymphocyte proliferation, and initiate the production of other pro-inflammatory cytokines (e.g. TNF induces production of IL-1 and IL-6, and IL-1 induces production of IL-6). Thus, TNF, IL-1 and IL-6 are mediators of both natural and acquired immunity and are an important link between them. In addition, these cytokines mediate the systemic effects of inflammation such as fever, weight loss and acute-phase protein synthesis in the liver. Production of appropriate amounts of TNF, IL-1 and IL-6 is clearly important in response to infection, but inappropriate production or overproduction can be dangerous and these cytokines, particularly TNF, are implicated in causing some of the pathological responses that occur in chronic inflammatory conditions (e.g. rheumatoid arthritis and psoriasis).

Helper T-lymphocytes have traditionally been subdivided into two broad categories (Figure 13.2) according to the pattern of cytokines they produce; although a third category of T-cells (Th17 cells) has recently been identified, their functional relevance has yet to be determined. Helper T cells that have not previously encountered antigen produce mainly IL-2 on the initial encounter with an antigen. These cells may differentiate into a population, sometimes referred to as Th_0 cells, which differentiate further into either Th_1 or Th_2 cells (Figure 13.2). This differentiation is regulated by cytokines: IL-12 and IFN-γ promote the development of Th_1 cells, while IL-4 promotes the development of Th_2 cells (Figure 13.2). Th_1 and Th_2 cells have relatively restricted profiles of cytokine production: Th_1 cells produce IL-2 and IFN-γ, which activate macrophages, natural killer

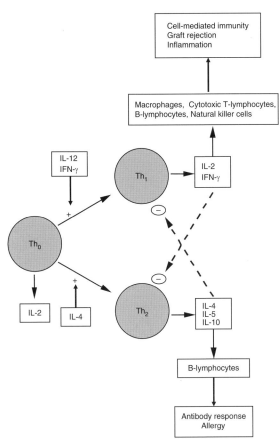

Figure 13.2 Development and cytokine profiles of Th$_1$ and Th$_2$ lymphocytes. IL, interleukin; IFN, interferon.

cells and cytotoxic T-lymphocytes, and are the principal effectors of cell-mediated immunity. Interactions with bacteria, viruses and fungi tend to induce Th$_1$ activity. Since Th$_1$ cytokines activate monocytes and macrophages, these cytokines may be regarded as proinflammatory. Th$_2$ cells produce IL-4, which stimulates IgE production, IL-5, an eosinophil-activating factor, and IL-10, which together with IL-4 suppresses cell-mediated immunity (Figure 13.2). Th$_2$ cells are responsible for defence against helminthic parasites, which is due to IgE-mediated activation of mast cells and basophils. Since Th$_2$ cytokines suppress Th$_1$ responses, these cytokines may be regarded as anti-inflammatory. The patterns of cytokine secretion by Th$_1$ and Th$_2$ lymphocytes were first demonstrated in mice. It has subsequently been demonstrated that while human helper T-lymphocytes do show differences in cytokine profile, the divisions are not clear and while some cells have a typical Th$_1$

or Th$_2$ profile, the majority secrete a mixture of Th$_1$ and Th$_2$ cytokines in differing proportions. Thus, the terms 'Th$_1$ dominant' and 'Th$_2$ dominant' are commonly used to describe the cytokine profiles of these cells. An interesting feature of Th$_1$/Th$_2$ dominance is that once a pattern of cytokine secretion has been established, the dominant arm is able to self-amplify and to antagonise the non-dominant arm. In this way, once a helper T-lymphocyte response has been established, it becomes increasingly polarised towards the dominant phenotype (inflammatory conditions for Th$_1$ and allergy for Th$_2$). The third, most recently characterised category of T helper cells is Th17, which appear to play an important role in autoimmunity (where the immune system attacks host tissues inappropriately). However, the range of activities of this class of T helper cells is not yet fully understood.

Inflammation

Inflammation is the body's immediate response to infection or injury. It is typified by redness, swelling, heat and pain. These occur as a result of increased blood flow, increased permeability across blood capillaries, which permits large molecules (e.g. complement, antibodies, cytokines) to leave the bloodstream and cross the endothelial wall, and increased movement of leukocytes from the bloodstream into the surrounding tissue. Thus, inflammation is an integral part of the innate immune response.

The immune system in health and disease

Clearly, a well-functioning immune system is essential to health and serves to protect the host from the effects of ever-present pathogenic organisms. Cells of the immune system also have a role in identifying and eliminating cancer cells. There are, however, some undesirable features of immune responses.

Firstly, in developing the ability to recognise and eliminate foreign antigens effectively, the immune system is responsible for the rejection of transplanted tissues.

Secondly, the ability to discriminate between 'self' and 'non-self' is an essential requirement of the immune system and is normally achieved by the destruction of self-recognising T- and B-lymphocytes before their maturation. However, since lymphocytes are unlikely to be exposed to all possible self-antigens in this way, a second mechanism termed clonal anergy exists, which ensures that an encounter with a self-antigen induces tolerance. In some individuals there is a breakdown of the mechanisms that normally preserve tolerance. A number of factors contribute to this, including a range of immunological abnormalities and a genetic predisposition in some individuals. As a result, an inappropriate immune response to host tissues is generated and this can lead to autoimmune and inflammatory diseases, which are typified by ongoing chronic inflammation and a dysregulated Th1 response. Examples of this type of disease include psoriasis, multiple sclerosis and rheumatoid arthritis.

Thirdly, the immune system of some individuals can become sensitised to usually benign antigens from the environment and can respond inappropriately to them. Such antigens can include components of foods or so-called allergens (e.g. cat or dog fur, house dust mites, some pollens), such that this response can lead to allergies, asthma and related atopic diseases. Although these diseases are often termed chronic inflammatory diseases and are typified by inappropriate recognition of and/or responses to antigens, they have a different immune basis from the diseases described above. Atopic diseases are typically initiated by the production of IgE by B-lymphocytes in response to exposure to an antigen for the first time (this can be present in a variety of forms, e.g. pollen, dust or in foods). Binding of IgE to specific receptors on the surfaces of mast cells and basophils then occurs (termed sensitisation). If the antigen is reintroduced, it will interact with the bound IgE, leading to activation of the cells and the release of both preformed and newly synthesised inflammatory mediators (particularly histamine and the Th_2 cytokines, IL-4, IL-5 and IL-10).

13.3 Factors influencing immune function

Many factors influence immune function and resistance to infection, leading to great variability within the normal adult population. They include genetics, gender, early life events, age and hormonal status. Immunological 'history' also plays a role in the form of previous exposure to pathogens, vaccination history and chronic disease burden (accumulating conditions over time). Environmental factors influencing immune function include stress (environmental,

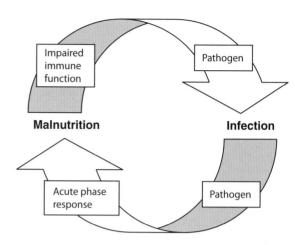

Figure 13.3 Cyclic relationships between malnutrition and infection. Undernutrition impairs immune defences, lowering resistance to invading pathogens. In turn, infection alters nutrient status and contributes to the undernourished state.

physiological and psychological), exercise (acute and chronic), obesity, smoking, alcohol consumption, gut microbiota and nutritional status. In a newborn baby, immunologic competence is gained as the immune system encounters new antigens and so matures and expands. Some of these early encounters with antigens play an important role in assuring tolerance and a breakdown in this system can lead to increased likelihood of childhood atopic diseases and perhaps also to certain inflammatory conditions later in life. At the other end of the lifecycle, older people experience a progressive dysregulation of the immune system, leading to decreased cell-mediated immunity and a greater susceptibility to infection. Innate immunity appears to be less affected by ageing; indeed, there is a progressive increase in chronic inflammation during ageing.

13.4 Impact of infection on nutrient status

Undernutrition decreases immune defences against invading pathogens and makes an individual more susceptible to infections. However, the immune response to an infection can itself impair nutritional status and body composition. Thus, there is a bidirectional interaction between nutrition, infection and immunity (Figure 13.3).

Infection impairs nutritional status and body composition in the following ways.

Infection is characterised by anorexia

Reduction in food intake (anorexia) can range from as little as 5% to almost complete loss of appetite. This can lead to nutrient deficiencies even if the host is not deficient before the infection and may make apparent existing borderline deficiencies.

Infection is characterised by nutrient malabsorption and loss

The range of infections associated with nutrient malabsorption is wide and includes bacteria, viruses, protozoa and intestinal helminths. Infections that cause diarrhoea or vomiting will result in nutrient loss. Apart from malabsorption, nutrients may also be lost through the faeces as a result of damage to the intestinal wall caused by some infectious agents.

Infection is characterised by increased resting energy expenditure

Infection increases the basal metabolic rate during fever: each 1°C increase in body temperature is associated with a 13% increase in metabolic rate, which significantly increases energy requirements. This places a significant demand on nutrient supply, particularly when coupled with anorexia, diarrhoea and other nutrient losses (e.g. in urine and sweat).

Infection is characterised by altered metabolism and redistribution of nutrients

The acute-phase response is the name given to the metabolic response to infections and it includes the onset of fever and anorexia, the production of specific acute-phase reactants, and the activation and proliferation of immune cells. This catabolic response occurs with all infections, even when they are subclinical, and serves to bring about a redistribution of nutrients away from skeletal muscle and adipose tissue and towards the host immune system. This redistribution is mediated by the production of proinflammatory cytokines by leukocytes and associated endocrine changes. Amino acids, mobilised from skeletal muscle, are used by the liver for the synthesis of acute-phase proteins (e.g. C-reactive protein) and by leukocytes for the synthesis of immunoglobulin and cytokines. The average loss of protein over a range of infections has been estimated to be 0.6–1.2 g/kg body weight per day.

It is clear that the inflammatory cytokines mediate many of the effects that lead to compromised nutritional status following an infection, including anorexia, increased energy expenditure and redistribution of nutrients, while malabsorption and maldigestion are brought about by the pathogen itself. The result is that an increased nutrient requirement coincides with reduced nutrient intake, reduced nutrient absorption and nutrient losses (Figure 13.4).

13.5 Why should nutrients affect immune function?

Although the immune system is functioning at all times, specific immunity becomes activated when the host is challenged by pathogens. This activation is associated with a marked increase in the demand of the immune system for substrates and nutrients to provide a ready source of energy, which can be supplied from exogenous sources (i.e. from the diet) and/or from endogenous pools. The cells of the immune system are metabolically active and are able to utilise glucose, amino acids and fatty acids as fuels.

Energy generation involves electron carriers, which are nucleotide derivatives, for example nicotinamide adenine dinucleotide (NAD), flavin adenine dinucleotide (FAD), and a range of coenzymes. The electron carriers and coenzymes are usually derivatives of vitamins: thiamine pyrophosphate is derived from thiamin (vitamin B_1), FAD and flavin mononucleotide from riboflavin (vitamin B_2), NAD from nicotinate (niacin), pyridoxal phosphate from pyridoxine (vitamin B_6), coenzyme A from pantothenate, tetrahydrofolate from folate and cobamide from cobalamin (vitamin B_{12}). In addition, biotin is required by some enzymes for activity. The final component of the pathway for energy generation (the mitochondrial electron transfer chain) includes electron carriers that have iron or copper at their active site.

Activation of the immune response gives rise to the production of proteins (immunoglobulins, cytokines, cytokine receptors, adhesion molecules, acute-phase proteins) and lipid-derived mediators (prostaglandins, leukotrienes). To respond optimally there must be the appropriate enzymic machinery in place (for RNA synthesis and protein synthesis and their regulation) and ample substrate available [nucleotides for RNA synthesis, the correct mix of

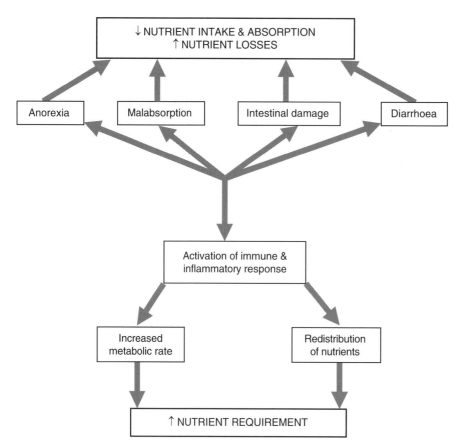

Figure 13.4 Impact of infection on nutritional status.

amino acids for protein synthesis, polyunsaturated fatty acids (PUFA) for eicosanoid synthesis].

An important component of the immune response is oxidative burst, during which superoxide anion radicals are produced from oxygen in a reaction linked to the oxidation of NADPH. The reactive oxygen species produced can be damaging to host tissues and thus antioxidant protective mechanisms are necessary. Among these are the classic antioxidant vitamins, α-tocopherol (vitamin E) and ascorbic acid (vitamin C), glutathione, a tripeptide composed of glutamate, cysteine and glycine, the antioxidant enzymes superoxide dismutase and catalase, and the glutathione recycling enzyme glutathione peroxidase. Superoxide dismutase has two forms, a mitochondrial form and a cytosolic form; the mitochondrial form includes manganese at its active site, whereas the cytosolic form includes copper and zinc. Catalase contains iron at its active site, whereas glutathione peroxidase contains selenium.

Cellular proliferation is a key component of the immune response, providing amplification and memory: before division there must be replication of DNA and then of all cellular components (proteins, membranes, intracellular organelles, etc.). In addition to energy, this clearly needs a supply of nucleotides (for DNA and RNA synthesis), amino acids (for protein synthesis), fatty acids, bases and phosphate (for phospholipid synthesis), and other lipids (e.g. cholesterol) and cellular components. Although nucleotides are synthesised mainly from amino acids, some of the cellular building blocks cannot be synthesised in mammalian cells and must come from the diet (e.g. essential fatty acids, essential amino acids, minerals). Amino acids (e.g. arginine) are precursors for the synthesis of polyamines, which have roles in the regulation of DNA replication and cell division. Various micronutrients (e.g. iron, folic, zinc, magnesium) are also involved in nucleotide and nucleic acid synthesis.

Thus, the roles for nutrients in immune function are many and varied, and it is easy to appreciate that an adequate and balanced supply of these is essential if an appropriate immune response is to be maintained.

13.6 Assessment of the effect of nutrition on immune function

There is a wide range of methodologies by which to assess the impact of nutrients on immune function. Assessments can be made of cell functions *ex vivo* (i.e. of the cells isolated from animals or humans subjected to dietary manipulation and studied in short- or long-term culture) or of indicators of immune function *in vivo* (e.g. by measuring the concentrations of proteins relevant to immune function in the bloodstream or the response to an immunological challenge). Table 13.2 lists some examples of methods used for the assessment of immune function. The biological relevance of these markers of immune function remains unclear. An Expert Task Force on Nutrition and Immunity in Man published a report in 2005 (see further reading), which classified markers into three categories with high, medium or low suitability for assessment of immune function. Those in the 'high suitability' category include the DTH response, vaccination response and production of secretory IgA. These were deemed to be suitable because they are *in vivo* measures, which involve no manipulation of cells outside the body. Those in the 'medium suitability' category include *ex vivo* markers, such as natural killer cell activity and cytokine production. The Task Force concluded that no single marker should be used to draw conclusions about modulation of the whole immune system, except for those studies which have infection as a clinical outcome, and that combining markers with high and medium suitability is currently the best approach is to measure immunomodulation in human nutritional studies.

13.7 Malnutrition and immune function

Protein–energy malnutrition

Protein–energy malnutrition, although often considered a problem solely of developing countries, has been described in even the most affluent of countries. Moderate malnutrition in the developed world is encountered among the elderly, anorexics and bulimics, premature babies, hospitalised patients and

Table 13.2 Assessment of the effect of nutrition on immune function

In vivo measures
  Size of lymphoid organs
  Cellularity of lymphoid organs
  Numbers and types of immune cells circulating in bloodstream
  Cell-surface expression of molecules involved in immune response (e.g. antigen presentation)
  Circulating concentrations of Ig specific for antigens after an antigen challenge
  Concentration of secretory IgA in saliva, tears and intestinal washings
  Delayed-type hypersensitivity response to intradermal application of antigen
  Response to challenge with live pathogens (mainly animal studies; outcome usually survival)
  Incidence and severity of infectious diseases (can be used in human studies)
Ex vivo measures
  Phagocytosis by neutrophils and macrophages
  Oxidative burst by neutrophils and macrophages
  Natural killer cell activity against specific target cells (usually tumour cells)
  Cytotoxic T-lymphocyte activity
  Lymphocyte proliferation (following stimulation with an antigen or mitogen)
  Production of cytokines by lymphocytes and macrophages
  Production of immunoglobulins by lymphocytes
  Cell-surface expression of molecules involved in cellular activation

patients with various disease conditions [e.g. cystic fibrosis, acquired immunodeficiency syndrome (AIDS) and some cancers]. It is important to recognise that protein–energy malnutrition often coexists with micronutrient deficiencies, and poor outcome of intervention can result from a lack of awareness of multiple deficiencies.

Practically all forms of immunity may be affected by protein–energy malnutrition but non-specific defences and cell-mediated immunity are more severely affected than humoral (antibody) responses. Protein–energy malnutrition causes atrophy of the lymphoid organs (thymus, spleen, lymph nodes, tonsils) in laboratory animals and humans. There is a decline in the number of circulating lymphocytes, which is proportional to the extent of malnutrition, and the proliferative responses of T-lymphocytes to mitogens and antigens is decreased by malnutrition, as is the synthesis of IL-2 and IFN-γ and the activity of natural killer cells. Production of cytokines by monocytes (TNF-α, IL-6 and IL-1β) is also decreased by malnutrition, although their phagocytic capacity appears to be unaffected. The *in vivo* skin DTH response to challenge with specific antigens is reduced by malnutrition. However, numbers of circulating B-lymphocytes and immunoglobulin levels do not seem to be affected or may even be increased by malnutrition; it has been suggested that underlying infections may influence these observations.

Low birthweight

The foetus accumulates several nutrients, including zinc, copper, iron and vitamin A, during the last trimester of pregnancy, particularly during the last 6–8 weeks. Premature babies are therefore born with lower nutrient reserves than term infants. There is transfer of IgG from mother to foetus beyond 32 weeks of gestation, which means that babies delivered prematurely have low serum IgG concentrations. This is thought to contribute to the high frequency of respiratory infections and sepsis in low birthweight babies, which may be exacerbated by their poor nutritional status.

Anorexia nervosa and bulimia nervosa

Anorexia nervosa is characterised by a marked fear of fatness, a disturbed perception of body size and image, and an obsessive desire to lose increasing amounts of weight. In anorexia nervosa the appetite will often remain normal until late in the course of the illness; binge eating and purging may be a characteristic. Patients with bulimia nervosa also obsessively pursue thinness, but in this disease there is often rapid consumption of a large quantity of food usually followed by purging; periods of fasting and excessive exercise may also be used.

Although impairment of immune function does exist in anorectic patients, it appears to be less severe than that seen in protein–energy malnutrition. This may be because, in contrast to subjects with protein–energy malnutrition, anorectics usually consume sufficient levels of protein and fat (although not carbohydrate or energy) and have only moderate vitamin and mineral deficiencies. The degree and nature of immune impairment seen in patients with anorexia nervosa and bulimia nervosa differ widely between patients and this may reflect the extent of the nutritional deprivation, the

stage of the disease and the precise nature of the hormonal abnormalities induced.

13.8 The influence of individual micronutrients on immune function

Much of what is known about the impact of single nutrients on immune function comes from studies of deficiency states in animals and humans, and from controlled animal studies in which the nutrients are included in the diet at known levels. There is now overwhelming evidence from these studies that particular nutrients are required for an efficient immune response and that deficiencies in one or more of these nutrients diminish immune function and provide a window of opportunity for infectious agents. It is logical that multiple nutrient deficiencies might have a more significant impact on immune function, and therefore resistance to infection, than a single nutrient deficiency. What is also apparent is that excess amounts of some nutrients also impair immune function and decrease resistance to pathogens. Thus, for some nutrients there may be a relatively narrow range of intake that is associated with optimal immune function.

Vitamin A

The vitamin A (or retinoid) family includes retinol, retinal, retinoic acid and esters of retinoic acid. Not long after its discovery, vitamin A was described as the 'anti-infective vitamin'. This is probably no longer an accurate title, however, because vitamin A tends to enhance recovery from infection rather than prevent it. The discovery and characterisation of nuclear receptors for vitamin A in the 1980s has done much to help elucidate its functions. There is a transitory decrease in serum retinol during the acute-phase response that follows a trauma or infection, which is likely to be due to decreased synthesis of retinol binding protein (RBP) by the liver, and therefore decreased release of retinol-RBP by the liver, and also to increased vascular permeability at sites of inflammation, allowing leakage into the extravascular space. For these reasons, serum retinol cannot be used as an indicator of vitamin A status in individuals with an active acute phase response.

Vitamin A is essential for maintaining epidermal and mucosal integrity; vitamin A-deficient mice have histopathological changes in the gut mucosa consistent with a breakdown in gut barrier integrity and impaired mucous secretion, both of which would facilitate entry of pathogens through this route. One of the key changes caused by vitamin A deficiency is the loss of mucus-producing goblet cells; the resulting lack of mucus diminishes resistance to infection by pathogens that would otherwise be trapped and washed away. Vitamin A regulates keratinocyte differentiation, and vitamin A deficiency induces changes in skin keratinisation, which may explain the observed increased incidence of skin infection. Many aspects of innate immunity, in addition to barrier function, are affected by vitamin A. It modulates gene expression to control the maturation of neutrophils; in vitamin A deficiency there are increased neutrophil numbers, but decreased phagocytic function. Macrophage-mediated inflammation is increased by vitamin A deficiency, but the ability to ingest and kill bacteria is impaired. Vitamin A deficiency may therefore lead to more severe infections, coupled with excessive inflammation. NK cell activity is diminished by vitamin A deficiency. The impact of vitamin A on acquired/specific immunity is less clear, but there is some evidence that vitamin A deficiency alters the Th1/Th2 balance, decreasing the Th2 response, but often without affecting the Th1 response. This area requires further research. There is very little evidence for effects of vitamin A supplements on the proliferation or activation of B-lymphocytes.

The impact of vitamin A deficiency on infectious disease has been studied widely in the developing world. Vitamin A deficiency is associated with increased morbidity and mortality in children, and appears to predispose to respiratory infections, diarrhoea and severe measles. Although vitamin A deficiency increases the risk of infectious disease, the interaction is bidirectional such that infections can lead to vitamin A deficiency: diarrhoea, respiratory infections, measles, chickenpox and human immunodeficiency virus (HIV) infection are all associated with the development of vitamin A deficiency.

Replenishment of vitamin A in deficient individuals by provision of supplements decreases mortality by approximately 30% in children aged 6 months to 5 years in areas of the world where deficiency is a problem. In general, frequent, small doses tend to decrease mortality more dramatically than infrequent high doses. Vitamin A supplements improve recovery from measles and decrease the duration, risk of complications and mortality from the disease. Because measles is an acute, immunosuppressive viral infection, it is often associated with secondary, opportunistic bacterial infections and it is not clear whether vitamin A improves recovery from the measles itself, the secondary infection or both. The ability of vitamin A to promote the regeneration of damaged mucosal epithelium and phagocytic activity of neutrophils and macrophages results in a reduction in the incidence and duration of diarrhoea, which may be of particular benefit to infants who are not breast-fed.

The effect of vitamin A on respiratory infections is particularly interesting. In community studies, vitamin A supplements increased the risk of respiratory infection, while in most clinical studies vitamin A simply failed to improve recovery. There is some evidence that low-dose supplements given frequently can reduce the severity of respiratory infections in children with underlying protein-energy malnutrition, but not in those that are not malnourished; indeed several studies indicate that vitamin A increases the severity of respiratory infections in the non-malnourished. The apparently undesirable effects of vitamin A supplements in community and clinical studies are puzzling and cannot be easily explained, but may be related to induction of excessive inflammation in the airways.

Carotenoids

The carotenoids are a group of over 600 naturally occurring pigmented compounds that are widespread in plants, although fewer than 30 carotenoids occur commonly in human foodstuffs. Some of the carotenoids possess vitamin A activity and most effectively quench free radicals, which could be useful in counteracting the damaging effects of reactive oxygen species (ROS) generated by respiratory burst. Early studies reported that providing carotenoids to children improved severe ear infections, and that dietary carotenoids appeared to protect against lung and skin cancers. However, detailed studies investigating the effects of carotenoids on parameters of immune function (e.g. lymphocyte proliferation, natural killer cell activity, cytotoxic T-cell activity, expression of cell-surface molecules on monocytes,

DTH) have generally not been consistent, with some studies showing benefit and others showing no effect. Further confusion in the area arose when three major intervention trials showed no benefit or an increase in lung cancer in smokers receiving β-carotene supplementation. This area requires further research.

Folic acid and B vitamins

Folic acid and the B vitamins participate as coenzymes in the synthesis of nucleic acids and proteins, which is crucial for many aspects of immune function. There is some suggestion that folate supplementation of elderly individuals improves immune function and in particular NK cell activity, although this is not entirely conclusive. However, elderly subjects supplemented with a combination of folic acid, vitamin E and vitamin B_{12} were reported to have fewer infections. Elderly individuals tend to be at risk of vitamin B_{12} deficiency and studies have shown that subjects over 65 years with low serum vitamin B_{12} concentrations have impaired antibody responses to a vaccine. Patients with vitamin B_{12} deficiency also have decreased numbers of lymphocytes and suppressed NK cell activity, which may be reversed with supplementation.

Vitamin B_6 deficiency in laboratory animals causes thymus and spleen atrophy, and decreases lymphocyte proliferation and the DTH response. In a study in healthy elderly humans a vitamin B_6-deficient diet (3 μg/kg body weight per day or about 0.17 and 0.1 mg/day for men and women, respectively) for 21 days resulted in a decreased percentage and total number of circulating lymphocytes, decreased T- and B-cell proliferation in response to mitogens and decreased IL-2 production. Repletion at 15 or 22.5 μg/kg body weight per day for 21 days did not return the immune functions to starting values, but repletion at 33.75 μg/kg body weight per day (about 1.9 and 1.1 mg/day for men and women, respectively) returned immune parameters to starting values. Providing a larger dose of 41 mg vitamin B_6/day for 4 days caused a further increase in lymphocyte proliferation and IL-2 production. This comprehensive study indicates that vitamin B_6 deficiency impairs human immune function, that the impairment is reversible by repletion and that lymphocyte functions are enhanced at levels of vitamin B_6 above those typical of habitual consumption.

Vitamin C

Vitamin C is a water-soluble antioxidant found in high concentrations in circulating leukocytes and appears to be utilised during infections. High circulating levels of vitamin C are associated with enhanced antibody response, neutrophil function and antiviral activity in animal studies. In humans, supplementation studies have mainly been conducted in athletes and populations with chronic illnesses. The interest in athletes is due to the fact that exercise induces an increase in the numbers of neutrophils and their capacity to produce ROS, which, if prolonged, can be immunosuppressive and reduce neutrophil activity in the recovery period following exercise. Since neutrophils form an important part of the defence against viruses, the suppression of neutrophil activity after strenuous exercise may explain why upper respiratory tract infections are often noted to coincide with this. Because of its antioxidant capacity, vitamin C could potentially counteract the exercise-induced generation of ROS and limit the post-exercise immunosuppression. However, randomised controlled trials (RCTs) have often been limited by lack of statistical power and do not conclusively show an effect of vitamin C on cell numbers, neutrophil function or ROS production. Similarly, RCT evidence for effects of vitamin C on immune function in chronic illnesses is lacking, although they do support a role for reducing trauma-induced increases in serum concentrations of pro-inflammatory cytokines.

Several studies suggest a modest benefit of vitamin C supplementation at doses ranging 1000–8000 mg/day in reducing the duration, but not the incidence, of respiratory infections. However, the incidence of common colds and pneumonia has been shown to be reduced in those individuals who regularly engage in strenuous physical activity, and also in those who live in crowded conditions. The potential benefits and risks of vitamin C supplementation at doses above 8000 mg/day and the role of vitamin C in non-respiratory infections have not been investigated.

Vitamin D

The active form of vitamin D is 1,25-dihydroxy vitamin D_3 and is referred to here as vitamin D. Vitamin D receptors have been identified in most immune cells, suggesting that it has immunoregulatory properties. In addition to this, there are a small number of reports suggesting immune defects in vitamin D-deficient patients and experimental animals, and anecdotal evidence that individuals with rickets are particularly prone to infection. However, there is, paradoxically, a large body of literature supporting an immunosuppressive role of vitamin D and related analogues. The current view is that under physiological conditions vitamin D probably facilitates immune responses, but that it may also play an active role in the prevention of autoimmunity and that there may be a therapeutic role for vitamin D in some immune-mediated diseases.

Vitamin D acts by binding to its receptor and regulating gene expression in target cells. Its effects include promotion of phagocytosis, superoxide synthesis and bacterial killing, but it is also reported to inhibit T-cell proliferation, production of Th1 cytokines and B-cell antibody production, highlighting the paradoxical nature of its effects. The role of vitamin D in autoimmunity is particularly interesting. There is increasing evidence, mainly from animal studies, that vitamin D deficiency is linked with autoimmune diseases such as multiple sclerosis, rheumatoid arthritis and inflammatory bowel disease. The inhibition of Th1 activity by vitamin D is thought to be involved in this link. In addition, a polymorphism in the vitamin D receptor gene has been associated with increased risk of Crohn's disease.

Taken together, the evidence suggests that vitamin D is a selective regulator of immune function and the effects of vitamin D deficiency, vitamin D receptor deficiency and vitamin D supplementation depend on the immunological situation (e.g. health, infectious disease, autoimmune disease).

Vitamin E

Vitamin E is the major lipid-soluble antioxidant in the body and is required for protection of membrane lipids from peroxidation. Free radicals and lipid peroxidation are immunosuppressive, thus it is thought that vitamin E should act to optimise and even enhance the immune response. Except in premature infants and the elderly, clinical vitamin E deficiency is rare in humans, although many individuals have vitamin E intakes below the recommended daily intake in many countries. Cigarette smoking imposes free radical damage and smokers have increased levels of indicators of free radical damage to lipids, low levels of lung and serum vitamin E, increased numbers of neutrophils and macrophages in the lung, increased reactive oxygen species production by phagocytes and depressed immune responses. Thus, cigarette smokers have a higher vitamin E requirement than non-smokers.

A positive association exists between plasma vitamin E levels and DTH responses, and a negative association has been demonstrated between plasma vitamin E levels and the incidence of infections in healthy adults over 60 years of age. There appears to be particular benefit of vitamin E supplementation for the elderly, with studies demonstrating enhanced Th1 cell-mediated immunity at high doses. However, randomised controlled trials do not consistently support a role for vitamin E supplementation in reducing the incidence, duration or severity of respiratory infections in elderly populations or smokers, although one large study did show benefit specifically for upper respiratory tract infections. A comprehensive study demonstrated increased DTH responses in elderly subjects supplemented with 60, 200 and 800 mg vitamin E/day, with maximal effect at a dose of 200 mg/day. This dose also increased the antibody responses to hepatitis B, tetanus toxoid and pneumococcus vaccinations. This 'optimal' dose of 200 mg vitamin E/day is well in excess of a typical recommended dose, thus it appears that adding vitamin E to the diet at levels beyond those normally recommended enhances some immune functions above normal, and it has even been argued that the recommended intake for vitamin E is not adequate for optimal immune function. However, as with many other micronutrients, doses that are hugely in excess of normal requirements may suppress the immune response; indeed, the 800 mg vitamin E/day supplement decreased some of the antibody responses to below those of the placebo group.

Zinc

Zinc is important for DNA synthesis and cellular growth, differentiation and antioxidant defence, and is therefore an important candidate for potential modulation of immune function. Zinc deficiency impairs many aspects of innate immunity, including phagocytosis by macrophages and neutrophils, natural killer cell activity, respiratory burst and complement activity, all of which could be important contributors to increased susceptibility to infection. Zinc deficiency has a marked impact on bone marrow, decreasing the number of nucleated cells and the number and proportion of cells that are lymphoid precursors. In patients with zinc deficiency related to sickle-cell disease, natural killer cell activity is decreased, but can be returned to normal by zinc supplementation. In acrodermatitis enteropathica, which is characterised by reduced intestinal zinc absorption, thymic atrophy, impaired lymphocyte development and reduced lymphocyte responsiveness and DTH are observed. Moderate or mild zinc deficiency or experimental zinc deficiency (induced by consumption of <3.5 mg zinc/day) in humans results in decreased thymulin activity, natural killer cell activity, lymphocyte proliferation, IL-2 production and DTH response; all can be corrected by zinc repletion.

Low plasma zinc levels can be used to predict the subsequent development of lower respiratory tract infections and diarrhoea in malnourished populations. Indeed, diarrhoea is considered a symptom of zinc deficiency and several studies show that zinc supplementation decreases the incidence, duration and severity of childhood diarrhoea. However, most (but not all) studies fail to show a benefit of zinc supplementation in respiratory disease in malnourished populations and available trials on the effect of zinc on the common cold in non-malnourished populations report conflicting results. Very high zinc intakes can result in copper depletion, and copper deficiency impairs immune function (see below).

Copper

Although overt copper deficiency is believed to be rare in humans, modest deficiency is likely to be present among some populations. Zinc and iron impair copper uptake, so that taking high doses of these might induce mild copper deficiency. Copper deficiency has been described in premature infants and in patients receiving total parenteral nutrition. The classic example of copper deficiency is Menkes syndrome, a rare congenital disease which results in the complete absence of ceruloplasmin, the copper-carrying protein in the blood. Children with Menkes syndrome have increased susceptibility to bacterial infections, diarrhoea and pneumonia.

Copper participates as a cofactor in the formation of ROS and appears to have an important role in innate immunity, particularly in respiratory burst. However, as with many other micronutrients,

high intakes over long periods can have a negative impact on immune function.

Iron

Iron deficiency has multiple effects on immune function in laboratory animals and humans. However, the relationship between iron deficiency and susceptibility to infection remains controversial. Furthermore, evidence suggests that infections caused by organisms that spend part of their life cycle intracellularly, such as plasmodia, mycobacteria and invasive salmonellae, may actually be enhanced by iron therapy. In the tropics, in children of all ages, at doses of >2 mg/kg/day iron has been associated with increased risk of malaria and other infections, including pneumonia. For these reasons, iron intervention in malaria-endemic areas is not advised, particularly high doses in the young, those with compromised immunity (e.g. HIV) and during the peak malaria transmission season. Iron treatment for anaemia in a malarious area must be preceded by effective antimalarial therapy and should be oral, rather than parenteral. The detrimental effects of iron administration may occur because microorganisms require iron and providing it may favour the growth and replication of the pathogen. Indeed, it has been argued that the decline in circulating iron concentrations that accompanies infection is an attempt by the host to 'starve' the infectious agent of iron. There are several mechanisms for withholding iron from a pathogen in this way. Lactoferrin has a higher binding affinity for iron than do bacterial siderospores, making bound iron unavailable to the pathogen. Furthermore, once lactoferrin reaches 40% saturation with iron, it is sequestered by macrophages. It is notable that breast milk contains lactoferrin, which may protect against the use of free iron by pathogens transferred to an infant.

It is important to note that oral iron supplementation has not been shown to increase risk of infection in non-malarious countries.

Selenium

Selemium is essential for an effectively functioning immune system. Deficiency in laboratory animals affects both innate and adaptive immunity, particularly neutrophil function. It also increases susceptibility to bacterial, viral, fungal and parasitic challenges. Lower selenium concentrations in humans have also been linked with increased virulence, diminished NK cell activity, increased mycobacterial disease and HIV progression. A study conducted in the UK demonstrated that selenium supplementation to adults with low selenium status improved some aspects of their immune response to a poliovirus vaccination.

Low dietary intakes of selenium are often associated with concurrent vitamin E deficiency, which has led to the conclusion that selenium deficiency has a significant impact on oxidant/antioxidant processes. This occurs mainly through glutathione peroxidases and explains why neutrophils and macrophages from selenium-deficient animals are able to ingest pathogens, but are unable to generate the respiratory burst to destroy them.

Supplementation with micronutrients in combination

Supplementation with combinations of vitamins may be particularly beneficial to athletes, since the combined antioxidant activity could enhance protection against free radical damage and reduce exercise-induced immunosuppression. Studies have indeed shown that supplementation with combined antioxidants increased respiratory burst, upregulated the antioxidant system of neutrophils and reduced the production of pro-inflammatory cytokines from exercising muscles. In contrast, in elderly individuals, combinations of vitamins do not appear to affect innate or adaptive immunity, DTH or the incidence of respiratory or urogenital infections. However, it should be noted that in the combined supplementation studies, the doses of vitamins used were lower than in the single vitamin studies showing benefits in respiratory infections. This is also the case for studies using combined multivitamin and multimineral supplements, which have tended to be small and to vary greatly in the doses of micronutrients provided. A recent systematic review concluded that there was no effect of such an approach on episodes of infection, number of days of infection or antibiotic use in those supplemented compared with those not supplemented, but given the lack of consistent methodology and study design this remains an important topic for study. It is also pertinent to note that most studies investigating the effects of multivitamin supplements on immune function and infection have been conducted in elderly or immunocompromised individuals and there is little or no information from studies conducted in children or populations in developing countries.

Micronutrients and human immunodeficiency virus infection

Many individuals with HIV infection consume less than the recommended daily allowance for a range of micronutrients. Nutrient intake by patients with HIV infection may be decreased as a result of loss of appetite, aversion to food and throat infections, while vomiting, diarrhoea and malabsorption may also contribute to deficiencies. The prevalence of micronutrient deficiencies (based largely on concentrations in the plasma or serum) varies widely depending on the population and the stage of the disease, but it appears that deficiencies in vitamins A, B_6, B_{12}, C, D and E, β-carotene, selenium and zinc are common.

Micronutrient deficiencies may increase oxidative stress and compromise host immunity, so contributing to HIV disease progression. In HIV patients, combined antioxidant supplements do appear to reduce oxidative stress and viral load and increase lymphocyte counts. These improved immune parameters may correlate with the observed benefits of multivitamins on HIV-associated clinical outcomes, such as opportunistic infections, disease progression and mortality. It is, of course, difficult to know whether any benefits are derived from individual nutrients or to synergistic effects between them.

Micronutrients and asthma and allergy

Respiratory diseases such as asthma impose oxidant stress on the individual as a result of inappropriate production of reactive oxygen species (e.g. superoxide and hydroxyl radicals, hydrogen peroxide, hypochlorous acid). These reactive species damage host tissues and up-regulate the production of inflammatory cytokines and adhesion molecules, thereby amplifying the inflammation, inducing bronchoconstriction, elevating mucus secretion and causing microvascular leakage. Oxidant stress can deplete cells and tissues of antioxidants if they are not replenished sufficiently through the diet. Furthermore, a low dietary intake of antioxidants may exacerbate the problem by allowing reactive species generation to proceed unchecked. Among the important antioxidants to consider are vitamins C and E (vitamin C is the major antioxidant present in the airway surface of the lung), glutathione, the glutathione recycling enzyme glutathione peroxidase, and the enzymes that remove superoxide and hydrogen peroxide (superoxide dismutase and catalase, respectively); glutathione peroxidase, superoxide dismutase and catalase contain selenium, copper and zinc, and iron, respectively. Low dietary intakes of selenium, vitamin C and vitamin E have been shown to increase the risk of asthma. The use of vitamin C in asthma and allergy has been investigated in a number of studies, half of which support its use while the other half demonstrate no benefit. The effects of selenium are similarly unclear, and while vitamin E has been shown to improve symptoms in animal models of asthma, human studies to verify this are lacking.

The roles that micronutrients play in immunity are summarised in Box 13.2.

13.9 Dietary fat and immune function

Fatty acids in the diet

Fatty acids consist of hydrocarbon chains, which may be saturated (no double bonds), monounsaturated (one double bond) or polyunsaturated (more than one double bond), with a terminal carboxyl group. Fatty acids have systematic names, but most also have common names and are also described by a shorthand nomenclature. This nomenclature indicates the number of carbon atoms in the chain, the number of double bonds in the chain and the position of the first double bond from the methyl-terminus of the chain. The position of the first double bond in the hydrocarbon chain is indicated by the n-7, n-9, n-6 or n-3 portion of the shorthand notation for a fatty acid. Thus, in an n-6 fatty acid the first double bond is located on carbon number 6 counted from the methyl-terminus and in an n-3 fatty acid the first double bond is located on carbon number 3 counted from the methyl-terminus. Note that the n notation is sometimes referred to as ω or omega.

Saturated fatty acids and most monounsaturated fatty acids can be synthesised in mammalian tissues from non-fat precursors, such as glucose or amino acids. However, mammals cannot insert double bonds before carbon number 9 in oleic acid. Thus, mammals cannot convert oleic acid (18:1n-9) into linoleic acid (18:2n-6). Likewise, mammals cannot convert linoleic acid into α-linolenic acid (18:3n-3). It is because linoleic acid and α-linolenic acid cannot be synthesised by mammals that they are termed essential fatty acids. Furthermore, mammalian cells cannot interconvert n-6 and n-3 fatty acids. However, desaturases and elongases, which are present in mammalian cells, are able to extend and insert further double bonds into linoleic and α-linolenic acids that have been consumed in the diet, generating families of n-6 and n-3 fatty acids (Figure 13.5). Derivatives of the essential fatty acids formed in this way are described as conditionally essential. The major product of n-6 fatty acid metabolism is arachidonic acid (20:4n-6), while the major end-products of n-3 fatty acid metabolism are eicosapentaenoic acid (EPA; 20:5n-3) and docosahexaenoic acid (DHA; 22:6n-3); these fatty acids are incorporated into cell membranes to a significant extent.

Plant tissues and plant oils tend to be rich sources of linoleic and α-linolenic acids. For example, linoleic acid comprises over 50%, and often up to 80%, of the fatty acids found in corn, sunflower, safflower and soybean oils. Rapeseed and soybean oils are good sources of α-linolenic acid, since this fatty

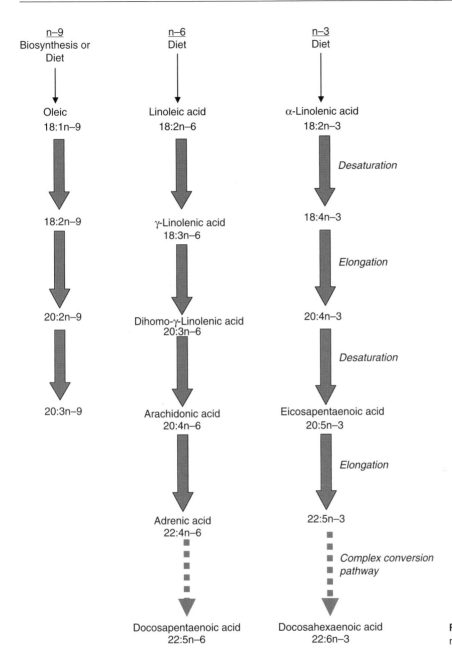

n–9
Biosynthesis or
Diet

Oleic
18:1n–9

18:2n–9

20:2n–9

20:3n–9

n–6
Diet

Linoleic acid
18:2n–6

γ-Linolenic acid
18:3n–6

Dihomo-γ-Linolenic acid
20:3n–6

Arachidonic acid
20:4n–6

Adrenic acid
22:4n–6

Docosapentaenoic acid
22:5n–6

n–3
Diet

α-Linolenic acid
18:2n–3

Desaturation

18:4n–3

Elongation

20:4n–3

Desaturation

Eicosapentaenoic acid
20:5n–3

Elongation

22:5n–3

Complex conversion pathway

Docosahexaenoic acid
22:6n–3

Figure 13.5 Metabolism of n-6 and n-3 polyunsaturated fatty acids.

acid contributes between 5 and 15% of total fatty acids. The intake of longer chain PUFA is not known precisely, but EPA and DHA are found in relatively high proportions in the tissues of oily fish (e.g. herring, mackerel, tuna, sardines) and in the commercial products 'fish oils', which are a preparation of the body oils of oily fish or liver oils of lean fish. Note that in the absence of significant consumption of oily fish, α-linolenic acid is the major dietary n-3 fatty acid.

Essential fatty acid deficiency and immune function

Animal studies have shown that deficiencies in both linoleic and α-linolenic acids result in decreased thymus and spleen weight, lymphocyte proliferation,

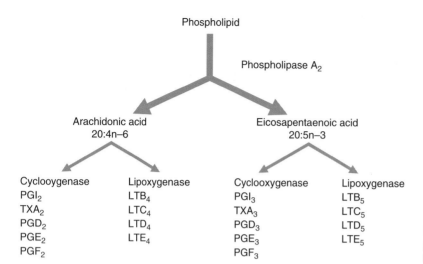

Figure 13.6 Synthesis of eicosanoids from polyunsaturated fatty acids. PG, prostaglandin; TX, thromboxane; LT, leukotriene.

neutrophil chemotaxis, macrophage-mediated cytotoxicity and DTH response compared with animals fed diets containing adequate amounts of these fatty acids. Thus, the immunological effects of essential fatty acid deficiency appear to be similar to the effects of single micronutrient deficiencies, although there are no human studies to confirm this (essential fatty acid deficiency is very rare in humans). However, essential fatty acid deficiency would be expected to have a similar effect because cells of the immune system require PUFA for membrane synthesis and as precursors for the synthesis of eicosanoids (see below).

Amount of dietary fat and immune function

High-fat diets have been reported to result in diminished immune cell functions (both natural and cell-mediated immunity) compared with low-fat diets, but the precise effect depends on the exact level of fat used in the high-fat diet and its source. Furthermore, reductions in total dietary fat intake to below 30% of total energy enhance many immune responses, including lymphocyte proliferation, natural killer cell activity and cytokine production.

Eicosanoids: a link between fatty acids and the immune system

The conversion of 20-carbon atom PUFA to a group of mediators termed eicosanoids provides the key link between fatty acids and immune function. The membranes of most cells contain large amounts of arachidonic acid, which is the principal precursor for eicosanoid synthesis. Arachidonic acid in cell membranes can be mobilised by various phospholipase enzymes, most notably phospholipase A_2, and the free arachidonic acid can subsequently act as a substrate for cyclooxygenase enzymes (COX), forming prostaglandins (PG) and related compounds, or for one of the lipoxygenase (LOX) enzymes, forming leukotrienes (LT) and related compounds (Figure 13.6). There are many different compounds belonging to each class of eicosanoid and they are each formed in a cell-specific manner. For example, monocytes and macrophages produce large amounts of PGE_2 and PGF_2, neutrophils produce moderate amounts of PGE_2 and mast cells produce PGD_2. The LOX enzymes have different tissue distributions, with 5-LOX being found mainly in mast cells, monocytes, macrophages and granulocytes, and 12- and 15-LOX being found mainly in epithelial cells.

Prostaglandins are involved in modulating the intensity and duration of inflammatory and immune responses. PGE_2 has a number of proinflammatory effects, including the induction of fever and erythema, increasing vascular permeability and vasodilatation, and enhancing pain and oedema caused by other agents such as histamine. However, PGE_2 also suppresses lymphocyte proliferation and natural killer cell activity, and inhibits the production of TNF-α, IL-1, IL-6, IL-2 and IFN-γ; thus, in these respects PGE_2 is immunosuppressive and anti-inflammatory.

LTB_4 increases vascular permeability, enhances local blood flow, is a potent chemotactic agent for leukocytes, induces the release of lysosomal enzymes, enhances the generation of reactive oxygen species, inhibits lymphocyte proliferation, promotes natural killer cell activity and can enhance the production of inflammatory cytokines. Thus, arachidonic acid gives rise to a range of mediators that may have opposing effects to one another, so the overall physiological effect will be governed by the nature of the cells producing the eicosanoids, the concentrations of the mediators, the timing of their production and the sensitivities of target cells to their effects.

Consumption of fish oil results in a decrease in the amount of arachidonic acid in the membranes of most cells in the body, including those involved in inflammation and immunity. This means that there is less substrate available for synthesis of eicosanoids from arachidonic acid. Furthermore, EPA competitively inhibits the oxygenation of arachidonic acid by COX. Thus, fish oil feeding results in a decreased capacity of immune cells to synthesise eicosanoids from arachidonic acid. In addition, EPA is itself able to act as a substrate for both COX and 5-LOX (Figure 13.7), giving rise to derivatives that have a different structure from those produced from arachidonic acid (i.e. 3-series PG and thromboxanes and 5-series LT). Thus, the EPA-induced suppression of the production of arachidonic-acid derived eicosanoids is mirrored by an elevation of the production of EPA-derived eicosanoids. The eicosanoids produced from EPA are often less biologically potent than the analogues synthesised from arachidonic acid, although the full range of biological activities of these compounds has not been investigated. LTB_5 is only about 10% as potent as a chemotactic agent and in promoting lysosomal enzyme release as LTB_4. LTB_5 can partially inhibit LTB_4-mediated superoxide formation and chemotaxis. The reduction in the generation of arachidonic acid-derived mediators that accompanies fish oil consumption has led to the idea that fish oil is anti-inflammatory and may affect immune function in general.

Linoleic acid, α-linolenic acid and immune function

Saturated fatty acids have little impact on immune function, whereas linoleic acid has the potential to suppress lymphocyte and natural killer cell activities.

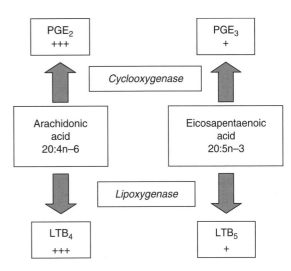

Figure 13.7 Potency of eicosanoids synthesised from arachidonic acid versus eicosapentaenoic acid. PG, prostaglandin; LT, leukotriene.

These effects may be exerted via the production of PGE_2 from arachidonic acid, which is derived from linoleic acid. Although PGE_2 is well known for its proinflammatory properties, it has several immunosuppressive activities. It is apparent, however, that both a deficiency and an excess of linoleic acid can lead to suppressed immune function, depending on the absolute level of fat in the diet (essential fatty acid deficiency leads to impaired immune function, but high-fat diets also suppress immunity).

The precise effect of α-linolenic acid on lymphocyte functions depends on the level of linoleic acid and the total PUFA content of the diet. Adding linseed oil (providing about 15 g α-linolenic acid/day) to a low-fat diet (total fat provided 29% energy) has been shown to result in a significant decrease in human blood lymphocyte proliferation and in the DTH response after 6 weeks. Thus, as for linoleic acid, it appears that both a deficiency and an excess of α-linolenic acid can lead to suppressed immune function.

Fish oil and immune function

Since EPA leads to decreased PGE_2 production (see above), it is often stated that fish oil consumption should reverse the effects of PGE_2. However, the situation is likely to be more complex than this because PGE_2 is not the sole mediator produced from arachidonic acid and the ranges of mediators produced have varying, sometimes opposite, actions (see above).

Furthermore, EPA will give rise to mediators, which also have varying actions. Thus, the overall effect of fish oil feeding cannot be predicted solely on the basis of an abrogation of PGE_2-mediated effects. The recognition of this complexity appears to be borne out by experimental observations. A large number of animal studies on the effects of fish oil on inflammation and immunity indicate that fish oil decreases a wide range of immune cell responses when fed at high levels. It has become clear that the observed effects of fish oil are different to those that are predicted solely on the basis of a decrease in PGE_2 production or indeed on production of eicosanoids *per se*. Thus, there are likely to be other mechanisms of action of fish oil that do not involve eicosanoids and have not yet been fully defined. It is also worth noting that most animal studies investigating the effects of fish oil have used amounts far in excess of those that would be consumed by humans.

Supplementation of the diet of healthy human volunteers with fish oil-derived n-3 PUFA has been shown, in general, to support the idea that fish oil (at the levels used experimentally) exerts a range of immunological effects, although not all studies agree. The most consistent effects of fish oil include diminished recognition of, and response to, host antigen, decreased movement of leukocytes towards sites of inflammatory activity, decreased binding of leukocytes to endothelial cells and their movement from the bloodstream to the subendothelial space, and decreased cellular activation and the release of chemoattractants, cytokines, eicosanoids and reactive species. Fish oil is clearly anti-inflammatory at levels provided in human studies, but these levels would require the consumption of at least six standard 1 g fish oil capsules per day (this would provide approximately 2 g EPA plus DHA). There is a considerable lack of human studies that seek to determine the dose dependence of fish oil on immune function.

Fish oil and infection

If fish oil were immunosuppressive it would be expected to diminish host defence. Some animal studies support this suggestion, while others do not. Since the response to microbial infections is predominantly a Th_1-mediated response (or at least requires Th_1-type cytokines such as IFN-γ), the reduced survival of laboratory animals fed large amounts of fish oil to bacterial challenges suggests that fish oil suppresses the Th1 response *in vivo*. However, fish oil also decreases the metabolic responses to bacterial infection, including fever, anorexia and weight loss, and can, in some situations, increase survival following a challenge by limiting inflammatory damage (mainly the action of proinflammatory cytokines) to the host. The outcome of fish oil supplementation in infections is therefore complex and will depend on the balance between effects on the immunological response to the pathogen and effects on the metabolic response to infection in the host.

Dietary fat and Th_1 skewed immunological diseases

Chronic inflammatory diseases are characterised by a dysregulated Th_1-type response and often by an inappropriate production of arachidonic acid-derived eicosanoids, especially PGE_2 and LTB_4. The effects of fish oil outlined above suggest that it might have a role in the prevention and therapy of chronic inflammatory diseases. There have been a number of clinical trials assessing the benefits of dietary supplementation with fish oils in several chronic inflammatory diseases in humans. In some of these studies, in particular clinical trials of rheumatoid arthritis, anti-inflammatory effects of fish oil were observed (e.g. lowered LTB_4, IL-1 and C-reactive protein production), which were associated with clinical improvements and a lower requirement of anti-inflammatory drugs. However, other chronic inflammatory conditions, such as multiple sclerosis and systemic lupus erythematosus, are unaffected or only marginally affected by fish oil treatment, suggesting that the therapeutic effect of fish oil in inflammatory conditions is not universal.

Dietary fat and Th_2 skewed immunological diseases

Eicosanoids synthesised from arachidonic acid play a role in atopic diseases: PGD_2, LTC_4, D_4 and E_4 are produced by the cells that mediate pulmonary inflammation in asthma, such as mast cells, and are believed to be the major mediators of asthmatic bronchoconstriction. The role of arachidonic acid as a precursor for eicosanoid synthesis has highlighted its significance in the aetiology of asthma. However, arachidonic acid appears to have a dual role in asthma, since PGE_2 regulates the activities of macrophages and lymphocytes; its actions in this context inhibit the production of the Th1-type cytokines IL-2 and IFN-γ without affecting the production of the Th_2-type cytokines IL-4 and IL-5, and stimulate B cells to produce IgE. These observations are important since they suggest that PGE_2 is involved the development of the allergic disease.

Linoleic acid consumption has increased dramatically in developed countries since the mid-1960s and this period of increased intake coincides with the period over which the incidence of childhood allergy has increased. There has therefore been speculation that increased vegetable oil (and hence linoleic acid) consumption results in increased cellular arachidonic acid levels, which increases the capacity for PGE_2 production, which in turn alters the balance of Th_1 and Th_2 cytokines to encourage the development of asthma and other allergic diseases.

The notion that elevated arachidonic acid levels are associated with allergic disease is opposed by the frequently reported abnormalities in fatty acid composition of blood, cells and milk from atopic mothers and/or their offspring. Lowered proportions of arachidonic acid have been observed in plasma, epidermal and erythrocyte phospholipids, and adipose tissue of patients with atopic dermatitis, in cord blood T cells and mononuclear cells of newborn infants at risk of atopy, and in the breast milk and colostrum of mothers with a history of atopic dermatitis. These observations have been taken to suggest that a deficiency in δ6-desaturase plays a role in these diseases. Such a deficiency would result in an imbalance between different members of the n-6 PUFA family and between the n-6 and the n-3 PUFA families. Rather than atopic disease being driven by an excess of arachidonic acid, an alternative suggestion is that PGE_2 plays a role in thymic T-cell development and in controlling T-cell activity, and that this regulation is diminished in atopics, owing to a decreased availability of arachidonic acid. This area has not yet been resolved and requires further work.

The roles that dietary fats play in immunity are summarised in Box 13.3.

Box 13.3 Key points: fatty acids and immune function

- Some fatty acids cannot be synthesised in the human body; these are termed essential fatty acids.
- Key physiological roles of fatty acids are as components of membranes and as precursors for hormone-like compounds termed eicosanoids.
- Essential fatty acid deficiency impairs cell-mediated immunity.
- Cell-mediated immunity and natural killer cell activity decrease as the fat content of the diet increases.
- Within a high-fat diet, different fatty acids can exert different effects.
- Saturated fatty acids appear to have less influence on immune function than polyunsaturated fatty acids.
- Increasing linoleic acid intake decreases cell-mediated immunity.
- Eicosanoids synthesised from arachidonic acid influence inflammation and immunity, and regulate the Th1 versus Th2 balance.
- The n-3 fatty acids found in fish oil replace arachidonic acid in cell membranes and therefore can oppose some of the effects of arachidonic acid.
- The n-3 fatty acids found in fish oil are anti-inflammatory and may regulate the Th1 versus Th2 balance.
- There is a theoretical basis for the use of the n-3 fatty acids found in fish oil in some immunologically based diseases.
- Fish oil has been shown to improve symptoms in rheumatoid arthritis, but there is limited evidence for its benefit in other chronic inflammatory diseases.

13.10 Dietary amino acids and related compounds and immune function

Sulphur amino acids and related compounds

Sulphur amino acids are essential in humans. Deficiency in methionine and cysteine results in atrophy of the thymus, spleen and lymph nodes, and prevents recovery from protein–energy malnutrition. When combined with a deficiency of isoleucine and valine, also essential amino acids, sulphur amino acid deficiency results in severe depletion of gut lymphoid tissue, very similar to the effect of protein deprivation.

Glutathione is a tripeptide that consists of glycine, cysteine and glutamate (from glutamine), and is recognised to have antioxidant properties. Glutathione concentrations in the liver, lung, small intestine and immune cells fall in response to inflammatory stimuli (probably as a result of oxidative stress), and this fall can be prevented in some organs by the provision of cysteine in the diet. Although the limiting precursor for glutathione biosynthesis is usually cysteine, the ability of sulphur amino acids to replete glutathione stores is related to the protein level of the diet. Glutathione can enhance the activity of human cytotoxic T cells, while depletion of intracellular glutathione diminishes lymphocyte proliferation and the generation of cytotoxic T-lymphocytes.

Taurine is a sulphonated β-amino acid derived from methionine and cysteine metabolism, but is not a component of proteins. Taurine transfer to the foetus occurs throughout gestation, but especially over the last 4 weeks, and neonates have a reduced capacity to synthesise taurine. Thus, taurine levels are low in premature and low-birthweight babies. In humans, plasma taurine concentrations are decreased by trauma and sepsis. Taurine is present in high concentrations in most tissues and particularly in cells of the immune system; in lymphocytes it contributes 50% of the free amino acid pool. The role of taurine within lymphocytes is not clear. In neutrophils taurine appears to play a role in maintaining phagocytic capacity and microbicidal action through interaction with myeloperoxidase, an enzyme involved in respiratory burst. Taurinechloramine is formed by complexing of taurine with hypochlorous acid (HOCl) produced by myeloperoxidase. Hypochlorous acid, although toxic to bacteria, causes damage to host tissues and it has been proposed that the formation of taurinechloramine is a mechanism to protect the host from this damage. Although taurine appears not to affect mediator production by macrophages, taurinechloramine decreases PGE_2, TNF-α and IL-6 production by macrophages.

Arginine

Arginine is a non-essential amino acid in humans and is involved in protein, urea and nucleotide synthesis, and adenosine triphosphate (ATP) generation. It also serves as the precursor of nitric oxide, a potent immunoregulatory mediator that is cytotoxic to tumour cells and to some microorganisms. In laboratory animals arginine decreases the thymus involution associated with trauma, promotes thymus repopulation and cellularity, increases lymphocyte proliferation, natural killer cell activity and macrophage cytotoxicity, improves DTH, increases resistance to bacterial infections, increases survival to sepsis and burns, and promotes wound healing. There are indications that arginine may have similar effects in humans, although these have not been tested thoroughly. There is particular interest in the inclusion of arginine in enteral formulae given to patients hospitalised for surgery, trauma and burns, since it appears to reduce the severity of infectious complications and the length of hospital stay. However, in many of the clinical studies carried out in these patients, the enteral formulae used have contained a variety of nutrients with immunomodulatory actions, so it has been difficult to ascribe beneficial effects to any one nutrient alone.

Glutamine

Glutamine is the most abundant amino acid in the blood and in the free amino acid pool in the body; skeletal muscle is considered to be the most important glutamine producer in the body. Once released from skeletal muscle, glutamine acts as an interorgan nitrogen transporter. Important users of glutamine include the kidney, liver, small intestine and cells of the immune system. Plasma glutamine levels are lowered (by up to 50%) by sepsis, injury and burns, and following surgery. Furthermore, the skeletal muscle glutamine concentration is lowered by more than 50% in at least some of these situations. These observations indicate that a significant depletion of the skeletal muscle glutamine pool is characteristic of trauma. The lowered plasma glutamine concentrations that occur are likely to be the result of demand for glutamine (by the liver, kidney, gut and immune system) exceeding the supply, and it has been suggested that the lowered plasma glutamine contributes, at least in part, to the impaired immune function that accompanies such situations. It has been argued that restoring plasma glutamine concentrations in these situations should restore immune function. As with arginine, there are animal studies to support this. Clinical studies, mainly using intravenous infusions of solutions containing glutamine, have also reported beneficial effects for patients undergoing bone marrow transplantation and colorectal surgery, patients in intensive care and low-birthweight babies, all of whom are at risk from infection and sepsis. In some of these studies, improved outcome was associated with improved immune function. In addition to a direct immunological effect, glutamine, even provided parenterally, improves gut barrier function in patients at risk of infection. This would have the benefit of decreasing the translocation of bacteria from the gut and eliminating a key source of infection.

Box 13.4 Key points: amino acids and immunity

- Deficiencies in essential amino acids are likely to impair immune function.
- A key role of sulphur amino acids is in maintaining levels of the antioxidant glutathione and thus preventing oxidative stress.
- Some classically non-essential amino acids (arginine, glutamine) may become essential in stress situations.

Box 13.5 Key points: probiotics and immunity

- Probiotics is the name given to desirable bacteria that colonise the human gut.
- Probiotic bacteria help to maintain the gut barrier and prevent colonisation by pathogenic bacteria.
- Probiotic bacteria enhance some aspects of immune function in laboratory animals and in humans.
- Probiotic bacteria may decrease the incidence and severity of diarrhoea.
- Prebiotics increase numbers of beneficial bacteria in the gut and may affect immune function, but it is not clear whether their effect is direct or indirect.

The roles that dietary amino acids play in immunity are summarised in Box 13.4.

13.11 Probiotics and immune function

Indigenous bacteria are believed to contribute to the immunological protection of the host by creating a barrier against colonisation by pathogenic bacteria. This barrier can be disrupted by disease and by the use of antibiotics, so allowing easier access to the host gut by pathogens. It is now believed that this barrier can be maintained by providing supplements containing live 'desirable' bacteria; such supplements are termed probiotics. Probiotic organisms are found in fermented foods, including traditionally cultured dairy products and some fermented milks. The organisms included in commercial probiotics include lactic acid bacteria (*Lactobacillus acidophilus*, *Lactobacillus casei*, *Enterococcus faecium*) and *Bifidobacteria*. These organisms only colonise the gut temporarily, making regular consumption necessary. In addition to creating a barrier effect, some of the metabolic products of probiotic bacteria (e.g. lactic acid and a class of antibiotic proteins termed bacteriocins produced by some bacteria) may inhibit the growth of pathogenic organisms. Probiotic bacteria may also compete with pathogenic bacteria for nutrients and may enhance the gut immune response to pathogenic bacteria. Probiotics have various routes for internalisation by the gut epithelium and contact with underlying immune tissues; it is through these interactions that probiotics are thought to be able to influence immune function. However, the nature of this regulation is not well understood.

A number of studies have examined the influence of various probiotic organisms, either alone or in combination, on immune function, infection and inflammatory conditions in humans. Probiotics appear to enhance innate immunity (particularly phagocytosis and natural killer cell activity), but have lesser effects on adaptive immunity. In children, probiotics have been shown to reduce the incidence and duration of diarrhoea, although the effects depend on the nature of the condition. In adults, some studies demonstrate a reduction in the risk of traveller's diarrhoea. The effects on other infectious outcomes is much less clear. There is some evidence that probiotics could be beneficial in ulcerative colitis, irritable bowel syndrome and allergy, but this is not entirely consistent. One of the difficulties in interpreting results is that there may be significant species and strain differences in the effects of probiotics, as well as differences in doses used, duration of treatment, subject characteristics, sample size and technical considerations.

Prebiotics are selectively fermented by the gut microbiota, leading to increased numbers of beneficial bacteria within the gut, which interact with other members of the gut microbiota and the host immune system. Although there is growing evidence for potential immunomodulatory effects of prebiotics, it is not clear whether they are direct effects or simply manifested through alteration of the gut microbiota. Furthermore, it is notable that while there is considerable supporting literature for the immunomodulatory effects of probiotics, the data for prebiotics alone remains inconsistent.

The effects of probiotics and prebiotics on immune function are summarised in Box 13.5.

13.12 Breast-feeding and immune function

The composition of breast milk

Breast milk is the best example of a foodstuff with immune-enhancing properties. It contains a wide range of immunologically active components, including cells (macrophages, T- and B-lymphocytes, neutrophils), immunoglobulins (IgG, IgM, IgD, sIgA), lysozyme (which has direct antibacterial action), lactoferrin (which binds iron, so preventing its uptake by bacteria), cytokines (IL-1, IL-6, IL-10, IFN-γ, TNF-α, transforming growth factor-β), growth factors (epidermal growth factor, insulin-like growth factor), hormones (thyroxin), fat-soluble vitamins (vitamins A, D, E), amino acids (taurine, glutamine), fatty acids, amino sugars and nucleotides. Breast milk also contains factors that prevent the adhesion of some microorganisms to the gastrointestinal tract and so prevents bacterial colonisation. Human breast milk contains factors that promote the growth of useful bacteria (e.g. *Bifidobacteria*) in the gut; this factor is absent from the milk of all other species. The content of many factors varies among milks of different species, and is different between human breast milk and many infant formulae.

Breast-feeding, immune function and infection

Breast-feeding is thought to play a key role in the prevention of infectious disease, particularly diarrhoea and gastrointestinal and lower respiratory infections, in both developing and developed countries. In addition to preventing infectious disease, breast-feeding enhances the antibody responses to vaccination. Several studies have examined the effect of breast-feeding versus formula-feeding on risk of death due to infectious diseases in developing countries. A meta-analysis of these studies, published in the *Lancet* in 2000 (see Further reading), suggested that infants who are not breast-fed have a six-fold greater risk of dying from infectious diseases in the first 2 months of life than those who are breast-fed. However, it appears that this protection decreases steadily with age, as infants begin complementary feeding, so that by 6–11 months, the protection afforded by breast-feeding is no longer apparent. Breast-feeding may provide better protection against diarrhoea (up to 6 months of age) than against deaths due to respiratory infections. There are also geographical influences on the protection afforded by breast-feeding; in some continents protection can be observed throughout the first year of life, whereas in others it is much more short-lived.

The roles that breast-feeding plays in immunity are summarised in Box 13.6.

Box 13.6 Key points: breast milk and immunity

- Breast milk contains a variety of immunologically active factors.
- The factors in breast milk appear designed to protect the neonate from infection and to promote development of the neonatal immune response.
- Human breast milk has a different composition to other milks.
- Breast-feeding protects against some infectious diseases.

13.13 Perspectives on the future

Deficiencies of total energy or of one or more essential nutrients, including vitamins A, B_6, B_{12}, C and E, folic acid, zinc, iron, copper, selenium, essential amino acids and essential fatty acids, impair immune function and increase susceptibility to infectious pathogens. This occurs because each of these nutrients is involved in the molecular and cellular responses to challenge of the immune system. Providing these nutrients to deficient individuals restores immune function and improves resistance to infection. For several nutrients the dietary intakes that result in the greatest enhancement of immune function are greater than recommended intakes. However, excessive intake of some nutrients also impairs immune responses. Thus, four potential general relationships between the intake of a nutrient and immune function appear to exist (Figure 13.8). It is often assumed when defining the relationship between nutrient intake and immune function that all components of the immune system will respond in the same dose-dependent fashion to a given nutrient. This is not correct, at least as far as some nutrients are concerned, and it appears likely that different components of the immune system show an individual dose–response relationship to the availability of a given nutrient (Figure 13.9).

Although outside the scope of this chapter, it is important to consider the role of hormones in regulating immune function during malnutrition. An inadequate supply of nutrients to the body may cause physiological stress, leading to an elevation in the circulating concentrations of glucocorticoids and catecholamines. Both classes of hormones have an inhibitory effect on immune function and may therefore be important factors when considering the relationship between nutrient supply and immunological outcome.

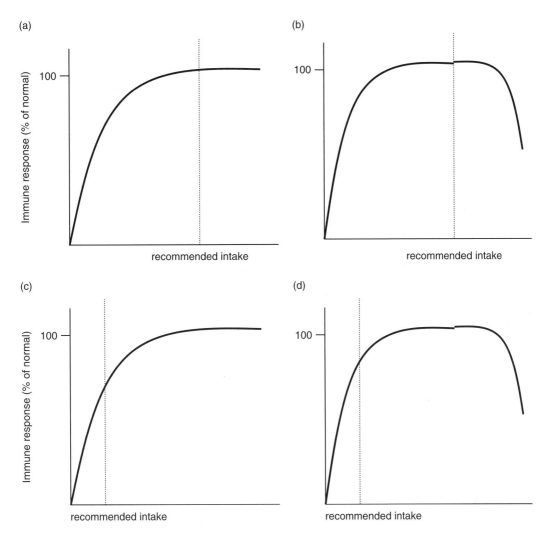

Figure 13.8 Four possible relationships between nutrient intake and immune function. All patterns assume that a deficiency of the nutrient impairs the immune response. In pattern (a) the immune response is maximal, in terms of relationship to the intake of the nutrient under study, at the recommended level of intake and intakes somewhat above the recommended intake do not impair immune function. In pattern (b) the immune response is maximal, in terms of relationship to the intake of the nutrient under study, at the recommended level of intake and intakes somewhat above the recommended intake impair immune function. In pattern (c) the immune response is submaximal, in terms of relationship to the intake of the nutrient under study, at the recommended level of intake and intakes somewhat above the recommended intake do not impair immune function. In pattern (d) the immune response is submaximal, in terms of relationship to the intake of the nutrient under study, at the recommended level of intake and intakes somewhat above the recommended intake impair immune function.

It is now appreciated that the supply of nutrients that are not considered to be essential according to traditional criteria may also influence immune function; this is particularly notable for the amino acids glutamine and arginine, and may indicate that a re-evaluation of the definitions of essentiality, nutrient requirements and nutrient status is required for some dietary components.

Finally, an early point of contact between nutrients and the immune system occurs within the intestinal tract. Relatively little is known about the relationship between nutrient status and the function of the gut-associated immune system. This is of particular relevance when considering adverse reactions to foods: the role of immunoregulatory nutrients in responses to food components and in sensitisation to food-borne

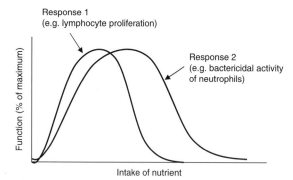

Figure 13.9 Dose–response relationships of different immune functions to the same nutrient may not be identical.

allergens is largely unknown. An understanding of the interaction between nutrients, the types of bacteria that inhabit the gut, and gut-associated and systemic immune responses is only now beginning to emerge.

The term 'optimal immune function' is often used in the literature without careful thought about its definition. An optimal immune response to any given nutrient measured by one marker will not necessarily be optimal according to a second marker of immune function. Furthermore, the effect of a given nutrient on immune response may be altered by levels of other nutrients. For these reasons, the natural desire to 'optimise' the immune response may not be realistic. At best, it is reasonable to expect that correction of marginal deficiencies will improve immunity, but further enhancement using micronutrient supplements cannot be guaranteed and in excessive doses is likely to be detrimental. At the other extreme, there is interest in the potential therapeutic effect of nutrients in diseases involving dysregulation of the immune system (e.g. n-3 fatty acids in rheumatoid arthritis). In some, but by no means all, cases there is supportive evidence for this approach. Between these extremes there are many unanswered questions, but it is clear that the study of the modulation of immune function by nutrients has important implications in both developing and developed countries.

Further reading

Albers R *et al*. Markers to measure immunomodulation in human nutrition intervention studies. Br J Nutr 2005; 94, 452–481.

Calder PC. N-3 polyunsaturated fatty acids, inflammation, and inflammatory diseases. Am J Clin Nutr, 2006; 83: 1505S–1519S.

Calder PC. The relationship between the fatty acid composition of immune cells and their function. PLEFA 2008; 79: 101–108.

Calder PC, Field CJ, Gill HS. Nutrition and Immune Function. Oxford: CABI, 2002.

Cummings JH *et al*. PASSCLAIM – Gut health and immunity. Eur J Nutr 2004; 43 (Suppl. 2): 118–73.

Li P *et al*. Amino acids and immune function. Br J Nutr 2007; 98: 237–252.

Lomax AR, Calder PC. Prebiotics, immune function, infection and inflammation: a review of the evidence. Br J Nutr 2009, 101: 633–658.

Lomax AR, Calder PC. Probiotics, immune function, infection and inflammation: a review of the evidence from studies conducted in humans. Curr Pharm Des 2009, 15, 1428–1518.

Scrimshaw NS, SanGiovanni JP. Synergism of nutrition, infection and immunity: an overview. Am J Clin Nutr 1997; 66: 464S–477S.

Tricon S *et al*. Nutrition and allergic disease. Clin Exp Allergy Rev 2006; 6: 117–188.

Webb AL, Villamor E. Update: Effects of antioxidant and non-antioxidant vitamin supplementation on immune function. Nutr Rev 2007; 65, 181–217.

14
Phytochemicals

Aedín Cassidy and Colin D Kay

Key messages

- Phytochemicals, often referred to as phytonutrients, are plant-based compounds that have physiological functions in mammalian systems.
- They can be classified as phenolic phytochemicals (flavonoids, tannins, lignans, stilbenes and phenolic acids), carotenoids, phytosterols and sulphur-containing compounds (sulphides and glucosinolates).
- Phytochemicals can have potential beneficial effects in a range of chronic diseases, including cardiovascular disease and cancer.
- For many classes of phytochemicals there is still incomplete knowledge about their metabolism, bioavailability, mechanisms of action and dose response.

14.1 Introduction

Fruits and vegetables are rich sources of micronutrients and dietary fibre, but they also contain a wide variety of secondary metabolites which provide the plant with colour, flavour, and antimicrobial, insecticidal and other such properties. Many of these potentially protective plant compounds, termed phytochemicals, may be important in disease prevention. Phytochemicals, also known as phytonutrients, are plant-based compounds with a number of physiological functions in mammalian systems. Phytonutrients are not thought to be essential for human/animal growth and development but may help maintain health throughout life, including the prevention of chronic disease. Many phytochemicals are ubiquitous throughout the plant kingdom and hence are present in our daily diet. Among the most important classes are the carotenoids, flavonoids, glucosinolates and phytosterols, which are classified based on their chemical and structural characteristics. This chapter will discuss the different classes of phytochemicals and their relationship to human diseases, with a specific focus on flavonoids.

14.2 Historical perspective

The belief that plants and plant foods hold properties beyond basic nutrition stems back to early civilisations. Egyptian culture, for example, used a number of teas and herbs for healing and treatment of disease. A report on diet and cancer from the Food and Nutrition Board of the US National Academy of Science in the early 1980s, together with other studies in the mid-1980s, highlighted the fact that there were compounds in our diet that protected us against cancer. In the early 1990s came a number of epidemiological studies which further emphasised the relationship between vegetable and fruit consumption and cancer. Since then, a large number of studies have strongly illustrated the possibility that phytochemicals in vegetables and fruits play a role in reducing the risk of cancer, as well as a number of other chronic health conditions such as cardiovascular disease.

Nutrition research is only beginning to understand the function of many of these naturally occurring compounds in the body. Like many nutrients, phytochemicals can have adverse effects as well as beneficial effects on human health, depending on the

Nutrition and Metabolism, Second Edition, edited by S. A. Lanham-New, I. A. Macdonald and H. M. Roche.   © 2011 The Nutrition Society.

biochemical nature of the compound (its reactivity, its metabolism or whether it is retained in the body or excreted rapidly in urine). When phytochemicals were first discovered, they were mainly considered to be toxic or as antinutrients. It is true that some phytochemicals are toxic or prevent the absorption of certain nutrients, but the focus has now changed to also examining the beneficial properties of many of these compounds.

To date, more than 30 000 phytochemicals have been identified, of which many are present in the foods that we consume. Although it is hard to quantify the dietary intake of phytochemicals, it has been estimated that the average diet contains a daily intake greater than 1 g.

Phytochemicals are classified based on their chemical structure and/or functional attributes. The list below is by no means exhaustive, but relates to phytochemicals that have been more commonly studied in cell, animal and human models, and consumed as part of our daily diet.

14.3 The phenolic phytochemicals

Flavonoids

Flavonoids form part of the largest category of phytochemicals, the phenolic phytochemicals. The term 'phenolic' encompasses a variety of plant compounds containing an aromatic ring with one or more hydroxyl groups. Many phenolics occur in nature with a sugar group attached to them, making them water soluble.

The phenolics are plant secondary metabolites, derived from the acetate and shikimate pathways. As will be discussed below, phenolics are partly responsible for the colour, taste and smell of many foods, be they desirable or undesirable. They are influenced by factors such as growing conditions, cultivar, ripeness, processing (i.e. fermentation and cooking) and storage.

Flavonoids have a 15-carbon structure made up of two phenolic rings connected by a three-carbon unit. Flavonoids are grouped into anthocyanins and anthoxanthins. Anthocyanins include molecules of red, blue and purple pigments, while anthoxanthins include colourless or white to yellow molecules such as flavonols and flavones. The six anthoxanthins are discussed first: flavonols, flavones, flavan-3-ols as one group; flavanones and chalcones as a second group; and isoflavones as a third group.

Dietary flavonoids represent a diverse range of polyphenolic compounds that occur naturally in plant foods. The range and structural complexity of flavonoids has led to their sub-classification as flavonols, flavones, flavanones, flavan-3-ols (and their oligomers, proanthocyanidins), isoflavones and anthocyanins. They are present in significant amounts in many commonly consumed fruits, vegetables, grains, herbs and drinks. These structurally diverse compounds exhibit a range of biological activities *in vitro* which may explain their potential cardioprotective and anti-cancer properties, including antioxidant, anti-inflammatory and apoptotic activity.

Flavonols, flavone and flavan-3-ols

Flavonols, together with flavones and flavan-3-ols (also referred to as flavanols), make up the three major subclasses of flavonoids and are the most widely distributed. Common flavonols include quercetin, kaempferol and myricetin, and they occur in relatively high levels in onions, apples, kale and some teas and wines (Figure 14.1 and Tables 14.1, 14.2). Two potentially important flavones include luteolin and apigenin, found in parsley and celery (Figure 14.1 and Tables 14.1, 14.2). The structural difference between flavonols and flavones is that flavones lack a hydroxyl group on the 3-position of the C ring. Flavan-3-ols differ from the above flavonoids in that they lack an oxygen molecule at the 4-position of the C ring. The principal flavan-3-ols include catechin, epicatechin and gallocatechin (Figure 14.2). These compounds are often found as esters with gallic acid and are known as epicatechin gallate and epigallocatechin gallate. Flavan-3-ols are also commonly referred to as catechins. They are found in many plant foods, notably chocolate, tea, red wine and apples (Table 14.1). Their current estimated intakes are around 150 mg/day and they have a relative bioavailability of less than 20% (Figure 14.3).

Improvements in analytical instrumentation and methodologies have made the analysis and identification of these compounds more reliable, precise and sensitive, but there are still no accepted standardised methods for the assessment of flavonoids in foods. Many of the flavonoids occur in plants bound to sugars as glycosides, with a minority also occurring in

Figure 14.1 Chemical structure of flavonols, flavones and flavan-3-ols.

Table 14.1 Main groups of flavonoids, the individual compounds in each sub-class and food sources

Flavonoid sub-class	Example	Major dietary sources	Estimated mean daily intakes (mg/day)
Flavonols	Quercetin, kaempferol, myricetin, isorhamnetin Important glycosides include rutin (quercetin rutinoside)	Onions, broccoli, leeks, tea, apples, red wine	13
Flavones	Apigenin, luteolin, tangeretin	Herbs (especially parsley), celery, chamomile tea, tangerines and some other citrus	<5
Flavanones	Naringenin, hesperetin Dietary forms are glycosides such as hesperidin and narirutin	Citrus fruit, including oranges, grapefruit	14
Flavan-3-ols including polymeric forms (esters, proanthocyanidins/ condensed tannins)	(+)-Catechin, (−)-epi-catechin, their polymers (e.g. pro-cyanidins B1, C1 etc.) and esters (e.g. epigallocatechin gallate; EGCG)	Cocoa/dark chocolate, apples, grapes and red wine, green tea and black tea to a lesser extent, berries, seeds, cereal grains	157
Anthocyanidins/ anthocyanins	Cyanidin, delphinidin, pelargonidin, peonidin, malvidin Glycosylated derivatives known as anthocyanins	Coloured berries, especially cranberries, blackcurrants, blueberries and elderberries, red wine, aubergine, blood orange juice	3–215
Isoflavones	Daidzein, genistein, glycitein Glycosylated forms are daidzin, genistin and glycitin	Soy products, including fermented products, e.g. tofu, tempeh, miso, soy protein isolate (ISP)	<5 in the USA and Europe 25–50 in Asia

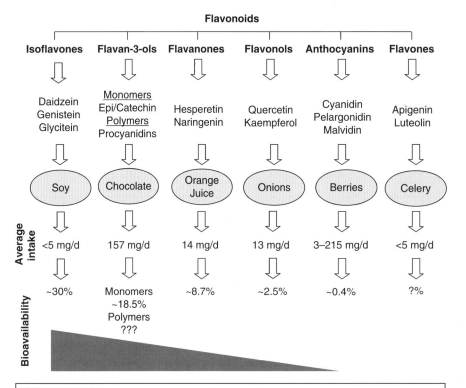

Figure 14.2 Chemical structure of the flavanols epicatechin, catechin and epigallocatechin.

Figure 14.3 Examples of foods containing flavonoids, their average dietary intake and their relative bioavailabilities.

the free unbound or aglycone form. For this reason, past extraction techniques have been developed to cleave the sugar group from the flavonoid before analysis by high performance liquid chromatography (HPLC) or liquid chromatography–mass spectrometry (LCMS). Various studies have analysed the flavonoid content of a number of vegetables, fruits and drinks, such as tea, wine and fruit juices. As mentioned previously, it is hard to estimate the relative average concentration of these compounds in food or their daily intake, given their complexity, their presence in so many foods and the fact that they are influenced by a number of other factors, such the matrix in which they occur, their various cultivars and the

Table 14.2 Concentrations of flavanols and flavones in various foods

Compound	Food or beverage	Concentration
Quercetin	Onions	300 mg/kg
	Kale	100 mg/kg
	Apples	20–70 mg/kg
	Black tea	10–25 mg/l
	Red wine	5–15 mg/l
	Fruit juices	≤5 mg/l
Kaempferol	Kale	211–470 mg/kg
Luteolin	Celery (stalks and leaves)	5–20 mg/kg
Apigenin	Celery (stalks and leaves)	15–60 mg/kg

environmental conditions in which they are grown. The formation of flavonols and flavones is dependent on many environmental factors, such as light, heat, water and predation. High concentrations of flavonols are found in the leaves and skin of fruits as these surfaces are more exposed to the environment.

Flavan-3-ols occur in a number of plant foods, but tea is probably the most substantial source in most countries based on its high level/volume of consumption. Tea, both black and green, contains small amounts of catechin, epicatechin and gallocatechin, and large amounts of epicatechin gallate, epigallocatechin and epigallocatechin gallate (Figure 14.2). Given the range of concentrations, it is hard to estimate the daily consumption of these compounds but total intake of phenolics (flavonoids and phenolic acids) is commonly estimated to be approximately 1 g/day. This level of intake is about 10 times higher than that of vitamin C and 100 times higher than that of vitamin E or β-carotene.

Several studies have examined the metabolism, bioavailability and health effects of flavonols, flavones and flavan-3-ols. The absorption, metabolism and urinary and bilary excretion are all separate physiological processes that contribute to levels in blood and determine a compound's bioavailability. The bioavailability of flavonoids shows great variation; isoflavones have the highest bioavailability (up to 30%), whereas the intact anthocyanins have very low bioavailability (0.1–1%) (Figure 14.3). Many flavonoids occur as glycosides in foods, and both flavonoid structure and the type of sugar moiety determine whether or not absorption in the small intestine is possible. Upon absorption of some flavonoid species in the small intestine, the glucosides, are hydrolysed by lactase phloridzin hydrolase located at the brush border membrane. Absorption from the small intestine results in peak plasma concentrations within 1–3 h after ingestion, which is the case for most flavonoids. The impact of the type of glycoside on bioavailability is demonstrated by the large differences between quercetin glucoside absorbed from the small intestine and quercetin rutinoside, which is a disaccharide that requires hydrolysis from colonic bacteria before it can be absorbed. In addition, the absorption of isoflavones (glycosides) requires prior hydrolysis of the sugar moiety by colonic bacteria prior to absorption. The bioavailability of flavan-3-ols differs markedly depending on the chemical complexity of the species, for example the bioavailability of the dimers and polymers is much less than that of the monomers.

Following absorption, flavonoids are readily metabolised in intestinal cells to form glucuronide and sulphate conjugates that appear in portal blood. In the liver additional conjugation and methylation can occur and these processes can significantly change the structure and biological activity of the flavonoids/polyphenols. Flavonoids for the most part are processed in the body in much the same way as drugs and their bioavailability is affected by such factors as food matrix, chemical composition, age, gender and genetics.

Flavonoids that are not absorbed from the small intestine are transported to the colon, where they are subjected to further metabolism by microbiota. Glycosides may be hydrolysed in the colon, which enables absorption, resulting in peak concentrations generally reaching the systemic circulation about 4–6 h after ingestion or even longer. In addition, flavonoids are broken down to a range of smaller molecules, including the phenolic acids and various lower molecular weight products of ring fission. These products may be subsequently reabsorbed and are an active area of current research.

There is significant interest in the health effects of these compounds, with growing evidence from intervention studies on the cardiovascular benefits of flavan-3-ols and flavonols; including beneficial effects on blood pressure and measures of blood flow, in addition to anticancer properties. For the flavone subclass (apigenin and luteolin) there is currently limited data on their bioavailability or bioactivity in humans. Current and emerging research is now beginning to focus on examining the mechanisms of action of both parent flavonoids and their metabolites relative to observed vascular and cancer activities.

Figure 14.4 Chemical structure of the flavanones hesperetin and naringenin.

Flavanones and chalcones

Flavanones and chalcones are described as minor flavonoids because of their limited occurrence, even though they are sometimes present in significant concentrations in specific foods. These two flavonoid sub-groups are closely related because flavanones can be converted to chalcones in alkaline media and the opposite can occur in acidic environments.

Flavanones are commonly found in citrus fruits. Examples include hesperidin (orange juice) and naringin (grapefruit) (Figure 14.4). Neohesperidin and naringin are responsible for much of the bitter taste of oranges and grapefruits. In terms of levels, these compounds are found in higher concentrations in the skin of the fruits than in the flesh or juice. Given the easy conversion of chalcones to flavanones, chalcones are limited in nature. Naringenin chalcone, for example, is present in tomato skin, juice, paste and sauce.

Similar to the flavonoids described previously, flavanones and chalcones occur mostly as glycosides in plants. Hesperetin and naringenin are aglycone flavanones, while their glycoside counterparts are called hesperidin, naringin, narirutin and rhamnoglucosides. Like other flavonoids, aglycones and some monoglycosides can be absorbed in the small intestine while more structurally complex diglycosides or rhamnoglucosides tend not to be absorbed until the aglycones are liberated by the action of the gut microflora. Studies measuring the urinary excretion of naringenin have demonstrated that individuals consuming grapefruit juice containing 200 mg of naringin excreted 30 mg of naringenin glucuronide daily. These flavanone aglycones have also been shown to be degraded by human and animal intestinal microflora to simpler phenols and phenolic acids, as discussed later.

Given that lipid peroxidation and oxygen free radicals are thought to be involved in conditions such as atherosclerosis, cancer and inflammation, and the flavonoids hydroxylated benzoid ring structure lends itself to radical scavenging, the primary health focus for flavonoids was traditionally their antioxidant properties. Indeed *in vitro* studies have shown that flavonoids are efficient scavengers of lipid peroxy radicals, superoxide anions and singlet oxygen. Additionally, many flavonoids have been shown to inhibit low-density lipoprotein (LDL) oxidation following consumption. However, based on the bioavailability of flavonoids and their blood concentrations relative to other endogenous antioxidants, their mechanisms of action are unlikely to be the result of global radical scavenging. For this reason many researchers have suggested that their mechanistic actions must be associated with cell signalling and receptor and/or enzyme regulation. This is currently an active area of research. One recent example of this is their ability to inhibit cyclooxygenase, which in turn reduces platelet aggregation and thrombosis. Other studies have shown that flavonoids can inhibit NADPH oxidase and regulate nitric oxide synthase, which are involved with inflammation and vascular function.

Anticancer activities of flavonoids have also been studied. In colon cancer-induced rats, the flavonone hesperidin has been shown to decrease the incidence of tumours and inhibit the development of aberrant crypt foci, although the mechanisms behind this are not fully understood.

Isoflavones

Isoflavones (also referred to as isoflavonoids) are flavonoids, but are also called phytoestrogens because of their oestrogenic activity. Structurally, they exhibit a similarity to mammalian oestrogens and bind to oestrogen receptors, including oestrogen receptor α and β. Apart from basic structural similarities, the

Figure 14.5 Chemical structure of the isoflavones genistein, daidzein and glycitein.

key to their oestrogenic effect is the presence and the distance between the hydroxyl groups on the A and B rings. They are weakly oestrogenic and as such have the potential to act as both oestrogen agonists and antagonists depending on the background oestrogenic environment. They have also demonstrated mechanisms that are independent of the oestrogen receptors.

Isoflavones are found in legumes, with soy being the principal dietary source. Like most flavonoids, they are present in plants mainly as glycosides (malonyl, acetyl or β-glycosides), with concentrations ranging from 0.1 to 3.0 mg/g. The main aglycones present following ingestion are genistein, daidzein and glycitein (Figure 14.5). Consumption levels of isoflavones are hard to estimate, but recent data suggest that populations that consume high levels of soy, such as the Japanese, ingest between 20 and 50 mg/day.

The metabolism and absorption of isoflavones require hydrolysation by intestinal glycosidases, which in turn release the aglycones. These are absorbed or further metabolised to other oestrogenic or non-oestrogenic compounds. The plasma half-life of these compounds is about 7–8 h, with levels ranging from 50 to 800 ng/ml in adults consuming soy foods. Isoflavones are mainly excreted in the urine conjugated to glucuronic acid or sulphate.

In humans, various factors affect the biological activity of isoflavones, such as the medium of administration (i.e. food matrix), chemical form, metabolism, bioavailability, level and duration of exposure, and the hormonal and dietary state of the individual. Isoflavones have potential health beneficial effects in relation to cardiovascular disease, cancer, osteoporosis and the menopause. These have been illustrated in many *in vitro* and animal studies, but to date results in human studies are inconsistent, possibly for the reasons listed above. Whether the isoflavones are the

active components responsible for these effects remains to be elucidated, but to a certain extent it seems that they have actions of their own and also act together with other components in soy. Like other flavonoids, isoflavones also have anti-inflammatory and antioxidant activity, adding to their potential beneficial cardiovascular effects.

Given their oestrogenic activity, it has been hypothesised that isoflavones may act similarly to hormone replacement therapy (HRT). Studies have examined the role of high soy-based diets and isoflavones in isolation on hot flushes and other menopausal symptoms but there is currently no consensus on the optimal dose or source of isoflavones for reduction of menopausal symptoms. The evidence suggests that the health effects cannot be attributed to isolated isoflavones alone. In addition, to date no firm conclusion can be drawn on the potential bone-preserving effects of isoflavones in menopausal women. Human data on the effects of isoflavones on cancer are scarce, and because of their oestrogenic activity there is some concern over their effects on oestrogen-dependent cancers such as breast cancer, but available human data do not support an oestrogenic effect of these compounds in women.

Anthocyanins

Anthocyanins are one of the most important groups of water-soluble pigments in plants (Figure 14.6). Like other flavonoids, they occur principally as glycosides and are responsible for red, blue, purple and shades in between. Their colour and intensity is dependent on the pH and other pigments present in the plant/food. It has been difficult to quantify the levels of anthocyanins in plants/foods and especially humans as a result of the effects of pH on their chemical form and relative instability in certain environments. Alkaline pH, processing, cooking and physical damage to the food can result in structural transformation

Figure 14.6 Chemical structure of the anthocyanins cyanidin, pelargonidin, delphinidin.

and even degradation of anthocyanins, making quantification even more difficult. This effect is compounded in the body as metabolism of the altered structures can produce numerous individual compounds that are difficult to identify.

Anthocyanins have been identified in over 27 families of food plants. The consumption of anthocyanins has been estimated to be between 80 and 215 mg/day, with higher intakes reported in the summer months. However, a single serving of blueberries, blackcurrants or blood orange juice can provide levels of anthocyanins exceeding 500 mg. Since the 'French paradox' suggested that components of red wine may be responsible for protection against cardiovascular disease, there has been increased interest in anthocyanins, but until recently very little was known of their absorption and metabolism. Data on their bioavailability in humans have grown over the past 5 years, and evidence has suggested they have limited bioavailability and are extensively metabolised in the body. Many argue that anthocyanins' relative bioavailability contradicts their perceived bioactivity and new evidence suggests that levels of potentially bioactive degradation products could exist in the circulation at much higher levels than their parent forms. Given the analytical limitations of high-performance liquid chromatography (HPLC) as commonly used for identification in the past, the identification of these products of degradation has been limited. The use of labelled compounds along with tandem mass spectrometry (MS/MS) as an adjunct to HPLC should solve these issues in the future.

At present, epidemiological and experimental evidence supports the contribution of dietary anthocyanins to improving cardiovascular health,

with specific indications for improvements in hypertension. Intervention studies using anthocyanin-rich extracts and foods suggest they have effects on vascular blood flow, although the mechanism is not fully understood. Current research is focusing on their activities on immune cell and NO activity.

Other phenolic phytochemicals

Tannins

Tannins differ from the phenolics in that they are compounds of high molecular weight. They are highly hydroxylated and can form insoluble complexes with carbohydrates and proteins. The term 'tannin' is derived from its tanning properties; it forms stable tannin–protein complexes in animal hides, as in leather. Over the past 30 years, much of the literature on tannins has been on their antinutritive effects, but the evidence below illustrates that they may also have health benefits.

Tannins can be divided into two major groups: hydrolysable tannins and condensed tannins. Hydrolysable tannins are readily hydrolysed with acid, alkali, enzymes and hot water. The principal hydrolysable tannins are esters of gallic acid or ellagic acid (Figure 14.7), referred to as gallotannins and ellagitannins. Condensed tannins, also known as proanthocyanidins, are oligomers or polymers of flavan-3-ols that are of high molecular weight and are far more common in the diet than the hydrolysable tannins. One of the key features of condensed tannins is that they yield anthocyanidins when heated in acidic media, hence the name proanthocyanidins. Proanthocyanidins that consist exclusively of catechins are often

Figure 14.7 Chemical structure of the tannin esters gallic and ellagic acid and procyanidin.

referred to as procyanidins and are the most abundant proanthocyanidin in plants.

Tannins are estimated to be consumed at twice the amount of other flavonoids and are found in relatively high concentrations in a wide range of cereals, fruits, berries, beans, nuts, wine and cocoa. Structurally, they possess over 10 phenolic groups and 5–7 aromatic rings per 1000 units of relative molecular mass. In foods levels of the highly polymerised proanthocyanidins rarely exceed those of the monomers, dimers and trimers. The complex polymer structure of tannins makes them hard to analyse, therefore making it difficult to estimate the amounts consumed, their digestibility, bioavailability and their physiological effects. It has been shown, however, that tannins are extensively recovered in faeces and their indigestibility may work in favour of tannins for their health effects, as new evidence suggests that colonic bacteria may break the tannins down into more bioactive and bioavailable forms, such as procyanidin monomers, dimmers and simpler phenolic structures.

The biological effects of tannins or their by-products of biodegradation on processes involved in atherosclerosis is an area of increasing focus, where proanthocyanidins have been shown to mediate anti-inflammatory activity, vascular endothelial function and platelet aggregation.

Figure 14.8 Chemical structure of the stilbenes cinnamic acid and resveratrol.

Stilbenes

Stilbenes are present in a wide range of plants and are synthesised from cinnamic acid derivatives. Their production in plants is positively associated with resistance to mould and they are produced in response to microbial infection or stress. A known major active compound in this family is *trans*-resveratrol and most studies to date have concentrated on its potential biological effects (Figure 14.8).

In folk medicine, including Chinese medicine, humans have used medicinal plants containing resveratrol. Based on the quantitative data currently available, the major dietary sources of stilbenes are grapes, grape juices, wine, peanuts and peanut butter. They are predominantly located in the skin and in general are absent or only present in low amounts in fruit flesh. In wines the levels of resveratrol depend on the grape variety, climatic and ecological conditions, and the harvesting procedures used, but studies suggest that the levels in red and white grape skins are comparable. The extent of maceration of skins and seeds during fermentation is the key determinant of the final stilbene concentration in the wine, but the yeast strains and fining agents used and the time spent in oak barrels also alter their levels. Red wines contain the highest levels of *trans*-resveratrol, with approximately 8 mg/l, but levels vary depending on the grape variety. Levels in rose wines generally range between 1.38 and 2.93 mg/l, while levels in white wines are generally low since during the wine-making process minimal contact is made with the grape skins, which are the main source of resveratrol.

Previously resveratrol was extensively studied for its effects on vascular activity, but more recent research is examining its effects on increasing longevity and reducing cellular degeneration.

Lignans

Lignans are phenolic compounds that are present in many plant species. Although they are present in high concentrations in linseed (flaxseed) they are also present in measurable amounts in many of the cereals, pulses, fruits and vegetables commonly consumed in the Western world. Although the levels of lignans are generally low on an individual food basis, their ubiquity in the plant kingdom suggests that they may well be an important source of phytoestrogens, particularly to consumers of high plant-based diets (e.g. vegans and vegetarians). The structure of lignans in plants is different to the structure of the mammalian lignans, which are formed as a result of microbial metabolism in the gut. The lignan precursors (including secoisolariciresinol, matairesinol, pinoresinol and sesamin) are present in plants as glycoside conjugates, but following ingestion microbial enzymes convert these precursors to the enterolignans, enterodiol and enterolactone (Figure 14.9). Confirmation of a bacterial source for the production of the mammalian lignans (including enterodiol and enterolactone) was provided many years ago when humans administered selective antibiotic therapy over a 6–8 day period which immediately showed a decrease in enterodiol and enterolactone excretion; after just 2–3 days the urinary excretion of the metabolites was undetectable.

Figure 14.9 Chemical structure of the mammalian lignans enterodiol and enterolactone.

Levels of enterolignans in humans are much lower than those of flavonoids and range from <0.1 to 180 nmol/l, but in vegetarians levels of up to 1000 nmol/l have been measured. In common with oestrogens and isoflavones, the lignans undergo efficient enterohepatic circulation: they are absorbed from the intestinal tract, and then transported via the portal vein to the liver, where they may undergo conjugation with glucuronic acid. These water-soluble conjugates are then excreted in the urine via the kidneys while non-glucuronide conjugates follow the biliary route of excreation.

To date, numerous animal studies have addressed the potential anticancer effects of these compounds, and there is growing interest in their potential role to reduce cardiovascular risk and preserve bone health.

14.4 Carotenoids

Carotenoids are the most abundant pigments responsible for the bright red, orange and yellow colours in many of the fruits and vegetables that we eat. They also provide coloration in certain species of insects, birds and crustaceans, such as the orange of lobster shells. Carotenoids are, however, not synthesised by animals, so the colours they provide to animals are the result of cumulative ingestion of plants and microorganisms that do synthesise them. Carotenoids protect cells against photosensitisation and act as light-absorbing pigments during photosynthesis, and some classes of carotenoid, such as β-carotene, can be converted to vitamin A, which plays a role in many physiological functions, including gene transcription, vision, immune function and skin health. Approximately 600 carotenoids have been identified in nature, of which about 50 contain provitamin A activity. Carotenoids such as the

Figure 14.10 Chemical structure of the carotenoids β-carotene, lycopene and lutein.

carotenes are hydrocarbons which contain oxygenated xanthophylls consisting of eight isoprenoid units. They have a high number of double bonds in their polyisoprenoid structure, thus making isomerisation possible to produce mono- or poly-*cis* isomers, even though most carotenoids occur in the *trans* configuration. Humans cannot synthesise carotenoids and are thus dependent on dietary sources. Carotenoids are usually fat soluble and once ingested are released from complex proteins, incorporated into micelles and transported to the intestinal mucosa. Provitamin A carotenoids are then cleaved to produce vitamin A, while unconverted carotenoids are absorbed directly into the blood. Carotenoids are transported in the circulation by lipoproteins. The major circulating carotenoids include β-carotene, α-carotene, lycopene, β-cryptoxanthin, lutein and zeaxanthin (Figure 14.10).

Epidemiological studies suggest a positive link between high dietary intakes and tissue accumulation of carotenoids with the reduction in the risk of chronic degenerative disease. While the epidemiological association between β-carotene and lung cancer has been strong, results of randomised, placebo-controlled trials have been inconsistent, but the evidence regarding other carotenoids and other

diseases such as cardiovascular disease, cancer and other age-related degenerative disorders is growing. Evidence for the health-beneficial effects of carotenoids established from epidemiological studies also suggests they may serve as useful markers of a healthy lifestyle or indicators of fruit and vegetable intake.

Lycopene is a type of cartenoid found in high concentrations in tomato sauce and ketchup, and has received much attention in recent years. It does not have provitamin A properties and as a result of its unsaturated nature is a potent antioxidant.

The antioxidant properties of carotenoids have been suggested in the past to be their main mechanism of action, but more recent evidence favours effects on cell signalling and growth regulation, modulation of immune response and detoxification enzyme activity, in addition to α- and β-carotenes provitamin A capacity.

14.5 Phytosterols

Over 250 plants have been reported to contain measurable levels of phytosterols. The nutritional interest in these compounds relates to the fact that they have

Figure 14.11 Chemical structure of the phytosterols sitosterol, stigmasterol, campesterol.

a similar structure to cholesterol, with differences in side-chain configuration, and therefore have the potential to act as 'natural' dietary cholesterol-lowering agents. Sitosterol is the major sterol in plant materials, but stigmasterol, campesterol, brassica and avena sterols also occur in many plant materials (Figure 14.11). Similar in structure to cholesterol in mammalian cells, they play an important role in the structure and function of cell membranes, where they regulate the fluidity of membranes and may play a role in the adaptation of membranes to temperature. Within the plant they also play a key role in cell differentiation and proliferation, and their accumulation in seeds and oils suggests that they are important in the growth of new cells and shoots.

The richest natural sources of these compounds are vegetable oils (and products derived from oils) but cereal grains (cereal-based products) and nuts also contain measurable amounts. Recent studies suggest that total estimated intake ranges from 146 to 405 mg/day, but intake in vegetarians may be up to three times higher. This difference has been reflected in serum levels, 350 µg/dl in vegetarians versus 270 µg/dl in non-vegetarians, and with studies suggesting that biliary clearance is higher in vegetarians.

In the 1950s large amounts of plant sterols (up to 50 g/day) were fed to patients with hypercholesterolaemia to lower their serum cholesterol levels. However, interest in their clinical use declined because they were poorly soluble and concerns were expressed over the potential causation of phytosterolaemia from increased intake. The development of fat-soluble plant stanol esters in the early 1990s unmasked the potential for relatively small (1.5 g/day) and safe doses to have hypocholesterolaemic effects in human studies. The popularity of stanol esters for cholesterol lowering renewed the interest in using plant sterols for that purpose, and clinical data showed that the addition of phytosterols to the diet lowered cholesterol even in normochlolesterolaemic subjects. Studies suggest that the dose of plant sterols is important, with 2 g/day offering the ideal dose for cholesterol lowering; higher doses do not appear to enhance efficacy. However, higher doses seem to interfere with the absorption of other phytochemicals such as carotenoids and other lipid-soluble compounds.

One of the major metabolic effects of consuming dietary plant sterols relates to reduced intestinal cholesterol absorption, leading to decreased blood LDL-cholesterol levels and lower cardiovascular disease risk. More recently other biological roles for phytosterols have been proposed, in particular in relation to potential inhibitory actions of phytosterols on several cancers.

14.6 Sulphur-containing compounds: sulphides and glucosinolates

Sulphides

Sulphur-containing compounds (the allium family) may have a number of beneficial health properties. Sulphides are found in large quantities in garlic and other bulbous plants. The main component, which is believed to be the active component, is allicin (Figure 14.12), formed by the combination of its precursor, alliin, with the enzyme allinase. These compounds are volatile and are responsible for the well-known garlic odour. Garlic cloves can contain up to 4g of alliin per kilogram of fresh weight, but no exact dosage is known for its health benefits. A large amount of work has been carried out on the metabolism of allicin in animal models and in humans, and to date there is still debate on the mode of action of these compounds. Although the evidence regarding the hypolipidaemic and hypoglycaemic effects of allium vegetables is inconsistent, there is a significant amount of data indicating their anticancer properties; including activities on a number of cellular events involved in cell cycle regulation, angiogenesis and apoptosis. More work is still needed to fully establish the extent to which these compounds contribute to the activity of allium vegetables, as plants such as garlic also contain a number of other bioactive compounds.

Glucosinolates

Glucosinolates are a large group of sulphur-containing compounds present in brassica vegetables. When the plant tissue is damaged by food preparation or chewing, the glucosinolates are hydrolysed by endogenous enzymes (myrosinase) to release a range of breakdown products, including isothiocyanates, thiocyanates and indoles. Isothiocyanates, also referred to as 'mustard oils', are hot and bitter compounds with an acrid smell.

Humans are sensitive to the strong flavours associated with glucosinolate breakdown products and these compounds are therefore important determinants of flavour in many important brassicas. Allyl isothiocyanate (Figure 14.12) is largely responsible for the characteristic hot flavours of mustard and horseradish, and the glucosinolates sinigrin and progoitrin are responsible for the bitterness of brussel sprouts and other brassica vegetables. Glucosinolate breakdown products exert a variety of toxic and antinutritional effects in several animal species; the adverse effects on thyroid metabolism are a noted example. They are goitrogenic in animals, but these effects can be mitigated to some extent by increasing levels of iodine in the diet. However, this goitrogenicity has limited the exploitation of brassica feedstuffs for domestic livestock. These compounds may induce goitrogenic effects in humans, but there is little epidemiological evidence to suggest that this is an important cause of human disease. In a study where 150g of Brussels sprouts was added to volunteer diets, there was no effect on thyroid hormone levels, presumably because cooking had inactivated the myrosinase and thus reduced the biological availability of the goitrogenic breakdown products to subclinical levels.

A great deal of evidence is emerging to suggest that brassica vegetables may have important anticarcinogenic effects associated with the biological activity of glucosinolate breakdown products. The World Cancer Research Fund review on the role of diet in cancer prevention concluded that diets rich in cruciferous vegetables probably protect humans specifically against cancers of the colon, rectum and thyroid and, when consumed as part of a diet rich in other types of vegetables, against cancers at other sites. This epidemiological evidence is consistent with a number of experimental studies, which from the 1960s onwards have indicated that glucosinolate breakdown products exert anti-carcinogenic effects in experimental animal models. The mechanism to explain these effects relates to the ability of glucosinolate breakdown products (e.g. the isothiocyanates and sulphurpane) to modulate the activities of phase I (e.g. cytochrome P450) and phase II (e.g. glutathione S-transferase, UDP-glucuronyl transferase) biotransformation enzymes, which together catalyse a variety

Figure 14.12 Chemical structure of the sulphur-containing compounds allicin and allyl isothiocyanate.

of hydrolytic, oxidation and reduction reactions (phase I), the products of which are then available for conjugation reactions (phase II).

14.7 Phytochemical toxicity

The concept that phytochemicals are potentially beneficial to human health is rapidly gaining both scientific and public credence. Although in the future sufficient convincing evidence may well be available to prove potential health benefits from the consumption of some of the phytochemicals addressed in this chapter, for several other phytochemicals there is clear evidence of toxicity to animals and occasionally to humans. For the majority of the currently identified phytochemicals there are limited data on safe levels or optimal levels of intake for health benefits, and it is critical that these margins are more clearly defined in future research.

14.8 Perspectives on the future

As illustrated throughout this chapter, phytochemicals in nutrition is a growing area of research. Phytochemicals are potentially involved as protective compounds for a number of chronic diseases, including cardiovascular disease, cancer and neurodegeneration. There is still much to be learnt about their metabolism, bioavailability, mode of action and dose–response effects and, in some cases, the actual compounds responsible for the health effects are still unknown.

Currently there are no recommended dietary intakes for phytochemicals, but consumers should eat a wide variety of foods that incorporate the various phytochemicals to maximise disease prevention. Further research is required to define optimal doses for potential health effects and to define 'safe' levels of intakes for many of these phytochemicals. Many of these compounds should be investigated with the same vigour as pharmaceuticals because, although they occur naturally, they still require the same levels of proof of efficacy and safety. With the current drive towards supplementation and the use of genetically modified technology to enhance levels of 'desirable' compounds in foods, it is paramount that further research is conducted to add to our knowledge of the importance of enhancing our diet with specific phytochemicals for potential health benefits.

Future work

(1) Improve analytical methods to more accurately assess the intakes and circulating levels of these compounds.
(2) Establish better characterisation of their metabolism and bioavailability.
(3) Conduct studies using specific compounds at physiologically attainable levels to better understand their mechanisms of action and, more importantly, studies using physiologically relevant metabolites.
(4) Define risks and benefits for human health and determine optimal level of intake.
(5) Focus research in humans using long-term intervention studies complimented by work in large established cohort studies.

Further reading

Chun OK, Chung SJ, Song WO, Estimated dietary flavonoid intake and major food sources of U.S. adults. J Nutr 2007; 137(5): 1244–1252.

D'Archivio M et al. Polyphenols, dietary sources and bioavailability. Ann Ist Super Sanita 2007; 43(4): 348–361.

Erdman JW Jr et al. Flavonoids and heart health: Proceedings of the ILSI North America Flavonoids Workshop, May 31–June 1, 2005, Washington, DC. J Nutr 2007; 137(3): 718S–737S.

Holst B, Williamson G. Nutrients and phytochemicals: from bioavailability to bioefficacy beyond antioxidants. Curr Opin Biotechnol 2008; 19(2): 73–82.

Hooper L et al. Flavonoids, flavonoid-rich foods, and cardiovascular risk: a meta-analysis of randomized controlled trials. Am J Clin Nutr 2008; 88(1): 38–50.

Manach C et al. Bioavailability and bioefficacy of polyphenols in humans. I. Review of 97 bioavailability studies. Am J Clin Nutr 2005; 81(1 Suppl): 230S–242S.

Milner JA. Preclinical perspectives on garlic and cancer. J Nutr 2006; 136 (3 Suppl): 827S–831S.

Rao AV, Rao LG. Carotenoids and human health. Pharmacol Res 2007; 55(3): 207–16.

Rasmussen SE et al. Dietary proanthocyanidins: occurrence, dietary intake, bioavailability, and protection against cardiovascular disease. Mol Nutr Food Res 2005; 49(2): 159–174.

Scalbert A., Williamson G. Dietary intake and bioavailability of polyphenols. J Nutr 2000; 130 (8S Suppl): 2073S–2085S.

USDA. USDA Database for the Flavonoid Content of Selected Foods – Release 2.1. 2007 [cited May 20, 2009]; Available from: http://www.nal.usda.gov/fnic/foodcomp/Data/Flav/Flav02-1.pdf.

Williamson G, Manach C. Bioavailability and bioefficacy of polyphenols in humans. II. Review of 93 intervention studies. Am J Clin Nutr 2005; 81(1 Suppl): 243S–255S.

Yang CS et al. Bioavailability issues in studying the health effects of plant polyphenolic compounds. Mol Nutr Food Res 2008; 52 Suppl 1: S139–S151.

15
The Control of Food Intake

Adam Drewnowski and France Bellisle

Key messages

- Food intake is a patterned activity governed by physiological signals and by factors in the environment.
- Physiological signals affecting food intake involve a feedback mechanism that responds to energy requirements to maintain energy homeostasis.
- In affluent societies where palatable food is overabundant, intake can be elicited by hedonic (pleasure) motivation that can override physiological homeostatic controls.

- Important motivational factors include hunger, satiety, satiation and palatability.
- Important descriptors of eating behaviour include meal size, meal frequency (meal pattern) and interval between eating occasions.
- Individual factors such as cognitive restraint and disinhibition are potent modulators of food intake.
- A greater understanding of the control of food intake is required in the context of the present epidemic of overweight and obesity.

15.1 Introduction

Food intake is a complex human behaviour, subject to many influences from within and outside the body. Internal physiological mechanisms, which influence when and how much we eat, regulate energy balance and help ensure our survival. External social, cultural and environmental factors guide food selection; shape the development of eating habits, and affect the types and amounts of foods consumed. Studying the interactions among the internal and external controls of food intake is needed to understand human nutrition and the management of body weight. Such studies can help us deal with diet-related diseases and the global obesity epidemic. However, deciding whether eating behaviours owe more to biology or to the food environment is no simple task.

Placing these complex interactions in a proper context requires a theoretical framework. Looking at how human food intake is organised over time is one place to start. One undisputed fact is that food intake in humans and in most animals is intermittent: people eat in spurts of varying duration, and then stop eating for varying periods of time. How individual eating behaviours are distributed over time is an important area of study. There is equal interest in knowing what happens in the course of an eating bout, immediately before and after eating, and during the longer periods of satiety before the next meal.

15.2 The underlying structure of eating behaviour

The 19th century French physiologist Claude Bernard noted that any living organism must continuously be able to satisfy a number of needs in order to maintain an independent life and survive. Behaviours of various types help the organism extract the materials of life from the environment. While the needs for energy, nutrients, and water are continuous, the behaviours required to satisfy them are intermittent. What is more, these discontinuous behaviours represent the adaptation of a species to a given environment. Eating, drinking and sleeping are all intermittent behaviours directed toward satisfying ongoing needs. Energy intakes for any one individual can vary considerably from day to day (Figure 15.1).

The diurnal cycle

The alternation between day and night defines the eating behaviour of humans and many animals. The day–night cycle is species specific: although humans mostly eat during the day, other species eat

Nutrition and Metabolism, Second Edition, edited by S. A. Lanham-New, I. A. Macdonald and H. M. Roche. © 2011 The Nutrition Society.

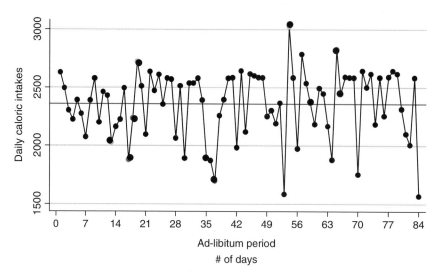

Figure 15.1   Energy intakes for 1 study participant over 85 consecutive days. (Data courtesy of Moz Benado, MS Thesis, University of Washington.)

mostly or exclusively at night. Little or no food intake occurs during the inactive resting phase.

Disturbances in the day–night cycle can signal an imbalance between energy consumption and energy needs. Genetically obese rats living in the laboratory eat both at night and during the day. Clinical observations in humans have shown that the 'night eating syndrome' can predict weight gain and the development of obesity (Stunkard *et al.*, 1996). What factors are responsible for altering the circadian patterns of food consumption in humans is not clear. Neuroendocrine disturbances brought about by depression and stress as well as irregular work patterns and sleep habits can threaten the day–night cycle of food consumption.

There are many other ways in which underlying biology can be in conflict with the demands of contemporary society. Humans are social animals that live in complex cultures. The diurnal distribution of meals is a behavioural adaptation to energy needs, but one that is shaped by culture and the food environment. In response to cultural demands, children can learn to be hungry at specific times of day, corresponding to culture-determined meal times. Laboratory animals can also learn to adapt to a fixed meal pattern and eat adequate amounts at each meal in order to minimise hunger between meals and meet their energy needs. Even physiological hunger signals such as glucose and insulin levels adapt to fixed meal patterns. However, such learning does not take place

when food is constantly available. By providing easy access to palatable food at all times of day, the Western culture is abandoning the fixed pattern of three meals per day in favour of grazing and snacking. If the control of food intake is partly learned, then a weakening of the regulatory mechanisms is likely to follow.

The meal cycle

During the waking hours, food is consumed in discrete episodes. Typically, humans consume three to four meals and snacks per day, whereas laboratory rats consume between 7 and 11. The total time spent eating over any 24-h period can be highly variable for humans, depending on age, custom and culture. For laboratory rodents it is less than 60 min, mostly at night.

Early studies in physiology suggested that energy deficits were a direct signal to start a meal. However, a look at human eating habits suggests that such a notion is much too simple to account for the many complexities of the timing and duration of meals. First, hunger is not the only trigger for eating. People (and animals) clearly eat even though they are not hungry and may not stop eating when full. Second, meals are generally finished well before the energy contained in the ingested food has been absorbed or metabolised to cover energy needs. Third, eating episodes can be timed to satisfy not only current but also

Figure 15.2   The typical preload study design used to test the impact of different beverages and foods on subsequent motivational ratings and energy intakes.

future energy needs. At culturally determined times of day; people eat meals and snacks in anticipation of future energy expenditures.

Immediately following the meal, a complex succession of events, described as a satiety cascade, inhibits further eating for a certain time – until the onset of the next meal. How long the period of satiety will last depends on the amount of energy consumed and on the volume and nutrient content of the just-eaten foods. The state of satiety is influenced by physiological processes such as stomach distension and emptying, but can also be affected by the sensory characteristics of the food itself and by the attitudes and beliefs of the consumer.

Studying how eating behaviours adapt to the provision of too much or too little energy is one way to understand the control of food intake. The usual expectation is that people will eat more in response to missing energy but will adjust their food consumption downwards after they are allowed (or compelled) to eat too much. Studies based on the so-called preload paradigm have examined the impact of different beverages or foods on hunger and satiety, and the amount of food eaten during the next meal (Figure 15.2).

Most such studies looked at the short-term adaptive responses following one single challenge. The food or beverage were given around breakfast time; the subjects were asked to record their sensations of hunger and fullness every 20 min until noon, at which time a copious lunch meal was offered on a tray. Subjects were instructed to eat until they were full and the amounts of uneaten foods and plate waste were measured later by researchers.

In many such studies, the provision of extra energy did not appreciably reduce energy consumption at the next meal. When energy-containing beverages were consumed at breakfast time, the amount of energy consumed at lunch was not correspondingly reduced. Together, the beverage and the lunch following it were higher in energy than if no beverage had been consumed. One popular theory tried to explain such findings by proposing that humans were incapable of perceiving dietary energy when presented in liquid form. However, preload studies have also shown that the consumption of a solid snack was not associated with less food at the next meal. Clearly, the mechanisms of the control of food intake can be imprecise and incomplete. In general, there was little downward adjustment following an energy-containing preload, and it mattered little whether the preload was liquid or solid.

Humans are much better at upward adjustment of energy intakes. Reducing preload energy was often followed by more food being consumed at the next eating occasion. Although results varied, growing children appeared to compensate for the missing energy better than adults and younger people better than older people. Arguably, responding to inadequate intakes by eating more is an important survival mechanism. By contrast, there are fewer control mechanisms to deal with the (once rare) episodes of overeating.

Whereas the size of meals and their number together determine energy intakes at the end of the day, longer term mechanisms take over when it comes to the long-term control of body weight. Here too, the amounts of food consumed from one day to the next can be highly variable. Eating a large amount of food on one day is not necessarily followed by an immediate reduction in energy intake on the next day. If energy compensation does occur, it occurs over a longer period of time.

15.3 Internal controls of food intake

The signals that trigger the beginning and the end of eating episodes are critical to survival. Researchers initially thought that eating would begin whenever triggered by physiological signals that were associated with energy deprivation. Theories of hunger were accordingly developed based on whatever nutrient the body was thought to be lacking at the time, be it glucose, protein or fat. One common feature of all theories was that they incorporated a feedback loop. Whereas a state of nutritional need was necessary and sufficient for eating or drinking behaviour to begin, satisfying this need through eating or drinking would cause the behaviour to stop. In other words, behaviours were driven directly by the shifting bodily needs of the organism.

Early concepts of control of food intake were all built around the notion of stability or homeostasis. The control mechanisms were there to ensure energy balance – that energy intakes met energy needs – and to regulate energy stores. The observation that body weights in adults were relatively stable over long periods of time suggested that some critical signalling mechanism also informed the brain of the current status of body weight. If body weights were stable, and at their physiological 'set-point', then energy intakes and energy expenditures were perfectly balanced. If body weights decreased below the set-point then food intake would increase to provide the body with needed energy. If body weights rose above the set-point, then physiological systems would act promptly to restrict further eating. Such theories depended on some regulated physiological parameter and the existence of a feedback loop. The physiological factor would provide information about the nutritional status of the body from the periphery to the brain.

A number of such physiological signals have been proposed over the years. The thermostatic theory suggested that heat generated during digestion led to a rise in body temperature that inhibited eating behaviour. The glucostatic theory posited that eating was triggered by a decrease in the availability of glucose to tissues. The increase in glucose levels after a meal was the factor that inhibited further eating. The lipostatic theory suggested that body fat was the key substance that determined eating behaviour. Linking to body fat stores, the lipostatic theory also tried to account for the fact that the amount of body fat was regulated and weight loss attempts were most often followed by weight regain until the pre-diet body weight was restored. The aminostatic theory suggested that amino acid and metabolites were the crucial agents determining satiety. This is reflected in current work on the high satiating value of protein-rich foods.

Homeostatic influences include short-term, episodic signals that trigger intake and inhibit it during satiety. Critical signals are blood glucose level as well as hormones secreted in the gastrointestinal tract. The level of ghrelin, a hormone secreted mainly in the stomach, is high before meals and falls after intake. Other substances, such as cholescystokinin (CCK), glucagon, glucagon-like peptide (GLP) and peptide YY (PYY), are generally viewed as satiety signals that inhibit intake for some time following an ingestion episode.

Superimposed on this episodic control, a longer-term control system modulates intake as a function of the size of the body fat stores. The lipostatic theory remained speculative until the discovery of leptin in 1995. This hormone is secreted by the adipose tissue itself and provides quantitative signals to the brain in proportion with the amount of body fat. These longer-term signals include not only leptin from the adipose tissue, but also insulin, a hormone secreted by the pancreas whose short-term peripheral action regulates the blood glucose level and acts directly in the brain to regulate body fat stores. A brain structure called the hypothalamus (particularly its arcuate nucleus) is recognised as a potent site of integration of signals that shape intake behaviour.

The episodic and long-term homeostatic control systems interact to influence intake. Their complex modes of interaction and their peripheral and brain substrates have been described in many excellent reviews. There are also multiple interactions between physiological mechanisms and the nature of the consumed food. The physiological signals that affect food intake are influenced by the ingestion of certain nutrients. Protein tends to induce more satiety than carbohydrate for a given energy load, and carbohydrate is more satiating than fat. Among other effects, the intake of proteins is critical to the release of the satiety hormone PYY, which has been reported to reduce appetite in humans and modulate neural responses in hypothalamic and cortical areas implicated in appetite control.

15.4 The pleasure response to foods

Whereas earlier theories of the control of food intake stressed physiological mechanisms, much of the recent focus has been on the nature of the foods themselves. Some researchers believe that certain foods, by virtue of their energy density, palatability or nutrient content, are able to override the body's regulatory systems. Among the many environmental influences, the pleasure derived from foods is said to be the most potent.

In human societies with easy access to palatable energy-dense foods, the pleasure response may be responsible for overeating. Many factors present in the environment can trigger eating in a satiated organism. While the present theoretical framework talks about pleasure, other researchers have talked about impulsive behaviours, cravings or even food addictions. In scientific terms, the pleasure response to modern foods can interact with homeostatic mechanisms to shape eating patterns in a way that no longer balances food consumption with energy expenditure.

In recent years, much research has been devoted to the neural substrate of the pleasure or hedonic response to foods. Anticipatory pleasure can strengthen appetite. In countering the effects of satiation, pleasure can prolong eating and so increase meal size. A brain network involving the limbic system and the cortex is responsible for organising eating behaviour in response to cognitive or affective influences. Endocannabinoids, serotonin and dopamine are important neurotransmitters in this system. Food intake can be triggered and maintained in the absence of need or hunger in response to a situation of stress or boredom, a social event or simply the presence of good-tasting foods in the environment. Recent research has distinguished between 'liking' a food and 'wanting' it. Liking and wanting are now considered two important but different aspects of the motivation to eat. Both can depend on homeostatic or hedonic mechanisms. Theoretically, excessive energy intake associated with such situations ought to be compensated for later, with the homeostatic mechanisms working to inhibit eating at the next eating occasion. The fact is that this happens rarely or never. Evolutionary mechanisms may be ill-equipped to deal with eating that is triggered by sensory, cognitive or emotional signals, or influenced by the food environment and unrelated to energy needs.

15.5 The psychology of eating

A vast literature has addressed the psychological determinants of food intake. However, early attempts to find out whether obese persons shared a common obese eating style were largely unsuccessful. One important insight was that concern with body weight, described as dietary restraint, was a potent influence on the short-term and long-term control of food intake. In early studies, dietary restraint was supposed to reflect the distance from the physiological set point and measure the amount of effort that dieters had to exert to keep their weight below where it was meant to be. Such studies stressed the paradoxical, counter-regulatory influence of dietary restraint, suggesting that overly restrained persons were also prone to over-eating and weight cycling.

Some experts now distinguish rigid restraint, which can indeed be associated with poor appetite control, from flexible restraint, which is a beneficial attitude facilitating dieting and weight loss. Based on responses to multiple questionnaires, studies have categorised people by such supposedly permanent psychological traits as disinhibition. People likely to lose control over eating in a variety of circumstances are said to show high levels of disinhibition. High disinhibition is associated with overweight and obesity, as well as with many metabolic disorders such as syndrome X and type 2 diabetes. The vulnerability to eat in response to situations of emotional or affective tension became known as emotionality whereas the vulnerability to overeat in response to food stimuli in the environment became known as externality.

Early life experiences have a major influence on the development of the individual hierarchy of likes and dislikes. Every child learns to enjoy the foods that are introduced to him/her during the first years of life and such attitudes survive even if the person later changes countries or cultural environments. Many aspects of the feeding experience in early life, such as exposure to certain foods, being offered food as a reward for various behaviours or associating foods with pleasurable social events, contribute to shape likes and dislikes.

Other foods can be rejected following aversive conditioning. If the consumption of a novel food is followed by gastric disorders and nausea, that food will become aversive even after only a single digestive disorder. This phenomenon, known as conditioned taste aversion, is a very potent mechanism. A very strong satiety effect can also reinforce avoidance of the food when the eater is next presented with it. The experience of satiety following ingestion of a food can thus have complex consequences and lead to either food acceptance or rejection.

15.6 Environmental determinants of food intake

The modern food supply provides us with foods that vary in their nutrient content, their physical form, their palatability and their sensory characteristics. The food environment can facilitate or counteract the physiological control of food intake.

The sensory characteristics of foods interact with the body's mechanisms. Food palatability and energy density are closely linked. The best-tasting or most palatable foods are those that are energy dense, i.e. provide the most energy per unit volume. Seeking out such foods in preference to lower-energy density foods was probably necessary for survival. Laboratory animals prefer energy-dense foods, some rich in added sugars and fats, to regular protein-rich laboratory chow. Human infants select the most intense sweet solutions and prefer sweeter sugars over less sweet ones. Young children select sugar and fat mixtures, and prefer the more energy-dense vegetables and fruit over broccoli or leeks.

The impact of food palatability on consumption has been amply demonstrated in a number of studies. Good taste can stimulate intake and better-tasting foods are often consumed in larger amounts than similar but less palatable alternatives. Given that satiety is often defined by the amounts of food consumed, good-tasting foods being consumed in larger amounts are – by definition – less satiating. The food industry's ongoing search for foods that are palatable yet at the same time highly satiating may be a contradiction in terms.

The food environment can also determine portion size. Food consumption studies among children and adults show that intake is a direct function of the amount of food or drink that is served. Larger portions stimulate larger intake, regardless of the intensity of hunger, but do not lead to a corresponding increase in post-ingestive satiety. Large portion sizes can induce what has been called passive over-consumption, which exceeds bodily needs and potentially facilitates weight gain. Large portion sizes combined with energy-dense foods are especially problematic. Unaware of their high energy density, the consumer is likely to overeat, given the weight of the food is low. Portion size and energy density have additive effects, so that large portions of high energy density foods are said to have low satiating power.

People generally consume meals or snacks of a relatively fixed weight or volume. Given that the meal volume is fixed, then the energy value of the meal or snack will depend critically on the energy density of the ingested foods. Another important factor could be the physical state of the ingested substance. However, studies on this topic are inconsistent: whereas soups seem to be more satiating than solid crackers and cheese, other studies have found conflicting results using whole fruit and fruit juices or milk and cheese. The difference in satiating power, if it does exist, seems to be in the order of 10%. Furthermore, all beverages seem to behave similarly – there was no difference in the satiety profile between pure fruit juice, 1% milk and regular cola. All three beverages have the same energy density but different nutrient content. In other studies, no difference in satiating power was observed between drinkable liquid yogurts and semi-solid yogurts that had to be eaten with a spoon. However, both types of yogurts were more satiating than beverages, whether by virtue of greater viscosity or higher levels of protein or fibre.

The variety of foods presented within a meal can also have an impact on total consumption. Sensory variety, regardless of nutrient content, can stimulate food consumption. The feeling of satiation is sensory-specific, such that the liking for the just-eaten food decreases relative to the about to be eaten foods. The attractiveness of foods that share similar sensory characteristics (taste, aroma, colour, shape) also decreases. This is why selecting or presenting foods with varied sensory characteristics is associated with larger intake.

Environmental stimuli and food consumption

In affluent societies, many food-related cues are present in the environment. The availability of foods at all times of day is an obvious stimulus of intake. The presence of food vending machines in the environment may trigger spontaneous food intake at any time of day or night. Environmental cues that have been associated with past eating bouts can reinstate consumption even in satiated children and adults. The experience of restriction imposed by well-meaning parents on the intake of favourite foods seems to be one potent facilitator of eating in the absence of hunger observed in young girls when the forbidden food becomes available.

Not all environmental stimuli need to be food related. The presence of television or music in the environment can stimulate meal size or meal frequency. As a general rule, the presence in the environment of factors that distract the consumer from the act of ingestion are likely to increase intake. One very potent factor in free-living conditions is the presence of others, especially friends and family. Social stimulation is a phenomenon found in free-living subjects and is a function of the number of persons present. Under laboratory or controlled environments, however, the stimulation effect is less clear. Eating with strangers can sometimes decrease intake. In free-living individuals who most often eat with familiar companions, a clear stimulation effect is observed, perhaps mediated by the duration of meals consumed in company.

Time of day affects food choices and the amount eaten. Food eaten in the early part of day usually has a higher satiety potency than food eaten in the afternoon or the evening. Food choices are also different. Children learn that some foods are more appropriate for breakfast while others are more appropriate for lunch, dinner or snack. The snacking pattern is also learned by experience of what is possible and acceptable in a given environment. While the potential influence of the daily number of meals and snacks on the control of body weight is still debated, it seems that eating early (as opposed to late) in the day is generally associated with lower body weight and a nutrient intake more in line with dietary recommendations.

15.7 Conclusions

The control of food intake in humans involves biology, the environment and behaviour. Physiological mechanisms, descended through evolution, help control energy balance and the maintenance of stable body weight. However, such mechanisms can come into conflict with modern lifestyles and the modern food supply. The control of food intake represents an adaptive process whereby eating behaviour is adjusted to energy and nutrients needs as well as to social and cultural norms. This delicate balance is easily disturbed, however, leading potentially to excess energy intakes and overweight.

Further reading

Blundell JE. A psychobiological system approach to appetite and weight control. In: Eating Disorders and Obesity: A Comprehensive Textbook. (Fairburn CG, Brownell KD, eds). New York: Guilford Press, 2002: pp. 43–49.

De Castro JM. Genes, the environment and the control of food intake. Br J Nutr 2004, 92 (Suppl 1): S59–S62.

Ello-Martin JA, Ledikwe JH, Rolls BJ. The influence of food portion size and energy density on energy intake: implications for weight management. Am J Clin Nutr 2005; 82 (suppl. 2): 236S–241S.

Savage JS, Fisher JO, Birch LL. Parental influence on eating behaviour: conception to adolescence. J Law Med Ethics 2007; 35: 22–34.

Sclafani A. Oral and postoral determinants of food reward. Physiol Behav 2004; 81: 773–779.

Yeomans MR, Blundell JE, Leshem M. Palatability: response to nutritional need or need-free stimulation of appetite? Br J Nutr 2004; 92 (suppl. 1): S3–S14.

16
Overnutrition

Linda Bandini, Albert Flynn and Renee Scampini

Key messages

Obesity

- The prevalence of obesity is increasing throughout the world in both developed and developing countries, and has become a worldwide health problem given its association with increased morbidity.
- Body mass index is the most widely used measure to assess obesity. Skinfold thicknesses and bioelectrical impedance are other clinical measures used to identify obesity.
- Obesity is the result of an energy imbalance where energy intake exceeds energy expenditure.
- The aetiology of obesity is complex and may be a result of genetic, metabolic, behavioural and environmental factors.

Vitamin and mineral overconsumption

- For a number of vitamins and minerals adverse health effects can result when the capacity for homeostasis is exceeded by continuing high dietary intakes.
- The tolerable upper intake level (UL) is a dietary reference standard that may be used to evaluate the risk of excessive intakes of vitamins and minerals in groups and as a guide to individuals for the maximum level of the usual intake of micronutrients.
- The UL for nutrients may be derived based on the principles of risk assessment, and ULs have been established for several vitamins and minerals by authorities in a number of countries.

Section I: Obesity

16.1 Introduction

The prevalence of obesity has been increasing throughout the world. The World Health Organization (WHO) estimated that in 2005, 1.5 billion adults (individuals over age 15) were overweight and 400 million were obese. Based on current worldwide trends, the WHO projects that 2.3 billion adults will be overweight and 700 million will be obese by the year 2015 (WHO, 2006). The aetiology of obesity is complex and may be attributed to genetic, metabolic, behavioural and environmental factors. In this chapter we will discuss the identification and assessment of obesity, how energy imbalance can lead to obesity, potential factors contributing to the development of obesity and the consequences of obesity.

16.2 Identification

Obesity is defined as an excess of body fat. Body fat can be measured precisely by laboratory methods such as dual-energy X-ray absorptiometry (DEXA), total body water and hydrodensitometry. These methods give an estimate of total body fat, or adipose tissue, in the body. Because people of different sizes will have different amounts of body fat, identification of obesity cannot be made on the basis of absolute amounts of fat.

For example, a person who has 20 kg of body fat and weighs 60 kg has a percentage body fat of 33%:

$$\frac{20}{60} \times 100 = 33\%$$

A second person who has 24 kg of fat but weighs 80 kg will have 30% body fat:

Nutrition and Metabolism, Second Edition, edited by S. A. Lanham-New, I. A. Macdonald and H. M. Roche.   © 2011 The Nutrition Society.

$$\frac{24}{80} \times 100 = 30\%$$

The first person has less total fat but a higher percentage body fat than the second person.

Although obesity is defined as an excess of body fat, laboratory techniques for directly assessing body fatness are not available for clinical use. Furthermore, there are no agreed cut-off points or defined criteria for identifying obesity from measures of body fatness. Studies developing these cut-offs are currently underway and will probably be gender and potentially age-specific. Thus, identifying obesity in clinical practice is not presently based on an individual's percentage of body fat but rather on measures that correlate with body fat. The most common methods used in clinical assessment are body mass index (BMI), skinfold thickness and bioelectrical impedance.

Body mass index

Adults

Body mass index (BMI) is the recommended international screening tool used to identify obesity. BMI is defined as weight in kilograms divided by height in metres squared.

A man who is 172 cm tall and weighs 89 kg will have a BMI of 30.1:

$$\frac{89}{(1.72)^2} = 30.1$$

Another man who is 172 cm tall and weighs 73 kg will have a BMI of 24.7:

$$\frac{73}{(1.72)^2} = 24.7$$

Studies have shown that BMI, although not a direct measure of fatness, is significantly correlated with body fat as measured by laboratory methods. One of the major advantages of using BMI to identify obesity is that it can be derived from measures of height and weight, which are much easier to obtain than measures of skinfold thickness. However, BMI cannot distinguish whether the excess weight is due to fat or muscle mass. Thus, the use of BMI to identify obese individuals may result in misclassification for

Table 16.1 The International classification of adult underweight, overweight and obesity according to BMI

Classification	BMI (kg/m²)	
	Principal cut-off points	Additional cut-off points
Underweight	<18.50	<18.50
Severe thinness	<16.00	<16.00
Moderate thinness	16.00–16.99	16.00–16.99
Mild thinness	17.00–18.49	17.00–18.49
Normal range	18.50–24.99	18.50–22.99
		23.00–24.99
Overweight	≥25.00	≥25.00
Pre-obese	25.00–29.99	25.00–27.49
		27.50–29.99
Obese	≥30.00	≥30.00
Obese class I	30.00–34.99	30.00–32.49
		32.50–34.99
Obese class II	35.00–39.99	35.00–37.49
		37.50–39.99
Obese class III	≥40.00	≥40.00

With kind permission from the World Health Organization, http:// apps.who.int/bmi/index.jsp?introPage=intro_3.html 2006 © WHO.

individuals with increased muscle mass, such as heavyweight boxers or wrestlers.

The WHO has classifications for overweight and obesity in adults based on BMI (WHO, 2006) (Table 16.1). However, recent studies suggest that percentage body fat at a specific BMI may be higher in some populations. These findings suggest that using BMI to identify obesity may require population specific cut-offs, for example body fat may be higher at a lower BMI in Asian populations. Research is underway to determine cut-points for BMI specific to various populations.

Children and adolescents

BMI is currently used to identify children who are overweight and obese. Because BMI changes with age in children, there is no specific numerical cut-off point for identifying overweight and obesity in children as there is for adults. Thus, BMI growth charts that are age and gender specific are used to identify obesity.

Cut-off points for overweight and obesity in children differ among countries. Several countries, such as the USA, France, Japan, the UK and Italy, have specific growth charts developed from populations within their countries. While many countries use their own reference population to define obesity, others may use reference populations from other countries. An international task force on obesity (IOTF) developed reference standards to identify obesity in children. These standards are based on pooled data from six countries, including Brazil, the UK, Hong Kong, The Netherlands, Singapore and the USA.

Skinfold thickness

The determination of clinical measures of overweight and obesity that accurately reflect body fat has been an area of much research and discussion. Measures of triceps skinfold (TSF) thickness provide an index of subcutaneous fatness (fat underneath the skin). Studies have shown that measures of TSF thickness correlate well with body fatness in both children and adults, and they are used to identify people who are obese. However, two assumptions are made when TSF thickness measures are used to assess body fatness. The first is that the TSF is representative of subcutaneous fatness and the second is that subcutaneous fatness is correlated with total body fat. However, these assumptions are not always valid. In disease states, or in individuals with significant amounts of visceral fat (fat around the internal organs), changes in body fat distribution may alter the relationship of TSF thickness with total body fat. Investigators have measured skinfold thickness at several subcutaneous sites, including the subscapular, suprailiac, abdominal, bicep and tricep areas. Equations have been developed to calculate body fatness from the sum of several skinfolds. Although the use of these equations is probably more representative of subcutaneous fat than TSF thickness alone, skinfold measurements cannot identify individuals with significant amounts of visceral fat.

A significant limitation of using skinfold thickness to measure body fatness is that extensive training is required to perform the measurement correctly. Furthermore, it is more difficult to measure skinfold thickness accurately in obese people, therefore as a person becomes fatter, the reliability of these measures decreases. These limitations make the method less useful for identifying obesity in a clinical setting.

Bioelectrical impedance

Bioelectrical impedance (BIA) is a method that can be used in the clinical setting to estimate body composition. BIA is based on the body's resistance to a harmless electrical current, which is related to total body water. The measure of resistance, as well as height and weight, are used to determine the percentage body fat from predictive equations. One concern with BIA is that the predictive equations were created based on data from specific populations. It is important that the predictive equations used to determine percentage body fat are derived from a population similar to the population being measured. Currently, studies to identify obesity based on percentage body fat are in progress.

16.3 Energy balance

Obesity is the result of a long-term energy imbalance where energy intake exceeds energy expenditure (Table 16.2). This leads to a positive energy imbalance and an increase in body fat stores. Small energy imbalances maintained over a long period can result in significant weight gain. For example, 1 kg of adipose tissue is 31 798 kilojoules (kJ). A small excess of 420 kJ every day over a year would result in a gain of approximately 5 kg of adipose tissue. This would equal, for example, eating only one additional slice of bread and jam (roughly 420 kJ) every day for a year:

$$420\,\text{kJ/day} \times 365\,\text{days/year} = 153\,300\,\text{kJ/year}$$

$$1\,\text{kg adipose} = 31\,798\,\text{kJ}$$

$$\frac{153300}{31798} = 4.8\,\text{kg adipose tissue per year}$$

Table 16.2 Energy balance

Energy balance	energy intake = energy expenditure	maintenance of fat stores
Positive energy imbalance	energy intake > energy expenditure	increase in fat stores
Negative energy imbalance	energy intake < energy expenditure	decrease in fat stores

Obesity ultimately results from a positive energy imbalance, which can result from any of the following:

- an increase in energy intake with no change in energy expenditure
- a decrease in energy expenditure with no change in energy intake
- an increase in energy intake and a decrease in energy expenditure

Efforts to understand the aetiology of obesity have focused on differences in energy intake and energy expenditures among obese and non-obese individuals. An increase in energy intake and/or a decrease in energy expenditure are potential factors that could contribute to a positive energy imbalance.

Energy intake

A considerable amount of research has examined whether people who are obese consume more energy than people who are not obese. The majority of studies of energy intake in obese and normal weight children and adults do not show differences in their energy intakes. The findings of these studies have been questioned because of the uncertainty about whether the subjects' self-reported energy intakes are accurate. It was not until the doubly labelled water (DLW) method for measuring energy expenditure was developed that it became possible to assess unobtrusively the validity of dietary reporting. Using the DLW technique, measures of daily energy expenditure can be made simultaneously with measures of energy intake. If an individual is in energy balance, energy expenditure should equal energy intake. However, studies using DLW to measure energy expenditure have revealed that both obese and non-obese people substantially underreport their energy intakes, and thus comparisons of self-reported energy intake among obese and non-obese individuals are often inaccurate and cannot be used to determine whether or not obese individuals eat more than non-obese individuals.

Energy expenditure

Energy expenditure comprises four components:

- resting metabolic rate (RMR)
- thermic effect of food (TEF)
- physical activity
- growth.

RMR accounts for a major proportion of daily energy expenditure. Its contribution to energy expenditure varies among individuals, but in sedentary adults it accounts for between 60 and 70% of daily energy expenditure. The remaining 30–40% of daily energy expenditure in sedentary adults is the energy spent on activity and the TEF. As physical activity increases, RMR's proportion of total energy expenditure decreases. Children and pregnant and lactating women also have increased energy needs to support growth and, in lactating women, milk production.

Variability in energy expenditure

Since the 1980s, many studies have been conducted to compare RMR, TEF and daily energy expenditure among obese and non-obese individuals. Studies have not shown significant differences in resting energy expenditure between obese and non-obese adults or children. Studies on the TEF are equivocal, with some suggesting that energy expenditure may be decreased in the obese and others showing no differences between obese and non-obese people. Although the TEF contributes only a small percentage to daily energy expenditure (6–10%), small differences over a long period could potentially lead to a significant energy imbalance, as highlighted above.

Studies of daily energy expenditure that include RMR, TEF and physical activity among obese and non-obese people have not found differences in total energy expenditure between the two groups. Although these studies have not found lower energy expenditure in obese individuals, it has been hypothesised that differences may exist among individuals before they become obese (preobese state). When an individual gains weight, RMR and daily energy expenditure increase, due to an increase in both fat and fat-free mass. It has been hypothesised that lower energy expenditure in the preobese state may be normalised with weight gain. Earlier studies by Ravussin et al. (1988) suggested that low energy expenditure may lead to increased weight gain as an adaptive mechanism to increase energy expenditure. However, most recent longitudinal studies in children and adults do not support the hypothesis that lower energy expenditure in the pre-obese state is associated with an increase in body fat.

Diet-induced thermogenesis (adaptive thermogenesis)

In the 1980s considerable research focused on the role of diet-induced thermogenesis (DIT) in maintaining energy balance. DIT refers to an increase in energy expenditure in response to overeating. If energy expenditure were increased in response to an excess intake of energy, the excess energy would be dissipated as heat and obesity could be prevented. It has been hypothesised that lean individuals compensate for excess energy intake by burning the excess energy as heat, whereas obese individuals are metabolically more efficient and store excess energy as fat. Results of overfeeding studies in which energy expenditure was measured have found little evidence for DIT in obese or non-obese individuals.

Stock (1999) suggested that the role of DIT in regulating energy balance is secondary to its role in eliminating non-essential energy for individuals consuming low nutrient-dense diets and that in our society only recently has food become so accessible that the role of DIT in maintaining energy balance has become significant. Stock calculated the theoretical cost of weight gain in many of these overfeeding studies that reported little evidence of DIT and argued that 84% of subjects in these studies exhibit some increase in DIT. Individual variability in adaptive thermogenesis has been hypothesised as a reason some individuals are more susceptible to weight gain and obesity in response to overeating.

Several mechanisms have been proposed for adaptive thermogenesis. The most widely studied is mitochondrial uncoupling through the action of uncoupling proteins (UCPs). UCPs provide heat without generating adenosine triphosphate (ATP) by uncoupling oxidation and phosphorylation. Thus, when food is oxidised, the energy is dissipated as heat rather than converted to ATP. In animals, DIT occurs in brown adipose tissue (BAT). Until recently it was thought that adult humans do not have significant amounts of BAT, and it was assumed that UCPs were not important for humans. However, BAT has been recently found in adults. Considerable research is presently underway to identify the role that UCPs may play in human body-weight regulation. Other possible mechanisms for adaptive thermogenesis that are presently under investigation include futile calcium cycling, protein turnover and substrate cycling.

Substrate oxidation

The three macronutrients carbohydrate, protein, and fat are oxidised to carbon dioxide and water and can provide energy for metabolic needs. Because the human body has a limited storage capacity for excess carbohydrate, a lack of storage capacity for excess protein and a large capacity to store excess fat, excess energy intakes of carbohydrate and protein will be oxidised preferentially to fat. Thus, fat oxidation is decreased and excess fat is stored. As shown in the energy balance equation (Table 16.2), when energy intake is greater than energy expenditure, body fat stores will increase. Thus, excess energy intake from any of the macronutrients will result in a positive gain of body fat stores.

The non-protein respiratory quotient (RQ) indicates the contribution of carbohydrate and fat being oxidised in the body. The RQ of carbohydrate is 1.0 and the RQ of fat is 0.71. An individual with a higher RQ is burning more carbohydrate than fat compared with a person with a lower RQ. Most people who are in energy balance and thus weight maintenance have a pattern of oxidation that reflects the amount of carbohydrate and fat obtained from the diet. However, studies which have examined substrate oxidation after weight loss have shown that fat oxidation is reduced in post-obese individuals. This suggests that reduced fat oxidation may be a risk factor for the development of obesity. Further research is needed to clarify the role of substrate oxidation in energy storage and the development of obesity.

16.4 Factors in the development of obesity

Medical conditions

Although obesity is rarely the result of a metabolic disorder, there are pathological syndromes in which this is the case. These syndromes account for only a small percentage of the obese population and include Prader–Willi syndrome, Laurence–Moon–Bardet Biedl syndrome, hypothyroidism, Alsrom–Hallgren syndrome, Carpenter syndrome, Cohen syndrome, Cushing's syndrome, growth hormone deficiency and polycystic ovary syndrome.

Genetic factors

Heritability of body fatness

Evidence suggests that there is a genetic component to obesity. Studies examining fatness similarities among twins and other biological siblings have shown that similarities are strongest for monozygotic twins (MZ), followed by dizygotic (DZ) twins and then other siblings. The heritability of fatness has been examined by measuring BMI in MZ and DZ twins living in similar or different environments and in adopted children separated from their biological parents. Studies of twins and adoptees both found that heredity was a major determinant of BMI. This observation supports a strong genetic component to fatness. In addition, overfeeding studies in twins have shown that genetics may influence the amount of weight that is gained as well as the amount of weight that is lost in response to exercise.

Genetic mutations and obesity

Recent improvements in genetic screening, as well as a cost reduction in the screens themselves have advanced the efforts to identify genetic mutations related to obesity. Research has uncovered at least 11 single gene mutations that may result in obesity. Many of these have been found through genetic screening of very obese individuals. Approximately 5% of obese persons are estimated to have a single-gene mutation, for example in the melanocortin-4-receptor gene (MC4R), which leads to increased energy intake.

Polygenes, that is multiple genes affecting the same trait, have also been positively associated with obesity. Using the Human Obesity Genome map, as many as 250 genes have been identified and 127 genes have been positively associated with obesity. Of those identified, 23 have been positively associated with obesity in more than five studies. The fat mass and obesity (FTO) associated gene is an example of a region of genes shown to have significant effect on BMI.

Single-gene mutations are much rarer, but typically have a larger effect on how much excess weight the person has. Polygenes are more common, but the effect size (i.e. the amount of excess weight) is smaller and can probably be mediated by many other factors.

Genetic factors influence energy intake and energy expenditure

A genetic basis of energy balance would be expected to show its effect on energy intake, energy expendi-

ture or both. In the 1950s it was suggested that body fat stores are regulated and that signals in the body provide feedback to the area of the brain controlling food intake and energy expenditure. These signals would be released in proportion to the body's adipose tissue stores. Therefore, if body fat stores increased, a compensatory mechanism would be initiated that would result in a decrease in energy intake. The discovery of leptin in 1994 provides a mechanism to support early theories of body-weight regulation. Leptin is a hormone secreted by adipose tissue that is involved in weight regulation through a series of complex interactions with other neurohormones that impact on energy intake and energy expenditure. Leptin plays a key role in a negative feedback loop to maintain adipose tissue stores. When adipose tissue decreases, leptin levels are reduced, resulting in an increase in food intake and a decrease in energy expenditure. Subsequent increases in adipose tissue are associated with an increase in leptin levels and a decrease in food intake. This homeostatic mechanism results in the maintenance of adipose tissue.

Studies in mice have shown that a defect in the gene for leptin is associated with obesity, resulting in increased food intake and reductions in metabolic rate. Although rare, mutations in the gene for leptin and the leptin receptor in humans are also associated with obesity. Plasma levels of leptin are positively associated with fat mass. In general, the more adipose tissue an individual has, the higher their leptin level will be. This suggests that human obesity is not associated with a decrease in leptin. It is hypothesised that obesity may be associated with a resistance to leptin. Thus, individuals with leptin resistance may have normal or high leptin levels, but may not be responsive to these levels of leptin.

Racial differences and obesity prevalence

Racial differences in the prevalence of obesity have led to speculation that such differences may be related to differences in energy expenditure. Because of the high prevalence of obesity reported in black individuals, many studies have been conducted to compare the energy expenditure between blacks and whites. These studies have examined RMR, total energy expenditure and substrate oxidation. Although most studies comparing RMR between the two groups report a reduced RMR in blacks, some do not. Even if these differences are established, these are cross-sectional studies so they cannot be interpreted to suggest that a low metabolic rate causes obesity. Longitudinal studies to date do not support the association between low a RMR and weight gain among blacks compared with whites. There are limited data on the relationship between RMR and weight gain in other ethnic groups.

Gene–environment interaction

Although genetic factors may increase the susceptibility of an individual to obesity, the significant increase in the prevalence of obesity in the past 30 years suggests that genetic factors alone could not be responsible for the obesity epidemic. Thus, it is likely that an interaction between genetics and an environment that promotes increased energy intake and/or decreased energy expenditure accounts for the development of obesity.

Twin studies take into account both familial and environmental factors, but the relationship is complicated. The degree of heritability of obesity varies among studies, so it is unknown how much influence one's genes and the environment have. Because families share the same environment, it is difficult to determine how much of the similarity in fatness is due to genetic factors and how much is due to environmental factors.

In an environment where energy intake is increased and energy expenditure is reduced, genetic factors that pre-dispose individuals to obesity may result in a positive energy balance. A good example of this can be seen in the Pima Indians living in Arizona, whose BMI is significantly higher than the BMI in a related group of Pima Indians living in Mexico. The diet of the Arizona Pima Indians is typical of a Western diet, that is it is higher in fat and lower in complex carbohydrates than the traditional diet of the Mexican Pimas. In addition, the Mexican Pimas engage in strenuous physical activity, whereas the Arizona Pimas are less physically active. This combination of a high-fat diet and decreased physical activity in this genetically susceptible population has contributed to a high prevalence of obesity.

Gene–environment interactions can also mediate the effect of a genetic predisposition to obesity. The aforementioned FTO gene region significantly increases the risk for overweight. However, emerging research suggests that this effect is nullified when persons with the FTO genotype are more physically active than average adults (Rampersaud et al., 2008), and the effect is intensified (i.e. there is a gain in adipose tissue) when they engage in little daily physical activity (Andreasen, 2008).

Factors affecting energy intake

Environmental factors

Lifestyle changes, including increased accessibility to food outside the home, increases in portion size and increased availability of high-energy, low-nutrient foods, may lead to increased energy intake. For example, in the USA high-energy food items are highly accessible in places like vending machines and small neighbourhood markets, and are less costly than fresh fruit and vegetables. Vending machines are located in recreational facilities, schools and office buildings and markets scattered throughout urban neighbourhoods. Neighbourhood markets in the USA have limited fruit and vegetable selections, and varied snack and sweet food options. Furthermore, vending machines are usually filled with high-energy, low-nutrient-dense foods or carbonated soft drinks and juices in 12–20 oz (560 ml) portions, providing 1.5–2.5 servings.

The availability of meals and food outside the home may also contribute to excess energy intake. Portion sizes in restaurants are often large and fast-food restaurants generally provide high-fat meals, resulting in increased energy intakes. Data from prospective studies in both adults and children reviewed in the *International Journal of Obesity* suggests that consuming fast food as a commonly-practiced meal pattern is associated with weight gain (Summerbell et al., 2009).

The way in which food is packaged and sold often makes it more economical to buy the larger size of an item, although the larger portion may provide more energy than the individual requires. For example, soft drinks are often purchased in 20 oz (560 ml) bottles, and although the nutrition label reads 2–2.5 servings, the consumer may not be aware of this.

Marketing strategies and advertising on television and billboards encourage the consumption of high-energy, low-nutrient-dense foods. Studies have shown that advertising these foods during typical television viewing hours increased childrens' requests for the specific food items.

Behavioural factors

Several dietary patterns have been hypothesised to increase energy intake and have been the focus of research. These include diets which are:

- high fat
- high energy density
- high glycaemic index
- low fibre.

Diets high in fat have been targeted as the culprit for excess energy intake owing to the high energy density and palatability of fat. However, there is considerable controversy regarding the relationship between high-fat diets and obesity.

Studies in metabolic units that have monitored the food intake of subjects support the hypothesis that energy intakes are higher on high-fat diets. Studies such as these are conducted in laboratory settings for short periods. However, these studies do not allow for generalisation to subjects living at home in an unrestricted environment. Thus, there may be additional factors that affect energy intake in free-living subjects that are not readily apparent in the laboratory, such as accessibility to food, social factors and opportunities for physical activity. Furthermore, changes occurring over a few days or weeks in the laboratory may not be maintained over longer periods.

The question of whether high-fat diets lead to increased energy intake is further complicated by the fact that fat has a higher energy density than carbohydrate. As a result, the energy content of food high in fat is greater than the energy content for the same weight of a food high in carbohydrate. Some researchers have suggested that energy-dense diets promote weight gain and that it is the energy density of food, not the fat content, that is associated with weight gain. Recently, a review conducted in the *International Journal of Obesity* looked at prospective studies that examined dietary factors related to weight gain from more than 125 countries (Summerbell *et al.*, 2009). They did not find evidence to suggest an association of either high fat diets or high-energy-dense diets with excessive weight gain, although it should be noted that there were only two studies available to assess the relationship of energy density with weight gain prospectively. Summerbell *et al.* also reviewed prospective observational studies on fibre intake and glycaemic index. Their results indicate that neither dietary fibre nor glycaemic index were consistently associated with obesity.

It should be noted, however, that findings from prospective studies have several limitations. Dietary intakes are based on self-reporting, which may be associated with both bias and measurement error. Additionally, many of the measures may not have been precise enough to detect small energy imbalances that, if maintained for long periods of time, may lead to weight gain. Although these studies did not find associations with some of these behavioural factors and obesity, it may be the combination of factors that leads to weight gain.

Factors affecting energy expenditure

Physical inactivity

The energy spent on physical activity is a significant determinant of daily energy expenditure, but accounts for less than 50% of total expenditure in most people. Decreases in physical activity will consequently decrease energy expenditure. If the energy spent on physical activity is decreased without a concomitant decrease in energy intake, a positive energy imbalance will result. Recent WHO data suggest that 60% of the world's population does not meet the recommended physical activity guidelines. Physical inactivity is a significant independent risk factor for obesity and chronic disease.

Environmental factors have resulted in decreased activity among individuals in both developed and developing countries. Technological advances in computers, labour-saving devices for food or goods production, and online shopping have decreased the time spent in activity at home and in the workplace. Automobile travel has reduced the amount of walking time, even for short distances. Living in an unsafe area can prohibit walking to and from work or school as well as outdoor play and exercise. All of these changes have contributed to a decrease in daily energy expenditure and potentially to weight gain.

Non-exercise activity thermogenesis (NEAT) may contribute to variable energy needs among individuals. NEAT describes any activity that is not a purposeful sport or exercise-type activity, for example fidgeting, walking to and from work or school, and gardening. Levine (2007) concluded that lean individuals spend about 2 h more a day walking and obese individuals spend 2.5 h more per day sitting.

However, people who are more likely to walk daily do have a propensity to continue walking even after having gained weight in overfeeding studies. Levine hypothesised that some people are biologically driven to move more in their daily lives. It is unknown whether there is a predisposition to sedentary activities that leads to obesity, or if obesity is the result of a tendency to engage in less physical activity and/or more sedentary activities.

Sedentary behaviour

Television viewing is a major sedentary behaviour in our current lifestyle. Much of the research on sedentary time has been on screen time (i.e. use of computers, video games and other electronic media) or television viewing. Total screen time has jumped in recent years, adding to time spent in sedentary activity. Studies suggest that increased time spent in sedentary behaviour increases the risk of obesity, but the mechanism is still unknown. Research on behaviour while watching television suggests that energy consumption (e.g. snacking) during viewing is increased, resulting in positive energy imbalance and potentially weight gain. One postulate is that individuals may fail to recognise or register their satiety signals while watching television, thus resulting in higher levels of energy intake. Furthermore, some studies have shown that food-related television commercials result in increased total energy intake during television viewing.

Sleep patterns

Epidemiologic evidence is accumulating to suggest an association between short sleep duration and increased body weight. Cross-sectional studies in both children and adults suggest an association between sleep duration and obesity. Experimental and observational studies have suggested several pathways to explain the link between short sleep duration and weight gain. Mechanisms currently under investigation are those that influence hunger and appetite; alterations in key energy intake hormones such as leptin and ghrelin are thought to play a role in the association of obesity with sleep quality and duration. The relationship of obesity to reduced sleep duration, the quality of sleep and the mechanisms responsible for this association are currently an area of active research.

16.5 Consequences of obesity

Physiological effects of excess fat

Obesity increases the risk of many chronic diseases, including:

- cardiovascular disease (e.g. stroke and hypertension)
- type II diabetes mellitus
- gallbladder disease
- some types of cancers
- respiratory illnesses
- reproductive problems.

Obesity is a risk factor for cardiovascular disease, including coronary heart disease, hypertension and stroke, and type II diabetes mellitus, development of gallbladder disease, some types of cancer, respiratory illnesses (i.e. sleep apnoea, Pickwickian syndrome) and reproductive problems. Obesity may result in osteoarthritis and low back pain, which may limit mobility and reduce independence in activities of daily living, thus impacting on the quality of life.

Obese children and adolescents show elevations in cardiovascular disease risk factors such as increases in cholesterol levels, blood glucose and blood pressure. These risk factors tend to cluster in individuals and track from childhood to adulthood. The incidence of type II diabetes, once thought to be an adult disease, is increasing in children and adolescents. This is concerning given the increasing prevalence of childhood obesity in many countries throughout the world and the co-morbidities associated with diabetes.

Not all obese people will develop these chronic diseases. The risk that an obese individual will develop any of the health consequences associated with obesity may be influenced by other factors, including genetics, behaviours such as drinking alcohol or smoking, and fat distribution and level of fitness.

Fat distribution

As early as the 1950s, an association between upper body fat obesity and metabolic complications such as diabetes and arteriosclerosis was recognised, with diabetes and arteriosclerosis being more common in individuals with upper body obesity than those with lower body obesity. In the 1980s, numerous studies showed a significant relationship between upper body obesity, assessed by the ratio of waist to hip circumference, and risk factors for cardiovascular disease and diabetes. This relationship, known as the metabolic syndrome (or the insulin resistance syndrome or syndrome X), describes the association of abdominal obesity with a cluster of metabolic abnormalities such as glucose intolerance, insulin resistance and abnormal triglyceride and cholesterol levels.

Individuals with upper body obesity have increased amounts of subcutaneous abdominal adipose tissue as well as increased amounts of visceral adipose tissue. The subcutaneous adipose tissue that is associated with upper body obesity is directly underneath the skin around the abdominal area. Visceral adipose tissue or intra-abdominal tissue surrounds the internal organs and can only be measured using computed tomographic (CT) scans and magnetic resonance imaging (MRI). Upper body obesity with increased amounts of subcutaneous and visceral fat is thought to be responsible for the metabolic abnormalities associated with upper body fatness. However, the relationship between visceral adiposity and metabolic abnormalities is not fully understood. Evidence suggests that increased levels of free fatty acids may have an important functional impact on these abnormalities. Further research is needed to understand the mechanisms associated with metabolic risk.

Risk assessment

Waist circumference is correlated with the amount of visceral fat in the body and appears to be a good marker for upper body obesity. Because fat distribution, like BMI, appears to be an independent risk factor for the morbidity of obesity, it is recommended that waist circumference be measured in addition to BMI to identify people at risk of obesity-related complications. Waist circumferences greater than 102 cm in men and 88 cm in women are associated with an increased risk of metabolic complications. More research is needed to determine the relationship between increased visceral adipose tissue and metabolic abnormalities, including lifestyle factors that may be beneficial in preventing the metabolic syndrome.

Psychological effects

The psychosocial effects of obesity on both children and adults can be substantial. Obese people are often viewed as lazy or lacking the willpower to diet and exercise. This misunderstanding of the causes of obesity leads to negative attitudes towards obese individuals. Obese children and adolescents often experience discrimination and teasing from other children. Research has documented that obese people are discriminated against in employment, housing, educational, earning and marital opportunities. There is considerable literature about the negative effects of stigma and the coping strategies that stigmatised individuals employ, which may include isolation, withdrawal, decreased achievement motivation, low self-esteem and depression.

16.6 Perspectives on the future

The study of obesity is a rapidly changing field. Future research will help to identify what factors increase an individual's susceptibility to obesity. The Human Obesity Genome map has just begun to unravel the puzzle of genetic factors related to obesity. Identifying the factors that influence food intake and energy expenditure will help to inform interventions for prevention and treatment.

Research has also suggested that early factors in growth and development may alter the risk for obesity. The developmental origins of chronic disease hypothesis suggests that early exposure to environmental influences may programme the foetus or infant to be more susceptible to obesity later in life. Further research is needed in this area to determine what factors during pregnancy, infancy and early childhood may impact on the risk for obesity.

The mechanisms associated with increased upper body obesity and metabolic abnormalities are not fully understood. Further research in this area is needed to determine the mechanisms linking abdominal fatness and the metabolic abnormalities observed.

Public health efforts are needed to promote physical activity and provide opportunities for daily regular physical activity. The WHO promotes 'Move for Health Day', a world initiative to increase physical activity. Efforts to increase the accessibility and affordability of fresh fruits and vegetables have been shown to improve health indicators. Using these foods to displace fast-food meals may have an important impact on energy intake and obesity.

Section II: Vitamin and mineral overconsumption

16.7 Introduction

The increased availability of fortified foods and the increased use of dietary supplements in many countries has led to increased interest in the adverse health effects that may arise from overconsumption of vitamins and minerals. It is well recognised that such adverse effects can occur with high intakes of some vitamins and minerals. While it is generally considered that the risk of such effects is low, the incidence of such occurrences in different populations is generally not known with any certainty. In some regions, for example in the European Union and North America, the need to protect consumer health through regulating the addition of vitamins and minerals to foods and nutritional supplements has led to the establishment of scientifically based upper limits of intake for these micronutrients.

16.8 Adverse effects of vitamins and minerals: concepts

Failure of homeostasis

Vitamins and essential minerals are subject to homeostatic control, through which body content is regulated. This reduces the risk of depletion of body pools, which could lead to deficiency when intakes are low. It also reduces the risk of excessive accumulation in tissues that could lead to adverse effects when intakes are high. A measure of protection against potential adverse effects of high intakes is provided by adaptation of homeostatic control mechanisms, for example limiting absorption efficiency, adaptation of metabolic processes or enhancing excretion in faeces, urine, skin or lungs (Box 16.1).

However, for a number of micronutrients the capacity for homeostasis may be exceeded by continuing high dietary intakes. This can lead to abnormal accumulation in tissues, or overloading of normal metabolic or transport pathways.

Threshold dose

For nutrients no risk of adverse health effects is expected unless a threshold dose (or intake) is exceeded. Thresholds for any given adverse effect

> **Box 16.1 Adaptive mechanisms that protect against adverse effects of continuing exposure to high dietary intakes of vitamins and minerals**
>
> - Reduced absorption efficiency with increasing dietary intake or body stores, for example for iron, zinc and calcium the mediated transport route of absorption in the small intestine mucosa is down-regulated.
> - Regulation of excretory pathways where excretion increases with increasing dietary intake or body stores, for example for calcium, increasing calcium ion concentration in plasma depresses parathyroid hormone and reduces the efficiency of calcium ion reabsorption in the renal tubule, leading to increased urinary calcium excretion; for selenium, high intakes lead to increased excretion of selenium as the volatile dimethyl selenide through the lungs or as the water-soluble trimethylselenonium ion in urine.
> - Increased endogenous secretion into the intestine occurs for some nutrients when intakes are high, for example increased secretion in pancreatic fluid (zinc) and bile (manganese), or increased losses by sloughing off of intestinal mucosal cells (iron, zinc).

vary among members of the population. In general, for nutrients there are insufficient data to establish the distribution of thresholds in the population for individual adverse effects.

Variation in the sensitivity of individuals

Sensitivity to the adverse effects of micronutrients is influenced by physiological changes and common conditions associated with growth and maturation that occur during an individual's lifespan. Even within relatively homogenous lifestage groups there is a range of sensitivities to adverse effects (e.g. sensitivity is influenced by body weight and lean body mass). Some sub-populations have extreme and distinct vulnerabilities owing to genetic predisposition or certain metabolic disorders or disease states (Box 16.2).

Effect of bioavailability

The bioavailability of a nutrient relates to its absorption and utilisation, and may be defined as its accessibility to normal metabolic and physiological processes. Bioavailability influences the usefulness of a nutrient for physiological functions at physiological levels of intake, and the nature and severity of adverse effects at excessive intakes. There is considerable variation in nutrient bioavailability in humans, for instance the chemical form of a nutrient may have a large influence on bioavailability. Other modulating factors include the nutritional status of the individual, nutrient intake level, interaction with other dietary components and the food matrix (e.g. consumption with or without food). For example, high zinc intakes increase the synthesis of intestinal mucosal cells of metallothionein, a protein that avidly binds copper and reduces its absorption.

Tolerable upper intake level

While dietary reference standards have been established over many years for evaluation of the nutritional adequacy of dietary intakes, it is only in recent years that the need for dietary reference standards for evaluating and managing the risk of excessive intakes of vitamins and minerals has been recognised. Such reference standards have been established for a number of vitamins and minerals and are referred to as tolerable upper intake levels (sometimes also called upper safe levels).

The tolerable upper intake level (UL) is the maximum level of total chronic daily intake of a nutrient (from all sources, including foods, water, nutrient supplements and medicines) judged to be unlikely to pose a risk of adverse health effects to almost all individuals in the general population. 'Tolerable' connotes a level of intake that can be tolerated physiologically by humans. ULs may be derived for various lifestage groups in the population (e.g. adults, pregnant and lactating women, infants and children). The UL is not a recommended level of intake but is an estimate of the highest (usual) level of intake that carries no appreciable risk of adverse health effects.

The UL is meant to apply to all groups of the general population, including sensitive individuals, throughout the lifestage. However, it is not meant to apply to individuals receiving the nutrient under medical supervision or to individuals with predisposing conditions that render them especially sensitive to one or more adverse effects of the nutrient, such as those with genetic predisposition or certain disease states.

The term 'adverse health effect' may be defined as any significant alteration in structure or function or any impairment of a physiologically important function that could lead to an adverse health effect in humans.

16.9 Derivation of the tolerable upper intake level

Risk assessment

ULs can be derived for nutrients using the principles of risk assessment that have been developed for biological and chemical agents. Risk assessment is a systematic means of evaluating the probability of occurrence of adverse health effects in humans from an excess exposure to an environmental agent (in this case nutrients in food and water, nutrient supplements and medicines). The hallmark of risk assessment is the requirement to be explicit in all of the evaluations and judgments that must be made to document conclusions.

In general, the same principles of risk assessment apply to nutrients as to other food chemicals, but it is recognised that vitamins and minerals possess some characteristics that distinguish them from other food chemicals (Box 16.3).

The steps involved in the application of risk assessment principles to the derivation of ULs for vitamins and minerals are summarised in Figure 16.1 and explained in more detail below.

Hazard identification

This involves the collection, organisation and evaluation of all information pertaining to the adverse health effects of a given nutrient, and summarises the evidence concerning the capacity of the nutrient to cause one or more types of adverse health effect in humans. Human studies provide the most relevant data for hazard identification and, when they are of sufficient

---

Box 16.3 Characteristics that distinguish vitamins and essential minerals from other food chemicals

- They are essential for human well-being within a certain range of intakes and there is a long history of safe consumption of nutrients at the levels found in balanced human diets.
- For some nutrients there may be experience of widespread chronic consumption (e.g. from dietary supplements) at levels significantly above those obtained from endogenous nutrients in foods without reported adverse health effects.
- Many nutrients are subject to homeostatic regulation of body content through adaptation of absorptive, excretory or metabolic processes, and this provides a measure of protection against exposures above usual intakes from balanced diets.
- Data on the adverse effects of nutrients are also often available from studies in humans, which helps to reduce the scientific uncertainties associated with extrapolation from the observed data to human populations.

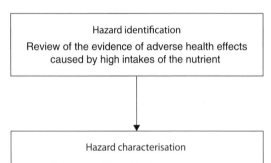

Figure 16.1 Steps in the development of the tolerable upper intake level (UL). NOAEL, no observed adverse effect level; LOAEL, lowest observed adverse effect level.

quality and extent, are given the greatest weight. Other experimental data (from experimental animals and *in vitro* studies) may also be used. Key issues that are addressed in the data evaluation include the extent to which there is evidence of adverse health effects on humans and whether or not the relationship established by the published human

data is causal, mechanisms of adverse effects, quality and completeness of the database, and identification of distinct and highly sensitive subpopulations.

Hazard characterisation

As intake of a nutrient increases, a threshold is reached above which increasing intake increases the risk of adverse health effects. This is illustrated diagrammatically in Figure 16.2.

Hazard characterisation involves the qualitative and quantitative evaluation of the nature of the adverse health effects associated with a nutrient. This includes a dose–response assessment, which involves determining the relationship between nutrient intake (dose) and adverse health effect (in terms of frequency and severity). Based on these evaluations, a UL is derived, taking into account the scientific uncertainties in the data. ULs may be derived for various lifestage groups within the population.

Dose–response assessment

The dose–response assessment involves a number of key components.

Selection of the critical data set

The data evaluation process results in the selection of the most appropriate or critical data set(s) for deriving the UL. The critical data set defines the dose–response relationship between intake and the extent of the adverse health effect known to be most relevant to humans. Data on bioavailability need to be considered and adjustments in expressions of dose–response are made to determine whether any apparent differences in dose–response between different forms of a nutrient can be explained. The critical data set should document the form of the nutrient investigated, the route of exposure, the magnitude and duration of intake, and the intake that does not produce adverse health effects, as well as the intake that produces adverse health effects.

Identification of the no observed adverse effect level or lowest observed adverse effect level and critical end-point

The no observed adverse effect level (NOAEL) is the highest intake of a nutrient at which no adverse effects have been observed. The NOAEL can be identified from evaluation of the critical data set. If there are no adequate data demonstrating a NOAEL,

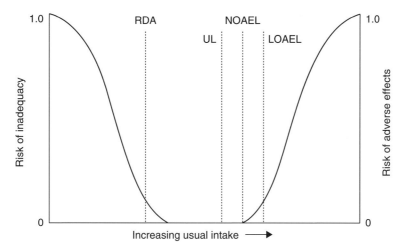

Figure 16.2 Theoretical description of health effects of a nutrient as a function of level of intake. As intakes increase above the tolerable upper intake level (UL) the risk of adverse effects increases. RDA, recommended daily allowance; NOAEL, no observed adverse effect level; LOAEL, lowest observed adverse effect level.

then a lowest observed adverse effect level (LOAEL, the lowest intake at which an adverse effect has been demonstrated) may be used. Where different adverse health effects (or end-points) occur for a nutrient, the NOAELs (or LOAELs) for these end-points will differ. The critical end-point is the adverse health effect exhibiting the lowest NOAEL (i.e. the most sensitive indicator of a nutrient's adverse effects). The derivation of a UL based on the most sensitive end-point will ensure protection against all other adverse health effects.

Uncertainty assessment

There are usually several scientific uncertainties associated with extrapolation from the observed data to the general population, and several judgments must be made in deriving uncertainty factors to account for the individual uncertainties. The individual uncertainty factors may be combined into a single composite uncertainty factor for each nutrient, and applying this (composite) uncertainty factor (UF) to a NOAEL (or LOAEL) will result in a value for the derived UL that is less than the experimentally derived NOAEL, unless the uncertainty factor is 1.0. The larger the uncertainty, the larger the UFs and the lower the UL.

UFs are used to account for imprecision of the data, lack of data and adequacy of the data on variability between individuals. There are several potential sources of uncertainty, including:

- interindividual variation and sensitivity with respect to the adverse effect
- extrapolation from experimental animal data to humans
- if a NOAEL is not available, a UF may be applied to account for the uncertainty in deriving a UL from the LOAEL
- using a subchronic NOAEL to predict chronic NOAEL.

The UFs are lower with higher quality data and when the adverse effects are extremely mild and reversible. For example, for magnesium a UF of 1.0 may be used since the adverse effect (osmotic diarrhoea) is relatively mild and reversible, there is a sufficiently large amount of data available relating magnesium intake level to this adverse effect in humans to cover adequately the range of interindividual variation in sensitivity, and a clear NOAEL can be established. In contrast, for vitamin B_6 a UF of 4 may be used since the adverse effect (neurotoxicity) is potentially severe, there are only limited data, mainly from inadequate studies of insufficient duration relating vitamin B_6 intake level to this adverse effect in humans, and no clear NOAEL can be established.

In the application of uncertainty factors there should be cognisance of nutritional needs, for example the derived UL should not be lower than the recommended intake.

Derivation of tolerable upper intake levels

The UL is derived by dividing the NOAEL (or LOAEL) by the (composite) UF. ULs are derived for different lifestage groups using relevant data. In the absence of data for a particular lifestage group, extrapolations are made from the UL for other groups on the basis of known differences in body size, physiology, metabolism, absorption and excretion of a nutrient. For example, when data are not available for children and adolescents, extrapolations are usually made on the basis of body weight using the reference weights for adults and children in the population.

Where possible, ULs are derived for separate lifestage groups (e.g. infants, children, adults, the elderly and women during pregnancy or lactation). Although within relatively homogeneous lifestage groups there is a range of sensitivities to adverse health effects due, for example, to differences in body weight and lean body mass, it is generally not possible to make a distinction between males and females in establishing ULs for adults or children.

The derivation of ULs for the normal healthy population, divided into various lifestage groups, accounts for normally expected variability in sensitivity, but it excludes sub-populations with extreme and distinct vulnerabilities due to genetic predisposition or other considerations. (Including these would result in ULs that are significantly lower than are needed to protect most people against the adverse effects of high intakes.) Sub-populations needing special protection are better served through the use of public health screening, healthcare providers, product labelling or other individualised strategies. The extent to which a sub-population becomes significant enough to be assumed to be representative of a general population is an area of judgment and risk management.

It should be noted that derivation of a UL does not take into account possible adverse effects of acute bolus dosages. In general, adverse effects from acute or short-term intake require much greater intake levels than those arising from long-term or chronic exposure.

ULs have been derived for a number of vitamins and minerals (Table 16.3) and examples of the derivation of UL for selenium and vitamin D are given in Boxes 16.4 and 16.5. Adverse effects associ-

Table 16.3 Examples of tolerable upper intake levels (ULs) for vitamins and minerals

Nutrient	UL (adults)	Adverse effect
Retinol	3000 µg	Teratogenicity, hepatotoxicity
Vitamin D	50 µg	Hypocalcaemia
Vitamin E	1000 mg	Hemorrhagic effects
Vitamin B_6	25 mg	Sensory neuropathy
Folic acid	1000 µg	Progression of neuropathy or masking of anaemia in B_{12} deficiency
Vitamin C	2000 mg	Osmotic diarrhoea, gastrointestinal disturbances
Calcium	2500 mg	Milk alkali syndrome
Magnesium	250 mg (supplemental)	Osmotic diarrhoea
Phosphorus	4000 mg	Hyperphosphataemia
Iron	45 mg (supplemental)	Gastrointestinal effects
Zinc	40 mg	Reduced copper status
Copper	10 mg	Hepatotoxicity
Manganese	11 mg	Neurotoxicity
Selenium	300 µg	Clinical selenosis: brittle nails, hair loss
Iodine	1100 µg	Thyrotoxicosis

From the US Food and Nutrition Board, European Food Safety Authority and EU Scientific Committee on Food.

Box 16.4 Derivation of UL for selenium

- Chronic selenosis has been described in regions of high soil selenium in China. Symptoms include hair and nail brittleness and loss, skin rash, mottled teeth, garlic-breath odour and neurological disturbances, including peripheral anaesthesia, with numbness, convulsions, paralysis and motor disturbances in more severe cases.

- The high prevalence of selenosis in Enshi, South China, provided an opportunity for the study of the dose–response relationship of selenium intake to selenosis in 350 adults during the 1980s. Toxic effects occurred with increasing frequency as selenium intake increased above 850 mg/day. Lowering selenium intake in affected individuals led to the disappearance of symptoms. The LOAEL for clinical symptoms of selenosis is about 900–1000 mg Se/day and a NOAEL of 850 mg/day can be established.

- A UF of 3 may be used to cover uncertainties in the data (the NOAEL used was derived from a study on a large number of subjects and is expected to include sensitive individuals; although the toxic effect is not severe, it may not be readily reversible). This leads to a UL of 300 mg/day for adults.

- This UL may also be applied to pregnant and lactating women as there is no evidence to indicate that there is increased sensitivity of the foetus or breast-fed infant to high levels of maternal selenium intake.

- Owing to insufficient data on the adverse effects of selenium in children, extrapolation from the UL for adults to children on a body-weight basis may be performed to derive a UL for children.

Box 16.5 Derivation of UL for vitamin D

- Vitamin D toxicity has been described in individuals consuming excessive amounts of vitamin D-containing supplements. The effects observed include damage to kidney and other soft tissues, such as blood vessels, heart and lungs, owing to calcification. This results from hypocalcaemia caused by a vitamin D-induced increase in calcium absorption in the gastrointestinal tract and calcium resorption from bone. Elevated serum 25-hydroxyvitamin D (an indicator of vitamin D status) levels may be used to confirm that the hypocalcaemia is vitamin D induced.
- Data from controlled studies of the response of serum 25-hydroxyvitamin D to increasing intakes of vitamin D intake in human subjects may be used to establish the dose–response relationship. A NOAEL of 100 μg/day can be established as the highest intake that does not result in elevation of serum 25-hydroxyvitamin D above the upper end of the reference range.
- A UF of 2 may be used to cover uncertainties in the data (i.e. to cover the range of interindividual sensitivity in the population). This leads to a UL of 50 μg/day for adults. This UL may also be applied to pregnant and lactating women as there is evidence to suggest that there is no increased sensitivity of the foetus or breast-fed infant to this level of maternal vitamin D intake.
- Although there are insufficient data for the adverse effects of vitamin D in children, a UL of 50 μg/day may be used for children of 10 years and older, and for children aged 1–9 years extrapolation from the UL for adults on a body-weight basis may be performed to derive a UL.

Box 16.6 Vitamin C high intakes: myths and facts

- Vitamin C is often taken in large amounts (500 mg/day or more) for presumed health benefits. Evidence to date does not support a role for high doses of vitamin C in prevention of the common cold, although there is a moderate benefit in terms of duration and severity of episodes in some groups. Although there is epidemiological evidence to suggest a protective effect of vitamin C against cardiovascular disease, some cancers (e.g. stomach, lung) and cataracts, such benefits have not been established unequivocally.
- It has been suggested that antioxidants such as vitamin C may act as pro-oxidants at high intake levels. This is partly based on *in vitro* observations that ascorbic acid may interact with free iron or copper to promote lipid peroxidation or oxidative damage to DNA. However, this hypothesis has not been substantiated *in vivo*, where both iron and copper are normally tightly bound to transport and storage proteins, and are unavailable to participate in such redox reactions.
- Reports of increased urinary oxalate excretion and kidney stone formation with high intakes of vitamin C have not been confirmed. Such effects are considered unlikely given the limited intestinal absorption of vitamin C at doses greater than 200 mg/day.
- A UL of 2000 mg/day may be derived based on osmotic diarrhoea and related gastrointestinal disturbances that arise from the osmotic effect of unabsorbed vitamin C passing through the intestine when the capacity of the saturable absorption system has been exceeded.

ated with high intakes of vitamin C, β-carotene and vitamin A are outlined in Boxes 16.6–16.8. While ULs are usually based on total intake of a nutrient, in some cases adverse health effects have been associated with intake from a particular source, such as supplements, rather than total intake, and in such cases the UL is based on intake from these sources only. For many nutrients there are no systematic studies of the adverse health effects of high intakes and the UL is derived from limited data. Experience has shown that it is not always possible to establish a UL for a micronutrient using the science-based risk-assessment approach. Such a situation can arise for different reasons:

- evidence of the absence of any adverse health effects at high intakes
- lack of evidence of any adverse effect; this does not necessarily mean that there is no potential for adverse effects resulting from high intake
- evidence of adverse effects but insufficient data on which to base a dose–response assessment.

16.10 Use of tolerable upper intake levels as dietary reference standards

The UL is a dietary reference standard that can be used for both the evaluation and management of risk of excessive intake of vitamins or minerals in individuals or populations. The UL is not in itself an indication of risk. However, the UL can be applied to data derived from intake assessment (e.g. the distribution of usual total daily nutrient intakes among members of the general population) to identify those individuals or population groups at risk and the circumstances in which risk is likely to occur. In general, risk is considered to be the probability of an adverse effect (and its severity) and will depend on the fraction of the population exceeding the UL and the magnitude and duration of such excesses.

Individuals

It is not possible to identify a single risk-free intake level for a nutrient that can be applied with certainty to all members of a population. However, if

---

Box 16.7 β-carotene supplementation and smoking

- Prospective epidemiological studies have shown that higher consumption of carotenoid-containing fruits and vegetables, and higher plasma levels of carotenoids, including β-carotene, are associated with a lower risk of a number of cancers and cardiovascular disease.
- Several long-term intervention studies with supplemental β-carotene have not shown a reduction in chronic disease risk. Indeed, two of the studies carried out in the 1990s reported an increase in lung cancer associated with supplemental β-carotene (20–30 mg/day for 4–8 years) in current smokers. However, another study reported that supplementation with 25 mg/day of β-carotene for up to 12 years (including smokers and non-smokers) showed no excess of lung cancer.
- No other adverse effects have been described for β-carotene. For example, no toxic effects have been reported from the therapeutic use of β-carotene at high doses (about 180 mg/day) over many years for the treatment of erythropoietic protoporphyria, a photosensitivity disorder. Carotenodermia, a yellowish discoloration of the skin, is a harmless and well-documented effect of excess intake of β-carotene and other carotenoids.
- At present the data on the potential for β-carotene to produce increased lung cancer are conflicting and not sufficient for a dose–response assessment and derivation of a UL. However, caution is advised in the use of β-carotene supplements.
- This does not conflict with dietary advice for fruit and vegetable consumption (e.g. five or more servings per day) since this provides much lower intakes of β-carotene (3–6 mg/day), which is also of lower bioavailability, than the supplemental intake levels associated with possible adverse effects (20 mg/day or more).

Box 16.8 Vitamin A toxicity

- High intakes [in excess of 3000 μg retinol equivalents (RE)/day] of preformed vitamin A (retinol and related compounds) appear to be teratogenic in humans, resulting in craniofacial malformations and abnormalities of the central nervous system (except for neural tube defects), thymus and heart. Evidence for this includes epidemiological studies on vitamin A intake level and pregnancy outcome, established teratogenicity in humans of therapeutic use of retinoic acid (a vitamin A metabolite), as well as established teratogenicity of vitamin A in a number of animal species.
- Hepatotoxicity is one of the most severe outcomes of chronic intake of high dosages of vitamin A (generally in excess of about 15 000 μg RE/day in supplements or in rich food sources such as liver and liver oils), arising from overload of the storage capacity of the liver for the vitamin.
- Some epidemiological studies have indicated that intakes of vitamin A in excess of 1500?μg RE/day may reduce bone mineral density and increase the risk of osteoporosis and hip fractures in some population groups, particularly in pre- and post-menopausal women. However, other studies have not found such an effect and this conflicting evidence is not adequate to establish a causal relationship or a UL.
- A UL of 3000 μg RE/day may be derived for women of reproductive age based on epidemiological data on the occurrence of birth defects in infants of exposed mothers. For other adults a UL of 3000 μg RE/day may be derived based on case reports of hepatoxicity arising from prolonged overconsumption of vitamin A.

---

an individual's usual nutrient intake remains below the UL there is no appreciable risk of adverse effects from excessive intake. At usual intakes above the UL the risk of adverse effects increases with increasing level of intake. However, the intake at which a given individual will develop adverse health effects as a result of taking large amounts of a nutrient is not known with certainty. The UL can be used as a guide for the maximum level of usual intake of individuals, although it is not a recommended intake. Occasional excursions above the UL are possible without an appreciable risk of adverse health effects.

Groups

The proportion of the population with usual intakes below the UL is likely to be at no appreciable risk of adverse health effects due to overconsumption, while the proportion above the UL may be at some risk, the magnitude of which depends on the magnitude and duration of the excess. The UL is derived to apply to the most sensitive members of the general population. Thus, many members of the population may regularly consume nutrients at or even somewhat above the UL without experiencing adverse effects. However, because it is not known which individuals are most sensitive, it is necessary to interpret the UL as applying to all individuals.

In the management of risk of excessive intake of vitamins or minerals in individuals or populations the UL can be used in several ways. For example, it may be used for setting maximum levels of addition of vitamins and minerals to foods or nutritional supplements such that the risk of excessive intake in the population is minimised. It is also a useful basis for providing information and advice to individuals or groups on maximum intake levels of nutrients, such as in the labelling of nutritional supplements.

16.11 Perspectives on the future

The application of science-based risk-assessment methods to the establishment of ULs for vitamins and minerals represents a significant advance in providing dietary reference standards for evaluating and managing the risk of overconsumption of these nutrients. These reference standards will be increasingly used in nutritional surveillance as studies on nutrient intakes in populations pay greater attention to the possibility of overconsumption of micronutrients resulting from the wider use of nutritional supplements and consumption of fortified foods in some countries.

This field is still limited by a lack of good data on dose–response relationships for the adverse health effects of micronutrients in humans. To improve the understanding of such effects research is needed to provide better knowledge of the physiological effects of micronutrients at the molecular, cellular and whole-body levels, and of the kinetics of their absorption, metabolism and excretion at different dietary levels of intake.

Further reading

Obesity

Andreasen CH *et al.* Low physical activity accentuates the effect of the FTO rs9939609 polymorphism on body fat accumulation. Diabetes 2008; 57: 95–101.

Levine, JA. Nonexercise activity thermogenesis – liberating the life-force. J Int Med 2007; 262: 273–287.

Rampersaud E *et al.* Physical activity and the association of common FTO gene variants with body mass index and obesity. Arch Int Med 2008; 168(16): 1791–1797.

Ravussin E *et al.* Reduced rate of energy expenditure as a risk factor for body-weight gain. New Eng J Med 1988 Feb 25; 318(8): 467–472.

Stock MJ. Gluttony and thermogenesis revisited. Int J Obes Relat Metab Disord 1999; 23(11): 1105–1117.

Summerbell CD *et al.* The association between diet and physical activity and subsequent excess weight gain and obesity assessed at 5 years of age or older: a systematic review of the epidemiological evidence. Int J Obes 2009; 33: S1–S88.

World Health Organization. http://www.who.int/

Vitamin and mineral overconsumption

European Food Safety Authority (2006) Tolerable upper intakes levels for vitamins and minerals. Parma, Italy: European Food Safety Authority. http://www.efsa.europa.eu/EFSA/efsa_locale-1178620753812_1178633962601.htm

FAO/WHO (Food and Agricultural Organization of the UN/World Health Organization, Expert Consultation) (2006) A model for establishing upper levels of intake for nutrients and related substances: report of a joint FAO/WHO technical workshop on nutrient risk assessment, Geneva, Switzerland, 2–6 May 2005. http://www.who.int/ipcs/highlights/full_report.pdf

Food and Nutrition Board, Institute of Medicine, National Academy of Sciences. Dietary Reference Intakes. Washington, DC: National Academy Press, 1997–2001. http://www.nap.edu/

Food and Nutrition Board, Institute of Medicine, National Academy of Sciences. Dietary Reference Intakes: Applications in Dietary Assessment: A report of the Subcommittees on Interpretation and Uses of Dietary Reference Intakes and Upper Reference Levels of Nutrients, and the Standing Committee on the Scientific Evaluation of Dietary Reference Intakes, Food and Nutrition Board. Washington, DC: National Academy Press, 2001. http://www.nap.edu/catalog/9956.html

17
Undernutrition

Paul Kelly

Key messages

- Undernutrition is a consequence of chronic energy deficiency (CED), which leads to reductive adaptation. This may lead to equilibrium at reduced body mass, but at a 'cost'.
- Classification of CED is based on the extent of the reduction of body mass index and physical activity level.
- To maintain homeostasis, the body adapts in CED to lower energy intake to ensure survival. Individuals with CED have lower body weights, fat-free mass and fat stores, accompanied by reduced resting metabolic rate, physical activity and thermogenesis.

- The nervous and endocrine systems are key regulatory mechanisms that favour energy conservation in CED.
- In humans the physiological or functional consequences of CED include reduced muscle strength and endurance, reduced immunity and altered autonomic nervous function. Each of these has important implications for lifestyle and health status.
- Undernutrition may be a consequence of food insecurity (poverty, crop failure, conflict) or disease (for example infectious disease, gastrointestinal or liver disease, cancer)

17.1 Introduction

Close to 800 million people in the world are believed to be undernourished. There are, however, large regional differences in the prevalence of undernutrition. The latest nutrition statistics from the World Bank suggest that in sub-Saharan Africa 27% of children under 5 years of age are wasted, 44% are stunted and 29% of the whole population is undernourished. This chapter will focus predominantly on adult undernutrition and its causes and consequences. Malnutrition in children is dealt with in the *Clinical Nutrition* textbook in this series.

17.2 Definition and classification of undernutrition

The term 'undernutrition' encompasses a wide range of macronutrient and micronutrient deficiencies. Micronutrient deficiencies, for instance, include those of water-soluble vitamins (thiamìn, riboflavin and niacin), fat-soluble vitamins (e.g. vitamin A and vitamin D) and minerals (e.g. iodine and iron).

Deficiencies of these micronutrients, if severe, lead to classic clinical presentations. Niacin deficiency, for instance, leads to pellagra, characterised by 'Casal's necklace', a typical skin lesion around the neck. Iodine deficiency is associated with a goitre, a swelling of the thyroid gland. Iron deficiency, which is widespread throughout the world and particularly in developing countries, is associated with anaemia. More subtle deficiencies of micronutrients may lead to ill-health in more complex, as yet ill-understood, ways. Detailed discussions of micronutrient deficiencies are dealt with in the relevant chapters dedicated to these nutrients in *Introduction to Human Nutrition*. This chapter deals primarily with energy deficiency.

In 1988, James, Ferro-Luzzi and Waterlow drew a distinction between acute energy deficiency (AED) and chronic energy deficiency (CED). AED was defined as 'a state of negative energy balance, i.e. a progressive loss of body energy'. This occurs in a variety of clinical conditions associated with acute weight loss, including anorexia nervosa, cancer and malabsorption disorders. In contrast, CED was defined as a 'steady state at which a person is in energy balance although at a "cost"'. Issues pertaining to AED are

Nutrition and Metabolism, Second Edition, edited by S. A. Lanham-New, I. A. Macdonald and H. M. Roche. © 2011 The Nutrition Society.

Table 17.1 Classification of chronic energy deficiency (CED) according to body mass index (BMI) and physical activity level (PAL)

	Normal		Chronic energy deficiency			
			Grade I		Grade II	Grade III
BMI	≥18.5	17.0–18.4	17.0–18.4	16.0–17.0	16.0–17.0	<16.0
PAL[a]	–	≥1.4	<1.4	≥1.4	<1.4	–

Modified from James *et al.* (1988).

[a] For this purpose PAL is calculated as the measured energy intake or expenditure divided by basal metabolic rate.

dealt with in Chapter 5, section 5.7, on the metabolic consequences of starvation.

Most definitions of undernutrition focus on reduced body mass, as this is a relatively easy thing to measure. However, it is likely that body mass is reduced only if the first processes of reductive adaptation still leave a negative energy balance. The idea of reductive adaptation is discussed further below, but initial reductions would include reduced energy expenditure through reduced physical activity and other behavioural adaptations. In sustained CED physiological adaptations occur. Undernutrition thus has functional consequences as well as structural consequences, and it is likely that borderline undernutrition impairs work capacity, school performance and quality of life. Good nutrition is required therefore in order to achieve the vision of health set out by the World Health Organization: 'Health is a state of complete physical, mental and social well-being'. The importance of body mass as an index of nutrition is apparent from the strong effect it has on mortality, with both overnutrition and undernutrition associated with increased mortality (a U-shaped relationship) (Whitlock *et al.*, 2009). There is a level of undernutrition, as measured by low BMI, that is incompatible with life (Collins, 1995).

Individuals of different body sizes have different basal metabolic rates (BMR), and BMRs can now be estimated using prediction equations. During the course of a day a sedentary individual expends a total amount of energy that is about 1.4 times the BMR. This multiplicative factor of BMR is called a physical activity level (PAL). The actual PAL of an individual can be computed as the daily energy intake divided by the BMR. Thus, individuals who have a PAL of <1.4 are clearly obtaining insufficient energy to support a sedentary lifestyle. Incidentally, studies have shown that a PAL of less than 1.4 is only seen in individuals who spend less than 4–5 h a day on their feet. In energy balance, energy intake is equal to the energy expended, and thus PAL can also be computed as the daily energy expenditure divided by the BMR. The identification of individuals with CED would be enhanced if we could combine the measurement of PAL with an additional, independent factor that reflects energy deficiency.

With energy deficiency there is a reduction in body weight and in energy stores [fat and fat-free mass (FFM)]. A simple index of body energy stores is the body mass index (BMI): weight in kg/(height in m)². Thus, BMI could be used to identify individuals who are energy deficient. The problem is to define the BMI cut-off, as in reality there is a gradation in severity. Based on the range of BMIs in healthy populations and on studies identifying the functional consequences of a low BMI, the lower limit of a desirable BMI has been fixed at 18.5 kg/m² (James *et al.*, 1988), and there is general agreement that BMI below this indicates undernutrition.

Table 17.1 provides a classification of CED based on the two principles outlined in the earlier paragraphs. It categorises CED based on a combination of a low PAL (signifying an inadequate energy intake) and a low BMI (signifying inadequate energy stores).

Individuals with marginally lower energy stores (BMI 17.0–18.4) but adequate energy intakes (PAL ≥ 1.4) are deemed normal. If, however, individuals have both marginally lower energy stores (BMI 17.0–18.4) and lower than adequate energy intakes (PAL < 1.4), they are categorised as grade I CED.

In several situations, the estimations of energy intake or energy expenditure become impractical. Under these circumstances, the combination of BMI with an index of socioeconomic status has been used to identify CED. The assumption is that individuals of a low socioeconomic status are more likely to be at risk of energy deprivation. The problems of this system in identifying CED are that local socioeconomic scales have to be devised, and these must be subjected to periodic revision to take into account changing economic and social conditions. There are unhelpful assumptions implicit in this concept, including the assumption that undernutrition is generally related to poverty, which neglects the often important role of ill-health, and this author does not recommend this approach.

In situations where a large population needs to be surveyed, BMI alone may be used as a simple but objective anthropometric indicator of the nutritional status of the adult population. When applied to large numbers of people (populations), BMI is sensitive to socioeconomic status and to seasonal fluctuations in food consumption levels, and has been recommended as the method of choice to assess the numbers of people who are undernourished worldwide. In situations where resources are very limited, such as in refugee camps in the midst of emergencies, mid upper arm circumference (MUAC) has been shown to be surprisingly effective as a tool for identifying people who are undernourished (Collins, 1996). MUAC, which is the simplest anthropometric index of all, can be applied to adults and children, obviously with different cut-offs, and is highly reproducible when carried out by trained observers, even those with no education. Although there may be some debate as to the correct cut-off to use, MUAC of 25 cm or less predicts poor outcome in hospitalised patients (Powell-Tuck & Hennessy, 2003).

To summarise, in different situations, CED may be identified on the basis of:

- a combination of BMI and PAL
- BMI alone
- MUAC.

17.3 Adaptation and chronic energy deficiency

When there is a sudden change in the internal environment of cells and tissues, the body calls on regulatory processes to maintain the constancy of the internal environment. This maintenance of internal constancy is called homeostasis. When the change in the internal or external environment is for a longer period, the body may need to evoke greater changes, in both structure and function, in order to survive. Adaptation is thus the process by which an organism maintains physiological activity and survives when there is a sustained alteration in the environment with respect to one or more parameters. These adaptive processes remain in place so long as the alteration in the environment persists. While this simplistic overview of adaptation may suggest that adaptation is without any detrimental consequences, this chapter will demonstrate that adaptation does indeed have a 'cost'. This cost is most clearly seen when the undernourished individual increases their energy intake again, the 're-feeding syndrome' (see below).

- Adaptation is the response of the body to a sustained perturbation in the environment, with the aim of ensuring function and survival.
- Adaptation persists for as long as the perturbation is maintained.
- Every adaptation has a cost.

In CED, the sustained environmental perturbation is a lower energy intake and the body adapts to this situation in order to ensure the survival of the individual. A suitable adaptation would be somehow to limit energy expenditure so that the individual remains in energy balance, albeit at a lower energy intake. In many situations, individuals with CED are involved in heavy physical activity (labourers, agricultural workers, etc.), despite their limited energy intakes. Their ability to work in this way despite CED suggests that CED subjects evoke energy-saving mechanisms to function adequately and to survive. The potential mechanisms that aid in the conservation of energy in CED are discussed below.

17.4 Changes in body composition in chronic energy deficiency

Before proceeding further, it is worthwhile getting a picture of what individuals with CED look like in terms of their body composition. This is illustrated in Table 17.2, which compares a typical male CED individual with his well-nourished counterpart.

Table 17.2 Anthropometric characteristics of a subject with chronic energy deficiency (CED) compared with a well-nourished subject

	CED	Well-nourished
Weight (kg)	42	69
Height (cm)	160	175
Body mass index (kg/m²)	**16.5**	**22.5**
Fat (%)	10	20
Fat mass (kg)	4	14
Fat-free mass (kg)	38	55

Table 17.2 indicates that individuals with CED have lower body weights, fat-free mass (FFM) and fat stores. In addition, individuals with CED may be shorter, which implies that energy deprivation began during the years of linear growth and had a limiting effect on growth. These changes in body composition help to conserve energy in CED. For instance, the lower body weight results in a lower energy cost of physical activity, particularly with weight-bearing activities. The reduction in metabolically active FFM ensures a lower BMR, in absolute terms. A reduction in these two major components of daily energy expenditure results in a considerable energy saving for the individual who is chronically energy deficient. Later, we shall see that the benefits of changes in body composition in the individual with CED which favour energy conservation are offset by some derangements in normal physiology. In contrast to the energy-saving benefit of a lower body weight and a lower FFM, the reduction in fat stores, and the attendant loss in heat insulation, would be expected, if anything, to enhance energy expenditure during cold exposure. This is discussed in greater detail later in this chapter.

17.5 Energy metabolism in chronic energy deficiency

Many researchers have attempted to determine whether CED subjects have energy-saving mechanisms that are independent of the loss in body weight and FFM. This inference could be made if the metabolic rate per unit of metabolically active tissue were lower than in well-nourished subjects. The most easily measurable form of metabolically active tissue is the FFM. Studies conducted so far have targeted most

components of daily energy expenditure and these are discussed in greater detail below.

Basal metabolic rate/resting metabolic rate

Classic studies on acute energy deprivation by Benedict, Keys *et al.* and Grande indicated that semi-starvation was associated with a reduction in resting metabolic rate (RMR). This reduction was explained both by a reduction in body weight and by a reduction in the metabolic activity of the tissues (metabolic efficiency). These findings have been replicated in more recent studies on obese subjects with restricted diets. The varying duration of energy restriction, however, makes comparisons between these studies difficult, particularly since there is some evidence that the reduction in RMR may occur in two phases. An initial phase of 2 or 3 weeks is associated with enhanced metabolic efficiency, while the further reduction in RMR with continued energy restriction beyond this period is largely accounted for by a loss of active tissue mass.

Chronically energy-deficient subjects also have reduced BMRs in absolute terms. In early studies, right up to the 1980s, 'metabolic efficiency' was essentially determined by dividing BMR by the active tissue mass (usually FFM). Some, but not all, studies showed a decrease in BMR/kg FFM. In recent years there have been detailed discussions on whether this computation of metabolic efficiency is appropriate. While the relationship between BMR and FFM is linear, there is a positive intercept, which means that smaller individuals have a higher BMR/kg FFM. This higher BMR/kg FFM may, in part, be related to the fact that the proportion of muscle mass lost from FFM is substantially more than the proportion of viscera. In undernutrition, it would make sense to think in terms of three or even four compartments (fat, bone, viscera, muscle and other connective tissue) but these are not yet easily measured and there is no consensus on this. Resting skeletal muscle mass is metabolically less active than viscera. Thus, the relatively higher viscera to muscle mass ratio in CED would be associated with a higher BMR/kg FFM.

A statistical method to adjust BMR for FFM is the analysis of covariance (ANCOVA). In this method it is assumed that since there is a linear relationship between FFM and BMR, changes in x (FFM) will affect the mean value of y (BMR). However, since x (FFM) is different between well-nourished and CED subjects, it follows that differences in y (BMR) between the two groups will be explained at least in part by the differences in x (FFM). The ANCOVA attempts a comparison of the BMRs of the two groups at the same FFM. More recent studies in CED that have used this statistical method have indicated that BMR is reduced in CED when adjusted for FFM using an ANCOVA.

Thus, CED subjects have a lower BMR, largely due to a lower body weight and a reduced active tissue mass. There is some evidence of increased metabolic efficiency in CED in terms of a reduced BMR when adjusted for FFM.

Physical activity

One of the ways in which an individual with CED could conserve energy is by being less physically active. This is, in fact, what has been observed in laboratory experiments involving semi-starvation for a long duration. It is more difficult to establish whether individuals with CED reduce their physical activity under free-living conditions. Earlier studies used the laborious method of time-and-motion analysis. In this method, trained observers accompany subjects and note their activities in a diary for the entire duration of a day or several days. The development of the doubly labelled water technique (see Chapter 2 of *Introduction to Human Nutrition*) has allowed for the estimation of free-living energy expenditure and, consequently, also of PALs. There are some data to suggest that individuals of low BMI can sustain high levels of physical activity at least over the periods of measurement. There is a possibility, however, particularly in largely agrarian societies, that CED subjects may show large seasonal variations in physical activity. One very clear example of the reduced physical activity is the example of human immunodeficiency virus (HIV) infection. Landmark studies in HIV have established that weight loss in most HIV-infected adults, and this is a major determinant of outcome in HIV, is due to anorexia. During periods of weight loss, physical activity decreases (Macallan, 1995).

Another way in which CED subjects may conserve energy is by an enhanced 'efficiency'. There are many ways in which efficiency is defined in exercise physiology. One of the more common terms is 'mechanical efficiency'. Mechanical efficiency is expressed as a percentage, and is the ratio of external work performed to the energy expended. The mechanical efficiency of performing activities such as climbing stairs and cycling is in the region of 20–25%. The rest of the energy expended is dissipated as heat. Several laboratory studies in CED subjects have assessed mechanical efficiency during stepping, treadmill walking and cycling. When viewed together, there is no compelling evidence, yet, to support the notion that CED subjects have a greater mechanical efficiency.

It is also conceivable that CED subjects may minimise the energy cost of physical activity by performing tasks in such a manner that reduces unnecessary movements or results in a better balance of loads ('ergonomic efficiency'). In Africa, for instance, women of the Luo and Kikuyu tribes can carry substantial loads with great economy. The possibility of an enhanced ergonomic efficiency in CED subjects needs to be investigated further.

Following strenuous, sustained physical exercise energy expenditure may be elevated for up to 24 h. This enhanced energy expenditure is sometimes called the excess postexercise oxygen consumption (EPOC). There is some evidence that EPOC is reduced in CED subjects, both in the immediate period following exercise and in the delayed period of about 12 h after exercise.

To summarise, CED subjects may potentially conserve energy in relation to physical activity by the following means:

- decreased physical activity
- increased mechanical efficiency
- enhanced ergonomic efficiency
- reduced EPOC.

A more detailed account of physical activity is provided in Chapter 18.

Thermogenesis

The thermic effect of food (TEF) comprises approximately 10% of daily energy expenditure and is defined as the rise in energy expenditure following the consumption of food. There are many factors that determine TEF, including the size and composition of the meal, the palatability of the food and the antecedent dietary intake. Because there is a very limited amount of data on TEF in CED, it is difficult to comment on whether TEF is reduced in this state.

There is some evidence that the TEF/kg FFM in CED subjects following a mixed meal is higher than in their well-nourished counterparts. Inter-country comparisons have demonstrated that Gambian men (not necessarily of low BMI) in the 'hungry' season have a lower TEF than Europeans.

On exposure to cold, individuals rely on both heat-conserving and heat-generating mechanisms to maintain body temperature. The heat-conserving mechanisms include the insulation provided by subcutaneous fat and vasoconstriction of peripheral blood vessels, particularly in skin and skeletal muscle. Vasoconstriction limits the amount of warm blood that is brought to the surface of the body. Thus, less heat is lost from the body. Heat-generating mechanisms include non-shivering thermogenesis (NST) and shivering. NST is largely mediated by the sympathetic nervous system, which enhances a whole host of metabolic processes, including glycogenolysis in liver and muscle, gluconeogenesis and lipolysis. NST has been studied under laboratory conditions by infusing either epinephrine (adrenaline) or norepinephrine (noradrenaline) intravenously into volunteers. These studies suggest that thermogenesis to exogenously administered catecholamines may be lower in CED subjects. On exposure to mild cold, CED subjects are able to thermoregulate adequately. Greater vasoconstriction of the peripheral blood vessels and an earlier onset of NST compensate for the lack of fat insulation. With more intense cold, however, undernourished subjects show reduced thermogenesis and are unable to thermoregulate adequately. Any energy conservation is therefore offset by their increased susceptibility to hypothermia in response to cold exposure. There is speculation that the high number of deaths during cold waves in developing countries may be related to this factor, and this is almost certainly true for elderly people in winter in temperate climates.

Protein metabolism in relation to energy expenditure

There have been a few studies in CED that have explored the relationship of protein metabolism and energy expenditure. The impetus for these investigations is the knowledge that protein synthesis contributes substantially to the BMR. Thus, a reduction in protein synthetic rates could conceivably reduce BMR and result in energy conservation. The studies demonstrate that while BMR and protein synthesis are both lower than in well-nourished subjects in absolute terms, there are no differences when protein turnover (synthesis and breakdown) is expressed per kilogram of FFM.

Energy expenditure during pregnancy

Pregnancy and lactation place increased energy demands on the mother. This is a situation where CED subjects are particularly vulnerable. Studies carried out on Gambian women have indicated that BMR is depressed during the first 18 weeks of gestation and that the total metabolic costs of pregnancy are far lower than in well-nourished women in Western populations. These results imply some energy-saving mechanisms. In this particular study, however, the vast majority of women had BMIs in excess of 18.5 kg/m^2. In contrast to the findings in the Gambia, studies on well-nourished pregnant Indian women, as well as Chinese and Malay women in Asia, failed to identify any conservation of energy during pregnancy. One of the consequences of a low BMI in pregnant women is the birth of babies of low birth weight. This is of importance because a low birth weight is associated with increased infant mortality. In addition, low birthweight babies may be more susceptible to chronic disease if they survive into adulthood. The metabolism of pregnancy and lactation is dealt with in greater detail in Chapter 6.

17.6 Regulatory processes in chronic energy deficiency

The two major regulatory systems in the body are the nervous system and the endocrine (hormonal) system, and both can modulate metabolic rate.

One of the components of the nervous system that has been studied fairly extensively in relation to metabolic activity is the sympathetic nervous system (SNS). Classic studies by Young and Landsberg demonstrated a reduction in SNS activity in animal models with underfeeding and an enhanced SNS activity with overfeeding. Pharmacological studies demonstrated that virtually all components of daily energy expenditure, including BMR, were reduced when SNS activity was blocked. Thus, a hypothesis has emerged that attempts to explain a putative reduction in metabolic activity in CED on the basis of diminished SNS activity. Short-term underfeeding experiments in humans support the hypothesis of a reduced SNS activity with reduced energy intakes. In CED too, there is evidence of reduced SNS activity. There have, however, been no studies that have measured metabolic rates in CED in the presence of SNS blockade.

Among the hormones, one that particularly stands out in terms of metabolic regulation is thyroid hormone (thyroxine). Indeed, there was a time before thyroxine levels could be measured in blood when hypothyroidism was diagnosed on the basis of a reduced BMR. Thyroid hormone exists in two forms, T_4 and T_3. Of these, active T_3 is biologically more active and is derived from T_4. Several studies have demonstrated that active T_3 is reduced with starvation and acute underfeeding experiments, and that this is, in part, due to a reduced conversion of T_4 to active T_3. Alteration in thyroid hormone status has been incompletely characterised in CED.

Several other hormones, such as glucagon, glucocorticoids, growth hormone, insulin-like growth factors and progesterone, could potentially modulate metabolic rate. The role of these hormones in CED has not been studied adequately.

17.7 Functional consequences of energy deficiency

This section explores some of the consequences of energy deficiency in terms of the cost of adaptation which was referred to above. Table 17.3 summarises this in terms of functional changes and real-life consequences.

Muscle function

Several laboratory studies have demonstrated that CED is associated with a reduction in muscle strength as well as muscle endurance. The reduction in muscle strength is to a large extent associated with a reduction in muscle mass. Some studies have, however, indicated that the loss in strength persists even after correcting for muscle mass. In other words, muscle strength per unit muscle area or mass is less than in well-nourished subjects. This suggests that there are functional changes in skeletal muscle with CED, and these may underlie the reduced grip strength observed in undernutrition.

Table 17.3 Real-life consequences of physiological functional changes that occur in chronic energy deficiency (CED)

Functional changes in CED	Real-life consequences
Reduced muscle strength and endurance	Decreased work performance and earning capacity
Reduced immunity	More infections, increased sickness
Altered autonomic nervous function	Possibly altered drug-dosage requirements
	Consequences with ageing not known

Skeletal muscle is made up of two large categories of muscle fibre types. Type I fibres are increased in marathon runners and are important for endurance. Type II muscle fibres are increased in weightlifters and are a determinant of muscle strength. In undernutrition there is a decline in type II fibres and this may account for the decline in muscle strength. There are also reports of a conversion of type II fibres to type I fibres. This has a benefit in energetic terms because the type I fibres use less adenosine triphosphate (ATP) during muscle contraction than type II fibres. In addition to the changes in muscle fibre type, undernutrition is associated with a reduction in sources of energy within skeletal muscle, such as glycogen, ATP and phosphocreatinine. A reduction in these energy sources could impair muscle function.

In real life, the consequence of diminished skeletal muscle function in CED is reduced work performance and physical work capacity. Thus, for instance, sugarcane cutters in Colombia who are taller and heavier and have higher FFMs are more productive.

Immune function

There are good grounds for thinking that acute energy deficiency is associated with diminished immune function, but actually the evidence is far from clear-cut. Immune function is of three types: cellular, humoral and innate. Cellular immunity, which is mediated by T-lymphocytes, is involved predominantly in defence against viruses, fungi and protozoa. Antibodies produced by B-lymphocytes mediate humoral immunity to bacteria and some viruses. Several studies suggest that cellular immunity is more affected than humoral immunity in children with protein–energy malnutrition, but since some evidence regarding T-cell behaviour has been discredited there is a paucity of direct evidence to explain how this might happen (Hughes & Kelly, 2006). Curiously, in anorexia nervosa, which is the purest form of undernutrition seen in current nutrition practice in the UK, there is little if any increase in susceptibility to infection (Golla *et al.*, 1981). In addition, mortality increases sharply in those individuals who are of low BMI, especially below a BMI of 16 kg/ m². Recent evidence suggests that innate immunity, notably dendritic cells, may be an important contributor to the immune dysfunction in undernourished children (Hughes *et al.*, 2009). The difficulty with understanding the link between undernutrition and infection is that infection itself can produce some of the immune defects which we often attribute to malnutrition, so establishing causality is not easy. The strongest evidence suggests the occurrence of thymolymphatic atrophy in severe undernutrition, and overall the evidence suggests that T-cell responses are impaired (Hughes & Kelly, 2006).

Autonomic nervous function

Earlier in this chapter we discussed how changes in sympathetic nervous function could help in the conservation of energy in CED. In CED there is evidence that sympathetic nervous activity is reduced. There is also some evidence that parasympathetic nervous activity (the other arm of the autonomic nervous system) is increased. Nerves act by releasing chemical messengers called neurotransmitters. These neurotransmitters in turn act on certain proteins on cell membranes called receptors, which then produce a cellular response. When the level of a neurotransmitter is high, the number of receptors reduces to maintain a constant cellular response. Conversely, when the neurotransmitter level is low, the number of receptors increases. Many drugs used in clinical practice act on the receptors of the autonomic nervous system. Because autonomic nervous activity (both sympathetic and parasympathetic) is altered in CED, the receptor number is also altered. If drugs are administered that act on these receptors, the response to the drug is likely to be higher or lower than normal, depending on whether the receptor number is increased or decreased. Thus, the required dose of drugs acting on the autonomic nervous system may be altered in CED.

Re-feeding syndrome

When prisoners in concentration camps were liberated at the end of World War II, Allied troops were horrified at the extreme malnutrition they encountered and understandably encouraged these starving individuals to take generous amounts of food. Unfortunately, many prisoners died on re-feeding and this has become known as the re-feeding syndrome (Solomon & Kirby, 1990). One of the consequences of muscle wasting in severe undernutrition is the loss (permanently, in the urine) of bulk minerals such as phosphate, potassium and magnesium. Re-feeding syndrome is characterised by severe hypophosphataemia, which may lead to sudden death and there are major disturbances of sodium distribution (Patrick, 1977). This cost of reductive adaptation has major implications for the treatment of severe undernutrition in both children and adults. Generally we assume that the greatest risk of re-feeding syndrome is over when appetite returns (severe undernutrition is usually accompanied by marked anorexia) but the validity of this belief is not absolutely clear and further work is needed.

In summary, therefore, the conservation of energy in the CED subject is largely due to a reduction in body size and in metabolically active tissue. Metabolic efficiency in CED contributes to energy saving in a rather small way. The adaptation of the CED subject to lowered energy intakes is not, however, without its costs, as highlighted in the preceding section.

17.8 Perspectives on the future

This chapter has highlighted some issues in CED for which we have an incomplete understanding. This section raises some of the issues that healthcare professionals will have to deal with in the future. Much of what follows is speculative, and the reader is encouraged to pick up the leads and delve further into the issues that have been raised.

Population changes and inequalities in nutrition

One adverse trend we are seeing in global health as the twenty-first century unfolds is the widening of inequalities in wealth, health and access to health care. While a large proportion of the world's population is undernourished, there is a large and growing proportion which is obese. As populations in developing countries abandon their traditional diets and consume foods which contain more meat (this is a rapid trend in China) and are more energy-dense, the number of people with the 'metabolic syndrome' is increasing rapidly. These two trends may be taking place in parallel simultaneously in the same country (e.g. India). Earlier in the chapter a typical CED subject with a BMI of 16.5 kg/m^2 was described. If this same individual were to gain weight to achieve a BMI of 25, his body weight at this BMI would be 64 kg, a gain of almost 22 kg. A substantial portion of this is likely to be fat. Individuals with a BMI near 25 kg/m^2 are conventionally considered to be at the upper end of the normal BMI range. How should this CED individual be evaluated? Should he be considered at higher risk of developing heart disease and diabetes because of his weight and fat gain, despite his normal BMI? What are the consequences for HIV-infected people who have been severely wasted and who regain weight (even to the point of obesity) thanks to anti-retroviral drugs and lipid-rich diets? While rescue therapy for severe undernutrition has been revolutionised thanks to the introduction of lipid-based ready-to-use food (RTUF), does this run the risk of metabolic syndrome after a certain threshold of weight has been gained? These questions are as yet unanswered.

Small babies now, larger problems later?

As mentioned earlier, low birthweight babies are seen more often in mothers with a low BMI. These babies also have a higher mortality. What happens to babies of low birth weight who survive into adulthood? Barker has shown that low birthweight babies in the UK had a higher prevalence of high blood pressure, diabetes and coronary heart disease when they grew up to be adults (Barker, 1993). The mechanism by which this happens is not fully understood. The increased prevalence of diabetes has been linked to poor foetal growth, resulting in a reduced number of pancreatic β-cells, which produce insulin. Will developing countries where low birth weights are fairly common have to face the increased burden of diabetes, hypertension and so on, as life spans increase? How can we dissect out the contributions of poor foetal growth from environmental factors that are operative after birth? Will continued CED into adulthood be protective against these diseases? The intriguing possibility of foetal undernutrition

affecting health in adulthood remains to be elucidated, particularly within the context of CED. For much of the world's population, this is already a question which urgently needs an answer.

References

Barker DJP, ed. Fetal and infant origins of adult disease. London: BMJ Publishing Group, 1993.

Collins S. The limit of human adaptation to starvation. Nat Med 1995; 1: 810–814.

Collins S. Using middle upper arm circumference to assess severe adult malnutrition during famine. JAMA 1996; 276: 391–395.

Golla JA, Larson LA, Anderson CF, Lucas AR, Wilson WR, Tomasi TB. An immunological assessment of patients with anorexia nervosa. Am J Clin Nutr 1981; 34: 2756–2762.

Hughes S, Kelly P. Interactions of malnutrition and immune impairment, with special reference to immunity against parasites. Parasite Immunol 2006; 28: 577–588.

Hughes S et al., Dendritic cell anergy results from endotoxemia in severe malnutrition. J Immunol 2009; 183: 2818–2826.

James WPT, Ferro-Luzzi A, Waterlow JC. Definition of chronic energy deficiency in adults. Report of a working party of the International Dietary Energy Consultative Group. Eur J Clin Nutr 1988; 42: 969–981.

Macallan DC et al. Energy expenditure and wasting in HIV infection. New Engl J Med 1995; 333: 83–88.

Patrick J. Death during recovery from severe malnutrition and its possible relationship to sodium pump activity in the leucocyte. BMJ 1977; i: 1051–1054.

Powell-Tuck J, Hennessy EM. A comparison of mid upper arm circumference, body mass index and weight loss as indices of undernutrition in acutely hospitalized patients. Clin Nutr 2003; 22: 307–312.

Solomon SM, Kirby DF. The refeeding syndrome: a review. J Parenteral Enteral Nutr 1990; 14: 90–97.

Whitlock G et al., for the Prospective Studies Collaboration. Body mass index and cause-specific mortality in 900,000 adults: collaborative analyses of 57 prospective studies. Lancet 2009; 373: 1083–1096.

Further reading

Della Bianca P, Jequier E, Schutz Y. Lack of metabolic and behavioural adaptation in rural Gambian men with low body mass index. Am J Clin Nutr 1994; 60: 37–42.

Norgan NG, Ferro-Luzzi A. Human adaptation to energy undernutrition. In Handbook of Physiology Section 4. Environmental Physiology Vol. II (Fregly MJ, Blatteis CM, eds). New York: Oxford University Press for The American Physiological Society, 1996: pp. 1391–1409.

Soares MJS, Shetty PS. Basal metabolic rates and metabolic economy in chronic undernutrition. Eur J Clin Nutr 1991; 45: 363–373.

Soares MJ et al., Whole body protein turnover in chronically undernourished individuals. Clin Sci 1994; 86: 441–446.

Waterlow JC. Protein energy malnutrition. London: Edward Arnold. 1992.

Waterlow JC. Metabolic adaptation of low intakes of energy and protein. Annu Rev Nutr 1986; 6: 495–526.

18
Exercise Performance

Asker E Jeukendrup and Louise M Burke

Key messages

- The most important component of energy expenditure for athletes is the energy cost of their training or competition workloads. Energy expenditure can amount to 36 MJ/day for endurance athletes undertaking the most strenuous exercise schedules, such as competing in the Tour de France.
- Carbohydrate plays a crucial role in the diet of most athletes as it restores muscle and liver glycogen to provide a key fuel for exercise. Carbohydrate intake in the everyday diet should be individualised for each athlete to meet their specific fuel requirements for training and recovery. Training with high carbohydrate availability will help the athlete to train harder, especially during 'quality' workouts involving high-intensity exercise. Carbohydrate loading to increase muscle glycogen stores has been shown to improve endurance capacity and performance in prolonged events involving sustained or intermittent exercise >90 min duration.
- Carbohydrate feeding in the hours before the start of prolonged exercise can enhance performance. Carbohydrate ingested during prolonged exercise (longer than ~60–90 min) improves exercise performance by maintaining blood glucose concentration and high rates of carbohydrate oxidation, spares liver glycogen and may in some conditions spare muscle glycogen. Carbohydrate intake also benefits the brain and central nervous system, and in shorter sustained events (~60 min) even rinsing the mouth with a carbohydrate drink may be enough to stimulate the brain to 'feel better' and work harder during exercise.
- Muscle glycogen stores can be increased effectively by eating a high-carbohydrate meal or snack providing at least 1 g/kg carbohydrate within 15–30 min of finishing the exercise session. This is important when the schedule calls for rapid recovery between prolonged training sessions (<8 h recovery).
- A diet containing 7–12 g carbohydrate/kg body weight usually results in maintenance of muscle glycogen stores on a 24 h basis in trained athletes.
- Several 'dietary periodisation' strategies are popular, including 'training low' (training with low carbohydrate availability to enhance the training stimulus) or 'fat loading' (adapting to a high-fat diet prior to carbohydrate loading for competition to increase the ability to use fat as an exercise fuel). However, there is no clear evidence that these strategies lead to better competition performance.

- Consuming a small amount of high-quality protein (20–25 g) soon after the end of a strenuous workout or competition enhances adaptation or recovery from the session. Although it is suggested that both endurance and strength athletes may have increased protein requirements (~1.2–1.8 g/kg body mass per day), these targets are normally easily met by the high energy intake of these athletes and it is likely that the timing of intake of protein is the most important factor.
- Low body fat and low body weight are important in many sports, especially at the elite level. If loss of body fat is required, a realistic rate loss of about 0.5 kg/week should be chosen and both short-term and long-term goals should be set.
- Low iron status in athletes is overdiagnosed from single measures of low haemoglobin and ferritin levels. A major problem is the failure to recognise that the increase in blood volume that accompanies training will cause a dilution of all the blood contents. This haemodilution, often termed 'sports anaemia', does not impair exercise performance.
- Dehydration can have dramatic effects on performance. Endurance performance is reduced but dehydration also affects sports with short duration, high-intensity exercise and skill sports. Severe dehydration can result in heat injury, characterised by excessive sweating, headache, nausea, dizziness, and reduced consciousness and mental function. When the core temperature rises to over 40°C, heat stroke may develop, characterised by hot, dry skin, confusion and loss of consciousness.
- Hyperhydration can reduce the thermal and cardiovascular strain of exercise. Hyperhydration can be induced by having subjects drink large volumes of water or water–electrolyte solutions for 1–3 h before exercise. However, much of the fluid overload is rapidly excreted and so expansions of the body water and blood volume are only transient.
- Fluid intake may be useful during exercise longer than 30–60 min, but there is no advantage during strenuous exercise of less than 30 min in duration.
- Plasma volume is more rapidly and completely restored in the post-exercise period if salt (sodium chloride) is added to rehydration drinks or if salt-rich foods are consumed with this fluid. The sodium concentration of oral rehydration solutions is optimal for promoting the retention of fluids (~50–60 mmol/l) and is similar

Nutrition and Metabolism, Second Edition, edited by S. A. Lanham-New, I. A. Macdonald and H. M. Roche.   © 2011 The Nutrition Society.

to the sodium concentration found in sweat, but is considerably higher than the sodium concentration of many commercially available sports drinks, which usually contain 10–25 mmol/l (60–150 mg/l).
• Fluid intake equal to 125–150% of the volume of the post-exercise fluid deficit is required to re-establish normal hydration within 6 h following exercise.
• The nutrition supplement market has grown incredibly in the last few years. However, there is little or no evidence to support the use of the vast majority of these supplements in sport.

• Oral creatine supplementation of 20 g/day for 5–6 days increases the muscle total creatine content in men by about 20% (30–40% of the increase is phosphocreatine). A subsequent daily dose of 2 g is enough for maintenance of this increased concentration. Creatine loading increases the amount of work performed during single and repeated bouts of short-lasting, high-intensity exercise. Besides weight gain, creatine does not seem to have major side-effects. However, the long-term effects of creatine ingestion are unknown and therefore caution must be exercised.

18.1 Introduction

The relationship between nutrition and physical performance has fascinated people for a long time. In Ancient Greece athletes had special nutrition regimes to prepare for the Olympic Games. It has become clear that different types of exercise and different sports will have different energy and nutrient requirements and therefore food intake must be adjusted accordingly. Certain nutritional strategies can enhance performance, improve recovery and result in more profound training adaptations. More recently, special drinks and energy bars have been developed and these have been marketed as sports foods. There is also a considerable amount of quackery in sports nutrition and there are a large number of nutrition supplements on the market with claims to improve performance and recovery. This chapter will first review the nutritional demands of exercise in relation to the physiological demands. Strategies to improve exercise performance are then discussed. Finally, practical applications will be discussed and detailed advice will be provided where possible.

18.2 Energy expenditure during physical activity

In resting conditions cells need energy to function: ionic pumps in membranes need energy to transport ions across cell membranes and the muscle fibres of the heart need energy to contract. During exercise the energy expenditure may increase several-fold, mainly because skeletal muscle requires energy to contract. In some cases the energy provision can become critical and continuation of the exercise is dependent on the availability of energy reserves. Most of these reserves must be obtained through nutrition.

In endurance athletes, for example, energy depletion (carbohydrate depletion) is one of the most common causes of fatigue. Carbohydrate intake is essential to prevent early fatigue as a result of carbohydrate depletion.

Definition and assessment methods

There are several ways to measure (or estimate) human energy expenditure:

• direct calorimetry
• indirect calorimetry:
  – closed circuit spirometry
  – open circuit spirometry (douglas bag technique, breath-by-breath technique, portable spirometry)
• doubly labelled water
• labelled bicarbonate
• heart-rate monitoring
• accelerometry
• observations, records of physical activity, activity diaries, recall.

The methods range from direct but complex measurements of heat production (direct calorimetry) to relatively simple indirect metabolic measurements (indirect calorimetry), and from very expensive tracer methods (doubly labelled water) to relatively cheap and convenient rough estimations of energy expenditure (heart-rate monitoring and accelerometry). For a detailed analysis of these methods the reader is referred to Chapter 2 of the *Introduction to Human Nutrition* textbook in this series.

The most important component of energy expenditure for athletes who are in training is exercise. Basal metabolic rate (BMR) and diet-induced thermogenesis (DIT) become relatively less important (accounting for less than 50% of total energy expenditure) when athletes train for 2 h/day or more. Energy expenditure during physical activity ranges from 20 kJ/min for very light activities to 100 kJ/min for very high-intensity exercise.

Energy expenditure and substrate use

Energy can be defined as the potential for performing work or producing force. Force production by skeletal muscles requires adenosine triphosphate (ATP). This compound contains energy in its phosphate bonds and on hydrolysis of ATP this energy is released and used to power all forms of biological work. In muscle, energy from the hydrolysis of ATP by myosin ATPase is used for muscle contraction. The hydrolysis of ATP yields approximately 31 kJ of free energy per mole of ATP degraded to ADP and inorganic phosphate (Pi):

$$ATP + H_2O \rightarrow ADP + H^+ + Pi$$
$$31 kJ \text{ per mole of ATP}$$

The stores of ATP are very small and would only be sufficient for about 2 s of maximal exercise. The body therefore has various ways to resynthesise ATP. The different mechanisms involved in the resynthesis of ATP for muscle force generation include:

- phosphocreatine breakdown
- glycolysis, which involves metabolism of glucose-6-phosphate, derived from muscle glycogen or blood-borne glucose
- the products of carbohydrate, fat, protein and alcohol metabolism can enter the tricarboxylic acid (TCA) cycle in the mitochondria and be oxidised to carbon dioxide and water (aerobic metabolism). This process is known as oxidative phosphorylation and yields energy for the synthesis of ATP.

The rate of energy delivery from phosphocreatine is very fast, somewhat slower from glycolysis and much slower from aerobic metabolism. Within the muscle fibre, the concentration of phosphocreatine is about three or four times greater than the concentration of ATP. When phosphocreatine is broken down to creatine and inorganic phosphate by the action of the enzyme creatine kinase, a large amount of free energy is released. The phosphocreatine can be regarded as a back-up energy store: when the ATP content begins to fall during exercise, the phosphocreatine is broken down, releasing energy for

restoration of ATP. During very intense exercise (8–10 s maximal exercise) the phosphocreatine (PCr) store can be almost completely depleted.

$$PCr + ADP + H^+ \leftrightarrow ATP + Cr$$
$$43 kJ \text{ per mole of PCr}$$

Under normal conditions, muscle clearly does not fatigue after only a few seconds of effort, so a source of energy other than ATP and phosphocreatine must be available. This is derived from glycolysis, which is the name given to the pathway involving the breakdown of glucose (or glycogen), the end-product of this series of chemical reactions being pyruvate. This process does not require oxygen, but does result in energy in the form of ATP. In order for the reactions to proceed, however, the pyruvate must be removed; in low-intensity exercise when adequate oxygen is available to the muscle, pyruvate is converted to carbon dioxide and water by an oxidative metabolism in the mitochondria. In some situations the pyruvate is removed by conversion to lactate, a reaction that does not involve oxygen. The net effect of glycolysis can thus be seen to be the conversion of one molecule of glucose to two molecules of pyruvate, with the net formation of two molecules of ATP and the conversion of two molecules of NAD^+ to NADH. If glycogen rather than glucose is the starting point, three molecules of ATP are produced, as there is no initial investment of ATP when the first phosphorylation step occurs. An 800-m runner, for example, obtains about 60% of the total energy requirement from anaerobic metabolism, and may convert about 100 g of carbohydrate (mostly glycogen, and equivalent to about 550 mmoles of glucose) to lactate in less than 2 min. The amount of ATP released in this way (three ATP molecules per glucose molecule degraded, about 1667 mmol of ATP in total) far exceeds that available from phosphocreatine hydrolysis. This high rate of anaerobic metabolism not only allows a faster steady-state speed than would be possible if aerobic metabolism alone had to be relied on, but also allows a faster pace in the early stages before the cardiovascular system has adjusted to the demands, and the delivery and utilisation of oxygen have increased in response to the exercise stimulus.

During exercise lasting for several minutes up to several hours carbohydrate and fat are the most important fuels. These two energy sources are stored in the human body and can be mobilised from these stores when the demand increases. Both carbohydrate and fat are broken down to acetyl-coenzyme A (acetyl-CoA), which will then enter a series of reactions referred to as the tricarboxylic acid (TCA) cycle or Krebs cycle. In essence, the most important function of the TCA cycle is to generate hydrogen atoms for their subsequent passage to the electron transport chain by means of NADH and $FADH_2$. The aerobic process of electron transport–oxidative phosphorylation regenerates ATP from ADP, thus conserving some of the chemical potential energy contained within the original substrates in the form of high-energy phosphates. As long as there is an adequate supply of oxygen and substrate is available, NAD^+ and FAD are continuously regenerated and TCA metabolism proceeds. This system cannot function without the use of oxygen.

Carbohydrate is stored in the liver and muscle (Table 18.1). The liver contains approximately 80 g of carbohydrate in the form of glycogen and skeletal muscle contains approximately 300–800 g (depending on muscle mass and diet). These stores are relatively small compared with the very large fat stores (mainly in subcutaneous adipose tissues). Even a lean athlete will have 4–7 kg of fat. Every gram of glycogen stored in liver or muscle is stored with 2.7 g of water. In addition, fat contains more than twice as much energy per gram as carbohydrate (37 kJ versus 17 kJ), therefore fat provides far more fuel per unit of weight than carbohydrate. In fact if we could only use the available carbohydrate as a substrate, we would probably only run between 20 and 30 km, whereas with fat as the only fuel, we could theoretically run between 1000 and 2000 km.

At rest and during low-intensity exercise, fat is often the substrate of choice. As the exercise intensity increases carbohydrate, and in particular muscle, glycogen will become more and more important. Figure 18.1 displays the most important sources of fuel utilised during exercise. During low-intensity exercise, plasma fatty acids provide approximately one-third of the total energy. Glucose derived from the liver accounts for approximately 10% at low intensities but becomes more and more important at higher exercise intensities. Muscle glycogen is relatively unimportant at low intensities [40% maximal aerobic power ($Vo_{2\,max}$)] but is by far the most important fuel during high-intensity exercise

Table 18.1 Availability of substrates in the human body (estimated energy stores of fat and carbohydrate in an 80 kg man with 15% body fat)

Substrate		Weight (kg)	Energy (kcal)
Carbohydrates	Plasma glucose	0.02	78
	Liver glycogen	0.1	388
	Muscle glycogen	0.4	1550
	Total (approximately)	0.52	2000
Fat	Plasma fatty acid	0.0004	4
	Plasma triacylglycerols	0.004	39
	Adipose tissue	12.0	100 000
	Intramuscular triacylglycerols	0.3	2616
	Total (approximately)	12.3	106 500

Adapted from Jeukendrup *et al.* (1998). Values given are estimates for a 'normal' man and not those of an athlete, who might be leaner and have more stored glycogen. The amount of protein in the body is not mentioned, but this would be about 10 kg (40 000 kcal); mainly located in the muscles.

Figure 18.1 Substrate utilisation at different exercise intensities. (AMERICAN JOURNAL OF PHYSIOLOGY: ENDOCRINOLOGY AND METABOLISM by JA Romijn, EF Coyle, LS Sidossis, A Gastaldelli, JF Horowitz, E Endert and RR Wolfe. Copyright © 1993 by AMERICAN PHYSIOLOGY SOCIETY. Reproduced with permission of AMERICAN PHYSIOLOGY SOCIETY in the format Textbook via Copyright Clearance Center.)

(70–90% $Vo_{2\,max}$). Fat oxidation is usually the predominant fuel at low exercise intensities, whereas during high exercise intensities carbohydrate is the major fuel.

In absolute terms, fat oxidation increases as the exercise intensity increases from low to moderate intensities, even though the percentage contribution of fat may actually decrease (Figure 18.2). For the transition

Figure 18.2 Fat oxidation as a function of exercise intensity in trained men. (Reprinted from Acten J, Gleeson M, Jeukendrup AE, Determination of the exercise intensity that elicits maximal fat oxidation. Med Sci Sports Exerc. 2002; 34: 92–99.)

from light to moderate-intensity exercise, the increased fat oxidation is a direct result of the increased energy expenditure. At higher intensities of exercise (>75% Vo_{2max}) fat oxidation will be inhibited and both the relative and absolute rates of fat oxidation will decrease to negligible values. Above approximately 65% $Vo_{2\,max}$, fat oxidation decreases despite high rates of lipolysis. The blood flow to the adipose tissue may be decreased (owing to sympathetic vasoconstriction) and this may result in a decreased removal of fatty acids from adipose tissue. During high-intensity exercise, lactate accumulation may also increase the re-esterification and inhibit the oxidation of fatty acids.

Carbohydrate and fat are always oxidised as a mixture, and whether carbohydrate or fat is the predominant fuel depends on a variety of factors.

Exercise intensity

At higher exercise intensities more carbohydrate and less fat will be utilised. Carbohydrate can be utilised aerobically at rates up to about 4 g/min. The breakdown during very high-intensity exercise can amount to 7 g/min.

Duration of exercise

Fat oxidation increases and carbohydrate oxidation decreases as the exercise duration increases. Typical fat oxidation rates are between 0.2 and 0.5 g/min, but values of over 1.0–1.5 g/min have been reported after 6 h of running. The contribution of fat to energy expenditure can even increase to as much as 90%. This increased fat oxidation is likely to be caused by a reduction in muscle glycogen stores towards the later stages of prolonged exercise.

Level of aerobic fitness

After endurance training the capacity to oxidise fatty acids increases and fat oxidation at the same absolute and relative exercise intensity is higher.

Diet

Substrate utilisation usually reflects the diet. A high-carbohydrate diet will promote carbohydrate oxidation, whereas a low-carbohydrate diet will reduce body carbohydrate stores and result in lower rates of carbohydrate oxidation.

Carbohydrate intake before or during exercise

After an overnight fast most of the energy requirement is covered by the oxidation of fatty acids derived from adipose tissue. Lipolysis in adipose tissue is mostly dependent on the concentrations of hormones (epinephrine (adrenaline) to stimulate lipolysis and insulin to inhibit lipolysis). At rest a large percentage (about 70%) of the fatty acids liberated after lipolysis will be re-esterified within the adipocyte and approximately 30% of the fatty acids will be released into the systemic circulation. Resting plasma fatty acids concentrations are typically between 0.2 and 0.4 mmol/l. As soon as exercise is initiated, the rate of lipolysis and the rate of fatty acid release from adipose tissue are increased. During moderate-intensity exercise lipolysis increases approximately three-fold, mainly because of an increased β-adrenergic stimulation and reduced plasma insulin concentration. In addition, during moderate-intensity exercise the blood flow to adipose tissue is doubled and the rate of re-esterification is halved. Blood flow in skeletal muscle is increased dramatically and therefore the delivery of fatty acids to muscle is increased.

18.3 Carbohydrate and performance

Carbohydrate fuel plays a major role in the performance of many types of exercise and sport. The depletion of body carbohydrate stores is a cause of fatigue or performance impairment during exercise, particularly during prolonged (>90 min) sessions of submaximal or intermittent high-intensity activity. This fatigue may be seen both in the muscle (peripheral fatigue) and in the brain and nervous system (central fatigue). Unfortunately, total body carbohydrate stores are limited, and are often substantially less than the fuel requirements of the training and competition sessions undertaken by athletes. Sports nutrition guidelines therefore promote a variety of options for increasing carbohydrate availability for an exercise session. These strategies include consuming carbohydrate before, during and in the recovery period between prolonged exercise bouts.

Many studies show that exercise is improved by strategies that enhance or maintain carbohydrate status during exercise. Exercise scientists find it convenient to measure performance by having the athlete exercise in a laboratory, often on a bike or running treadmill, at a steady workrate. They measure the time for which the athlete can exercise until they fatigue, or the point at which they fail to keep up with this workrate. Technically, this measurement should be called exercise capacity or endurance. Although these studies are relatively easy to conduct and can show the beneficial effects of a dietary intervention, they do not necessarily mimic the real demands of a sporting event. After all, in most races, the athlete tries to cover a set distance as fast as possible rather than exercise until they are exhausted. Studies that try to simulate a real event, especially in the field rather than in the laboratory, are harder to conduct. The most complicated types of performance belong to unpredictable team games or sports involving complex decision-making and motor skills. It is hard to find a way to measure adequately all the components of performance, and it is complicated to organise a protocol in which the same event is conducted twice, before and after an intervention, or with a treatment and a placebo. Despite the difficulties in conducting studies, strategies that enhance carbohydrate availability have been shown to enhance cycling and running endurance, cycling and running performance, and the performance of complex games such as tennis, soccer and ice hockey. There is also some evidence that the benefits of combining two strategies that enhance carbohydrate availability, for example a combination of eating a high-carbohydrate meal before the event and consuming carbohydrate during the event, are additive. Studies of single-carbohydrate strategies or combinations of strategies need to be conducted over a greater range of sports and exercise events so that scientists can give more detailed and specific advice to athletes.

Recent studies have provided evidence that there are other benefits from high-carbohydrate eating strategies apart from increasing muscle fuel for exercise. For example, a growing number of investigations have reported performance benefits when carbohydrate is consumed before and during high-intensity exercise of around 1 h. In these situations, the athlete's muscle carbohydrate stores should already be sufficient to fuel the event, so another mechanism to explain the findings has been investigated. It now seems clear that carbohydrate intake improves the function of the brain and central nervous system, which makes the athlete feel better during the exercise task and work harder. In fact, some studies have shown that even rinsing the mouth out with a carbohydrate drink can produce performance benefits, at least when an athlete undertakes exercise without having had a pre-event meal. The swishing of carbohydrate around the mouth is picked up by sensors which relay the message to the brain that fuel is on the way.

Finally, carbohydrate intake, during and after exercise, appears to assist the immune response to exercise. Cellular immune parameters are often reduced or compromised after a prolonged workout. However, some studies have shown that carbohydrate intake can decrease or prevent this outcome. Whether this actually leads to an improvement in the immune status and health of athletes (e.g. fever sick days) remains to be seen and would require a sophisticated long-term study.

Fuelling up before exercise

Carbohydrate stores in the muscle and liver should be well-filled prior to exercise, particularly in the competition setting, where the athlete wants to perform at their best. The key factors in glycogen storage are dietary carbohydrate intake and, in the case of muscle stores, tapered exercise or rest. In the absence of muscle damage, muscle glycogen stores can be returned to normal resting levels (to 350–500 mmol/kg dry weight muscle) with 24–36 h of rest and an adequate carbohydrate intake (7–12/kg body weight per day). Normalised stores appear adequate for the fuel needs of events of less than 60–90 min in duration (e.g. a soccer game, half-marathon or basketball game). Supercompensated glycogen levels do not enhance performance in these events.

Carbohydrate loading is a special practice that aims to maximise or supercompensate muscle glycogen stores up to twice the normal resting level (e.g. ~500–900 mmol/kg dry weight). The first protocol was devised in the late 1960s by Scandinavian sports scientists who found, using muscle biopsy techniques, that the size of pre-exercise muscle glycogen stores affected endurance during submaximal exercise. Their series of studies found that several days of a low-carbohydrate diet depleted muscle glycogen stores and reduced cycling endurance compared with a mixed diet. However, following up with a high-carbohydrate intake over several days caused a supercompensation of muscle glycogen stores and prolonged the cycling time to exhaustion. These pioneering studies produced the 'classical' 7-day model of carbohydrate loading. This model consists of a 3–4 day depletion phase of hard training and low carbohydrate intake, finishing with a 3–4 day loading phase of high carbohydrate eating and exercise taper (i.e. decreased amounts of training). Early field studies of prolonged running events showed that carbohydrate loading enhanced sports performance, not by allowing the athlete to run faster, but by prolonging the time for which race pace could be maintained.

Further studies undertaken on trained subjects have produced a modified carbohydrate loading strategy. The muscle of well-trained athletes has been found to be able to supercompensate its glycogen stores without a prior depletion or glycogen-stripping phase. Furthermore, a recent study has shown, for well-trained athletes at least, that a loading phase of rest and high carbohydrate intake may maximise muscle glycogen stores in as little as 36 h. These modifications offer a more practical strategy for competition preparation at several levels. Firstly, they avoid the fatigue and complexity of the extreme diet and training protocols associated with the previous depletion phase. Secondly, they can be achieved and repeated in a short time frame, making it possible for athletes to regularly fuel up for prolonged events such as weekly races in the triathlon calendar or games in the tournament fixture. Typically, carbohydrate loading will postpone fatigue and extend the duration of steady-state exercise by around 20%, and improve performance over a set distance or workload by 2–3%.

Pre-event meal

Food and fluids consumed in the 4 h before an event may help to achieve the following sports nutrition goals:

- to continue to fill muscle glycogen stores if they have not fully restored or loaded since the last exercise session
- to restore liver glycogen levels, especially for events undertaken in the morning where liver stores are depleted from an overnight fast
- to ensure that the athlete is well hydrated
- to prevent hunger, yet avoid gastrointestinal discomfort and upset during exercise
- to include foods and practices that are important to the athlete's psychology or superstitions.

Consuming carbohydrate-rich foods and drinks in the pre-event meal is especially important in situations where body carbohydrate stores have not been fully restored and/or where the event is of sufficient duration and intensity to deplete these stores. The intake of a substantial amount of carbohydrate (~200–300 g) in the 2–4 h before exercise has been shown to enhance various measures of exercise performance compared with performance undertaken after an overnight fast.

However, some experts have suggested that carbohydrate intake before exercise may have negative consequences for performance, especially in the hour before exercise. Carbohydrate intake causes a rise in plasma insulin concentrations, which in turn suppresses the availability and oxidation of fat as an exercise fuel. The final result is an increased reliance on carbohydrate oxidation at the onset of exercise, leading to faster depletion of muscle glycogen stores and a decline in plasma glucose concentration. There has been considerable publicity surrounding one study from the 1970s, which found that subjects performed worse after consuming carbohydrate in the hour before exercise than when they cycled without consuming anything. This has led to warnings that carbohydrate should not be consumed in the hour before exercise. However, a far greater number of studies have shown that any metabolic disturbances following pre-exercise carbohydrate feedings are short-lived or unimportant. These studies show that carbohydrate intake in the hour before exercise is associated with a neutral effect or a beneficial performance outcome.

Nevertheless, there is a small subgroup of athletes who experience a true fatigue, associated with a decline in blood glucose levels, if they start to exercise within the hour after consuming a carbohydrate snack. This problem can be avoided or diminished by a number of dietary strategies:

- Consume a substantial amount of carbohydrate (>75 g) rather than a small amount, so that the additional carbohydrate more than compensates for the increased rate of carbohydrate oxidation during the exercise.
- Choose a carbohydrate-rich food or drink that produces a low glycaemic index (GI) response (that is, a low blood glucose and insulin response) rather than a carbohydrate source that has a high GI (producing a large and rapid blood glucose and insulin response).
- Consume carbohydrate throughout the exercise session.

Some sports scientists have suggested that all athletes will benefit from the choice of low GI rather than high GI carbohydrate foods in the pre-event meal. This theory is based on the idea that low GI foods will provide a more sustained release of carbohydrate energy throughout the exercise session, and create less of a metabolic disturbance during exercise because of a reduced insulin response. However, the balance of studies has failed to find performance benefits following the intake of a low GI pre-exercise meal compared with an equal amount of high GI carbohydrate, even when metabolic differences between low GI and high GI meals were noted. Furthermore, it has been shown that when carbohydrate is ingested during exercise according to sports nutrition guidelines, any metabolic or performance effects arising from the choice of a low GI or high GI pre-event meal are overridden.

Each athlete must judge the benefits and the practical issues associated with pre-exercise meals in their particular sport or situation. The type, timing and quantity of pre-event meals should be chosen according to the athlete's individual circumstances and experiences. Foods with a low-fat, low-fibre and low to moderate protein content are the preferred choice for the pre-event menu since they are less likely to cause gastrointestinal upsets. Liquid meal supplements or carbohydrate-containing drinks and bars are a simple snack for athletes who suffer from pre-event nerves or have an uncertain competition timetable. Examples of carbohydrate-rich foods and drinks that are often used in pre-event meals are listed in Box 18.1.

Box 18.1 Examples of suitable pre-event meal choices

- Breakfast cereal + low-fat milk + fresh/canned fruit
- Muffins or crumpets + jam/honey
- Pancakes + syrup
- Toast + baked beans (NB: this is a high-fibre choice)
- Creamed rice
- Rolls or sandwiches with banana filling
- Fruit salad + low-fat fruit yogurt
- Spaghetti with tomato or low-fat sauce
- Baked potatoes with low-fat filling
- Fruit smoothie (low-fat milk + fruit + yogurt/ice cream)
- Liquid meal supplement (e.g. Sustagen Sport, Powerbar Protein Plus or Recovery)
- Cereal bars or sports bars

Carbohydrate intake during exercise

Numerous studies show that the intake of carbohydrate during prolonged sessions of moderate-intensity or intermittent high-intensity exercise can improve endurance (i.e. prolong time to exhaustion) and performance. As reviewed above, there is also some evidence that carbohydrate intake may benefit shorter duration high-intensity sports, or the immune response to prolonged exercise. Even when there is no significant benefit from consuming carbohydrate during exercise, performance is not adversely affected. Although there is some evidence that increasing carbohydrate availability causes glycogen sparing in slow-twitch muscle fibres during running, the major mechanisms to explain the benefits of carbohydrate feeding during prolonged exercise are the maintenance of plasma glucose concentration (sustaining brain function) and the provision of an additional carbohydrate supply to allow the muscle to continue high rates of carbohydrate oxidation.

Investigations into different types of carbohydrate show that there are no important differences in the oxidation of moderate to high GI carbohydrate sources consumed during prolonged, moderate-intensity exercise. Carbohydrate consumed during exercise is oxidised in small amounts during the first hour of exercise (~20 g) and thereafter reaches a peak rate of around 1 g/min, at least when a single form of carbohydrate, like glucose, is consumed. However, when multiple forms of carbohydrate which use different transport routes for uptake in the intestines

Table 18.2 Overview of recommendations for various events based on a number of studies reviewed in Jeukendrup *et al.* (2004, 2008)

Event	Choice of carbohydrate			
	Energy expenditure	Carbohydrate required for optimal performance and minimising negative energy balance	Recommended intake	Carbohydrate type
Exercise of <45 min duration	>18 kcal/min	No CHO required	NA	NA
Exercise of 1 h duration	14–18 kcal/min	Very small amounts of CHO	NA	NA
Exercise >2 h Low to moderate intensity	5–7 kcal/min	Small amounts of CHO	Up to 30 g/h	Can be achieved with most forms of CHO
Exercise >2 h Moderate to high intensity	7–10 kcal/min	Moderate amounts of CHO	Up to 60 g/h	Can be achieved with CHO that are rapidly oxidised
Exercise >3 h, Ironman, Tour de France stage races	10–14 kcal/min	Large amounts of CHO	Up to 90 g/h	Can only be achieved by intakes of multiple transportable CHO

NA, not applicable.

are consumed together (e.g. glucose and fructose), higher intakes of carbohydrate intake can lead to higher rates of carbohydrate use by the muscles. In most endurance events a carbohydrate intake of 30–60 g/h, starting well in advance of fatigue/depletion of body carbohydrate stores, will enhance performance. In ultra-endurance events, ingestion of higher rates of carbohydrate mixtures can provide additional fuel and further enhance performance. A recent study showed that ingestion of 90 g/h of glucose plus fructose improved performance more than the ingestion of a similar amount of glucose. The glucose already improved endurance exercise performance compared with placebo. A suggested carbohydrate intake schedule for various events can be found in Table 18.2.

In the world of sport, athletes consume carbohydrate during exercise using a variety of foods and drinks, and a variety of feeding schedules. Sports drinks [commercial solutions providing 4–8% carbohydrate (4–8 g carbohydrate/100 ml), electrolytes and palatable flavours) are particularly valuable since these allow the athlete to replace their fluid and carbohydrate needs simultaneously. Such drinks will be discussed in greater detail in the section below. Each sport or exercise activity offers particular opportunities for fluid and carbohydrate to be consumed throughout the session, whether it be from aid stations, supplies carried by the athlete, or at formal stoppages in play such as time-outs or half-time breaks. The athlete should be creative in making use of these opportunities.

Post-exercise refuelling

Restoration of muscle glycogen concentrations is an important component of post-exercise recovery and is challenging for athletes who train or compete more than once each day. The main dietary issue in refuelling is the amount of carbohydrate consumed, with requirements being within the range of 7–12 g/kg body weight per day, depending on the workload and amount of muscle mass involved. Glycogen storage occurs at a slightly faster rate during the first couple of hours after exercise, but the main reason for encouraging an athlete to consume carbohydrate-rich meals or snacks soon after exercise is that effective refuelling does not start until a substantial amount of carbohydrate (~1 g/kg body weight) is consumed, therefore when there is limited time between workouts or events (e.g. 8 h or less) it makes sense to turn every minute into effective recovery time by consuming carbohydrate as soon as possible after the first session. However, when recovery time is longer, immediate carbohydrate intake after exercise is unnecessary and the athlete can afford to follow their preferred and practical eating schedule as long as goals for total carbohydrate intake are met over the day.

Certain amino acids have a potent effect on the secretion of insulin, which is a stimulator of glycogen resynthesis. For this reason the effects of adding amino acids and proteins to a carbohydrate solution have been investigated. While the evidence that protein–carbohydrate combinations enhance refuelling is unclear, there are other good reasons to provide protein in recovery meals and snacks. The timely intake of a source of high-quality protein after a workout or event will enhance protein synthesis in response to the exercise stimulus. As we will see later, the amount of protein needed is only small (20–25 g). Depending on the type of exercise, this may lead to increases in muscle size and strength (e.g. response to resistance exercise), repair of damaged tissues and increases in functional proteins such as the enzymes and other factors involved in exercise metabolism.

Everyday eating for recovery

Although strategies to promote carbohydrate availability have been shown to enhance performance and recovery after a single bout of exercise, it has been difficult to demonstrate that a long-term period of high-carbohydrate eating will promote better training adaptations and long-term performance than a moderate carbohydrate diet. Theoretically, inadequate carbohydrate intake during repeated days of exercise will lead to gradual depletion of muscle glycogen stores and impairment of exercise endurance. This theory, based on observations of reduced muscle glycogen levels following successive days of running, is summarised in Figure 18.3. Several studies have been undertaken to compare refuelling and performance on high-carbohydrate diets and moderate carbohydrate diets for periods of 7 days to 4 weeks. Although these studies show that high-carbohydrate diets are better at promoting muscle glycogen restoration, superior performance has not been clearly demonstrated. Some scientists have suggested that this means that high-carbohydrate diets are not really needed by endurance athletes. Others feel that the lack of clear evidence is a reflection of problems with the design of the studies, for example not being conducted over sufficient time to see a separation in performance or not having a measurement of performance that is sensitive enough to detect small but real differences.

Figure 18.3 Muscle glycogen concentration after 3 days of hard training with a high-carbohydrate (CHO) or a mixed diet. (JOURNAL OF APPLIED PHYSIOLOGY by DL Costill, R Bowers, G Branam & K Sparks. Copyright © 1971 AMERICAN PHYSIOLOGY SOCIETY. Reproduced with the permission by AMERICAN PHYSIOLOGY SOCIETY in the format Textbook via Copyright Clearance Center.)

A 'hot issue' in sports nutrition is the idea that deliberately training in a low-glycogen or low-carbohydrate environment might enhance the outcomes of a training programme. This is part of a dietary periodisation concept, where the athlete might 'train low' to enhance the effectiveness of their training response then refuel for competition situations ('compete high'). Training with low carbohydrate availability can be achieved by scheduling a second workout soon after a session that reduced muscle glycogen stores or by training after an overnight fast and without any carbohydrate intake during the session. Such training has been shown to enhance the cellular signals that promote the adaptations to an exercise stimulus. Studies of this 'train low' strategy are relatively new. So far, despite reasonably consistent evidence that muscle adaptation can be increased by training in a low glycogen state, there is a lack of evidence that it results in a better performance outcome. In fact, training low reduces the intensity and volume of the workouts that can be performed by the athlete – this is contradictory to the philosophy of optimal training. There may be other disadvantages to forced sessions of low carbohydrate training, such as an increased risk of injury and illness. Further carefully conducted studies are needed. In the meantime, in view of the evidence of the benefits of high carbohydrate availability on acute exercise performance, it is sensible for athletes to employ good fuelling strategies during key phases or sessions of their training programmes, particularly to support high-intensity workouts or events, or during periods of prolonged strenuous training competition.

Dietary guidelines for the general population make recommendations for carbohydrate intake as a percentage of dietary energy intake (e.g. to increase carbohydrate to >55% of total energy intake). Sports nutrition guidelines used to follow this terminology. However, athletes undertaking strenuous exercise have carbohydrate requirements based principally on muscle fuel needs, which are quantifiable according to the size of the athlete and the duration of their exercise programme. It therefore makes sense, and is more practical, to be consist in describing carbohydrate goals in terms of grams per kilogram of the athlete's body weight. This allows the athlete to work out their carbohydrate requirement for a given situation (e.g. 7 g/kg for a 70 kg athlete = 490 g). Meals and menus can then be constructed using information on food labels or in food composition tables to achieve this carbohydrate target. General eating patterns that help the athlete to meet the fuel targets are summarised in Box 18.2.

Box 18.2 Guidelines for meeting the fuel needs of training, competition and recovery

- Set carbohydrate intake targets based on the predicted fuel requirements of workouts, events and recovery. A range of targets has been suggested as a starting point – experiment to find the carbohydrate intake that is consistent with good performance and allows the athletes to meet their energy needs and total nutritional goals.
  - Light exercise programme (low intensity or skill-based exercise) – 3–5 g/kg body mass/day.
  - Moderate exercise programme (e.g. 1 h/day) – 3–5 g/kg/day.
  - Heavy exercise programme (e.g. 1–3 h/day) – 6–10 g/kg/day.
  - Very heavy exercise programme (>4–5 h/day) – 10–12 g/kg/day.
  - Base meals and snacks around nutrient-rich carbohydrate foods so that they can supply additional nutrients while meeting fuel needs: whole-grain breads and breakfast cereals, rice, pasta, noodles and other grain foods, fruits, starchy vegetables (e.g. potatoes, corn), legumes (lentils, beans, soy-based products) and sweetened dairy products (e.g. fruit-flavoured yogurt, fruit smoothies).
- Use sugar and sugar-rich foods as a palatable and compact source of carbohydrate when total fuel needs are high or when this is a more practical way to supply fuel needs. This may be especially important before, during and after exercise.
- Lower fibre choices of carbohydrate-rich foods may also be preferable sources when fuel needs are high or to provide a better tolerated pre-event meal.

- When carbohydrate and energy needs are high, increase the *number* of meals and snacks, rather than the *size* of meals. Be organised to have snacks on hand in a busy day.
- Note that carbohydrate-rich drinks (e.g. fruit juices, soft drinks, fruit/milk smoothies) are also a compact source for special situations or high-carbohydrate diets. This category includes many of the supplements made specially for athletes (e.g. sports drinks, liquid meal supplements, carbohydrate gels, sports bars).
- Fuel up for competition with 24–36 h of exercise taper and high carbohydrate intake (7–12 g/kg per day). Where practical, extend this preparation to 48 or even 72 h, to 'carbohydrate load' in preparation for endurance events (>90 min duration). Specialist dietary advice from a sports dietitian may be needed to achieve high-carbohydrate intake goals.
- Consume carbohydrates during training and competition sessions of greater than 90 min duration, and experiment to see whether this helps during high-intensity sessions of 60 min. Sports drinks will look after fluid and carbohydrate needs simultaneously, being specially designed to deliver these nutrients rapidly. Design a feeding protocol that provides 30–60 g carbohydrate per hour for most events, but be prepared to increase intake to more than 60 g/h for ultra-endurance events. Feeding protocols need to balance the fuel requirements of the event, opportunities to consume carbohydrate-rich foods, drinks and sports products, and the risk of gastrointestinal distress.
- Begin effective recovery of muscle glycogen stores by eating a high-carbohydrate meal or snack providing at least 1 g/kg carbohydrate within 15–30 min of finishing the exercise session. This is important when the schedule calls for rapid recovery between prolonged training sessions (<8 h recovery).
- Combine other foods with carbohydrate-rich choices to provide other needs for recovery, for example carbohydrate-protein combinations include:
  - cereal with milk
  - sandwiches with meat/cheese/dairy fillings
  - sweetened dairy products (e.g. flavoured milk, fruit flavoured yoghurt and milkshakes/fruit smoothies)
  - rice or pasta based main meals
  - pizza with lean meat/cheese topping.

18.4 Fat metabolism and performance

At rest and during exercise skeletal muscle is the main site of oxidation of fatty acids. In resting conditions, and especially after fasting, fatty acids are the predominant fuel used by skeletal muscle. During low-intensity exercise, metabolism is elevated several-fold compared with resting conditions and fat oxidation is increased. When the exercise intensity increases, fat oxidation increases further, until exercise intensities of about 65% $Vo_{2\,max}$, after which a decline in the rate of fat oxidation is observed. In contrast to carbohydrate metabolism, which increases as a function of the aerobic workrate, fat oxidation is reduced at high exercise intensities (Figure 18.2).

Fat oxidation and diet

Diet has marked effects on fat oxidation. In general, a high-carbohydrate, low-fat diet will reduce fat oxidation, whereas a high-fat, low-carbohydrate diet will increase fat oxidation. It might be argued that in most of these studies the effects were seen because of the effects of the last meal, which is known to have a marked effect on substrate utilisation. However, 5 days of a high-fat, low-carbohydrate diet has been shown to retool the muscle and increase fat utilisation during exercise. These changes in substrate use during subsequent exercise are apparently robust, since they persisted even when the fat loading period was followed by a day of high-carbohydrate meals and further carbohydrate intake during exercise. The performance outcomes of such 'fat adaptation' or 'fat loading' protocols will be discussed below, but show that there are chronic effects of diet on substrate use during exercise that cannot directly be explained by immediate substrate availability.

Fat intake during exercise

Long-chain triglycerides

Nutritional fats include triglycerides (containing mostly C16 and C18 fatty acids), phospholipids and cholesterol, of which only triglycerides can contribute to any extent to energy provision during exercise. In contrast to carbohydrates, nutritional fats reach the circulation only slowly since they are potent inhibitors of gastric emptying. Furthermore, the digestion in the gut and absorption of fat are also rather slow processes compared with the digestion and absorption of carbohydrates. Bile salts, produced by the liver, and lipase secreted by the pancreas are needed for the breakdown of the long-chain triglycerides (LCT) into glycerol and three long-chain fatty acids. The fatty acids are then transported in chylomicrons via the lymphatic system, which ultimately drains into the systemic circulation. Long-chain dietary fatty acids typically enter the blood 3–4 h after ingestion.

The fact that these long-chain fatty acids enter the circulation in chylomicrons is also important, and it is generally believed that the rate of breakdown of chylomicron-bound triglycerides by muscle is relatively slow. It has been suggested that the primary role of these triglycerides in chylomicrons is the replenishment of intramuscular fat stores after exercise. The usual advice, therefore, is to reduce the intake of fat during exercise to a minimum. Many 'sports bars' or 'energy bars', however, contain significant amounts of fat and it is therefore advisable to check the food label before choosing an energy bar.

In summary, LCT ingestion during exercise is not desirable because it slows gastric emptying and because the triglycerides only slowly appear in the systemic circulation in chylomicrons, which are believed to be a less important fuel source during exercise.

Medium-chain triglycerides

Medium-chain fatty acids have different properties to long-chain fatty acids and it has been suggested that medium-chain fatty acids could be a useful energy source during exercise. Medium-chain fatty acids contain 8–10 carbons, whereas long-chain fatty acids contain 12 or more carbons. Medium-chain triglycerides (MCT) are more polar and therefore more soluble in water, and they are more rapidly digested and absorbed in the intestine than LCT. Furthermore, medium-chain fatty acids follow the portal venous system and enter the liver directly, while long-chain fatty acids are passed into the systemic circulation slowly via the lymphatic system. MCT is normally present in our diet in very small quantities, with few natural sources. MCT is usually synthesised from coconut oil.

Unlike LCT, MCT are rapidly emptied from the stomach, rapidly absorbed and metabolised, and may be a valuable exogenous energy source during exercise, in addition to carbohydrates. It has been suggested that MCT ingestion may improve exercise performance by elevating plasma fatty acid levels and sparing muscle glycogen. However, the ingestion of 30 g of MCT has no effect on plasma fatty acid concentration, glycogen sparing or exercise performance. Ingestion of larger amounts of MCT is likely to cause gastrointestinal distress and therefore cannot be recommended, therefore MCT do not appear to have the positive effects on performance that are often claimed.

Fasting

Fasting has been proposed as a way to increase fat utilisation, spare muscle glycogen and improve exercise performance. In rats, short-term fasting increases plasma epinephrine (adrenaline) and norepinephrine (noradrenaline) concentrations, stimulates lipolysis and increases the concentration of circulating plasma fatty acids. This, in turn, increases fat oxidation and 'spares' muscle glycogen, leading to a similar, or even increased, running time to exhaustion in rats. In humans, fasting also results in an increased concentration of circulating catecholamines, increased lipolysis, increased concentration of plasma fatty acids and a decreased glucose turnover. Muscle glycogen concentrations, however, are unaffected by fasting for 24h when no strenuous exercise is performed. Although it has been reported that fasting had no effect on endurance capacity at low exercise intensities (45% $Vo_{2\,max}$), performance may be significantly impaired at intensities higher than 50% $Vo_{2\,max}$. The observed decrease in performance was not reversible by carbohydrate ingestion during exercise. Liver glycogen stores will be substantially depleted after a 24h fast and therefore euglycaemia may not be as well maintained during exercise, compromising brain function.

In summary, fasting increases the availability of lipid substrates, resulting in increased oxidation of fatty acids at rest and during exercise. However, since the liver glycogen stores are not maintained, exercise performance is impaired.

High-fat diets

In 1939, Christensen and Hansen demonstrated that a high-fat diet for 3–5 days resulted in impaired exercise capacity. This is likely to be related to the decreased muscle glycogen concentrations that can be expected after a high-fat, low-carbohydrate diet. Fat oxidation increases with such a diet, but this may merely be the result of the lack of availability of carbohydrate as an energy source.

Early studies reported that adaptation to a high-fat diet for 4–6 weeks resulted in increased fat oxidation and a maintenance of endurance capacity. However, these studies are difficult to interpret because of the small subject numbers and the variation in the results.

Nevertheless, it is remarkable that performance was not reduced in all subjects, even though muscle glycogen levels measured before exercise were decreased by almost 50%. In at least some cases it appears that the increased capacity for fat oxidation can compensate for the low availability of muscle glycogen. However, other studies have shown that a fat-adaptation period beyond 4 weeks causes a decrease in subsequent capacity for exercise, which cannot be reversed by a week on a high-carbohydrate diet. These results indicate that the reduction in performance might be caused by an impairment of the adaptations achieved by the training programme.

More recent research has shown that worthwhile adaptations to a high-fat diet occur in as little as 5–6 days, providing a more practical period for undertaking major dietary changes, and perhaps an opportunity to gain benefits without causing long-term inhibition of the training process. This has been investigated in another example of a 'dietary periodisation' strategy, whereby the athlete could adapt to a high-fat diet just prior to an endurance or ultra-endurance event followed by acute carbohydrate feeding strategies in the day prior to, and during, the event. This strategy might induce enzymic adaptations in the muscle to promote the use of fat as an exercise fuel, while also making carbohydrate fuels available. A series of studies has been performed to test this possibility, with cyclists undertaking high volume training while consuming a high-fat diet for a relatively short period (5–6 days), followed by a variety of strategies to restore for a performance test. These studies have shown clear evidence that the fat adaptation strategy enhanced fat use during exercise with a 'sparing' of glycogen use. However, this did not lead to an improvement in endurance or ultra-endurance performance. Further investigation revealed that the fat adaptation protocol down-regulated key pathways for the utilisation of carbohydrate during exercise – impairing rather than sparing utilisation of glycogen stores. In fact, one study reported an impairment of the ability to perform high-intensity exercise, which is reliant on high rates of carbohydrate oxidation. Because the outcome of even prolonged events can be determined by high-intensity exercise (a sprint to the line, a surge up a hill etc.), therefore, fat adaptation strategies cannot be recommended to athletes in conventional sports.

18.5 Effect of exercise on protein requirements

There is still considerable debate about how much dietary protein is required for optimal athletic performance. This interest in protein (meat) probably dates back to Ancient Greece. There are reports that athletes in Ancient Greece, in preparation for the Olympic Games, consumed large amounts of meat. This belief stems partly from the large amount of muscle in the human body (40% of body weight) containing 10–15% of bodyweight in protein. Muscle also accounts for 30–50% of all protein turnover in the body. Both the structural proteins that make up the myofibrillar proteins and the proteins which act as enzymes within a muscle cell change as an adaptation to exercise training. Indeed, muscle mass, muscle protein composition and muscle protein content will change in response to training, therefore it is not surprising that meat has been popular as a protein source for athletes, especially strength athletes.

Non-essential amino acids can be synthesised from essential and non-essential amino acids. This is important in situations with inadequate dietary protein intake. In muscle, the majority of amino acids are incorporated into tissue proteins, with a small pool of free amino acids. This pool undergoes turnover, receiving free amino acids from the breakdown of protein and contributing amino acids for protein synthesis. Protein breakdown in skeletal muscle serves two main purposes:

- to provide essential amino acids when individual amino acids are converted to acetyl-CoA or TCA cycle intermediates
- to provide individual amino acids that can be used elsewhere in the body for the synthesis of neurotransmitters, hormones, glucose and proteins.

Clearly, if protein degradation rates are greater than the rates of synthesis, there will be a reduction in protein content; conversely, muscle protein content can only increase if the rate of synthesis exceeds that of degradation.

Increased protein requirements

Exercise, especially endurance exercise, results in increased oxidation of the branched chain amino acids (BCAA), which are essential amino acids and cannot be synthesised in the body. Increased oxidation would imply that the dietary protein requirements are increased. Some studies in which the nitrogen balance technique was used showed that the dietary protein requirements for athletes involved in prolonged endurance training were higher than those for sedentary individuals. However, these results have been questioned.

It has been estimated that protein may contribute up to about 15% to energy expenditure in resting conditions. During exercise this relative contribution is likely to decrease because energy expenditure is increased and most of this energy is provided by carbohydrate and fat. During very prolonged exercise, when carbohydrate availability becomes limited, the contribution of protein to energy expenditure may amount up to about 10% of total energy expenditure. Thus, although protein oxidation is increased during endurance exercise, the relative contribution of protein to energy expenditure remains small. Protein requirements may be increased somewhat, but this increased need may be met easily by a moderate protein intake. The research groups that advocate an increased protein intake for endurance athletes in heavy training usually recommend a daily intake of 1.2–1.8 g/kg body weight. This is about twice the level of protein intake that is recommended for sedentary populations.

There are reports of increased protein breakdown after resistance exercise. The suggested increased dietary protein requirements with resistance training are related to increased muscle bulk (hypertrophy) rather than increased oxidation of amino acids. Muscle protein breakdown is increased after resistance training, but to a smaller degree than muscle protein synthesis. The elevations in protein degradation and synthesis are transient. Protein breakdown and synthesis after exercise are elevated at 3 and 24 h after exercise, but return to baseline levels after 48 h. These results seem to apply to resistance exercise and high-intensity dynamic exercise.

There is controversy as to whether strength athletes really need to eat large amounts of protein. The nitrogen balance studies that have been conducted on such athletes have been criticised because they generally have been of short duration and a steady-state situation may not be established. The recommendation for protein intakes for strength athletes is therefore generally 1.6–1.7 g/kg body weight per day. Again this seems to be met easily with a normal diet and no extra attention to protein intake is needed. Protein supplements are often used, but are not necessary to meet the recommended protein intake.

Timing of protein intake

Although athletes have long been focused on the importance of the amount of protein in their diets, recent studies using techniques to monitor changes in protein synthesis in response to training have found that the timing of intake of protein in relation to a training session is probably more important. A bout of exercise stimulates an increase in protein synthesis during the recovery period, with an increase in the manufacture of various protein subfractions responding to the type of exercise stimulus (e.g. endurance, resistance or interval training). The provision of a source of essential amino acids during the recovery period enhances the net gain of such protein subfractions. There is still much work to be done to develop our understanding of optimal feeding for the protein response to exercise – that is, optimal amounts, types and timing of protein-rich sources. However, our present understanding is that maximal adaptation occurs when relatively small amounts of high-quality protein are consumed (e.g. 20–25 g protein, providing 6–8 g of essential amino acids). There are a range of food combinations that would allow an athlete to consume high protein in combination with carbohydrate to achieve recovery goals for refuelling and protein synthesis simultaneously. These are included in Box 18.2

18.6 Physique and sports performance

Physical characteristics, such as height, body weight, muscle mass and body fat levels, can all play a role in the performance of sport. An athlete's physique is determined by inherited characteristics, as well as the conditioning effects of their training programme and diet. Often, 'ideal' physiques for individual sports are set, based on a rigid set of characteristics of successful athletes. However, this process fails to take into account that there is considerable variability in the physical characteristics of sports people, even between elite athletes in the same sport. It is therefore dangerous to establish rigid prescriptions for individuals, particularly with regard to body composition. Instead, it is preferable to nominate a range of acceptable

values for body fat and body weight within each sport, and then monitor the health and performance of individual athletes within this range. These values may change over the athlete's career.

Some athletes easily achieve the body composition suited to their sport. However, others may need to manipulate characteristics such as muscle mass or body fat levels through changes in diet and training. It is important for an athlete to identify a suitable and realistic body-fat goal, and to achieve this desired change in a suitable period using sensible methods. Descriptions of the various methods of body composition assessment are found elsewhere in this text. For athletes, the criteria for choosing a certain technique should include the validity, reliability and sensitivity of the method. Some methods are best suited to laboratory studies, while methods that are accessible and inexpensive can be used in the field by athletes and coaches. In practice, useful information about body composition can be collected from anthropometric data such as skinfold (subcutaneous) fat measurements, and various body girths and circumferences. Coaches or sports scientists who make these assessments on athletes should be well trained so that they have a small degree of error in repeating measurements. Regular monitoring of the body composition of an athlete can determine their individual 'ideal' physique at different times of the training and competition calendar. It can also monitor their success in achieving these ideals.

18.7 Weight maintenance and other body-weight issues

Losing weight

Many sports dieticians note that losing body weight or, more precisely, losing body fat, is the most common reason for an athlete to seek nutrition counselling. A small body size is useful to reduce the energy cost of activity, to improve temperature regulation in hot conditions and to allow mobility to undertake twists and turns in a confined space. This physique is characteristic of athletes such as gymnasts, divers and marathon runners. A low level of body fat enhances the power to weight ratio over a range of body sizes, and is a desirable characteristic of many sports that require weight-bearing movement, particularly against gravity (e.g. distance running, mountain biking and uphill cycling, jumps and hurdles). However, low body-fat levels are also important for aesthetic sports such as diving, gymnastics and figure skating, where judging involves appearance as well as skill.

There are many common situations in which an athlete's body-fat level increases above their healthy or ideal range. A common example is the athlete who comes back from an injury or a break from training several kilograms of body fat in excess of their usual competing weight. Where it is warranted, loss of body fat by an athlete should be achieved by a gradual programme of sustained and moderate energy deficit, achieved by a decrease in dietary energy intake and, perhaps, an increase in energy expenditure through aerobic exercise or activity (see Box 18.3). However, many athletes in weight- or fat-conscious sports strive to achieve very low body-fat levels or to reduce body-fat levels below what seems to be their natural or healthy level. Although weight-loss efforts often produce a short-term improvement in performance, this must be balanced against the disadvantages related to having very low body-fat stores or following unsafe weight-loss methods. Excessive training, chronic low energy and nutrient intake, and psychological distress are often involved in fat-loss strategies and may cause long-term damage to health, happiness or performance. We now realise that periods of low energy availability – where total daily intake of energy is below the level needed to cover both the energy cost of training/competition and requirements for full health/function – impair bone health, reproductive health and other body functions.

Athletes should be encouraged to set realistic goals for body weight and body fat. These are specific to each individual and must be judged by trial and error over a period of time. 'Ideal' weight and body-fat targets should be set in terms of ranges, and should consider measures of long-term health and performance rather than short-term benefits alone. In addition, athletes should be able to achieve their targets while eating a diet that is adequate in energy and nutrients, and free of unreasonable food-related stress. Some racial groups or individuals naturally carry very low levels of body fat or can achieve these without paying a substantial penalty. Furthermore, some athletes vary their body-fat levels over a season, so that very low levels are achieved only for a specific and short time. In general, however, athletes should not undertake strategies to minimise body-fat levels unless they

---

Box 18.3 Strategies for eating to lose body fat

- Identify individual 'ideal' body-fat and body weight targets that are consistent with good health and performance, and are achievable.
- If loss of body fat is required, plan for a realistic rate loss of about 0.5 kg/week, and set both short-term and long-term goals.
- Examine current exercise and activity plans. If training is primarily skill or technique based, or a sedentary lifestyle between training sessions is observed, the athlete may benefit from scheduling in some aerobic exercise activities. This should always be done in conjunction with the coach.
- Take an objective look at what the athlete is really eating by arranging to keep a food diary for a period (e.g. a week). Many athletes who feel that they 'hardly eat anything' will be amazed at their hidden eating activities.
- Reduce typical energy intake by an amount that is appropriate to produce loss of body fat (e.g. 2–4 MJ or 500–1000 kcal/day) but still ensures adequate food and nutrient intake. An athlete should not reduce their energy intake below 5–6 MJ or 1200–1500 kcal/day unless supervised by a sports dietitian. Meals should not be skipped, rather food should be spread over the day, particularly to allow for efficient refuelling after training sessions.
- Target occasions of overeating for special attention. Useful techniques include making meals filling by choosing high-fibre and low glycaemic index forms of foods, fighting the need to finish everything on the plate and spreading food intake over the day so that there is no need to approach meals feeling extreme hunger.
- Focus on opportunities to reduce intake of fats and oils. Such strategies include choosing low-fat versions of nutritious protein foods, minimising added fats and oils in cooking and food preparation, and enjoying high-fat snack and sweet foods as occasional treats rather than everyday foods.
- Be moderate with alcohol intake (and perhaps sugar), since these may represent 'empty' kilojoules. Since alcohol intake is associated with relaxation, it is often associated with unwise eating.
- Focus on nutrient-rich foods so that nutrient needs can be met from a lower energy intake. A broad-range, low-dose vitamin/mineral supplement should be considered if daily energy intake is to be restricted below 6 MJ or 1500 kcal for prolonged periods.
- Be aware of inappropriate eating behaviour. This includes eating when bored or upset, or eating too quickly. Stress or boredom should be handled using alternative activities.
- Be wary of supplements that promise weight loss. There are no special pills, potions or products that produce safe and effective weight loss. If something sounds too good to be true, it probably is.
- Note that a sports dietitian can assist athletes who are having difficulties with weight-loss goals or would like a supervised programme. Expert advice is needed for those who are struggling with an eating disorder or disordered eating behaviour.

can be sure there are no side-effects or disadvantages. Most importantly, the low body-fat levels of elite athletes should not be considered natural or necessary for recreational and subelite performers.

It is suggested that there is a higher risk of eating disorders, or disordered eating behaviours and body perceptions, among athletes in weight-division sports or sports in which success is associated with lower body-fat levels than might be expected in the general community. Females seem at greater risk than males, reflecting the general dissatisfaction of females in the community with their body shape, as well as the biological predisposition for female athletes to have higher body-fat levels than male athletes, despite undertaking the same training programme. Even where clinical eating disorders do not exist, many athletes appear to be restrained eaters, reporting energy intakes that are considerably less than their expected energy requirements. An adequate intake of energy is a prerequisite for many of the goals of sports nutrition.

Recently, the female athlete triad, the coexistence of disordered eating, disturbed menstrual function and suboptimal bone density, has received considerable publicity. This will be discussed in greater detail in the section below. Expert advice from sports medicine professionals, including dieticians, psychologists and physicians, is important in the early detection and management of problems related to body composition and nutrition.

Making weight

Some sports involve weight divisions in competition, with the goal of matching opponents of equal size and strength. Examples include combative sports (boxing, judo and wrestling), light-weight rowing and weight-lifting. Unfortunately, the culture and common practice in these sports is to try to compete in a weight division that is considerably lighter than normal training body weight. Athletes then 'make weight' over the days before the competition by dehydrating (via saunas, exercising in 'sweat clothes' and diuretics), and restricting food and fluid intake. The short-term penalties of these behaviours include the effect of dehydration and inadequate fuel status on performance. Long-term penalties include psychological stress, chronic inadequate nutrition and effects on hormone status. In 1997 three deaths were recorded among college wrestlers in the USA as a result of severe weight-making practices. Athletes in

these sports should be guided to make better choice of the appropriate competition weight division and to achieve necessary weight loss by safe and long-term strategies to reduce body-fat levels.

Gaining muscle mass

Gain of muscle mass is desired by many athletes whose performance is linked to size, strength or power. Increases in muscle mass and strength occur during adolescence, particularly in males. In addition, many athletes pursue specific muscle hypertrophy gains through a programme of progressive muscle overload. The main nutritional requirement for gain of muscle mass while undertaking a strength-training programme is additional energy intake. This is required for the manufacture of new muscle tissue and other tissues needed to support it, as well as to provide fuel for the training programme that supplied the stimulus for this muscle growth. Many athletes do not achieve an adequate energy intake to support these goals. Box 18.4 provides some practical strategies to address this challenge.

18.8 Vitamins and minerals

The daily requirement for at least some vitamins and minerals is increased beyond population levels in people undertaking a strenuous exercise programme. The potential reasons for this increased requirement are increased loss through sweat, urine and perhaps faeces, and through increased production of free radicals. Unfortunately, at present the additional micronutrient requirements of athletes cannot be quantified. The key factors ensuring an adequate intake of vitamins and minerals are a moderate to high energy intake and a varied diet based on nutritious foods. Dietary surveys show that most athletes report dietary practices that easily supply vitamins and minerals in excess of recommended daily allowances (RDAs) and are likely to meet any increases in micronutrient demand caused by training. However, not all athletes eat varied diets of adequate energy intake and some may need help to improve both the quality and quantity of their food selections.

Studies of the micronutrient status of athletes have not revealed any significant differences between indices in athletes and sedentary controls. The results suggest

> **Box 18.4 Strategies for eating to increase muscle mass**
>
> - Ensure that the athlete is following a well-devised weight training programme that will stimulate muscle development and growth.
> - Set goals for weight and strength gain that are practical and achievable. Continued increases of 2–4 kg/month are generally considered a good return.
> - Be organised: apply the same dedication to the eating programme as is applied to training in order to increase the intake of nutrient-dense foods and supply a daily energy surplus of approximately 2–4 MJ (500–1000 kcal). This additional food should supply carbohydrate to fuel the training sessions, and adequate protein and micronutrients for the development and support of new tissue.
> - Be particularly vigilant to have appropriate foods and drinks available for recovery eating after workouts, supplying protein and carbohydrate needs for refuelling. This will provide additional energy over the day as well as promoting more effective recovery and adaptation following the exercise stimulus.
> - Increase the number of times that atheletes eat rather than the size of meals. This will enable greater intake of food with less risk of 'overfilling' and gastrointestinal discomfort.
> - Avoid excessive intake of fibre and include the use of 'white' cereals with less bulk (e.g. white rice, white bread). It is often impractical to consume a diet that is solely based on wholegrain and high-fibre foods.
> - Make use of high-energy fluids such as milkshakes, fruit smoothies or commercial liquid meal supplements. These drinks provide a compact and low-bulk source of energy and nutrients, and can be consumed with meals or as snacks, including before or after a training session.
> - Be aware that many athletes do not eat as much – or more importantly, as often – as they think. It is useful to examine the actual intake of athletes who fail to gain weight yet report 'constant eating'. Commitments such as training, sleep, medical/physiotherapy appointments, work or school often get in the way of eating opportunities. A food record will identify the hours and occasions of minimal food intake. This information should be used to reorganise the day or to find creative ways to make nutritious foods and drinks part of the activity.

that athletic training, *per se*, does not lead to micronutrient deficiency. These data should, however, be interpreted very carefully since most indices are not sensitive enough to detect marginal deficiencies. Overall, generalised vitamin and mineral supplementation for all athletes is not justified. Furthermore, studies do not support an increase in performance with such supplementation, except in the case where a pre-existing deficiency was corrected.

The best management for the athlete with a high risk of suboptimal intake of micronutrients is to provide nutrition education to improve their food intake.

However, a low-dose, broad-range multivitamin/mineral supplement may be useful where the athlete is unwilling or unable to make dietary changes, or when the athlete is travelling to places with an uncertain food supply and eating schedule.

Antioxidant vitamins

Exercise has been linked with an increased production of free oxygen radical species capable of causing cellular damage. A sudden increase in training stress (such as an increase in volume or intensity) or a stressful environment (e.g. training in hot conditions or at altitude) is believed to increase the production of these free oxygen radicals, leading to an increase in markers of cellular damage. Supplementation with antioxidant vitamins such as vitamin C or vitamin E has been suggested to increase antioxidant status and provide protection against this damage.

The literature on the effects of antioxidant supplementation on antioxidant status, cellular damage and performance is complex and confusing. Some, but not all, studies show that acute supplementation during periods of increased stress may provide bridging protection until the athlete is able to adapt his or her own antioxidant status to meet this stress. It is possible that subtle benefits occur at a cellular level but these are too small to translate into detectable performance outcomes. On the other hand, new research that shows that oxidative reactions provide a useful role in signalling the adaptations to an exercise stimulus. Antioxidant supplementation may therefore be harmful to the process of adaptation to exercise if it reduces the signalling stimulus. Again, any reduction in the training response may be too small to detect. At the present time it is unwise to make recommendations about whether antioxidant supplementation is useful or harmful. A more valuable approach may be to increase the antioxidant content of the diet by eating plenty of fruits, vegetables and wholegrain cereals. This way an increase in a range of antioxidants and plant phytochemicals can be achieved rather than upsetting the delicate balance of the body's antioxidant system by supplementing with large amount of a few compounds.

Iron

Minerals are the micronutrients at most risk of inadequate intake in the diets of athletes. Inadequate iron status can reduce exercise performance via suboptimal levels of haemoglobin, and perhaps iron-related muscle enzymes. Reductions in the haemoglobin levels of distance runners first alerted sports scientists to the issue of iron status of athletes. However, more recent research has raised the problem of distinguishing true iron deficiency from alterations in iron status measures that are caused by exercise itself. Low iron status in athletes is overdiagnosed from single measures of low haemoglobin and ferritin levels. A major problem is the failure to recognise that the increase in blood volume that accompanies training will cause a dilution of all the blood contents. This haemodilution, often termed sports anaemia, does not impair exercise performance.

Nevertheless, some athletes are at true risk of becoming iron deficient. The causes are essentially the same as for members of the general community: a lower than desirable intake of bioavailable iron and/or increased iron requirements or losses. Iron requirements may be increased in some athletes owing to growth needs or to increased losses of blood and red blood cell destruction. However, the most common risk factor among athletes is a low-energy and/or low-iron diet, with females, restricted eaters, vegetarians and athletes eating high-carbohydrate, low-meat diets being likely targets.

Iron is found in a range of plant and animal food sources in two forms. Haeme iron is found only in animal foods containing flesh or blood, whereas organic iron is found both in animal foods and plant foods. Whereas haeme iron is relatively well absorbed from single foods and mixed meals (15–35% bioavailability), the absorption of non-haeme iron from single plant sources is low and variable (2–8%). The bioavailability of non-haeme iron, and to a lesser extent haeme ion, is affected by other foods consumed in the same meal. Factors that enhance iron absorption include vitamin C, peptides from fish, meat/and chicken, alcohol and food acids, while factors that inhibit absorption include phytates, polyphenols, calcium and peptides from plant sources such as soy protein. The absorption of both haeme and non-haeme iron is increased as an adaptive response in people who are iron deficient or have increased iron requirements. While the iron bioavailability studies from which these observations have been made have not been undertaken on special groups such as athletes, it is generally assumed that the results can be applied across populations of healthy people.

The assessment of total dietary iron intake of athletes is not necessarily a good predictor of their iron status; the mixing and matching of foods at meals plays an important role by determining the bioavailability of dietary iron intake. For example, in two groups of female runners who reported similar intakes of total dietary iron, the group that reported regular intake of meat was estimated to have a greater intake of absorbable iron and showed higher iron status than a matched group of runners who ate meat only occasionally.

Low iron status, indicated by serum ferritin levels lower than 20 ng/ml, should be considered for further assessment and treatment. Present evidence does not support the belief that low iron status without anaemia reduces exercise performance. However, many athletes with such low iron stores, or a sudden drop in iron status, frequently complain of fatigue and an inability to recover after heavy training. Many of these respond to strategies that improve iron status or prevent a further decrease in iron stores.

Evaluation and management of iron status should be undertaken on an individual basis by a sports medicine expert. Prevention and treatment of iron deficiency may include iron supplementation, with a recommended therapeutic dose of 100 mg/day of elemental iron for 2–3 months. However, the management plan should include dietary counselling to increase the intake of bioavailable iron and appropriate strategies to reduce any unwarranted iron loss. Many athletes self-prescribe iron supplements, indeed mass supplementation of athletes with iron has been fashionable at various times. However, these practices do not provide the athlete with the opportunity for adequate assessment of iron losses and expert dietary counselling from a sports dietitian. A dietary guideline for increasing iron intake should be integrated with the athlete's other nutritional goals, such as a need for high carbohydrate intake or reduced energy intake (Box 18.5).

Calcium

Weight-bearing exercise is considered to be one of the best protectors of bone health, therefore it is puzzling to find reports of low body density in some female athletes, notably distance runners. However, a serious outcome of menstrual disturbances in female

Box 18.5 Strategies to meet iron and calcium needs

- Include haeme iron-rich foods (red meats, shellfish, liver) regularly in meals, at least three to five times per week. These can be added to a high-carbohydrate meal (e.g. meat sauce on a pasta dish, liver pâté in a sandwich).
- Enhance the absorption of non-haeme iron (found in wholegrains, cereal foods, eggs, leafy green vegetables, etc.) by including a vitamin C food or meat/fish/chicken at the same meal. For example, a glass of orange juice may be consumed with breakfast cereal or a small amount of lean meat can be added to beans to make a chilli con carne.
- Be aware that some foods (excess bran, strongly brewed tea) interfere with iron absorption from non-haeme iron foods. Athletes who are at risk of iron deficiency should avoid these items or separate them from meals.
- Take iron supplements only on the advice of a sports dietitian or doctor. They may be useful in the supervised treatment and prevention of iron deficiency, but are not a substitute for dietary improvements.
- Eat at least three servings of dairy foods a day, where one serving is equal to 200 ml of milk or a 200-g carton of yogurt. Low-fat and reduced-fat types are available. Dairy products can be added to a high-carbohydrate meal (e.g. milk on breakfast cereal, cheese in a sandwich).
- Use fortified soy products (soy milk, yogurts) when the athlete is unable to eat dairy products.
- Allow extra calcium for athletes who are growing, having a baby or breast-feeding. Dairy intake should be increased to four or five servings a day. Female athletes who are not having regular menstrual cycles also require extra calcium and should seek expert advice from a sports physician.
- Note that fish eaten with its bones (e.g. tinned salmon, sardines) is also a useful calcium source and can also accompany a high-carbohydrate meal (e.g. salmon casserole with rice).
- Athletes who are vegetarian, or unable to eat dairy or soy products and red meat in these amounts, should seek the advice of a sports dietitian. With assistance they may find creative ways to use other foods to meet iron and calcium needs, or to use mineral supplements correctly.

athletes is the high risk of either direct loss of bone density or failure to optimise the gaining of peak bone mass during early adulthood. Individually or in combination, the problems involved in the female athlete triad (disordered eating, menstrual dysfunction and reduced bone status) can directly impair athletic performance. Significantly, they will reduce the athlete's career span by increasing their risk of illness and injury, including stress fractures. Long-term problems may include an increased risk of osteoporosis in later life.

Optimal nutrition is important to correct factors that underpin the menstrual dysfunction, as well as those that contribute to suboptimal bone density. Adequate energy intake and the reversal of disordered eating or inadequate nutrient intake are important. A team approach involving a sports physician, sports dietician, psychologist and/or psychiatrist, a coach and the family may be needed to treat the athlete with disordered eating or eating disorders.

Adequate calcium intake is important for bone health and requirements may be increased to 1200–1500 mg/day in athletes with impaired menstrual function. Again, strategies to meet calcium needs must be integrated into the total nutrition goals of the athlete. Where adequate calcium intake cannot be met through dietary means, usually through the use of low-fat dairy foods or calcium-enriched soy alternatives, a calcium supplement may be considered (see Box 18.5).

18.9 Fluid and electrolyte loss and replacement in exercise

Water has many important functions in the human body. Approximately 55–60% of the body is comprised of water. The total water content of the human body is between 30 and 50 l. Every day we excrete water (sweat, urine, evaporative losses), while water intake may vary from 1 l to about 12 l per day. Water turnover can be very high in some conditions, but the total body water content is remarkably constant and rarely exceeds variations of 1 l. However, during exercise and especially during exercise in hot conditions, sweat rates (and thus water losses) may increase dramatically and dehydration may occur (i.e. the body is in negative fluid balance). Dehydration can have an enormous impact on physical and mental function, and increases the risk of heat illness. Even mild dehydration can result in reduced exercise capacity.

Fluid losses

Exercise (muscle contraction) causes an increase in heat production in the body. Muscle contraction during most activities is only about 15–20% efficient. This means that of all the energy produced only about 15–20% is used for the actual movement and the remainder is lost as heat. For every litre of oxygen consumed during exercise approximately 16 kJ of heat is produced and only 4 kJ is actually used to perform mechanical work. If this heat was not dissipated the body would soon overheat.

When a well-trained individual is exercising at 80–90% $Vo_{2\,max}$, the body's heat production may be more than 1000 W (i.e. 3.6 MJ/h). This could potentially cause the body core temperature to increase by 1°C every 5–8 min if no heat could be dissipated. As a result, body core temperature could approach dangerous levels in less than 20 min.

There are several mechanisms to dissipate this heat and to maintain body core temperature in a relatively narrow range: 36–38°C in resting conditions and 38–40°C during exercise and hot conditions. The most important cooling mechanism of the body is sweating, although radiation and convection can also contribute. Sweat must evaporate from the body surface to exert a cooling effect. Evaporation of 1 l of water from the skin will remove 2.4 MJ of heat from the body. Although sweating is a very effective way to dissipate heat, it may cause dehydration if sweat losses are not replenished. This may cause further problems for the athlete: progressive dehydration impairs the ability to sweat and, therefore, to regulate body temperature. Body temperature rises more rapidly in the dehydrated state and this is commonly accompanied by a higher heart rate during exercise.

Fluid losses are mainly dependent on three factors:

- the ambient environmental conditions (temperature, humidity)
- the exercise intensity
- the duration of exercise and the duration of the heat exposure.

The environmental heat stress is determined by the ambient temperature, relative humidity, wind velocity and solar radiation. The relative humidity is the most important of these factors, since a high humidity will severely compromise the evaporative loss of sweat. Often sweat will drip off the skin in such conditions, rather than evaporate. This means that heat loss via this route will be less effective.

It is important to note that problems of hyperthermia and heat injury are not restricted to prolonged exercise in a hot environment: heat production is directly proportional to exercise intensity, so very strenuous exercise, even in a cool environment, can cause a substantial rise in body temperature.

To maintain water balance, fluid intake must compensate for the fluid loss that occurs during exercise. Fluid intake is usually dependent on thirst feelings, but thirst (or the lack of thirst) can also be overridden by conscious control. It is important to note, however, that thirst is a poor indicator of fluid requirements or the degree of dehydration. In general, the sensation of feeling thirsty is not perceived until a person has lost at least 2% of body mass. As already mentioned, even this mild degree of dehydration is sufficient to impair exercise performance. It has also been shown that athletes tend to drink too little even when sufficient fluid is available.

Effects of dehydration

As the body becomes progressively dehydrated, a reduction in skin blood flow and sweat rate may occur. A high humidity may limit evaporative sweat loss, which will lead to further rises in core temperature, resulting in fatigue and possible heat injury to body tissues. The latter is potentially fatal.

Effect of dehydration on exercise performance

Several studies have shown that mild dehydration, equivalent to the loss of only 2% body weight, is sufficient to impair exercise performance significantly. In addition, it is often reported that losses of 4–5% of body weight or more can decrease the capacity for work by 20–30% (Figure 18.4). Even very low-intensity exercise (i.e. walking) is affected by dehydration. The capacity to perform high-intensity exercise which results in exhaustion within only a few minutes has been shown to be reduced by as much as 45% by prior dehydration (2.5% of body weight). Although there is little opportunity for sweat loss during such short-duration, high-intensity events, athletes who travel to compete in hot climates are likely to experience acute dehydration, which can persist for several days and can be of sufficient magnitude to have a detrimental effect on performance in competition. Although dehydration has detrimental effects, especially on performance in hot conditions, such effects can also be observed in cool conditions. Both decreases in maximal aerobic power ($Vo_{2\,max}$) and decreases in endurance capacity have been reported with dehydration in temperate conditions.

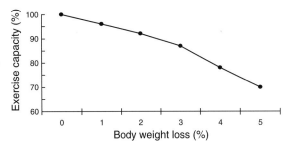

Figure 18.4 Effect of dehydration on exercise capacity.

There are several reasons why dehydration results in decreased exercise performance. First of all, a fall in plasma volume, decreased blood volume, increased blood viscosity and a lower central venous pressure can result in a reduced stroke volume and maximal cardiac output. In addition, during exercise in the heat, the dilatation of the skin blood vessels reduces the proportion of the cardiac output that is devoted to perfusion of the working muscles. Dehydration also impairs the ability of the body to lose heat. Both sweat rate and skin blood flow are lower at the same core temperature for the dehydrated compared with the euhydrated state. This means that body temperature rises more rapidly during exercise when the body is dehydrated. Finally, the larger rise in core temperature during exercise in the dehydrated state is associated with an increased rate of muscle glycogen breakdown. Depletion of these stores could also result in premature fatigue during prolonged exercise. In addition to the effects of dehydration on endurance, there are reported negative effects on coordination and cognitive functioning. This is likely to impact on all sports where skill and decision making are involved.

Heat illness

Dehydration poses a serious health risk in that it increases the risk of cramps, heat exhaustion and life-threatening heat stroke. Early symptoms of heat injury are excessive sweating, headache, nausea, dizziness, and reduced consciousness and mental function. When the core temperature rises to over 40°C, heat stroke may develop, characterised by hot, dry skin, confusion and loss of consciousness. There are several anecdotal reports of athletes and army recruits dying because of heat stroke. Most of these deaths have been explained by exercise in hot conditions,

often with insufficient fluid intake. These problems affect not only highly trained athletes, but also less well-trained people participating in sport. Although well-trained individuals will generally exercise at higher intensities and therefore produce more heat, less well-trained individuals have less effective thermoregulation during exercise and work less economically. Overweight, unacclimated and ill individuals are especially likely to develop heat stroke.

Box 18.6 provides some drinking strategies for exercise in hot environments.

Hyponatraemia

An electrolyte imbalance commonly referred to as hyponatraemia (low plasma sodium) or 'water intoxication' has occasionally been reported in endurance athletes due to excessive intake of fluid before and during an event. This appears to be most common among slow runners in marathon and ultra-marathon races who are able to drink at rates that are far greater than their sweat losses. High losses of sodium in sweat may add to this problem. The symptoms of hyponatraemia are similar to those associated with dehydration, and include mental confusion, weakness and fainting. Hyponatraemia can be fatal and has caused several deaths in marathons and ultra-endurance events. It is an avoidable problem if athletes are aware of their fluid requirements during sport and have a well-practised drinking plan that replaces most of, but not more than, their sweat losses during the session. There is also a danger of misdiagnosis of this condition when it occurs in individuals participating in sporting events. The usual treatment for dehydration is administration of fluid intravenously and orally. If this treatment were to be given to a hyponatraemic individual, the consequences could be fatal.

Fluid intake strategies

Fluid intake during exercise can help to maintain plasma volume and prevent the adverse effects of dehydration on muscle strength, endurance and coordination. When there is only little time in between two exercise bouts, rapid rehydration is crucial and drinking regimens need to be employed to optimise fluid delivery. Strategies for fluid replacement before, during and after exercise will be discussed in the following sections.

Box 18.6 Drinking strategies for exercise

- Be aware of factors that can affect heat accumulation during training or competition: time of day, duration and intensity of exercise, environmental conditions or the conditions in indoor venues, the suitability of uniforms or protective gear. It may be possible to adjust some of these factors if an unacceptable head load is anticipated.
- Begin the event properly hydrated. Fluid losses from previous events or training sessions need to be restored. Fluids should be included in the pre-event meal and during/after the warmp up, with the volume and timing of intake being chosen to allow time for excess fluid to be urinated before the start of the event.
- Gain an appreciation of typical sweat losses during workouts and events by monitoring weight loss over the session. Typically, a kilogram of fluid loss is equivalent to a fluid deficit of 1 l. If possible and practical, fluid intake during a session should keep the total fluid deficit to less than 2% of body mass. It may take practice and creativity to develop drinking practices that achieve this goal. Athletes should practice drinking strategies in training so that they can implement them successfully in competition.
- Make good use of the availability of fluids (e.g. access to aid stations, use of trainers) and the opportunities to drink (e.g. half-time, time outs, injury breaks) that occur in each specific sporting activity or exercise environment. These will allow each athlete to develop their own drinking plan. Generally it is best for fluid intake to occur early and regularly during the exercise to prevent a large fluid deficit from occurring.
- Do not drink at a rate that exceeds sweating rates so that weight is gained over the session. Excessive overhydration can cause the potentially fatal condition of hyponatraemia.
- Note that the voluntary intake of drinks that provide flavour, sweetness and salt is greater than that of plain water. Sports drinks can meet several goals of sports nutrition, since they supply fuel as well as assisting hydration needs. Cool fluids will also be appealing in warm conditions.
- Rehydrate after the session, knowing that most exercise situations will result in a fluid deficit (sweat losses are greater than fluid intake). An intake of fluid equal to 125–150% of the fluid deficit over the hours after exercise will be needed to accommodate further fluid losses (urine and sweat losses) and fully restore hydration levels. A plan of intake is useful when the fluid deficit exceeds 2% body mass since thirst may not cover immediate fluid needs.
  Promote fluid retention and overall fluid restoration by replacing the salt lost in sweat. This can be achieved by drinking salt-containing fluids (oral rehydration solutions or high-salt sports drinks developed for endurance sports) or by consuming salt-rich meals and foods at the same time as fluids. Avoid excessive intake of alcohol since it increases urine losses and interferes with rehydration.

Fluid intake during exercise

To avoid dehydration during prolonged exercise fluids must be consumed to match the sweat losses. By regularly measuring body weight before and after a training session it is possible to obtain a good indication of fluid loss. Ideally, the weight loss is compensated by a similar amount of fluid intake. However, it may not always be possible or necessary to prevent dehydration completely.

Sweat rates during strenuous exercise in the heat can amount up to 2–3 l/h. Such large volumes of fluid are difficult if not impossible to ingest without causing gastrointestinal discomfort, therefore it is often not practically possible to achieve fluid intakes that match sweat losses during exercise. Another factor that can make the ingestion of large amounts of fluid difficult is the fact that in some sports or disciplines the rules or practicalities of the specific sport may limit the opportunities for drinking during exercise.

Fluid intake may be useful during exercise longer than 30–60 min, but there is no advantage during strenuous exercise of less than 30 min in duration. During such high-intensity exercise gastric emptying is inhibited and the drink may cause gastrointestinal distress with no performance benefit.

Practice drinking during training

Although it is often difficult to tolerate the volumes of fluid needed to prevent dehydration, the volume of fluid that is tolerable is trainable and can be increased with frequent drinking in training. Often this is neglected during training. Training to drink will accustom athletes to the feeling of exercising with fluid in the stomach. It also gives the opportunity to experiment with different volumes and flavourings to determine how much fluid intake they can tolerate and which formulations suit them best.

Composition of sports drinks

Numerous studies have shown that regular water intake during prolonged exercise is effective in improving performance. Fluid intake during prolonged exercise also offers the opportunity to provide some fuel (carbohydrate). The addition of some carbohydrate to drinks consumed during exercise has been shown to have an additive independent effect in improving exercise performance (Figure 18.5). The ideal drink for fluid and energy replacement during exercise is one that tastes good to the athlete, does not

Small fluid

Small fluid + CHO

Large fluid

Large fluid + CHO

Time to complete the time trial (min)

Mean values ± SEM (n = 8)

Figure 18.5 The effect of carbohydrate (CHO) and fluid intake during exercise is additive. Subjects performed steady-state exercise followed by a performance measurement (time trial). The shorter the time to complete the time trial, the better the performance. They ingested a small amount of fluid (no carbohydrate), a small amount of fluid plus carbohydrate, a large amount of fluid with no carbohydrate, or a large amount of fluid with carbohydrate. (Reproduced with permission from Below PR, Mora-Rodriguez R, Gonzáles Alonso J, Coyle EF. Fluid and carbohydrate ingestion independently improve performance during 1 h of intense exercise. J. Med Sci Sports Exerc 1995; 27(2): 200–210.)

cause gastrointestinal discomfort when consumed in large volumes, is rapidly emptied from the stomach and absorbed in the intestine, and provides energy in the form of carbohydrate.

Sports drinks typically have three main ingredients: water, carbohydrate and sodium. The water and carbohydrate provide fluid and energy, respectively, while sodium is included to aid water absorption and retention.

Although carbohydrate is important, a too-concentrated carbohydrate solution may provide more fuel for the working muscles but will decrease the amount of water that can be absorbed owing to a slowing of gastric emptying. Water is absorbed into the body primarily through the small intestine, but the absorption of water is decreased if the concentration of dissolved carbohydrate (or other substances) in the drink is too high. In this situation, water will be drawn out of the interstitial fluid and plasma into the lumen of the small intestine by osmosis. As long as the fluid remains hypotonic with respect to plasma, the uptake of water from the small intestine is not adversely affected. The presence of small amounts of glucose and sodium tend to increase slightly the rate of water absorption compared with pure water. It must be emphasised here

that the addition of sodium and other electrolytes to sports drinks is to increase palatability, maintain thirst (and therefore promote drinking), prevent hyponatraemia and increase the rate of water uptake, rather than to replace the electrolyte losses through sweating. Replacement of the electrolytes lost in sweat can normally wait until the post-exercise recovery period.

Rehydration after exercise

When there is little time for recovery in between exercise bouts, the replacement of fluid and electrolytes in the post-exercise recovery period is of crucial importance. In the limited time available the athlete should strive to maximise rehydration. The main factors influencing the effectiveness of post-exercise dehydration are the volume and composition of the fluid consumed. Plain water is not the ideal post-exercise rehydration beverage when rapid and complete restoration of body fluid balance is necessary. Ingestion of water alone in the post-exercise period results in a rapid fall in the plasma sodium concentration and the plasma osmolarity. These changes have the effect of reducing the stimulation to drink (thirst) and increasing the urine output, both of which will delay the rehydration process. Plasma volume is more rapidly and completely restored in the post-exercise period if salt (sodium chloride) is added to the water consumed. The optimal sodium concentration of rehydration fluids (~50–60 mmol/l) is similar to the upper limit of the sodium concentration found in sweat, but is considerably higher than that of many commercially available sports drinks, which usually contain 10–25 mmol/l (60–150 mg/l).

Ingesting a beverage containing sodium not only promotes rapid fluid absorption in the small intestine, but also allows the plasma sodium concentration to remain elevated during the rehydration period and helps to maintain thirst while delaying stimulation of urine production. The inclusion of potassium in the beverage consumed after exercise would be expected to enhance the replacement of intracellular water and thus promote rehydration, but currently there is little experimental evidence to support this. The rehydration drink should also contain carbohydrate because the presence of glucose will also stimulate fluid absorption in the gut and improve beverage taste. Following exercise, the uptake of glucose into

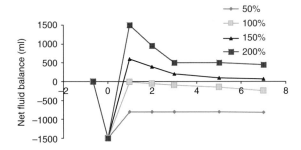

Figure 18.6 Net fluid balance after exercise with the ingestion of different volumes of a drink. Ingestion of 150% or more of weight loss is required to achieve normal hydration within 6 h after exercise. (Reproduced with permission from Shirreffs SM, Taylor AJ, Leiper JB, Maughan RJ. Post-exercise rehydration in man: effects of volume consumed and drink sodium content. Med Sci Sports Exerc 1996; 28(10): 1260–1271.)

the muscle for glycogen resynthesis should also promote intracellular rehydration.

Restoring fluid balance after exercise requires the intake of a greater volume of fluid than the deficit that was incurred during the session. This is because some of the ingested fluid will be excreted in urine. Recent studies indicate that ingestion of 125–150% or more of weight loss is required to achieve normal hydration within 6 h after exercise (Figure 18.6). Current American College of Sports Medicine (ACSM) guidelines on fluid ingestion before, during and after exercise, formulated and published in 2007, are shown in Box 18.7.

18.10 Nutritional ergogenics

The dietary supplement industry has grown enormously and annual sales were estimated to be US$ 12 billion in 1998. Up to US$ 800 million was spent on 'sports supplements'. Studies of the dietary practices of athletes report that nutritional supplements in one form or another are used by 40–100% of all athletes. There is also evidence that athletes use combinations of nutrition supplements and sometimes ingest very high doses. The claims and the experimental evidence for a selection of common supplements are reviewed here. Since there are now over 600 nutrition supplements on the market it is impossible to review them all, but here the focus is on the most common ones. The most important supplements are discussed below in alphabetical order.

Box 18.7 Summary of the American College of Sports Medicine Position Stand on Exercise and Fluid Replacement (2007)

The ACSM Position Stand provides guidance on fluid replacement to sustain appropriate hydration of individuals performing physical activity.
- Prehydrating with beverages, in addition to normal meals and fluid intake, should be initiated when needed at least several hours before the activity to enable fluid absorption and allow urine output to return to normal levels.
- The goal of drinking during exercise is to prevent excessive (>2% body weight loss from water deficit) dehydration and excessive changes in electrolyte balance to avert compromised performance.
- As there is considerable variability in sweating rates and sweat electrolyte content between individuals, customised fluid replacement programmes are recommended. Individual sweat rates can be estimated by measuring body weight before and after exercise.
- During exercise, consuming beverages containing electrolytes and carbohydrates can provide benefits over water alone under certain circumstances. After exercise, the goal is to replace any fluid electrolyte deficit.
- The speed with which rehydration is needed and the magnitude of fluid electrolyte deficits will determine if an aggressive replacement programme is merited.

Buffers

The effects of the excessive accumulation of H+ ions from anaerobic glycolysis are believed to limit the performance of high-intensity exercise lasting for 1–8 min, and perhaps repeated bouts of high-intensity work. There is good evidence that strategies that increase the blood capacity to buffer excess hydrogen ions can extend the time that such exercise can be undertaken, thus enhancing performance. Such strategies include the ingestion of well-known buffers such as bicarbonate and citrate with typical protocols being an intake of 0.3 mg/kg bicarbonate or 0.5 mg/kg citrate in the 1–2 h prior to the exercise task. Bicarbonate loading has been shown to enhance the performance of events such as middle distance swimming (200–400 m events), rowing and kayaking, and middle distance running (800–1500 m). Some studies have also reported benefits to the performance of protocols simulating the work patterns of team sports or high-intensity bouts at the end of an endurance bout, but the evidence for such benefits requires further confirmation. Citrate appears to be a less effective buffer.

Unfortunately, a disadvantage of bicarbonate loading protocols is the side-effect of gastrointestinal symptoms such as gut cramps and diarrhoea. This is likely to limit the practical use of bicarbonate loading by some individuals or for some events in which there is already an increased risk of gut problems. Further work is needed to test out the efficacy of bicarbonate loading strategies in elite competitors over the range of events in which it has theoretical benefits. However, there are practical issues that need to be addressed, such as the ability to repeat loading protocols in events which involved heats, semi-finals and finals to determine the eventual winner.

Another area of research that has gained recent attention is the ability to increase intracellular buffering capacity by increasing muscle levels of carnosine. The muscle concentration of the peptide carnosine can apparently be elevated by increasing the dietary intake of one of its amino acid precursors, β-alanine. We await the results of future studies which can document the protocols for optimising carnosine levels and confirm whether this transfers into performance benefits in high-intensity sports.

Caffeine

Caffeine originates naturally in 63 species of plants and is probably one of the most common drugs used by humans. The main sources of caffeine are coffee beans, tea leaves, cacao beans and cola nuts, and caffeine and caffeine-like substances can be found in a variety of foods and drinks (including special sports foods and 'energy drinks') as consumed by most adults as part of their daily diet. Caffeine has a large number of physiological and pharmacological effects on the body, including its well-known ability to mask fatigue or perceptions of effort.

Caffeine and exercise performance

Caffeine has been used to enhance the performance of sport or exercise for more than a century. It is unusual as an ergogenic aid in that it can aid performance across a wide variety of events, including endurance sports, intermittent activities resembling team sports, sustained high-intensity events lasting 1–20 min and prolonged skill-based activities. A variety of mechanisms have been proposed to explain the benefits of caffeine, including an increase in utilisation of fatty acids, effects on neuromuscular pathways

Figure 18.7 Effect of different dosages of caffeine or placebo 1 h before a ride on time to exhaustion at 75% of peak power output. With the lowest dose (5 mg/kg body weight) endurance capacity was improved by 20%, but a further increase in dosage had no further effect on performance. (Reprinted from Pasman WJ, van Baak MA, Jeukendrup AE, deHaan A. The effect of varied dosages of caffeine on endurance performance time. Int J Sports Med 1995; 16(4): 225–230. (c) Gerog Thieme Verlag KG.)

facilitating recruitment of muscle fibres or increasing the number of fibres recruited and direct effects of caffeine on muscle ion handling. Nevertheless, it appears that the most important effect of caffeine is to reduce fatigue and allow the athlete to continue for longer at their required pace or effort.

Although the traditional studies of caffeine supplementation and exercise used protocols in which 6 mg/kg body mass doses of caffeine were ingested an hour before exercise, newer studies have shown that equivalent benefits of caffeine are found with lower doses (2–3 mg/kg body mass) and when caffeine is ingested in a variety of protocols (before and during exercise, including just prior to the onset of fatigue). Indeed in one study, where subjects received three different doses of caffeine or placebo 1 h before a ride to exhaustion at 75% of peak power output, there were no further enhancements of performance with increasing caffeine doses (Figure 18.7). Caffeine was removed from the List of Prohibited Substances and Methods of the World Anti-Doping Agency in 2004, which makes sense because the levels of intake of caffeine which are shown to be ergogenic in sport cannot be distinguished from the caffeine intakes that are habitually consumed by most adults. Athletes who propose to use caffeine as an ergogenic aid for training or competition performance are advised to experiment to find the lowest dose at which benefits occur, since there is the possibility of side-effects such as interference with sleep, gastrointestinal upsets, and elevations of blood pressure and heart rate at higher doses. The response to caffeine is also individual. The widespread belief that caffeine is a dehydrating agent now seems poorly founded, especially since most people consume caffeine in the form of drinks which add to their fluid balance.

Carnitine

L-Carnitine is a natural substance, present in relatively high quantities in meat. Oral carnitine supplementation in humans for periods of 2–3 weeks does not increase the carnitine concentration in muscle and does not have an effect on muscle metabolism at rest or during exercise. In contrast to the claims made for carnitine supplements, there is little or no evidence that carnitine supplementation reduces body-fat mass, increases fat oxidation or reduces glycogen breakdown during prolonged exercise. In addition, carnitine supplementation does not increase $Vo_{2\,max}$ and does not reduce lactate accumulation during maximal and supramaximal exercise. It is likely that this is because carnitine supplementation does not normally increase the intracellular carnitine concentration. Although recent studies have demonstrated that elevating insulin by ingesting large amounts of carbohydrate can increase carnitine retention in the muscle, this practice would counteract any stimulating effect on fat metabolism or weight loss.

Chromium

Chromium is a trace element that is present in foods such as brewer's yeast, mushrooms and wheat-germ, and is considered an essential nutrient. Supplemental forms of chromium have become very popular in recent years, with claims that they increase muscle bulk and reduce body-fat levels. It has been reported that chromium increases insulin action, and insulin stimulates glucose and amino acid uptake by cells. It is thought that by stimulating amino acid uptake, there will be an increase in protein synthesis and muscle mass gain. Although there is some evidence that chromium supplements increase muscle mass and growth in animals, the effect on muscle mass in humans is less clear.

The vast majority of studies have not found effects of chromium on changes in body composition (percentage body fat, lean body mass). In a recent well-controlled study, the effect of 8 weeks of chromium supplementation or a placebo in untrained men who started a resistance-training programme was examined. Although chromium supplements increased urinary chromium excretion they had no effect on body composition. It must therefore be concluded that the vast majority of the studies demonstrate that chromium supplements are not effective in increasing lean body mass.

Coenzyme Q10

Coenzyme Q10 (CoQ10) or ubiquinone is an integral part of the electron transport chain of the mitochondria and therefore plays an important role in oxidative phosphorylation. CoQ10 is especially present in heart muscle and has been used therapeutically to treat cardiovascular disease and post-cardiac surgery. In these patients, CoQ10 supplementation improves oxidative metabolism and exercise capacity. Manufacturers have extrapolated the results of improved $Vo_{2\,max}$ in cardiac patients to healthy and trained athletes. It is claimed that coenzyme Q10 increases $Vo_{2\,max}$ and increases 'stamina' and 'energy'.

Few studies have investigated the effects of CoQ10 supplementation in athletes. Although most of these studies report elevated plasma CoQ10 levels, no changes were observed in $Vo_{2\,max}$, performance or lactate at submaximal workloads. CoQ10 is also marketed as an antioxidant.

Recently it was reported that ingestion of 120 mg CoQ10/day for 20 days resulted in marked increases in plasma CoQ10 concentrations, but the muscle CoQ10 concentration was unaltered. This observation leads us to conclude that most claims are unfounded. There may even be some negative effects of CoQ10. It has been reported that during high exercise intensity when there is an abundance of hydrogen ions in the cells, CoQ10 can even augment free radical production. Paradoxically, this is the opposite effect of what CoQ10 is claimed to do but agrees with the theory that antioxidant supplementation may actually reduce the adaptations to training.

Creatine

Creatine became a popular supplement in the early 1990s after several successful athletes supposedly used creatine supplements. Nearly two decades later, it has been the subject of more than 300 studies, and found to have benefits for exercise performance as well as clinical applications for several muscle disorders. Creatine is a naturally occurring compound synthesised from several amino acids and found in meat and fish. Our normal dietary intake is about 2 g of creatine/day, and creatine is broken down to creatinine and excreted in the urine at about the same rate. Strict vegetarians and vegans will have negligible creatine intake, because plants contain only trace amounts of creatine, and are therefore dependent on endogenous synthesis of creatine. Oral ingestion of creatine suppresses the biosynthesis. In a 70-kg man, the total body creatine pool is approximately 120 mg, most (95%) of which is found in muscle, with small amounts in the liver, brain, kidney and testes.

Functions of phosphocreatine

The role of creatine and phosphocreatine (PCr) was discussed at the beginning of this chapter. Briefly, the transfer of the phosphate group from creatine phosphate to ADP results in the regeneration of ATP:

$$PCr + ADP + H^+ \rightarrow Creatine + ATP$$

Phosphocreatine is present in resting muscle in a concentration that is three to four times that of ATP, and anaerobic degradation of phosphocreatine and glycogen is responsible for a significant rate of ATP resynthesis during the first seconds of high-intensity exercise. However, the phosphocreatine store in muscle is small and could be depleted within 4–5 s of supramaximal exercise. Elevated stores could potentially provide more energy. High phosphocreatine stores may also reduce the need for anaerobic glycolysis and lactic acid formation during intense exercise, and this might be another potential benefit of phosphocreatine. A third important function of creatine is its potential buffering capacity for hydrogen ions as these ions are used during ATP regeneration (see metabolic reaction above). The roles of creatine listed above suggest that elevating muscle creatine and phosphocreatine stores would benefit high-intensity exercise performance.

In 1992 Harris and colleagues were the first to suggest that ingesting creatine monohydrate could increase muscle total creatine stores (creatine and phosphocreatine). In that study ingesting 5 g of creatine four to six times per day for several days increased the total creatine concentration by an average of 20–25 mmol kg dry weight. This increase corresponded to about 20% of the basal muscle total creatine concentration of about 125 mmol/kg dry weight. About one-third of the increase in total creatine content was in the form of phosphocreatine. In a subsequent study, ingestion of 20 g of creatine/day for 5 days was shown to improve performance by about 6% during repeated bouts of maximal knee extensor exercise. Today, the evidence supports the positive effects of creatine supplementation on intermittent bouts of very high-intensity exercise with relatively short recovery periods (e.g. interval training, resistance training, team sports). Typically, performance improvements are found not in the first few sprints but after several repeated sprints. Creatine supplementation may allow more repetitions of repeated exercise and thus a better quality of training, including resistance training. Further studies have found that creatine loading can be achieved through a 'slower' loading protocol, with a daily dose of 3 g/day. In addition, creatine uptake and muscle total creatine can be increased more when creatine is ingested in combination with carbohydrate.

Not everyone may benefit from creatine supplementation. This may be related to the fact that there is considerable variation between subjects in the initial muscle total creatine concentration. The largest increase in muscle creatine concentration is observed in individuals with the lowest initial concentration, while individuals with an already high creatine concentration benefit only marginally (Figure 18.8). A concentration of 160 mmol/kg dry matter appears to be the maximal creatine concentration achievable as a result of creatine supplementation. The reasons for these individual differences are largely unknown, but may at least partly be related to the habitual diet. Studies have shown that individuals who display the largest increases in muscle total creatine concentration also exhibit the largest performance benefit. It has been suggested that a change in muscle creatine content of about 20 mmol/kg dry weight should be present before significant changes in performance can be observed. About 30% of all individuals will not display such large increases in muscle creatine and therefore will not benefit. These people are often referred to as non-responders.

Creatine supplementation is generally accompanied by increases in body weight of approximately 1 kg, although some individuals may gain minimal weight and others as much as 3.5 kg. This increase in body weight results from increases in intracellular water.

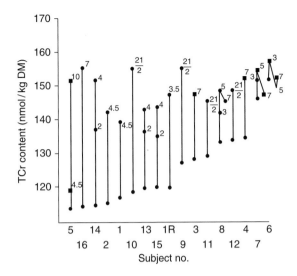

Figure 18.8 Effect of creatine loading on muscle total creatine (TCr) content. Individuals with low initial creatine concentrations seem to benefit more from supplementation than those with already high concentrations. There also seems to be an upper limit for total creatine content of about 160 mmol/kg day weight. (JOURNAL OF APPLIED PHYSIOLOGY by Hultman E, Soderlund K, Timmons A, Cederblad G, Greenhaff PL, Copyright © 1996 by AMERICAN PHYSIOLOGY SOCIETY. Reproduced with permission of AMERICAN PHYSIOLOGY SOCIETY in the format Texbook via Copyright Clearance Center.)

The increase in body weight may be beneficial or have no effect in some disciplines, but can be detrimental to performance in weight-bearing activities (such as running or gymnastics). There are numerous anecdotal reports that creatine supplementation caused gastrointestinal, cardiovascular and muscular problems, as well as nausea, vomiting and diarrhoea, but there are no scientific studies to confirm this. There is also no evidence of alterations in renal or liver function, the occurrence of muscle cramps or elevated blood pressure. However, as pointed out in a round-table discussion by the ACSM: 'The evidence is not definitive and/or it is incomplete to indict the practice of creatine supplementation as a health risk; at the same time, our lack of information cannot be taken as an assurance that creatine supplementation is free from health risks. Ignorance provides little comfort of untoward effects yet to be discovered.'

Fish oil

It has been suggested that by increasing the fraction of polyunsaturated fatty acids in the phospholipids of erythrocyte membranes, membrane fluidity would be improved and red blood cell deformability increased, resulting in improved peripheral oxygen supply. Such changes in red blood cell deformability and a change in the fatty acid composition of membranes towards a higher percentage of unsaturated fatty acids are also seen after exercise training. This could at least theoretically be accomplished by consuming a diet high in fish oil or by taking fish oil capsules.

Controlled studies supplemented trained cyclists for 3 weeks with placebo or fish oil (6 g/day). Fish oil did not alter red blood cell characteristics in this study and had no effect on $Vo_{2\,max}$, maximal power output or time trial performance. It can be concluded that fish oil could potentially have some long-term positive effects, but at present scientific evidence is lacking to support claims that fish oil improves maximal oxygen uptake and performance.

18.11 Dietary supplements and failed drug tests

Dietary supplements may cause a failed doping test. There have been several recent cases in which failed doping tests were ascribed to dietary supplement use. Most of the recent attention has been on nandrolone, but other banned substances have also been found in these supplements. There are many cases in which athletes tested positive for ephedrine or other stimulants after using herbal products. A ground-breaking study conducted over 10 years ago by an International Olympic Committee accredited laboratory found that 15% of supplements contained a banned substance (prohormone or testosterone) that was not declared on the product label. Despite the publicity given to this study, more recent testing shows that the problem of supplements that are contaminated or intentionally 'spiked' with banned stimulants or anabolic agents has not disappeared. When such supplements are given to volunteers and urine samples are collected the results often indicate a positive doping test. The regulations for nutrition supplements are less strict than those for medical products and therefore it is difficult to control the quality of a product. Even dietary supplements that are labelled as being safe for use by athletes may be contaminated.

At present there is little an athlete can do to ensure that the products used are safe. Reputable brands of common supplements produced by major food and drug companies that are normally manufactured with the highest standards are likely to be safer than products from small manufacturers. The athlete will have to make a decision as to whether the supposed effect of the supplement is worth the risk of a positive drug test.

18.12 Practical issues in nutrition for athletes

Despite the sports nutrition knowledge available to modern athletes and coaches, sports nutritionists report that athletes do not always achieve the practices of optimal sports nutrition. A number of factors may be involved:

- poor understanding of sports nutrition principles; reliance on myths and misconceptions
- failure to recognise the specific nutritional requirements of different sports and individuals within these sports
- apparent conflict of nutrition goals (e.g. how can an athlete achieve increased requirements for nutrients such as carbohydrate and iron while limiting energy intake to achieve loss of body fat?)
- lack of practical nutrition knowledge and skills (e.g. knowledge of food composition, domestic skills such as food purchasing, preparation and cooking)
- overcommitted lifestyle; inadequate time and opportunities to obtain or consume appropriate foods owing to heavy workload of sport, work, school, etc.
- inadequate finances
- the challenge of frequent travel.

Given the specific nutritional requirements of sports and individuals, according to age and gender, it is impossible to prepare a single set of nutrition guidelines for athletes. Nevertheless, education tools that address key issues of nutrition for athletes are an important resource for coaches, athletes and sports nutritionists. Education strategies that focus on practical areas of food choice and preparation, and guidelines that can address a number of key nutrition issues simultaneously are most valuable. In situations where nutritional goals can be achieved by modest changes to typical population eating patterns, it may be sufficient to provide a set of behavioural strategies to guide

---

Box 18.8 Strategies for eating well while travelling

- Investigate the food resources at the trip destination before leaving. People who have travelled previously to that country, competition or accommodation facility may be able to warn about likely problems and enable the preparation of a suitable plan in advance.
- Organise special menus and meals in restaurants, airplanes or hotels in advance.
- Find out about food hygiene and water safety in new countries. It may be necessary to restrict fluid intake to bottled or boiled drinks, and to avoid foods that are high risk for contamination (e.g. unpeeled fruits and vegetables).
- Take some food supplies on the trip if important foods are likely to be unavailable or expensive. Foods that are portable and low in perishability include breakfast cereals, milk powder, tinned and dehydrated foods, and special sports supplements.
- Be aware of special nutritional requirements in the new location. Be prepared to meet increased requirements for fluid, carbohydrate and other nutrients.

---

athletes to achieve such changes. However, in situations where the athlete has extreme nutrient requirements, where nutritional goals appear to conflict or where medical problems are present, the athlete should be directed to seek individualised and expert counselling from a sports nutritionist or dietician.

It should be appreciated that many of the practical challenges to achieving sports nutrition goals arise directly because of exercise or the environment in which it is undertaken. Goals of nutrition before, during and after a workout or training must often be compromised or modified because of the effects of exercise on gastrointestinal function and comfort. Access to foods and drinks is often restricted in the busy day of the athlete or in the exercise environment. The frequent travel schedules of the athlete must also be negotiated in dietary advice. In many cases the expertise of the sports dietician is required to provide creative ways to meet sports nutrition goals. Strategies for the travelling athlete are summarised in Box 18.8.

18.13 Perspectives for the future

A significant proportion of the future research in the area of sports nutrition will be focused on recovery. New strategies to improve glycogen and protein synthesis or to reduce protein breakdown will be explored. Thus far, the work in this area has been limited because the techniques for studying protein metabolism are complicated and very expensive. The work in this area will be important for all sports at high level where the amount of training that can be performed is often crucial to performance. All methods to reduce recovery time can be beneficial. In addition, refinements will be made to optimise the fluid and carbohydrate delivery from sports drinks. In addition nutritional strategies will be investigated to optimise training adaptations. Researchers are starting to unravel the complex mechanisms underlying these training adaptations and as the understanding increases it will be possible to develop nutritional strategies to maximise the factors that initiate the adaptation. It is also likely that more new supplements will be promoted and researched.

Further reading

Achten J, Gleeson M, Jeukendrup AE. Determination of the exercise intensity that elicits maximal fat oxidation. Med Sci Sports Exerc. 2002; 34: 92–99.

American College of Sports Medicine. Weight loss in wrestlers. Med Sci Sports Exerc 1996; 28: ix–xii.

American College of Sports Medicine. Roundtable: The physiological and health effects of oral creatine supplementation. Med Sci Sports Exerc 2000; 32: 706–717.

Below PR et al. Fluid and carbohydrate ingestion independently improve performance during 1 h of intense exercise. Med Sci Sports Exerc 1995; 27(2): 200–210.

Brownell KD, Rodin J. Prevalence of eating disorders in athletes. In: Eating Body Weight and Performance in Athletes: Disorders of Modern Society (Brownell KD, Rodin J, Wilmore JH, eds). Philadelphia, PA: Lea & Febiger, 2000: pp. 128–145.

Burke L, Practical Sports Nutrition, Ilinois, Human Kinetics, 2007.

Burke L, Deakin V, eds. Clinical Sports Nutrition, 4nd edn. Sydney: McGraw Hill, 2010.

Costill DL et al. Muscle glycogen utilization during prolonged exercise on successive days. J Appl Physiol 1971; 31: 834–838.

Geyer H et al. Analysis of non-hormonal nutritional supplements for anabolic-androgenic steroids – results of an international study. Int J Sports Med 2004; 25: 124–129.

Hultman E et al. Muscle creatine loading in men. J Appl Physiol 1996; 81(1): 232–237.

Jeukendrup AE. Carbohydrate intake during exercise and performance. Nutrition 2004; 20: 669–677.

Jeukendrup AE. Carbohydrate intake during exercise. Eur J Sport Sci, 2008; 8(2): 77–86.

Jeukendrup AE, ed. Sports Nutrition: from Lab to Kitchen. Aachen: Meyer and Meyer, 2010.

Jeukendrup AE, Gleeson M. Sport Nutrition. An Introduction into Energy Metabolism and Performance, 2nd edn. Champaign, IL, Human Kinetics, 2010.

Maughan RJ, ed. IOC Encyclopedia of Sports Medicine: Nutrition in Sport. Oxford: Blackwell Science, 2000.

Maughan RJ, Burke LM, Coyle EF. Food, nutrition and sports performance II. London: Routledge, 2004.

Pasman WJ et al. The effect of varied dosages of caffeine on endurance performance time. Int J Sports Med 1995; 16(4): 225–230.

Rodriguez NR, DiMarco NM, Langley S. Position of the American Dietetic Association, Dietitians of Canada, and the American College of Sports Medicine: Nutrition and athletic performance. J Am Diet Assoc. 2009; 109: 509–527.

Romijn JA et al. Regulation of endogenous fat and carbohydrate metabolism in relation to exercise intensity. Am J Physiol 1993; 265: E380–E391.

Sawka MN et al. American College of Sports Medicine position stand. Exercise and fluid replacement. Med Sci Sports Exerc 2007; 39: 377–390.

Shirreffs SM et al. Post-exercise rehydration in man: effects of volume consumed and drink sodium content. Med Sci Sports Exerc 1996; 28(10): 1260–1271.

Index

Nutrition and Metabolism, Second Edition, edited by S. A. Lanham-New, I. A. Macdonald and H. M. Roche. © 2011 The Nutrition Society.